Atlas of SPINAL SURGERY

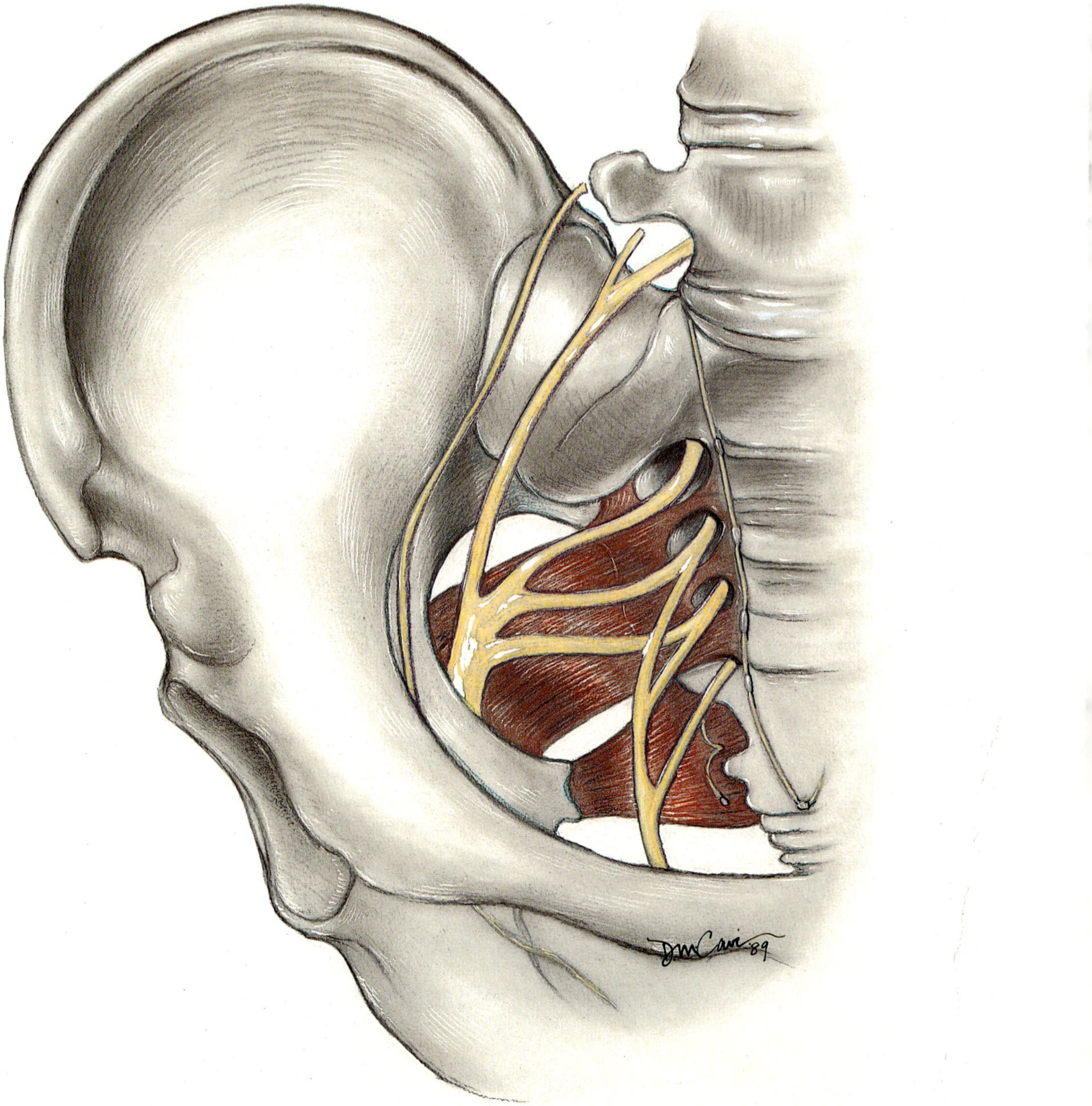

Atlas of SPINAL SURGERY

Donlin M. Long, M.D., Ph.D.

Professor and Director
Department of Neurological Surgery
The Johns Hopkins University School of Medicine
Baltimore, Maryland

Paul C. McAfee, M.D.

Associate Professor
Department of Orthopaedic Surgery
The Johns Hopkins University School of Medicine
Baltimore, Maryland
and
Chief of Spinal Reconstructive Surgery
St. Joseph's Hospital
Towson, Maryland

Illustrations by **Donna M. Cavi**

SANS TACHE
WILLIAMS & WILKINS
BALTIMORE • HONG KONG • LONDON • MUNICH
PHILADELPHIA • SYDNEY • TOKYO

Editor: Carol-Lynn Brown
Managing Editor: Victoria M. Vaughn
Copy Editor: Bill Cady
Designer: JoAnne Janowiak/Dan Pfisterer
Illustration Planner: Lorraine Wrzosek
Production Coordinator: Raymond E. Reter

Williams & Wilkins
428 East Preston Street
Baltimore, Maryland 21202, USA

Printed in the United States of America

ISBN 0-683-05149-0

91 92 93 94 95
1 2 3 4 5 6 7 8 9 10

This volume is dedicated to my teachers:

Lyle A. French, who emphasized the importance of spinal problems in neurosurgery and the need for meticulous surgical technique for all spinal operations;

Shelley Chou, who broadened the horizons of neurosurgeons with his innovative approaches to the spinal cord;

Robert Robinson, who introduced me to the biomechanical problems of the spine, their solutions, and the concept of restoration of function through spinal surgery; and

David Filtzer, whose exacting historical and physical evaluations of patients with spinal disease serve as a model for us all.

Preface

The importance of spinal surgery is growing rapidly. Surgical treatment of the herniated lumbar or cervical disc has long been recognized as an important part of both neurosurgical and orthopedic practice. Treatment of spinal tumors and infections of all kinds is fundamental to the practice of both specialties. Correction of congenital and some acquired anomalies has long been a part of the practice of spinal surgery. The enormous growth of surgery for the correction of degenerative disease represents the major change in spinal surgery in the past decade.

With this growth has come emphasis on the biomechanical function of the spine and restoration of that function. A steadily increasing number of prosthetic reparative and fixation devices are now available to the surgeon. Spinal surgery has moved from a relatively simple repertoire of standardized procedures done for a limited number of spinal diseases to an often-bewildering array of choices of approach and technique.

The dichotomy of spinal surgery between orthopedists and neurosurgeons has added to the complexity of the situation. Both specialties pursue research in spinal diseases and spinal surgical techniques independently. Lack of cooperation is frequently apparent at all levels in both specialties. Training has been separated in most institutions.

This book grew from a collaborative effort in a unified spine service in which both neurosurgeons and orthopedists met together to better understand and treat spinal diseases. Many patients were managed jointly in a team effort, and much of the surgery was done in a collaborative fashion. Young surgeons irrespective of their specialty were trained by all members of the team in most aspects of spinal surgery. A few procedures, because of their highly specialized nature requiring long periods of specialized training, clearly remain the province of one specialty or the other.

For the remainder, the atlas is meant to be a guide to a comprehensive practice of spinal surgery to which every spine surgeon can aspire with appropriate training and experience. While comprehensive, this atlas cannot be complete. The techniques of spinal fixation are evolving so rapidly that it is not possible to maintain a catalog of them. Furthermore, the place of these different systems in the management of spinal deformity is far from clear.

We have attempted to present the fundamental collection of what have been traditional neurosurgical and orthopedic procedures that should now be mastered by any spinal surgeon. Skilled application of these universal concepts will allow any new procedure to be understood and added to the surgeon's technical catalog of operations.

Of greater importance is the philosophical basis for this atlas. Our approach assumes that the spinal surgeon of the future will master all approaches for exposure of the spine while understanding and utilizing biomechanical principles for spinal reconstruction. The challenges of spinal surgery are many. Anatomy of the spine is not generally stressed in medical education. Biomechanics of spinal function, though much studied, has not played an important role in the development of operations for spinal reconstruction. Most such operations limit function rather than restoring it.

The future for those wishing to emphasize spinal surgery is to improve current operative techniques. This atlas emphasizes the diversity of approaches and techniques that are now available for the correction of spinal problems. Limited stereotyped procedures for all disease can be replaced by a spectrum of operations chosen to be most appropriate for an individual patient. Then our goal must be improved reconstruction. Restoration of normal spinal function, while not possible at present, should be the aim of every surgeon who operates on the spine.

We hope that this atlas will be instructive for those who wish to expand their repertoire of spinal operations and an inspiration for spinal surgeons to develop new and better procedures to benefit those suffering from diseases of the spine.

Acknowledgments

We would like to extend our thanks to several individuals without whom completion of this book would not have been possible.

Shawne Tubinis was responsible for typing the manuscripts, collating and maintaining the written materials, editing and correcting the initial efforts, and producing the final drafts. The book owes its form and shape to her hard work.

Donna Cavi was responsible for the art work. Ms. Cavi made original sketches in the operating room in every case and then worked with the authors to produce a coherent word/picture study.

Dr. James Zinreich was responsible for choosing and producing the radiographs used to illustrate the manuscript. Dr. Edward Oldfield produced the definitive chapter on surgery for arteriovenous malformations.

Our special thanks is due to the residents and fellows who collaborated in the production of several chapters that related to spinal fixation techniques.

Finally, we are all grateful to the skilled staff at Williams & Wilkins. Their advice in the formulation of the book was of help. Their editorial work was invaluable. The production staff has been particularly helpful in establishing the final format, finding and correcting all the errors, no matter how minor, to produce a book pleasing to all of us.

Contributors

Charles Carroll IV, M.D.
Assistant Professor of Clinical Orthopaedic Surgery
Northwestern University
Chicago, Illinois

Jeffrey D. Coe, M.D.
Director of Spinal Surgery
Orthopaedic Surgery Service
Brooke Army Medical Center
San Antonio, Texas
and
Clinical Assistant Professor of Orthopaedic Surgery
University of Texas Health Science Center at San Antonio
San Antonio, Texas

R. F. Davis, M.D.
Instructor
Department of Orthopaedic Surgery
Department of Neurosurgery
The Johns Hopkins University School of Medicine
Baltimore, Maryland

A. Alexander M. Jones, M.D.
Lieutenant Commander, Medical Corp, USNR
Director, Spine Clinic
Naval Hospital Oakland
Oakland, California

Donlin M. Long, M.D., Ph.D.
Professor and Director
Department of Neurological Surgery
The Johns Hopkins University School of Medicine
Baltimore, Maryland

David F. Martin, M.D.
Assistant Professor
Department of Orthopaedic Surgery
Bowman Gray School of Medicine
Winston-Salem, North Carolina

Paul C. McAfee, M.D.
Associate Professor
Department of Orthopaedic Surgery
The Johns Hopkins University School of Medicine
Baltimore, Maryland
and
Chief, Spinal Reconstructive Surgery
St. Joseph's Hospital
Towson, Maryland

Edward H. Oldfield, M.D.
Chief, Surgical Neurology Branch
National Institute of Neurological and Communicative Disorders and Stroke
Bethesda, Maryland

Lee H. Riley III, M.D.
Research Fellow
Department of Neurosurgery
The Johns Hopkins University School of Medicine
Baltimore, Maryland

Henry Wang, M.D.
Assistant Professor
Department of Radiology
The Johns Hopkins University School of Medicine
Baltimore, Maryland

S. James Zinreich, M.D.
Assistant Professor
Department of Radiology
The Johns Hopkins University School of Medicine
Baltimore, Maryland

Contents

Introduction

A Philosophy of Spinal Surgery

Spinal surgery has been the domain of two specialties, neurosurgery and orthopedics. Traditionally, neurosurgeons have dealt with all problems inside the dura and bony abnormalities that resulted in compromise of spinal cord or nerves, while orthopedists were principally concerned with skeletal deformity. The role of each specialty in degenerative disc disease and spinal trauma has been less well defined. The first article on the herniated lumbar disc was coauthored by an orthopedist and a neurosurgeon. Both specialties have claimed the herniated disc since, and both are actively involved in the evaluation and treatment of all forms of disc disease. In spinal trauma this situation was, at one time, more clear-cut. Neurosurgeons generally treated patients with neurological deficits, and orthopedists generally treated patients without neurological deficits. Increasingly this division is blurred, and members of both groups who specialize in spinal trauma deal with all aspects of spinal injury.

It is increasingly apparent that these traditional divisions no longer suffice. As a group, spinal abnormalities are the most prevalent health problem in the western world. Our greatly enhanced ability to image the spine has created a new understanding of spinal disease. Biomechanical and anatomical appreciation of spinal function have increased the potential to restore normal spinal function through surgical therapy. The spine is a complex organ. Patients with complaints of spinal pain are even more complex and heterogeneous. Understanding the spine, its function, and patients with complaints that relate to the spine is increasingly a full-time occupation that deserves subspecialization.

No area of medicine requires such introspection as does spinal surgery. In spite of the enormous advances in imaging, the clinical correlations of the abnormalities are not certain. The ubiquitous nature of degenerative disc disease makes it possible to find abnormalities in large numbers of patients when the surgical attack on these abnormalities may not be indicated. The results from much spinal surgery are less than optimal, and there are many uncertainties about both disc excision and stabilization. Psychosocial and economic factors play important roles in maintaining the complaint of low back pain. The relationship between patient complaints, the usual paucity of physical complaints, imaging evidence for structural abnormalities, and psychological, social, and economic factors remains to be defined. All of this means that the spinal surgeon must develop and maintain a philosophy of diagnosis and treatment that is dependent on the best techniques currently available and continues to incorporate new knowledge for the modification of surgical practice.

The first goal in evaluation is a careful history and physical examination. There are few completely typical diagnostic spinal syndromes, and most of these diagnoses can be made by history alone. The physical examination may be confirmatory, and physical findings rarely surprise the diagnostician. Acute spinal problems without obvious cause are almost always self-limited and disappear spontaneously. Those that persist or are associated with disturbing physical findings should be pursued through imaging studies. Weight bearing and dynamic films are still important. When the abnormalities are expected to be bony, the computed tomography (CT) scan should follow plain films. If soft tissues are expected to be the principal problem, then the magnetic resonance imaging (MRI) scan is superior as the next step. CT myelography can now be reserved for indeterminate problems and for those patients who have undergone previous surgery where the images may be more complex. Electrodiagnostics are of limited primary utility but may be very useful where spinal cord compression is a possibility and in patients who have undergone previous operations. To recommend a spinal operation, it is necessary that the history indicates a problem of sufficient magnitude that surgery is warranted and that the physical examination substantiates the history. The images should confirm the diagnosis. Furthermore, the images demonstrate the pathological anatomy and what must be corrected. The exact extent of disc herniation, canal narrowing, spinal narrowing, spur formation, and the like can now be known before surgery. This allows the surgeon to plan an operation that will both correct the abnormal anatomy and restore function insofar as possible.

The functional anatomy of the spine is much better understood than previously. The contribution of the different spinal elements and what follows their disruption are important for every spinal surgeon to know. Spinal anatomy is relatively simple, while spinal function is very complex. Every operation should be planned to restore functional anatomy. This means removal of the least amount of bone possible that is commensurate with an appropriate outcome for the patient, maintenance of joints, and restoration of the relationships between muscles and bone. It is particularly important that the lumbar, thoracic, and cervical fascial layers be returned to a normal configuration. These planes are critical to normal muscle function in the spine.

The spinal surgeon almost more than any other bears a responsibility for an accurate diagnosis of a disease competent to cause the patient's complaint. The operation must be planned to correct the problem and to maintain or restore the critical function of the spine. The armamentarium of spinal operations has greatly increased over the past decade. Much remains to be done, for there are still many patients who are not satisfactorily diagnosed or treated with what is currently available. The spinal surgeon bears the responsibility for precise diagnosis, cognizance of psychosocial factors that may influence the patient's complaint, a well-designed operation, and attention to the patient's postoperative rehabilitation. Good spinal surgery requires a thorough understanding of anatomy and biomechanics, meticulous surgical technique, and a commitment to return the patient to full function.

These ideals are often confounded by current issues, both political and surgical. Spine surgery for disc disease is much criticized. Low back pain is the most common disabling complaint, and the pressures from patients for surgical relief are significant. In litigation the complaint of back pain is hard to prove or disprove. Most patients heal spontaneously, and only a small number progress to the need for surgical therapy. The number of failures of back surgery are significant, and the so-called "failed back syndrome" occupies a good deal of the time of every spinal surgeon. All of this simply emphasizes the need for careful diagnosis, well-considered surgery, and ongoing exploration for better ways to do things in this highly challenging field.

REFERENCES

Louis R: *Surgery of the Spine: Surgical Anatomy and Operative Approaches.* Berlin, Springer-Verlag, 1983.

Rickenbacher J, Landolt AM, Theiler K: *Applied Anatomy of the Back.* Berlin, Springer-Verlag, 1985.

Rothman RH, Simeone FA: *The Spine.* Philadelphia, WB Saunders, 1982.

Seeger W: *Microsurgery of the Spinal Cord and Surrounding Structures: Anatomical and Technical Principles.* Berlin, Springer-Verlag, 1982.

Watkins R: *Surgical Approaches to the Spine.* Berlin, Springer-Verlag, 1983.

Imaging of Spinal Disorders

The addition of magnetic resonance imaging (MRI), computerized axial tomography, particularly with two-dimensional and three-dimensional reconstructions to augment plain x-rays, myelography, and angiography has greatly enhanced diagnostic capabilities in spinal disease. Nevertheless, the clinical correlations of these new studies are not well known, and in many patients the causes of the major spinal complaints cannot be defined. From a practical clinical point of view the physician is usually confronted with two main complaints: neck pain with or without arm pain, and back pain with or without leg pain. The problem is the parsimonious choice of diagnostic studies that are most appropriate and most likely to give the best diagnosis.

Examination of the Cervical Spine

The first question to be asked is whether the abnormalities sought are likely to be bony or soft tissue. Whichever the case, it is wise to begin with plain cervical spine x-rays with anterior, posterior, lateral, oblique, and dynamic views. In the typical situation of acute pain, which is likely to be self-limited, it is reasonable to defer any films until several weeks have elapsed. When the pain does not disappear spontaneously, has some unusual character, or is associated with a significant neurological deficit, proceeding to plain films, at least, is good practice. The decision about more sophisticated imaging will depend on the clinical presentation and the findings on the plain films. When these x-rays are abnormal, showing degenerative arthritis, subluxation, or bony lesions, the appropriate next study is usually the computer tomography (CT) scan. This will outline the bony detail and is most likely to give an appropriate diagnosis. The three-dimensional scan is rapidly evolving as the best way to look at overall bony detail, although serial sections still have an important role. The CT scan may also provide diagnosis of a herniated disc. With relatively normal plain films, the suspicion of intrinsic spinal cord disease, or the high likelihood of a soft tissue abnormality such as disc protrusion, the diagnostic study of choice is the MRI. When there is no obvious pathology of bones, it is important to examine soft tissues carefully, so MRI should follow nondiagnostic CT. This means that in some patients both studies will be needed, but it is redundant to do them unless one will contribute something obvious. In most patients with neurological problems, particularly myelopathy, MRI is the study of choice, even if the plain films are strikingly abnormal. If the diagnosis cannot be made by combinations of these three modalities, CT with intrathecal contrast is the next choice.

Examination of the Thoracic Spine

Thoracic spinal problems are best evaluated with plain x-rays. Anterior, posterior, and lateral views usually suffice. Dynamic views are indicated only if a subluxation is likely to be a problem. If there is no obvious diagnosis, the next appropriate study is MRI. This will allow the whole thoracic spine to be seen. CT of the entire thoracic spine is a formidable procedure and generally is carried out only over specific areas where the diagnosis is thought to be localized. For those patients without diagnosis by either study, CT myelography is the appropriate choice.

Examination of the Lumbar Spine

Most patients with back pain have spontaneous remission, and over half never have any x-ray or specific clinical diagnosis made. When the pain is entirely in the back, and there are no neurological complaints or findings, the most appropriate study is plain x-ray.

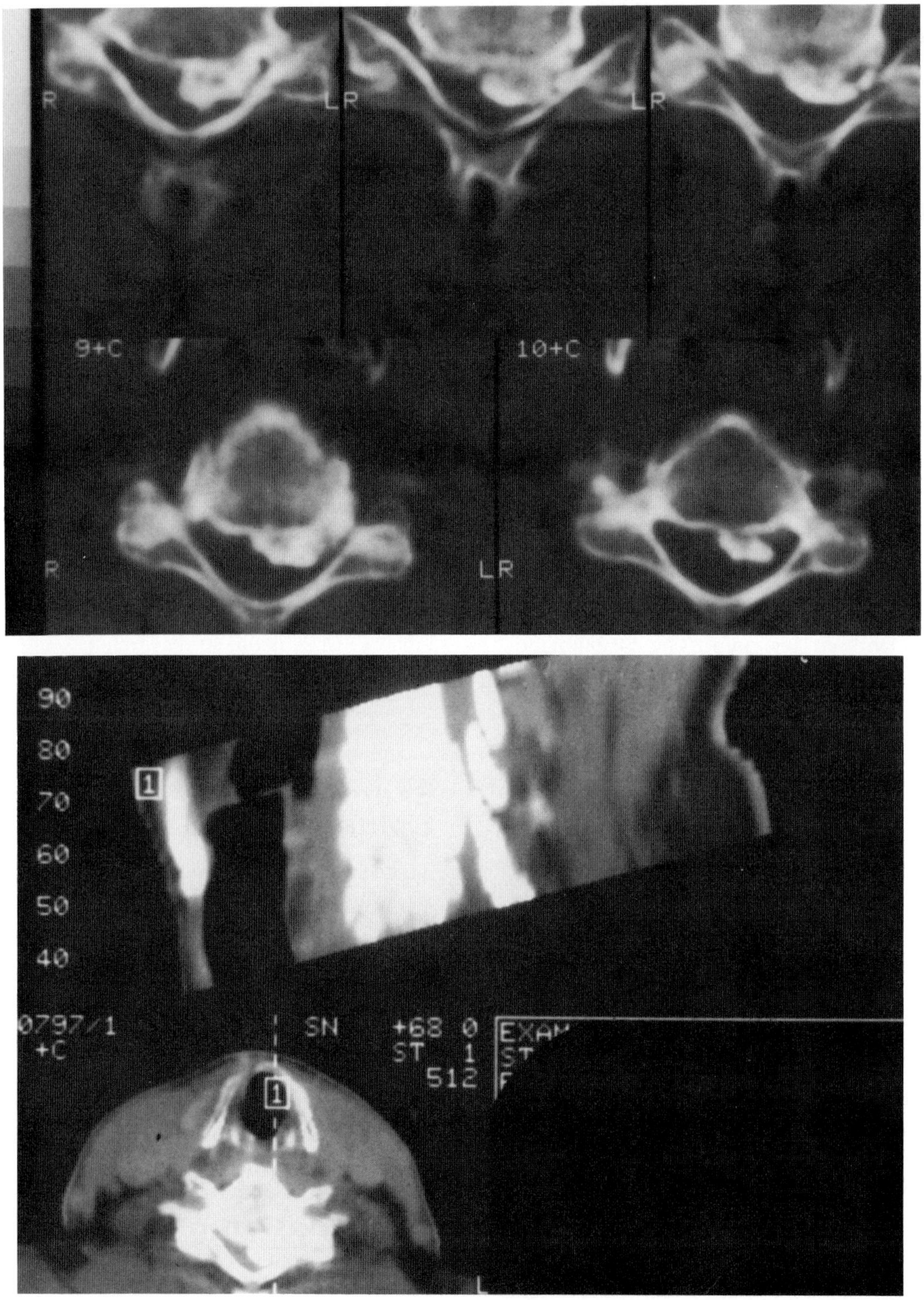

Figure I.1. Calcification of the posterior and longitudinal ligaments has greatly reduced the lumen of the cervical canal. Appropriate surgery will be radical resection of the bodies and the calcified ligament with anterior block graft.

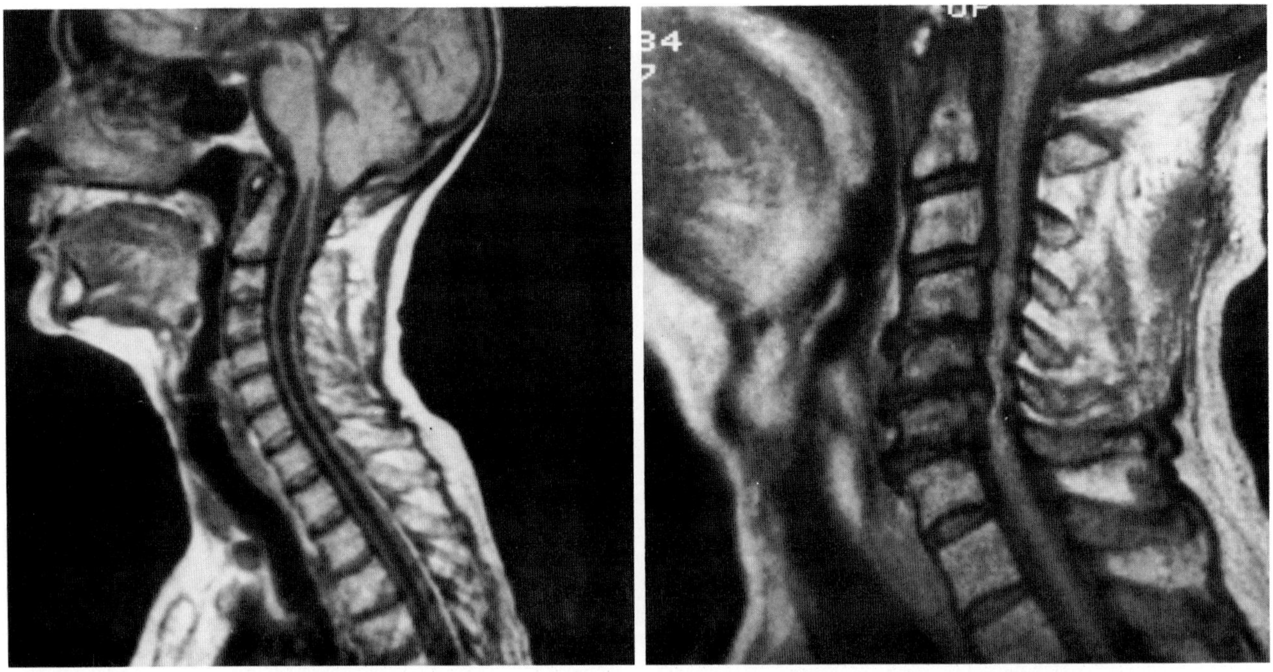

Figure I.2. MRI scan demonstrating multilevel degenerative disc disease with anterior herniations at the C3-C4, C4-C5, C5-C6 levels. There is a posterior herniation at the C5-C6 level, which was the symptomatic lesion.

Anterior, posterior, lateral, oblique, and dynamic views are required. These should be weight bearing. They need not be accomplished until after a trial of expectant conservative therapy unless the symptoms are extreme, there is some atypical component, or the patient fails to respond after a reasonable period of conservative care. When the problem is thought to be disc disease, MRI is the next choice. The CT scan will also show disc herniation but is less specific. If there is an expected significant bony component, then CT scanning is superior. When the diagnosis cannot be made by either modality, CT myelography is indicated. In most patients who have had previous surgery, a CT myelogram is required because it is not yet possible to differentiate postoperative scar from recurrent disc herniation, and the studies without contrast do not delimit the process. Three-dimensional reconstruction is invaluable in the postoperative patient and is a real adjunct with all patients with lumbar spondylosis. Canal size and foraminal stenosis can be estimated better with this technique than with any other.

The choice of studies is now difficult to make. It is important to remember that not all studies have to be done on every patient. Choose only those studies that are most likely to give a satisfactory diagnosis. Cost is a consideration. CT scanning is much less expensive than MRI, and CT myelography is more expensive than either, particularly when a 1-day hospitalization is required. There is no reason to continue repeated studies when the only reason for repetition is ongoing complaints by the patient. A study that was normal on one occasion is likely to remain so unless the patient's complaints have changed or new physical findings have appeared.

Radiography for Spinal Trauma

The plain films remain the basis for diagnosis. Anteroposterior lateral and oblique films are required on

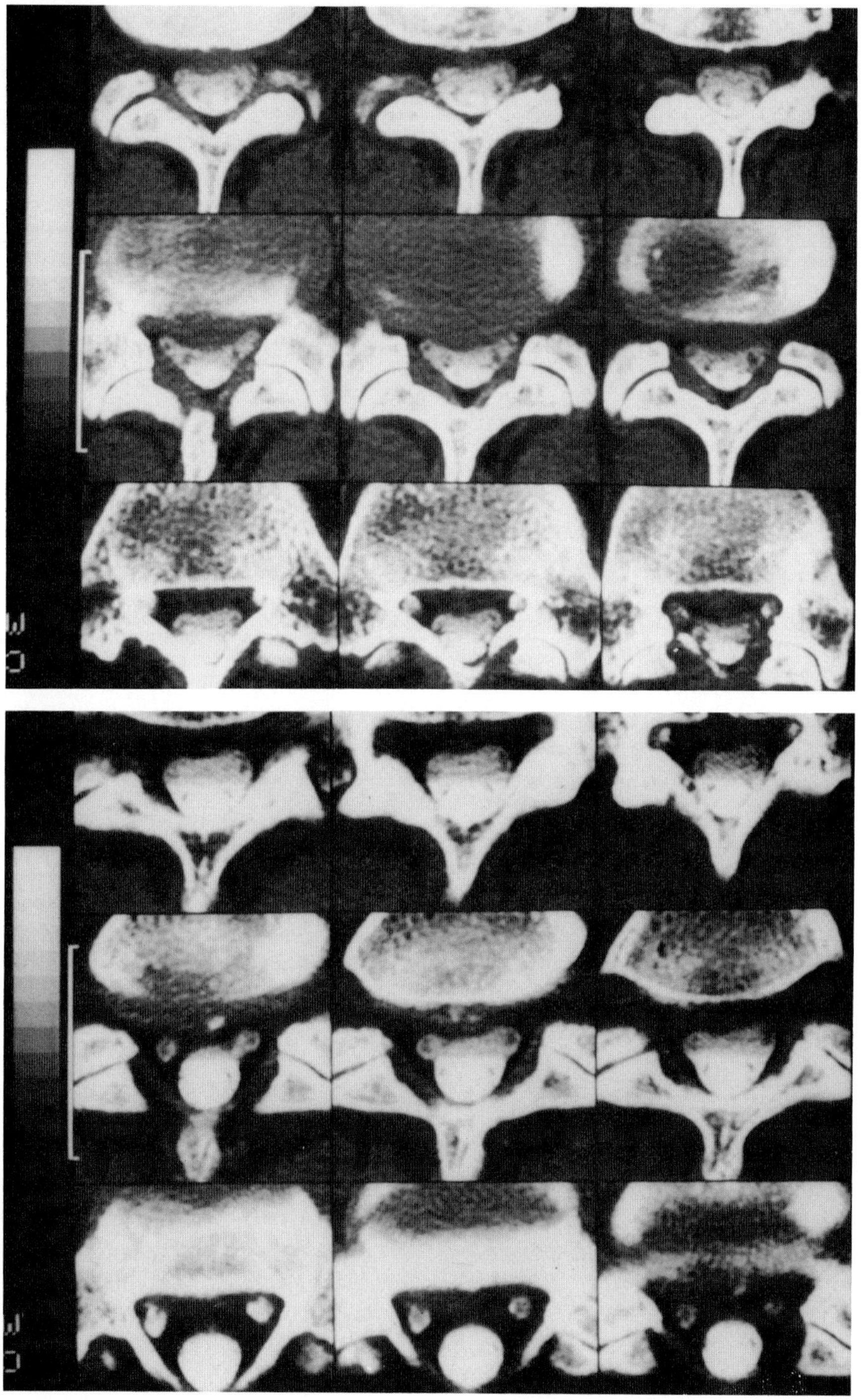

Figure I.3. Lumbar disc. Midline bulging disc is present with deformation of the sac but without obvious nerve root compression. In case 1 *(upper image)*, the patient's complaint was back pain only, no surgery was indicated, and the patient has improved with bracing and exercise. In case 2 *(lower image)*, a significant cauda equina syndrome was present. The disc was amenable to removal by a unilateral hemilaminectomy approach.

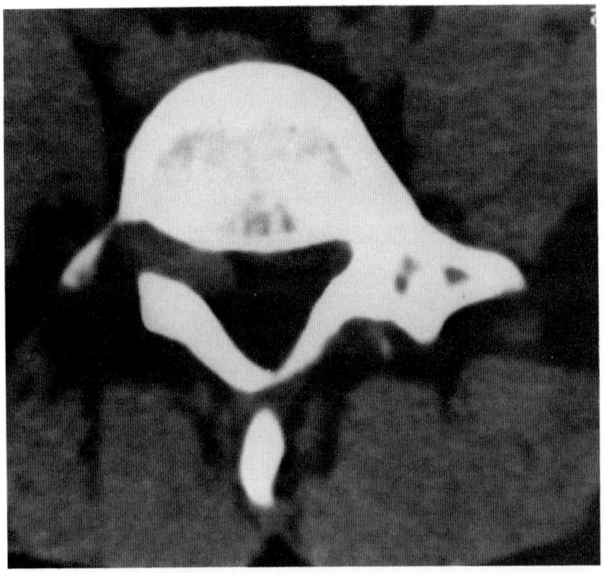

Figure I.4. CT scan demonstrates a typical laterally herniated lumbar disc with medial displacement of the nerve root. Such a lesion may be approached by either the lateral or the traditional midline surgery.

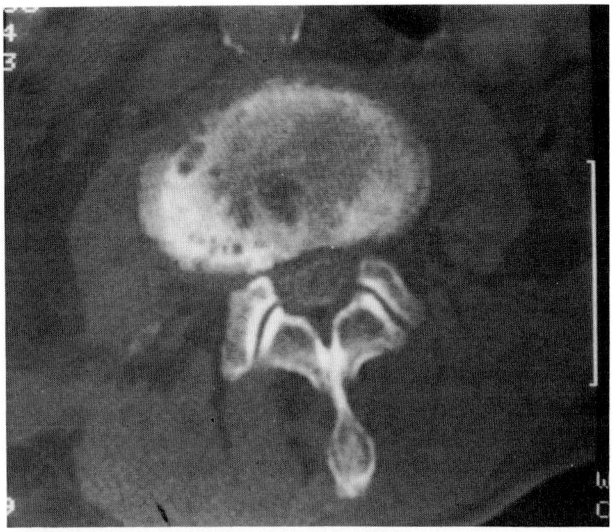

Figure I.5. Lumbar CT scan demonstrates obliteration of the lateral neural foramina. Decompression from the inferior surface of the superior articular process is obvious.

all cases of spinal trauma through the areas that are suspected. Remember that the entire spine where the suspected trauma may have occurred must be examined. Failure to examine the lower cervical spine, the upper lumbar spine, and the thoracic spine is, in general, the most common cause of a missed diagnosis in trauma. When the status of spinal cord compression is to be analyzed, MRI is the next choice. Plain CT plays a much smaller role. When MRI is not available or will not suffice, CT myelography is required.

Radiography for Spinal Cord Tumors and Related Spinal Cord Diseases

The MRI has revolutionized the evaluation of all of these kinds of spinal lesions. At one time, plain films and myelography were fundamental to the diagnosis. Now, both are unnecessary unless plain films have been taken for some other reason. When tumor is suspected, MRI scan is the study of choice. CT myelography may be required when the diagnosis is indeterminate, but increasingly it is not required.

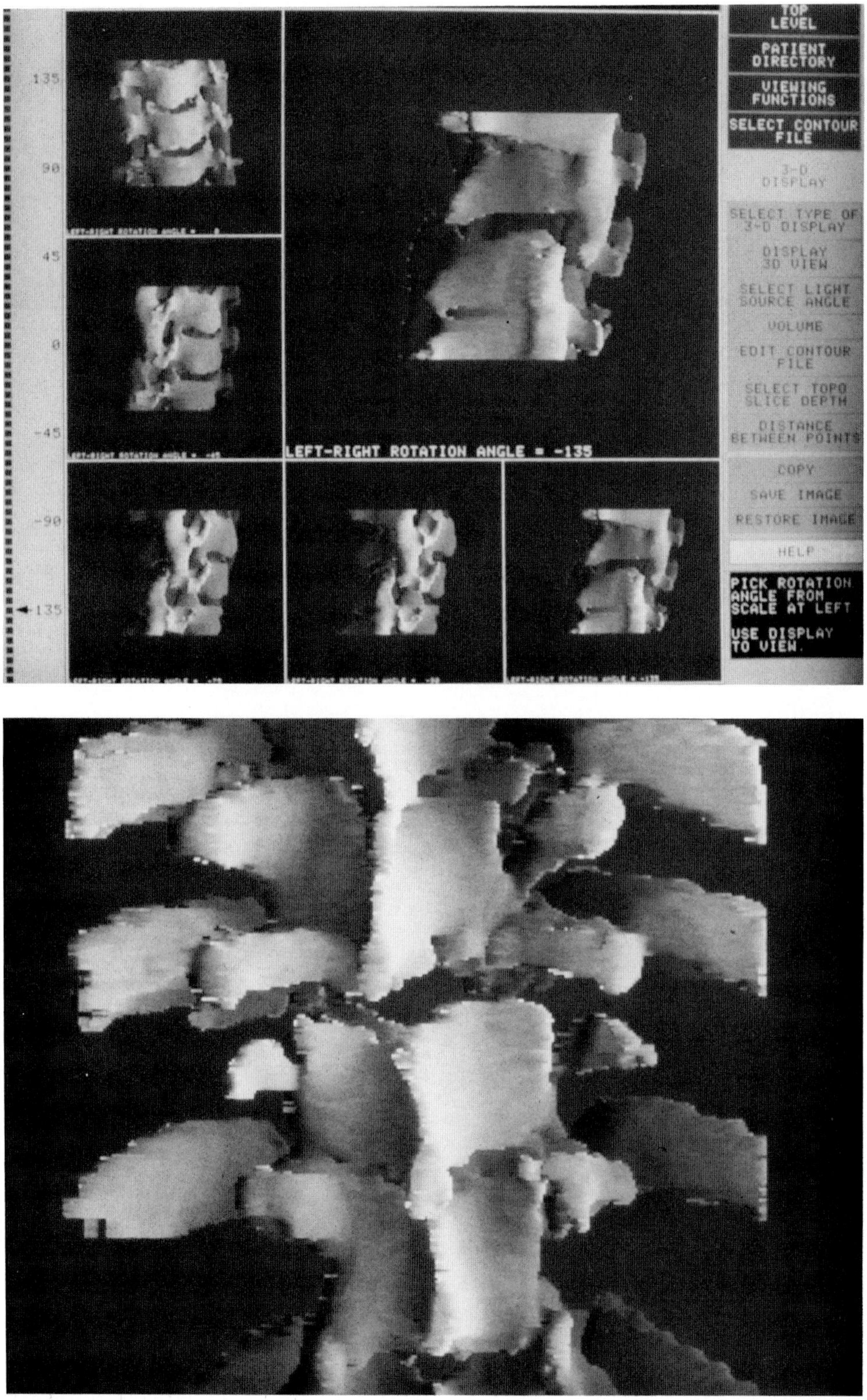

Figure I.6. Multiple-level views demonstrate a fracture with disruptions of both facets and lateral translation. Three-dimensional reconstructions produce an accurate picture of the fracture and allow appropriate planning for reconstruction.

Midline Spinal Incision

The skin incision should be made in the midline over the spinous processes (see Fig. 3.3, p. 61). It should be long enough to allow exposure of the expected pathology and for a margin of error in localization. For most diseases, one segment above and below provides adequate exposure. For diseases that are unisegmental, it is probable that only that segment needs to be exposed. In the cervical and lower lumbar region, anatomical localization is usually adequate. In other areas, an x-ray may be necessary. Division of the ligamentous and fascial layers should be exactly in the midline down to the level of the spinous processes. In the lumbar region the thick lumbar fascia is divided to bone and then undercut along the spinous process to provide a solid mass of fascia that can be closed exactly in the midline again. The thoracic fascia is much less well defined and is only cut away from the spinous processes laterally. The ligamentum nuchae provides the strength in the cervical region. It is divided to bone in the midline for later closure. The much thinner cervical fascia and the muscular attachments must be cut away from spinous processes. They do not provide adequate strength for closure. The posterior mass of muscle is attached to the spinous process, laminae, and zygapophyseal joints. This muscle mass must be raised with the least damage possible. The goal is a subperiosteal elevation of the muscles from the bone (see Fig. 3.4, p. 63). In practice this is rarely realized. Nevertheless, the goal is the least trauma possible to the muscles. Bony removal should be kept to a minimum, commensurate with what is required to solve the problem. The more normal the anatomy that remains, the better the function. There are two basic techniques of laminectomy. The time-honored method is piecemeal removal of bone with rongeurs. The bone is not replaced, and the muscles are simply allowed to resume their normal location without bony attachments. The second technique requires that the laminae be cut laterally near the zygapophyseal joints so that laminae and spinous processes can be removed as a single piece. They are later returned to their normal location and wired in position. No clear advantage for either method has yet been described. The zygapophyseal joints should be maintained whenever possible. When it is necessary to enter one, as much of it should be retained as commensurate with the necessities of the operative procedure. There is little evidence that partial or total removal of one or several joints has any deleterious effect, but preservation of function certainly dictates as little disruption to their anatomy as possible. When the muscles must be dissected from zygapophyseal joints and transverse processes as in posterolateral fusion, it is important to maintain the muscle mass in continuity and restore it to as near normal a position as possible.

Closing the Spinal Incision

The goals of closure in spinal incision are to eliminate the possibility of pseudomeningocele development, protect the neural elements, and approximate muscles and ligaments in their functional position. The dura should be closed with or without a patch whenever possible. Sometimes, it is undesirable to close the dura for fear of constriction of the neural elements, and a patch is not feasible. Covering the exposed dural incision with Gelfoam or fat is an acceptable alternative. The muscles are then approximated in the midline with sutures in the lumbar, dorsal fascia, or the ligamentum nuchae (see Fig. 3.8, p. 67). It is usually undesirable to put sutures in the muscle bellies themselves. They simply strangulate muscle and cause excessive fibrosis. Occasionally, there is enough oozing that it is better to bring the muscle edges together to aid in hemostasis. This should be done with large through-and-through disposable sutures, not tightly tied sutures, and then the ligaments should be closed tightly. When dural closure is not complete, the ligament sutures must achieve a watertight closure so that cerebrospinal fluid leak does not occur. The subcutaneous tissues and skin are then closed in the routine fashion.

SECTION 1

Lumbar Disc and Related Problems

1

Primary Operations on Lumbar Disc

Lumbar Discectomy

Patient positioning for lumbar discectomy is important; there are several acceptable positions that may be utilized according to the surgeon's experience. The most common position places the patient prone on one of the commercially available laminectomy frames or rolls that support the iliac crest and shoulders, leaving the abdomen and chest without compression. The lumbar spine should be parallel to the floor. A variation of this is the knee-chest position in which the patient is placed kneeling on the table or a frame. Again, the patient's lumbar spine is kept parallel to the floor. The goal of both of these positions is to reduce intraabdominal and intrathoracic pressure, thereby reducing epidural venous congestion. The third position in common use is the lateral. The patient is placed on one side and positioned so that the back is exactly at the edge of the table and the knees and head are both drawn up toward the abdomen without causing abdominal or thoracic compression. The operative side is up so that the muscle is easily retracted. The position chosen is certainly the surgeon's preference. There is no advantage to one position over the other except that of familiarity. The principle of position is unimpeded epidural venous return. These operations may be carried out with the patient under general or local anesthesia, according to the surgeon's

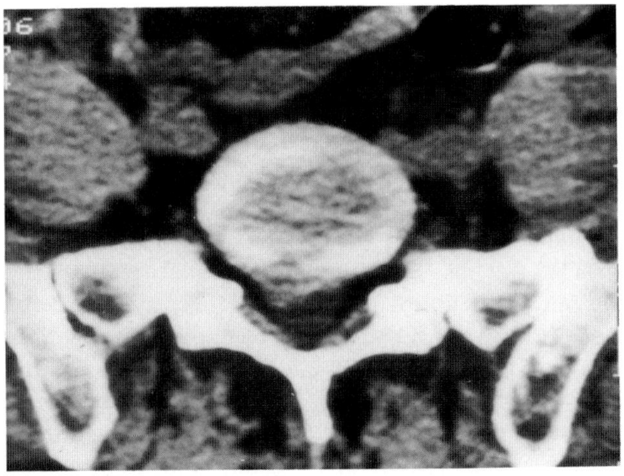

Figure 1.1. Computed tomography (CT) scan of typical herniated lumbar disc at L5-S1 level.

preference. It is feasible to carry out the procedure under local anesthesia in cooperative patients. Most surgeons use general anesthesia now, but local anesthesia is an attractive alternative for the surgeon skilled in its use.

Prone Position

After induction of general anesthesia while on the cart, the patient is rolled onto a laminectomy frame, and the frame is fitted so that it supports the iliac crest (both sides) and the shoulders, leaving the chest and abdomen free. The patient is carefully positioned so the back is parallel to the floor and the legs are elevated on a pillow to facilitate venous return through the procedure (see Fig. 3.2). The location of the skin incision should be estimated from the plain films. A small incision exposing one space is preferred by many surgeons. The usual incision for an experienced surgeon is 1–2 inches long. Some surgeons prefer to see at least two spaces, and sometimes three spaces will be necessary for accurate localization. If a small incision is used, it is important to obtain an intraoperative x-ray for localization *if* there is any doubt. With more experience an x-ray becomes less and less necessary. For the usual disc occurring at L4-L5 or L5-S1, a skin incision that exposes both spaces provides absolute certainty of localization. At higher levels a film is important and the smaller incisions are routine. Localization by anatomy or x-ray is a matter of personal preference, and the choice is of very little consequence.

The original skin incision is carried to the spinous processes in the midline, and a self-retaining retractor is used to retract the skin. There is no reason to coagulate the usual small skin bleeding points. They will stop spontaneously, and coagulation of the skin impairs the quality of wound healing. The next step is a careful section of the lumbar fascia and a subperiosteal dissection of the paravertebral muscle mass from the spines, the laminae, and the medial portion of zygapophyseal joints. The ligamentous section may be carried out with a knife or with cautery. The electric knife or cautery virtually eliminates bleeding. The lumbar ligaments should be divided in the midline down to the spinous processes and then undercut back to the muscle (Fig. 1.2). It is extremely important to have undisturbed ligament to close to restore normal biomechanics to the lumbar spine. It is also important to find a subperiosteal plane at the apex of the spinous process. In the proper plane the paravertebral muscle mass will be virtually undisturbed by the dissection. If the surgeon does not take the time to find this plane, then the muscles will be torn and bleeding at the close of the dissection. This produces unnecessary postoperative pain and probably impedes the restoration of normal back function. Once the lumbar fascia is divided and the muscle is exposed, the muscular attachments to the interspinous ligaments should be cut (Fig. 1.2). This attachment is wide, usually at least 1 cm, and will not strip easily unless it is divided sharply. The cautery knife is effective here. Osteotomes are used to complete the subperiosteal dissection of muscles from spines and lamina. The technique is important. The lumbar osteotomes preferably should be square and approximately the size of the laminae. Two osteotomes are used. Starting at any convenient place, the surgeon should make the first cut straight down the spinous process and out the lamina. Muscle retraction is maintained by tension on the osteotome, and the osteotome in the second hand is used to cut the muscles away from either the inferior or the superior margin of the lamina, depending on which hand has been used to make the first cut. Retraction is always maintained by one osteotome while the other is taken out and reinserted to make the next cut. On the left side, if the first cut is made with the left hand, the muscles are cut from the inferior margin with the right hand, and then the third cut at each space is made to remove the muscles from the superior margin of the lamina and the intralaminar space above. The process is then repeated at each level to be exposed. The process is reversed on the right. There is no need for more than three maneuvers with the osteotomes at each space. If a sponge is put in at this time, it will absorb any blood, and if the maneuvers are repeated over the sponge, all of the loose areolar tissue and fat will be wiped away with the sponge, so that the area will be completely clean. The sponge should be removed, and deep retractors put in place. There are a variety of laminectomy and hemilaminectomy retractors. The choice of the retractor is virtually the preference of the surgeon. Use of an angled cerebellar-type retractor with a post on one side, which is placed in the intraspinous space, and a flat-toothed plate on the opposite side, which holds the muscle back, works well. There is no need to expose more than one interspace unless you plan to explore more than one. The retractor should expose approximately half of the lamina above, half of the lamina below, and the entire intralaminar and intraspinous space out to the medial margin of the facet. The retractors should be posterior to the facet, and at least half the zygapophyseal joint should be exposed.

The intralaminar space should then be explored. It may be possible to remove the disc without removing any bone. If the space is large enough, this is quite feasible, especially at L5-S1. When the space is smaller, it may be necessary to remove bone. The Adson rongeur is an ideal instrument. One bite of the lamina above is usually sufficient to allow exposure of the nerve root (Fig. 1.2). It is unusual that more than half of the lamina needs to be removed (Fig. 1.3). This will expose a broad expanse of ligamentum flavum. The ligamentum flavum must be divided, and the epidural space entered, without injury to the dura and nerve root beneath. A window or flap can be cut, or a linear incision used (Figs. 1.4 and 1.5). Remember the nerve root and the dural sac may be pushed up tightly against the ligament by a large disc herniation and it is easy to enter the dura if this maneuver is not carefully done (Fig. 1.1). In elderly people, the dura and the ligament may be especially adherent. It is important to free the ligament from the dura by blunt dissection before additional ligament is removed with a punch. Next, gently probe the interspace to locate the disc fragment. The Olivecrona dissector is an ideal instrument for this purpose. Palpating the dura and the root will usually locate the disc herniation quickly. When the location of the herniation is determined, it is then necessary only to extend the ligament and bone removal with a Kerrison-type punch in the direction that will give adequate access to the disc fragment (Figs. 1.3 and 1.5). The disc should be removed from the direction in which it will come out most easily (Fig. 1.6). If the disc herniation is most visible in the axilla, then the dural sac can be retracted medially, and the nerve root laterally, to expose the disc. If the disc is more laterally placed, then the nerve root should be retracted medially over it. If the nerve root is stretched tightly by the disc herniation, it is best to carry out a small foraminotomy until the nerve root is sufficiently loose to be mobilized medially over the disc (Figs. 1.3 and 1.5). All of this should be carried out under direct vision, and there should be little or no blood loss. The operating microscope provides especially good definition. Excessive venous bleeding usually means less-than-optimal positioning with some compression of abdomen or chest. Be careful not to enter the zygapophyseal joint unnecessarily. There is scarcely ever a need to disrupt the joint when carrying out a simple discectomy. Leave the epidural fat compartments intact except over the root. Once the disc is adequately exposed, it may be necessary to place some packing in the epidural space to eliminate bleeding and allow the disc to be removed under direct vision. Cottonoid patties work well, as does the twisted end of a 4×4 sponge. Cotton balls are very easy to lose in the field. Packing the epidural space should provide a completely bloodless field for removal of the disc. A free fragment of disc may be loose in the canal or may still be contained by the ligament (Figs. 1.1 and 1.7). When the dural sac is adequately visualized and the nerve root is seen, the retractor can be placed either against the dural sac, when the axilla is to be the route of approach, or against the nerve root, when the nerve root is to be retracted medially. The broad dural root retractors provide excellent protection of dura and root disc during removal. When the disc is a free fragment, the only maneuver required is to grasp the disc fragment with the disc rongeur and gently to tease it out from under the nerve root and dura (Figs. 1.6 and 1.8). The disc will usually come out as a single piece, but often several fragments are out of the interspace, and each must be removed separately. If the ligament is still intact over the disc fragment, then it must be incised (Fig. 1.6). The veins should be dissected away until a glistening white ligament is seen. A cruciate

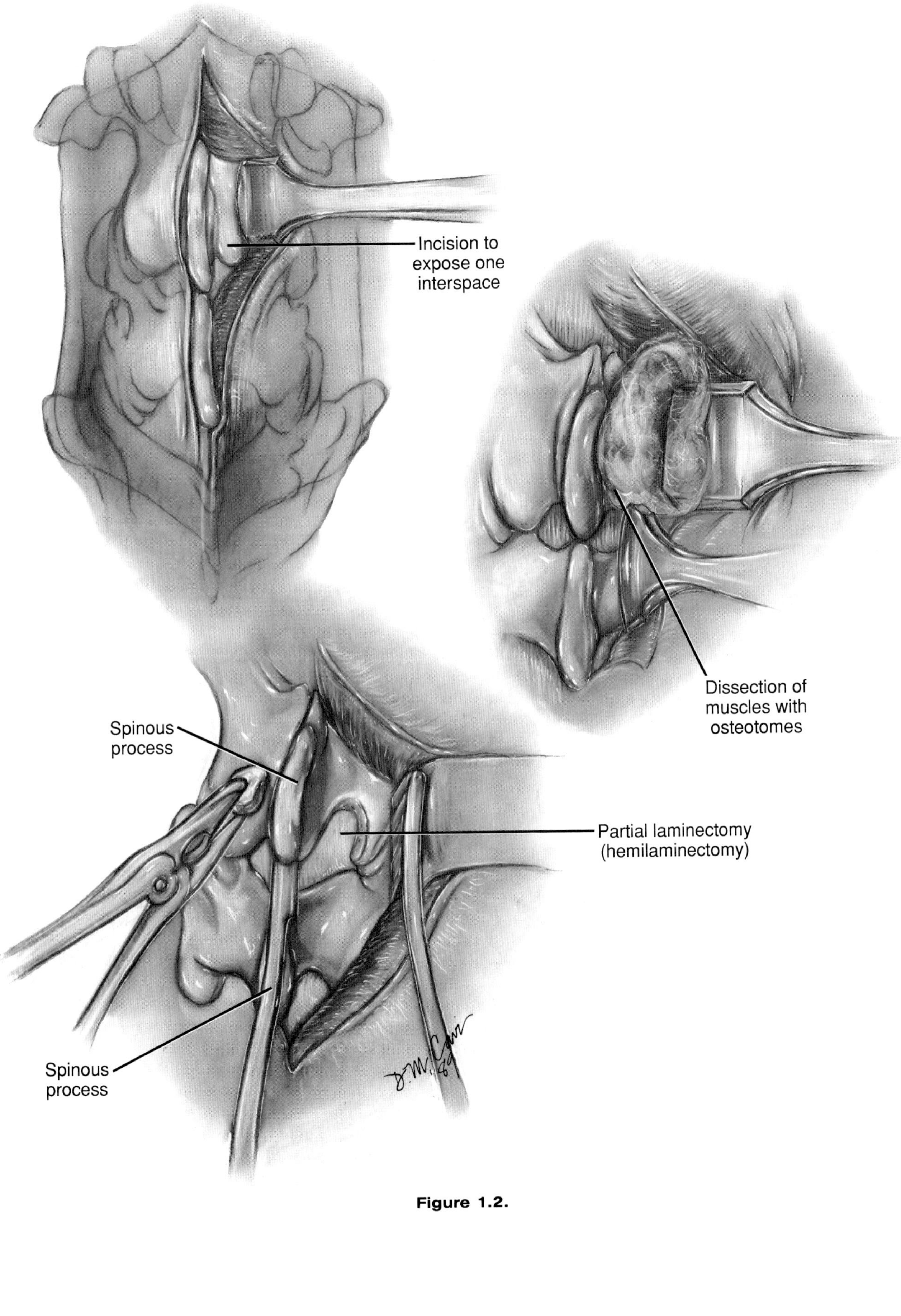
Incision to expose one interspace
Dissection of muscles with osteotomes
Spinous process
Partial laminectomy (hemilaminectomy)
Spinous process

Figure 1.2.

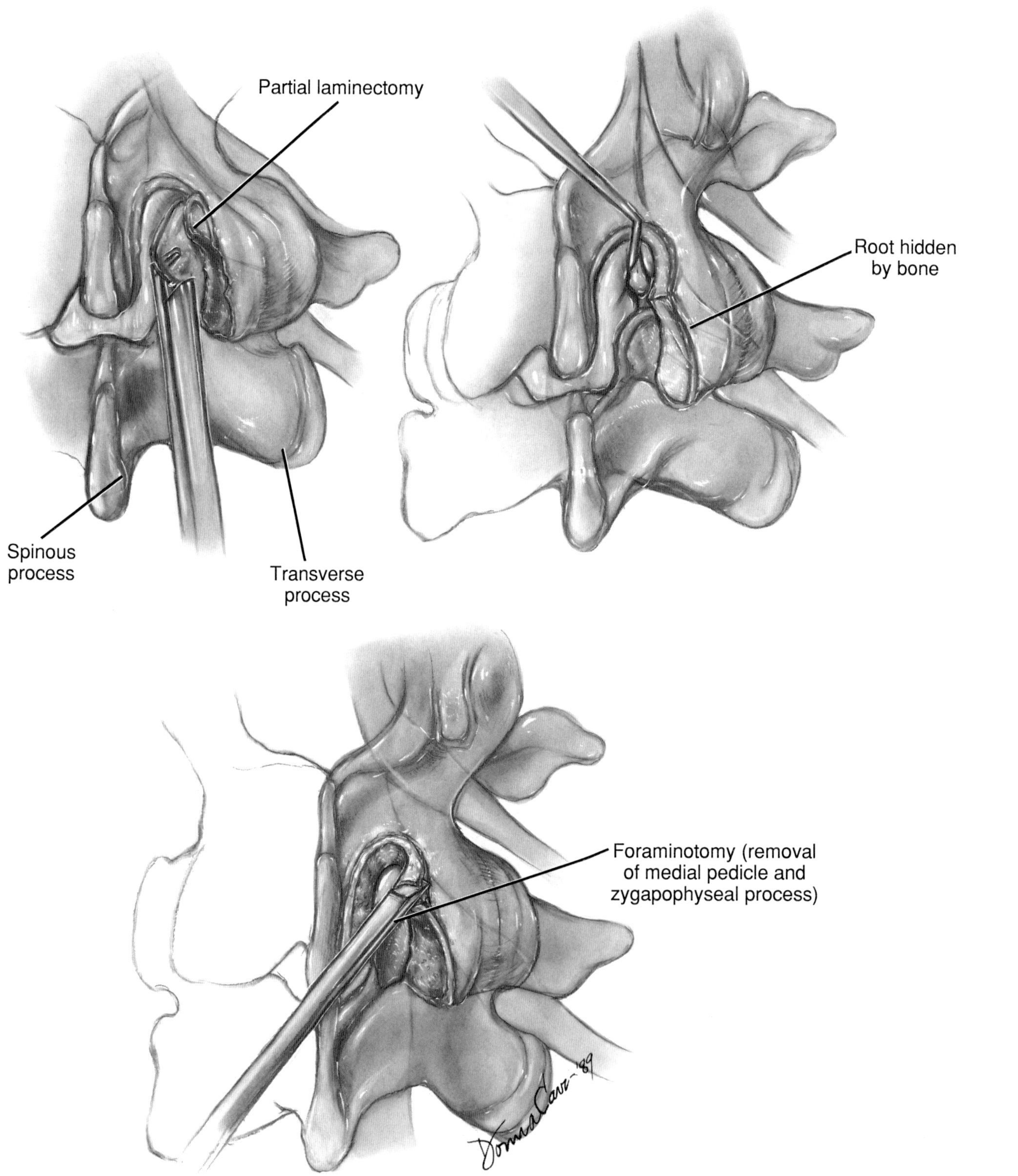
Partial laminectomy
Root hidden by bone
Spinous process
Transverse process
Foraminotomy (removal of medial pedicle and zygapophyseal process)

Figure 1.3.

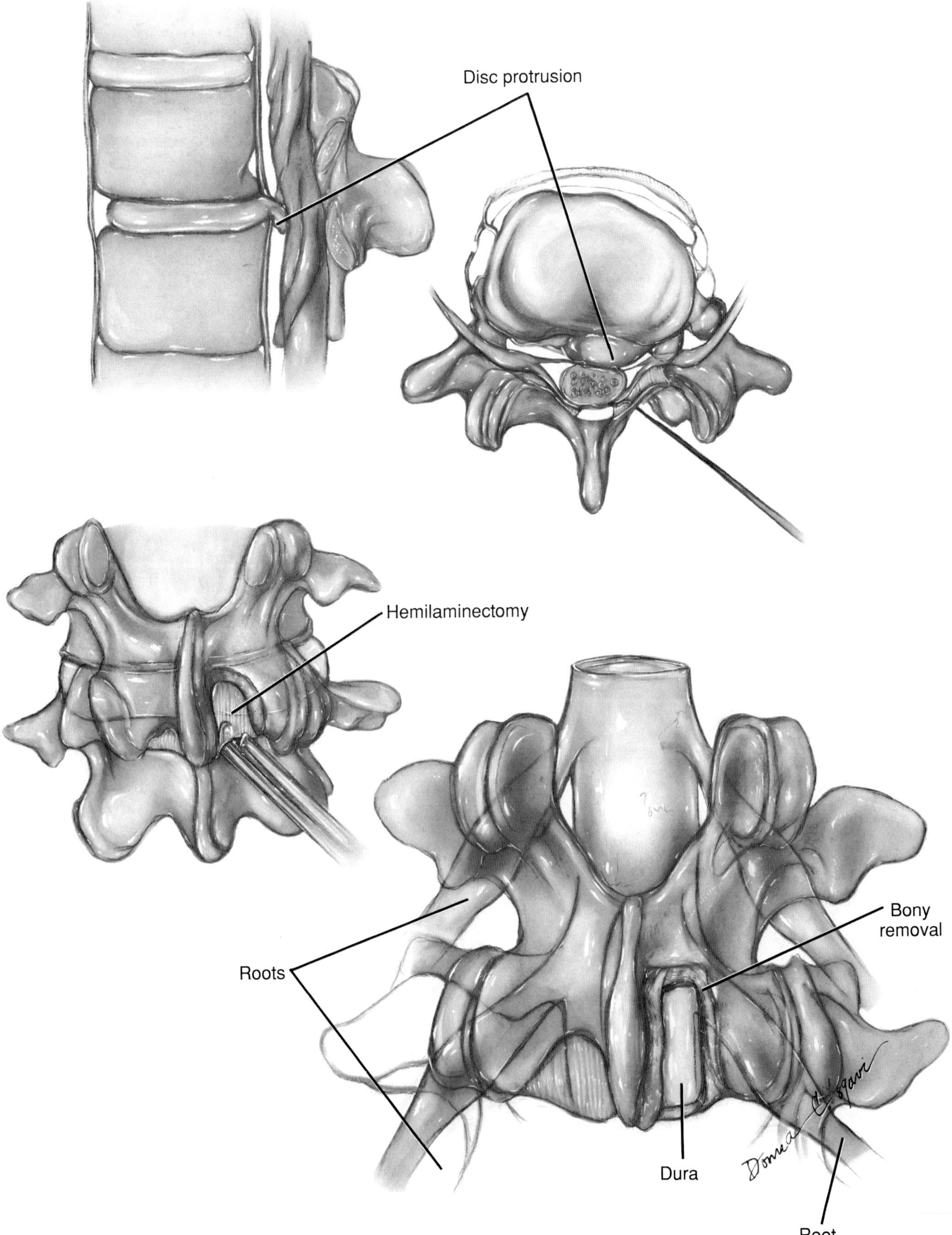
Disc protrusion
Hemilaminectomy
Bony removal
Roots
Dura
Root

Figure 1.4.

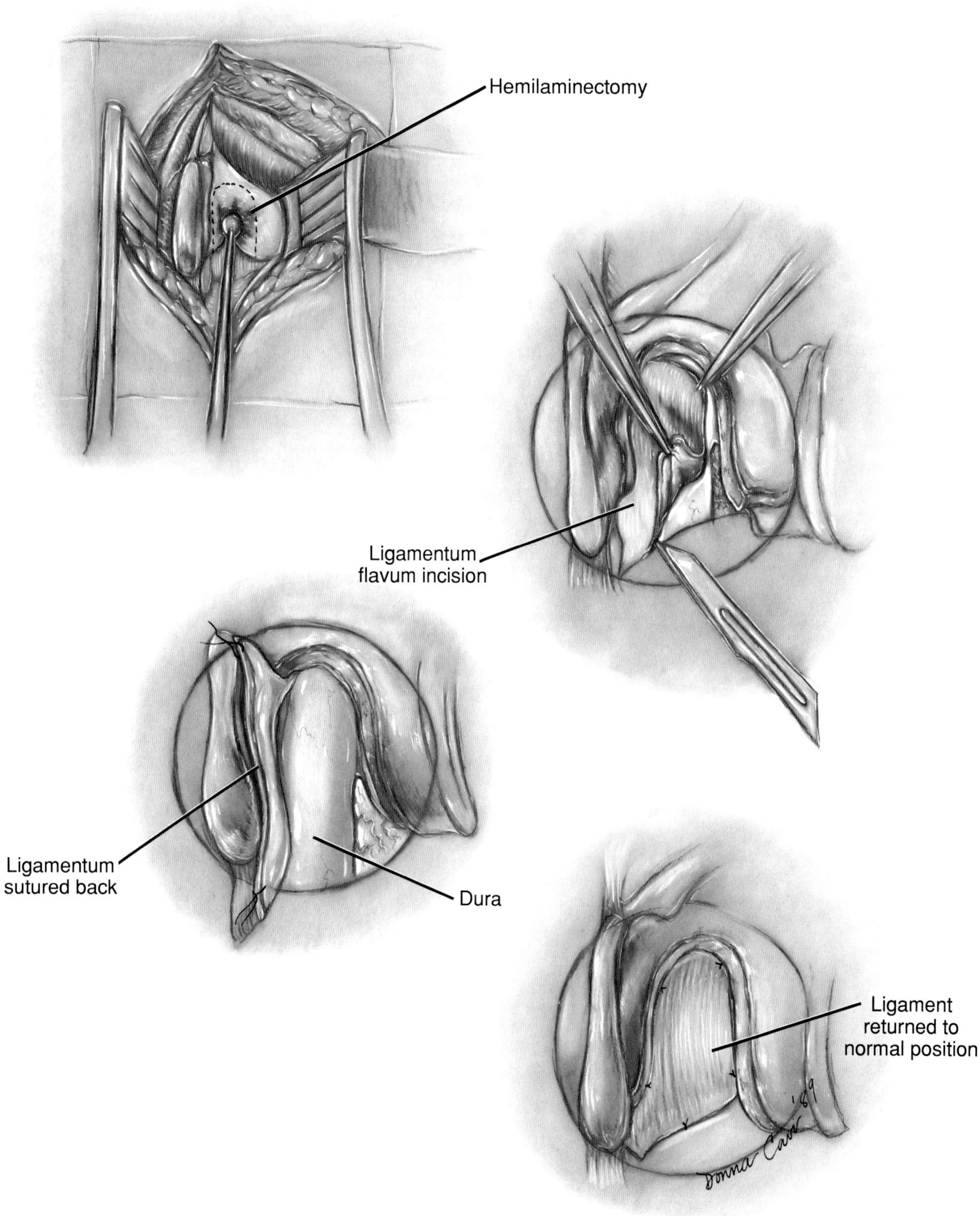
Hemilaminectomy
Ligamentum flavum incision
Ligamentum sutured back
Dura
Ligament returned to normal position
Donna Carr '89

Figure 1.5.

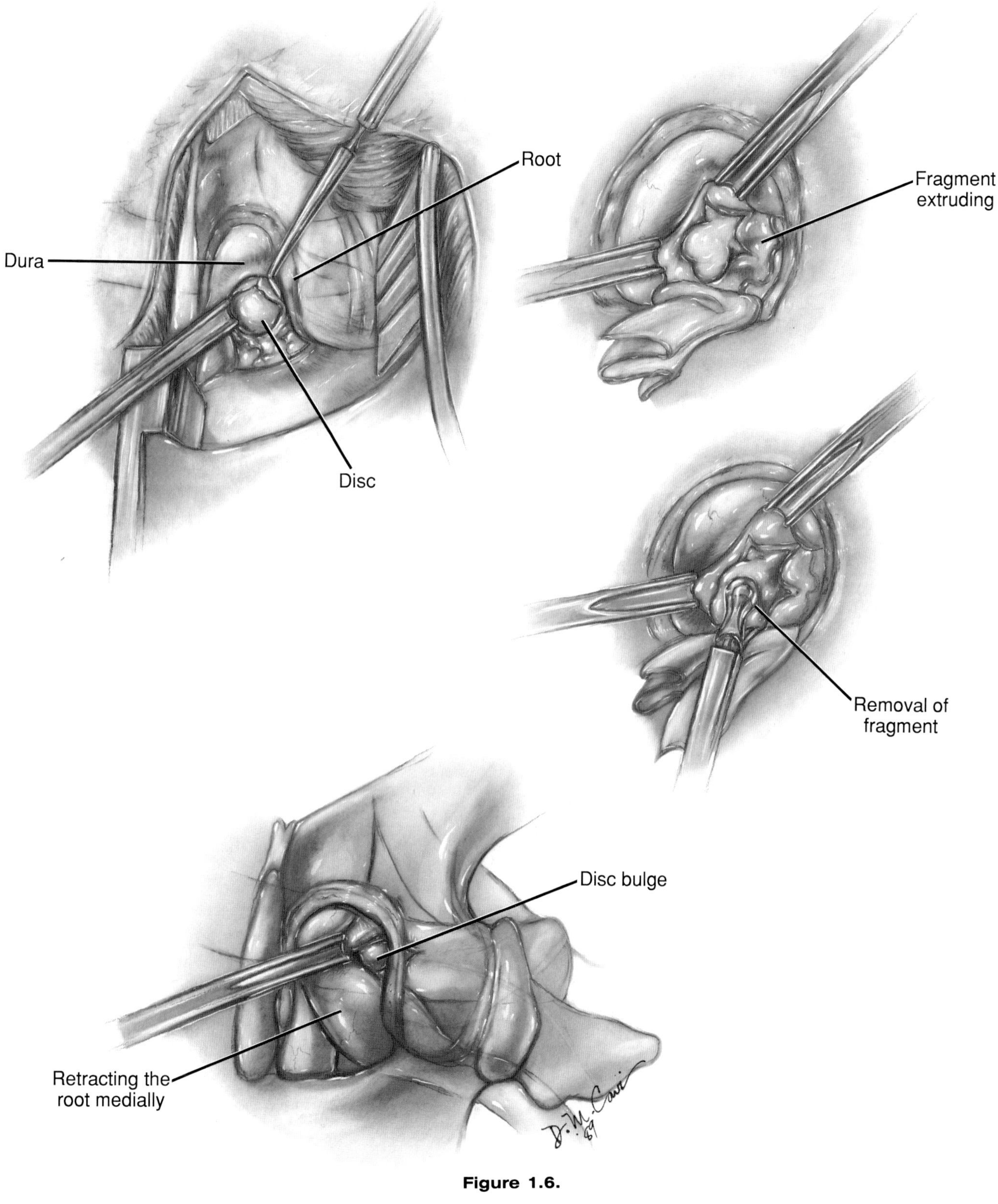
Root
Dura
Disc
Fragment
extruding
Removal of
fragment
Disc bulge
Retracting the
root medially

Figure 1.6.

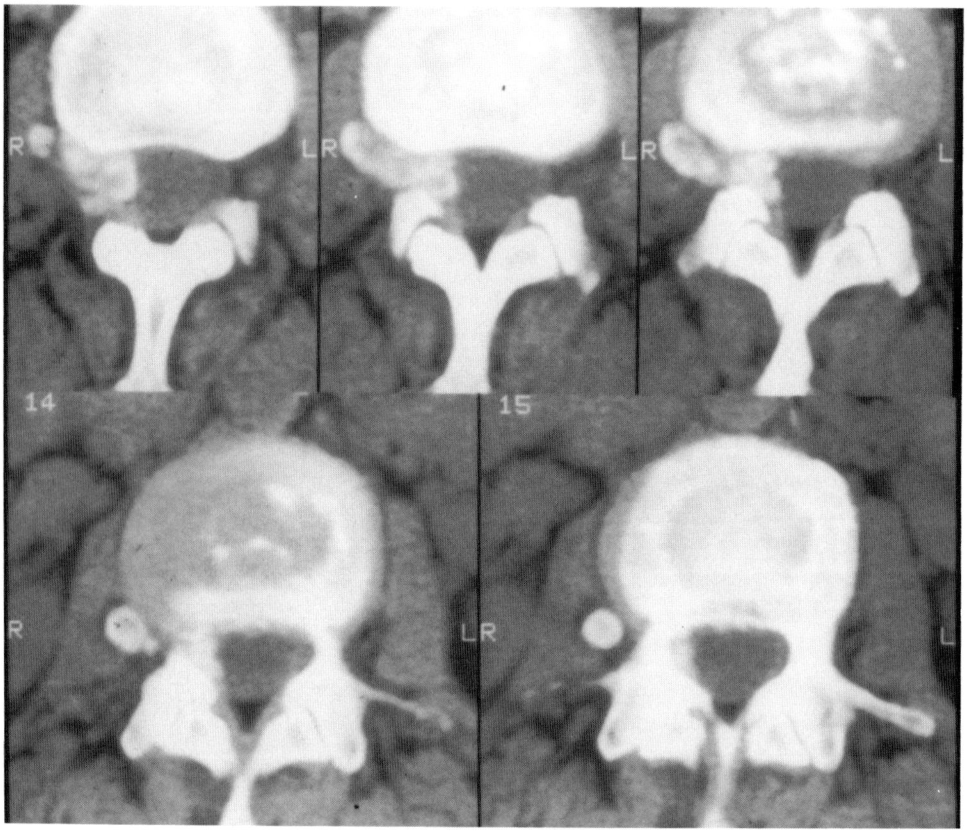

Figure 1.7. Typical picture of lateral herniated disc, which is approachable either from inside the spinal canal or laterally, which would be preferable.

incision in the ligament suffices. The disc fragment will immediately herniate into the field and can be grasped with the disc rongeur and removed. (Fig. 1.6). The interspace should then be entered (Fig. 1.8). The straight disc rongeur should be used to remove all easily available degenerated disc material from the interspace. It is important to have a repetitive technique for doing this. The depth of the interspace must be clearly kept in mind, and the instruments utilized in a way that always considers where the tip is located before any bite is taken. The disc rongeur should be placed through the ligament with the jaws closed. Then the jaws should be immediately opened, and the instrument inserted to the proper depth. Then the jaws are closed, and disc material that is easily removable will be extracted by multiple bites in this way. It is important to extend removal as far medially and as far laterally as possible so that all of the degenerated disc material is removed. Some surgeons make a point of a radical removal of disc material. Others do not, and there have never been data that indicate that one approach is superior to the other. Large curettes can be turned within the inner space to free any adherent degenerated portions of disc that then can be removed by the disc rongeur. The interspace should be irrigated so that any small fragments can be washed out. The root retractors are removed, and the tension on the nerve root is tested to be certain that it is relieved. Before closure, it is important to explore medially under the dural sac in the axilla and laterally along the nerve root to be sure that no fragment has been missed. If there is any question about tension on the root, a foraminotomy should be performed until the nerve root is free or until another fragment is found. If the findings are not those expected from the imaging study, an intraoperative film should be taken to be certain that localization of the interspace has been correct. There

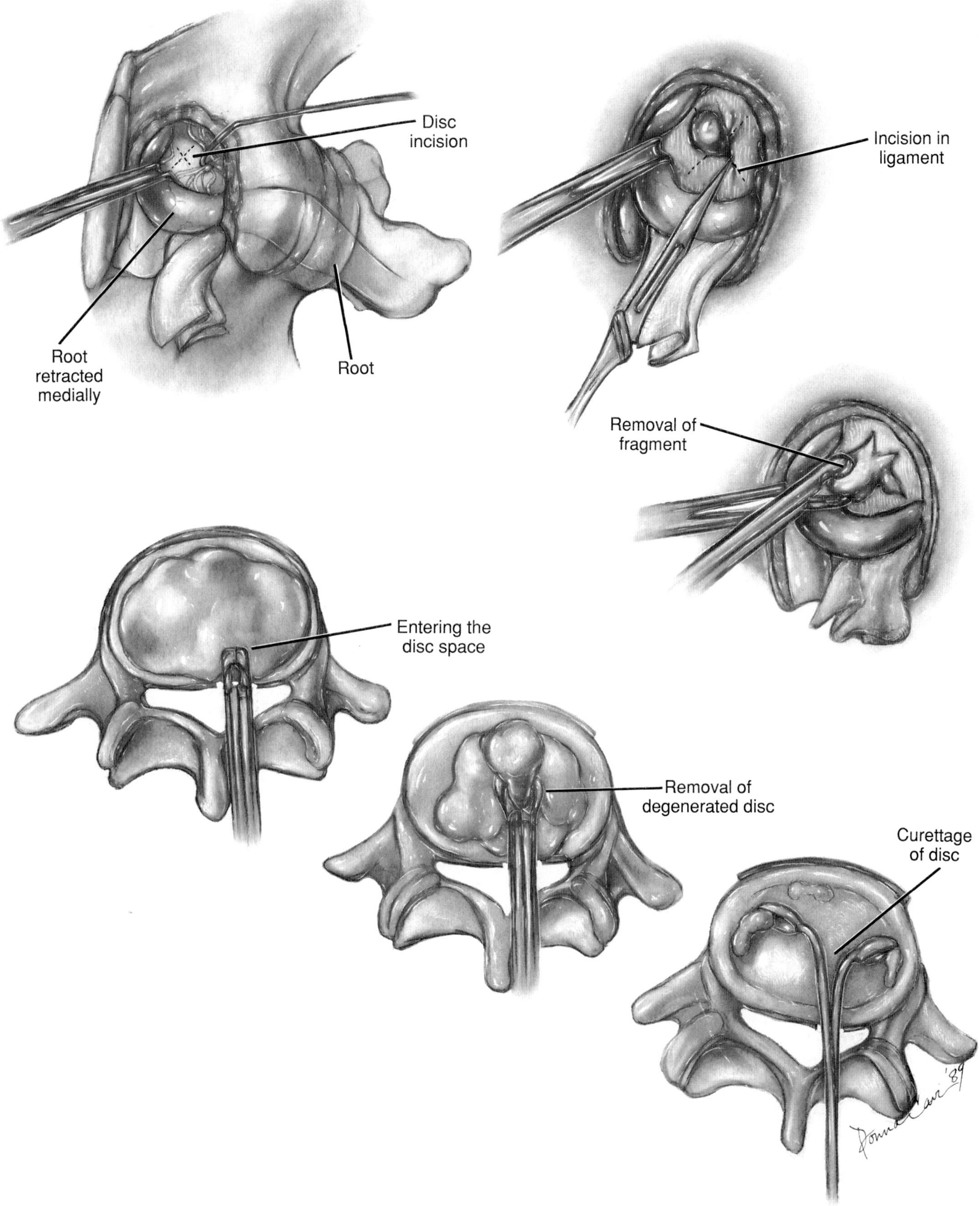
Disc
incision
Root
retracted
medially
Root
Incision in
ligament
Removal of
fragment
Entering the
disc space
Removal of
degenerated disc
Curettage
of disc

Figure 1.8.

should be no bleeding at closure. The environment is reconstituted with a small piece of subcutaneous fat that is carefully tucked around the nerve and replaces the excised ligamentum flavum. The operation can be done with a flap of ligamentum flavum used (Fig. 1.5). This approach is utilized particularly when the operating microscope is employed for discectomy. Nothing in the literature at present substantiates that any one of the variations in discectomy technique is superior to another. The principles are meticulous exposure, gentleness in handling the tissues, avoidance of nerve injury, and immaculate hemostasis. The results of surgery for the truly herniated lumbar disc are extremely good, and it is one of the most gratifying operations known to neurosurgery or orthopaedics. It is unlikely that any minor variations in technique significantly effect the outcome. The most common cause of a poor result in lumbar surgery is poor selection of the operative candidate, not surgical technique. Surgery for the degenerated, not the herniated, lumbar disc is not very rewarding, and surgery in the face of a major psychosocial disturbance is virtually guaranteed to fail.

The closure is simple. Stitches should be placed in the lumbar fascia alone. Heavy sutures that will not break are best, i.e., 0 or its equivalent. The subcutaneous tissue should be closed, and a subcuticular skin stitch will allow the patient to leave the hospital promptly without return for stitch removal. Staples also provide a cosmetically desirable incision. No stitches should be placed in the lumbar muscles so that there will be a minimum of scarring and disruption of the normal mechanics of the back.

Microdiscectomy

In the past few years much has been made of the value of the operating microscope for lumbar disc surgery. It is possible to do excellent disc surgery without the microscope and to achieve excellent results. However, there is no question that the techniques required by the operating microscope emphasize gentleness of tissue handling and hemostasis. For this reason, the microscope is an excellent adjunct for anyone newly learning disc surgery. There are some variations in the technique that the microdiscectomy requires. First, only a very small incision, no more than 1 inch, is required. This means preoperative localization is mandatory, and an intraoperative film is usually desirable. The exposure of the interspace is done in the same way as for traditional lumbar discectomy (Fig. 1.5). Then the microscope is brought into the field before the ligament is opened. When the microscope is employed, vision is good enough so that only a small flap of ligamentum flavum needs to be raised. This should be hinged on the midline; the ligament should be incised under direct vision around the margins of the bony confines of the exposure. It is sutured back to the interspinous ligament to keep it out of the way. The exploration of the interspace is carried out with the microscope. Use of the microscope means that hemostasis must be completely adequate or you will not be able to see at all. Otherwise, the exposure and the disc removal are exactly the same as described (Fig. 1.8). The small size of the microinstruments and the need for hemostasis make gentleness of dissection and atraumatic tissue handling virtually a necessity. It also allows the fat surrounding the root to be preserved. Once the disc is removed, the ligamentum flavum and the interspace are carefully explored, the ligamentum flavum is returned to position, and the wound is closed in usual fashion (Fig. 1.5).

There is one trick for use during microdiscectomy. Rather than use rongeurs for bone removal, it is much easier to carry out the hemilaminectomy and foraminotomy with the high-speed surgical drill (Fig. 1.5). This provides good hemostasis and excellent control. It is actually faster than working with traditional rongeurs. The accurate use of the drill is enhanced by the microscope. When the drill is used, it is necessary to dissect the ligamentum flavum from the laminae carefully, have the muscles retracted well back, and have all soft tissue removed from the bone.

Foraminotomy

Foraminotomy is an important procedure, the goal of which is decompression of the nerve root with minimal disruption of stability. The procedure is most commonly utilized for foraminal stenosis caused by pressure on the nerve root from the combined pedicle and both articular processes (see Fig. 1.1). Less commonly, there is an anterior spur. A third reason for foraminotomy is a laterally placed disc that is beyond the point that is easily reached by the usual hemilaminectomy exposure (Fig. 1.7). This is a different consideration from foraminal stenosis and is usually treated via an extraforaminal approach (Fig. 1.7). For the usual patient with bony stenosis, the goal must be to create a new neural foramen by removing part of the pedicle and the undersurface of the superior articular process without entering the joint itself; sometimes, facetectomy must be utilized, but pressure on the root can usually be relived by simple bone removal that does not necessarily include entering the joint. The exposure for the foraminotomy is the same as that utilized for simple discectomy until the nerve root is identified (Figs. 1.9 and 1.10). Then the dissection must be carried laterally out the foramen. First, remove all of the ligamentum flavum laterally as far as possible, using small angled punches. The nerve root can be pushed up into the lateral recess, and if the punches are not carefully placed, the nerve root can be grasped along with the bone in the lateral recess, either crushing it or avulsing it with the bit of the rongeur. Once the ligament is removed, it should be possible to see the root hooked around the pedicle and compressed in the neural foramen (Fig. 1.9). Frazier probes are ideal to assess the size of the foramen and root compression. The next step is to remove the underportion of the facet joints (Fig. 1.10). This can be carried out in several ways. Small angled punches will reach into the foramen and bite away the lower half of the superior articular process without entering the joint space (Fig. 1.3). A second way to remove the bone is to fashion a new foramen with small chisels, first removing the inferior one half to one third of the superior articular process and then chiseling away the pedicle until the compression of the nerve at its exit from the spinal canal is removed. The chiseling is done to remove thin sheets of bone. Otherwise, it is likely that the zygapophyseal joint will be fractured or the pedicle can actually be broken. Be careful not to break any portions of bone so as to compress the nerve root or to leave any broken fragments of bone in the foramen. As the bone is removed, the nerve root will migrate laterally, and the tension will become progressively less. Probing with the Frazier dissector will indicate when the foramen is open. When the dissector passes easily into the paravertebral muscles, then the foramen is satisfactorily enlarged. This part of the dissection can also be done with the high-speed drill (Figs. 1.9 and 1.10). There are guards that protect the dura and root beneath, allowing the surgeon simply to ream out the foramen by using a large cutting burr carefully inserted into the foramen. Both the pedicle and the articular process are drilled away until there is sufficient room for the nerve root (Fig. 1.10). When using chisels or rongeurs, the surgeon stands on the side of the pathology. When the drill is used, however, it is not possible to see well enough from the symptomatic side. For drilling, therefore, the surgeon should leave the side of pathology and carry out the procedure from the opposite side where vision will be better. The use of the operating microscope adds a degree of accuracy and protection to the drilling, but it is not absolutely necessary. Once the neural foramen is adequately decompressed, whatever the method used, the operative site is covered with a small pledget of fat. The closure is the same as for lumbar discectomy.

Lateral Disc Herniation

When the disc has herniated far laterally into the neural foramen, the technique differs somewhat from either of the approaches described (Fig. 1.7). Lateral discs may be exposed by foraminotomy or by the extraforaminal route. Exposure for the former is the same to the point where the hemilaminectomy is complete and the interspace can be explored. When it becomes apparent that the disc is placed too far laterally to be removed by the usual technique, it becomes necessary to open the foramen (Fig. 1.3). In this case, the drilling that would be done for bony foraminal stenosis will not suffice. A facetectomy, partial or total, is required. This may be carried out with a high-speed drill or with the Kerrison-type punches. The pedicle need not be approached, but the entire joint, both superior and inferior articular processes, must be entered. The bone simply is removed out the neural foramen, through the facet, whatever distance is required to visualize the nerve and the disc herniation. These lateral herniations are almost always free fragments, and a corner of the fragment can usually be seen under the splayed nerve. The fragments should be grasped with a small disc rongeur and gradually teased out from under the root. If it does not come easily, the facetectomy should be continued until it is complete. This will always allow the root to be mobilized enough to remove the disc. When the remainder of the spine is normal, a unilateral facetectomy is of little concern, and subsequent instability rarely occurs. Once the disc fragment is removed and the root is decompressed, return to the

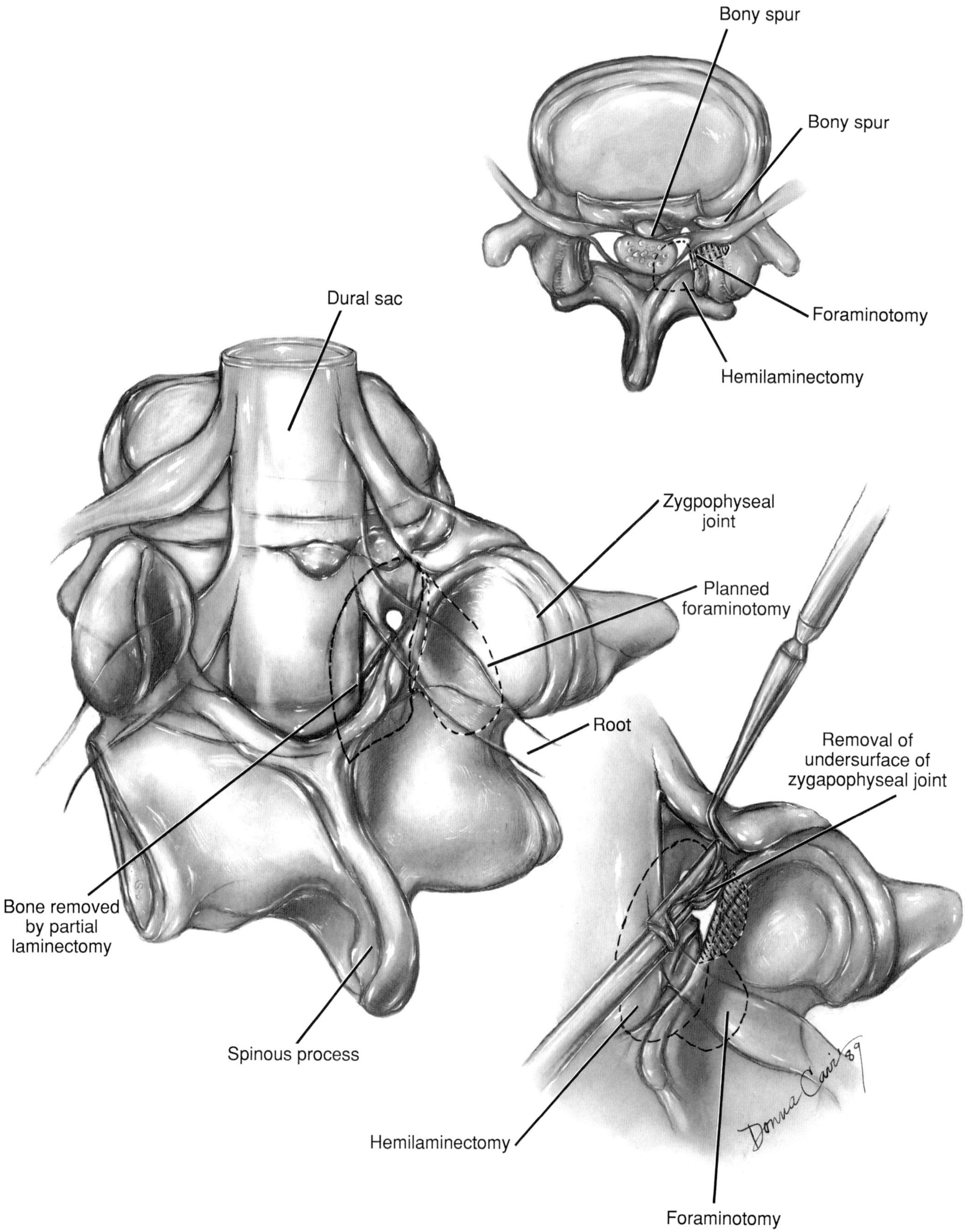
Bony spur
Bony spur
Foraminotomy
Hemilaminectomy
Dural sac
Zygpophyseal joint
Planned foraminotomy
Root
Removal of undersurface of zygapophyseal joint
Bone removed by partial laminectomy
Spinous process
Hemilaminectomy
Foraminotomy

Figure 1.9.

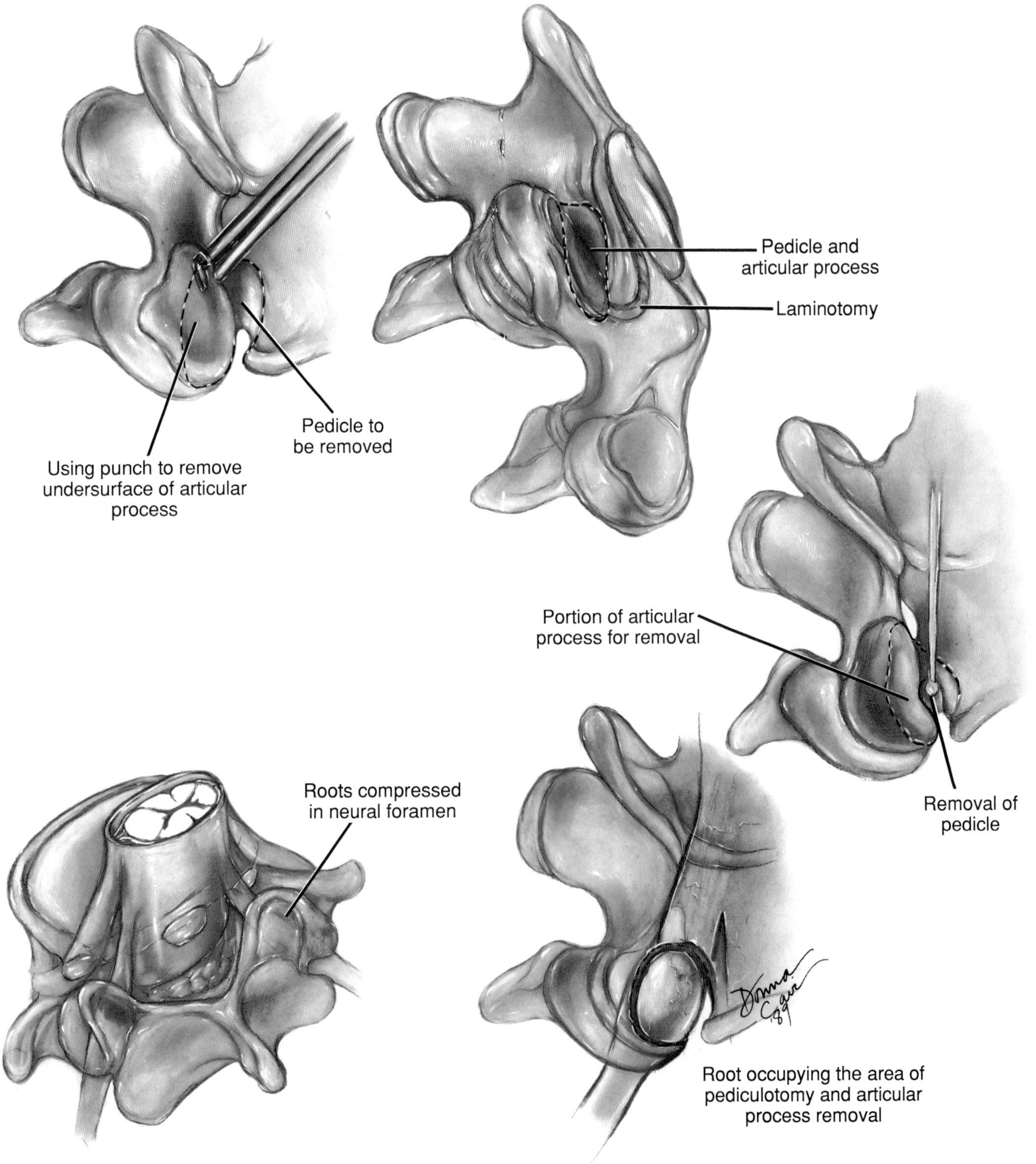
Pedicle and articular process
Laminotomy
Pedicle to be removed
Using punch to remove undersurface of articular process
Portion of articular process for removal
Removal of pedicle
Roots compressed in neural foramen
Root occupying the area of pediculotomy and articular process removal

Figure 1.10.

interspace. The nerve root should then be retracted medially or laterally, depending on which direction is easier, and the interspace exposed. The remainder of the degenerated material within the interspace should be removed in the manner described for simple discectomy. Closure with a laterally herniated disc does not require any special care.

Far Lateral Disc Herniation

Lumbar disc herniations that occur in the lateral half of the foramen or are extraforaminal can be excised through an approach that is lateral to the foramen and does not enter the spinal canal at all. Computed tomography (CT) imaging now demonstrates the location of these lateral disc herniations so precisely that the surgeon can make a decision whether traditional hemilaminotomy and excision from within the spinal canal or the lateral approach outside the spinal canal will be superior. For the disc herniations that are truly outside the foramen, the lateral approach is far superior. This approach is modified from that suggested by Dr. H. J. Reulen of Bern, Switzerland.

The goal of surgery is removal of the disc fragment without disruption of the zygapophyseal joint. The operation is carried out with the patient under general anesthesia in the prone position. Once the patient is in position, a skin marker is applied and an x-ray is taken to localize the appropriate interspace. The patient is prepared and draped, and then at the point of the skin incision, about 2½ cm from the midline, a sterile spinal needle is inserted to the transverse process above the involved root. For a disc at L4-L5 the needle is placed on the L4 transverse process, and for a disc at L5-S1 the L5 transverse process is identified. The sterile needle can be kept in place, and a skin incision 3–5 cm in length is made parallel to the midline and about 2½–3 cm lateral. The incision is carried down to the level of the transverse processes, and those structures above and below the herniated disc are identified. Of course, at L5-S1 the ala of the sacrum rather than another transverse process is exposed. The exposure should identify the transverse processes above the intertransverse ligament, the upper margins of the pedicles, and zygapophyseal joint medially (Fig. 1.11). Use of the Williams or Cloward retractor is excellent for maintaining this exposure. Via the medial exposure, muscle can be dissected off the zygapophyseal joint to the lamina if there is muscle overhang, but it is not necessary to do so (Fig. 1.12). The intertransverse ligament is cut away from the transverse process above and reflected out of the way, exposing the root anterior to it (Fig. 1.13). The affected root is usually pushed laterally, superiorly, and posteriorly. The anatomy will have been well defined by the CT scan, and exposure of the root follows the expected anatomical location. The root exits from the neural foramen in its superior portion and is usually tucked under the transverse process medially. Frequently, the fragment will become immediately apparent as soon as the ligament is opened (Fig. 1.14). If it is not apparent, the tissues surrounding the root are gently teased away until the root is found and the disc can be removed. As soon as the fragment is identified, it is grasped with a disc forceps and gently teased from beneath the root. The annulus may have to be incised. The decompression of the root should be ensured by careful exploration. There is no need for attempted radical excision of remaining disc tissue, but the exit of the disc through the annulus should be explored to be certain there are no additional medial fragments. The retractor is removed, allowing the muscle margins to fall together. The incision in the lumbar fascia should be closed to prevent a muscle hernia. Subcutaneous tissue and skin are closed in the routine fashion.

Transdural Approach to Herniated Lumbar Disc

Rarely a lumbar disc will herniate through the dura and appear as an intradural mass compressing the cauda equina. This most commonly occurs in patients who have undergone previous operation. The subsequent adhesions make the intradural herniation an easier route than lateral herniation. The patients often present with catastrophic neurological deficit. With CT myelography, the nature of the problem is usually known before surgery is undertaken. Removal of the intradural disc requires a very different technique than is utilized for the epidural free fragment. A complete laminectomy should be done immediately over the disc fragment. The dura should be opened in the midline, and the disc fragment enmeshed in the roots of the cauda will usually be apparent (Fig. 1.15). The operating microscope should be used and is brought into the field to open the dura. Sometimes, when the herniation is fresh, the disc fragment may

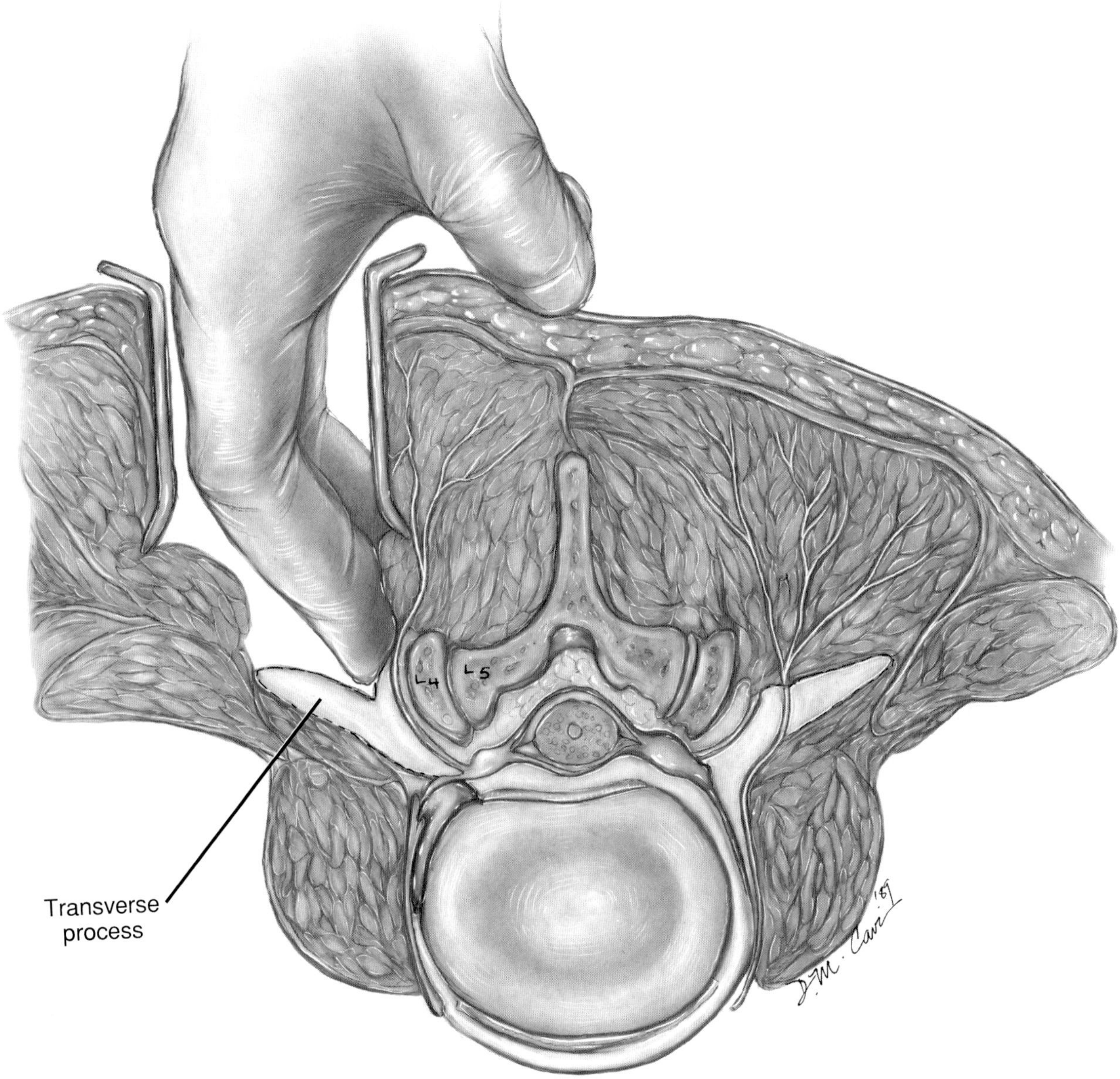

Figure 1.11. Paramedian approach to lateral disc herniation.

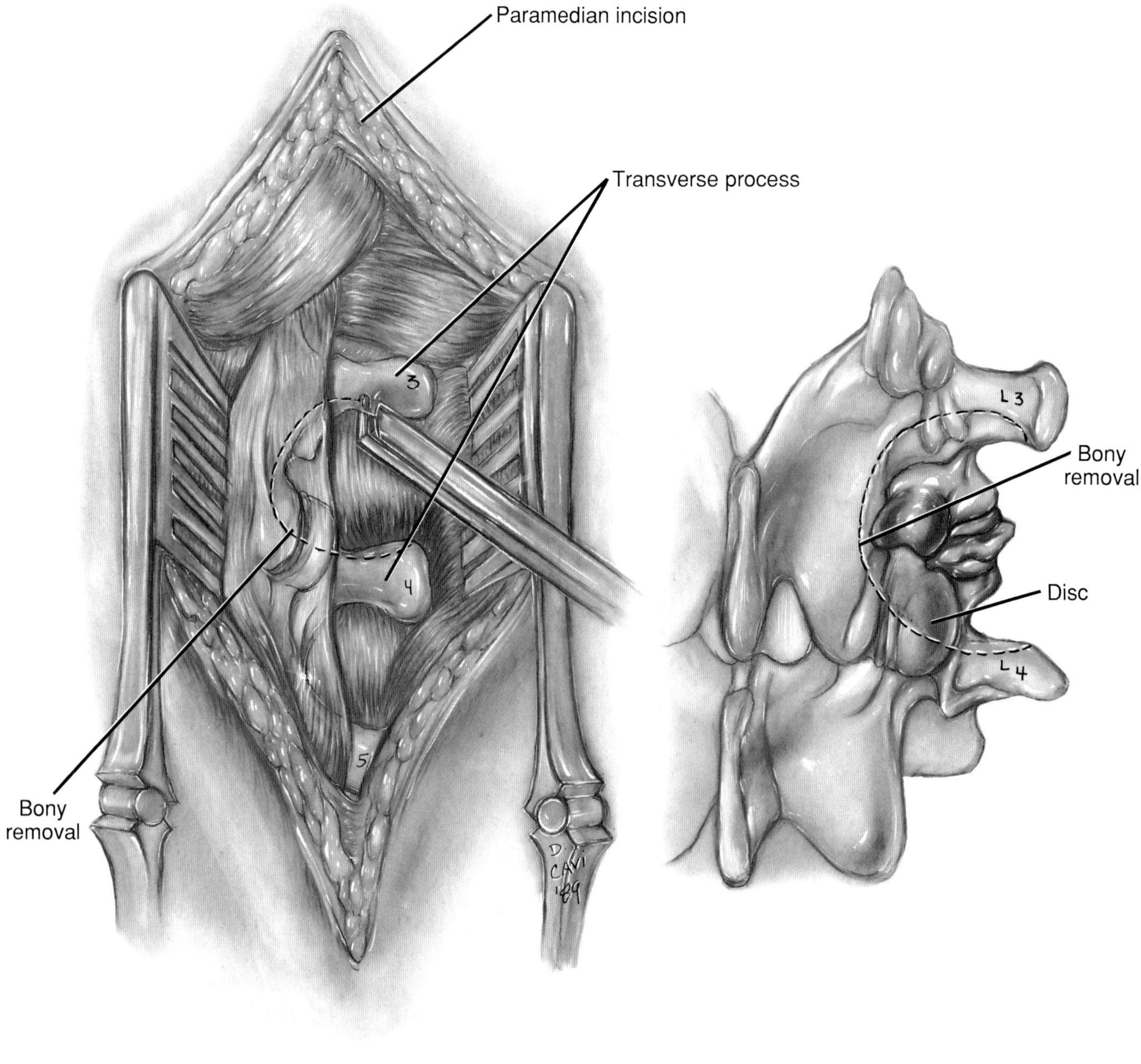
Paramedian incision
Transverse process
3
4
5
Bony
removal
L3
Bony
removal
Disc
L4

Figure 1.12.

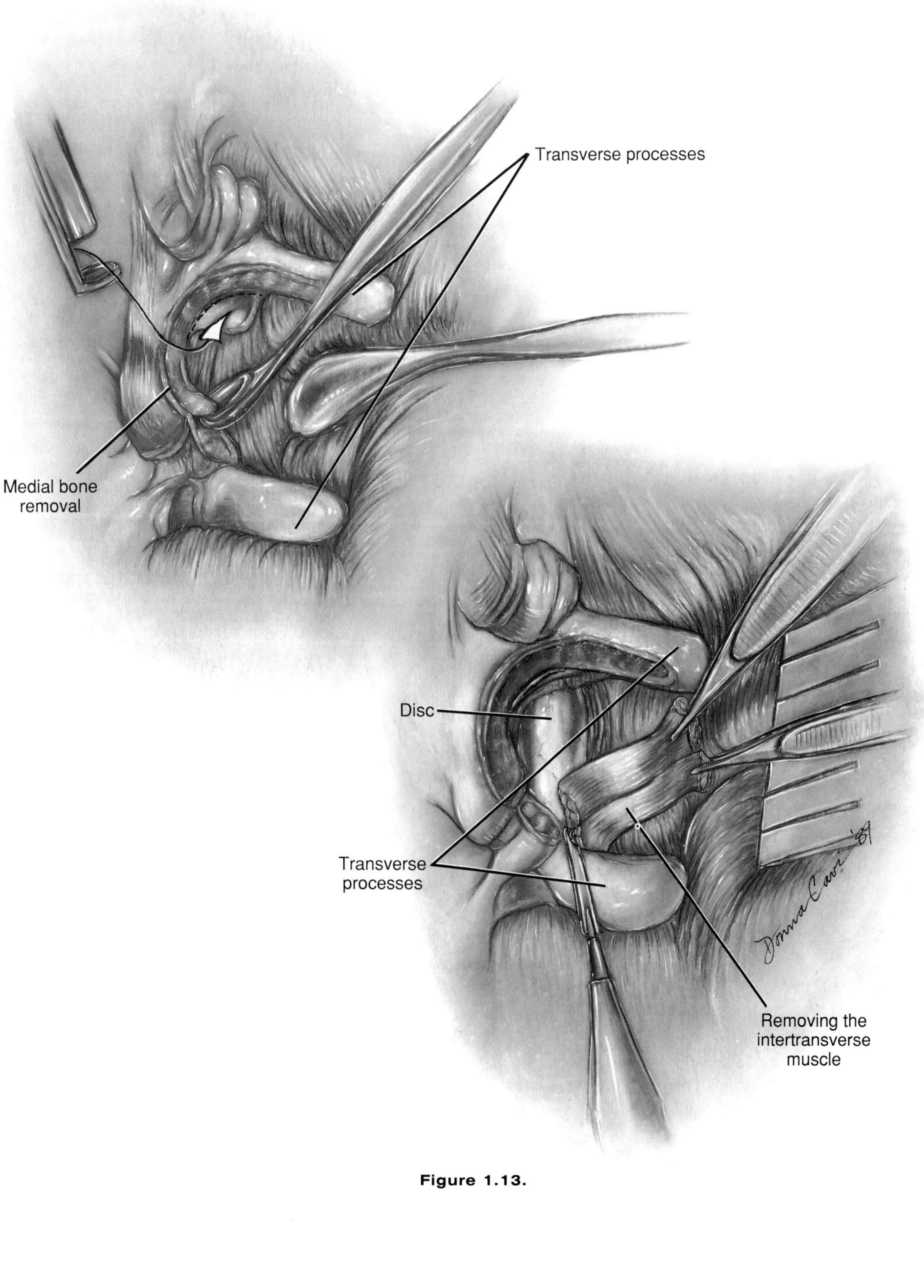
Transverse processes
Medial bone removal
Disc
Transverse processes
Removing the intertransverse muscle

Figure 1.13.

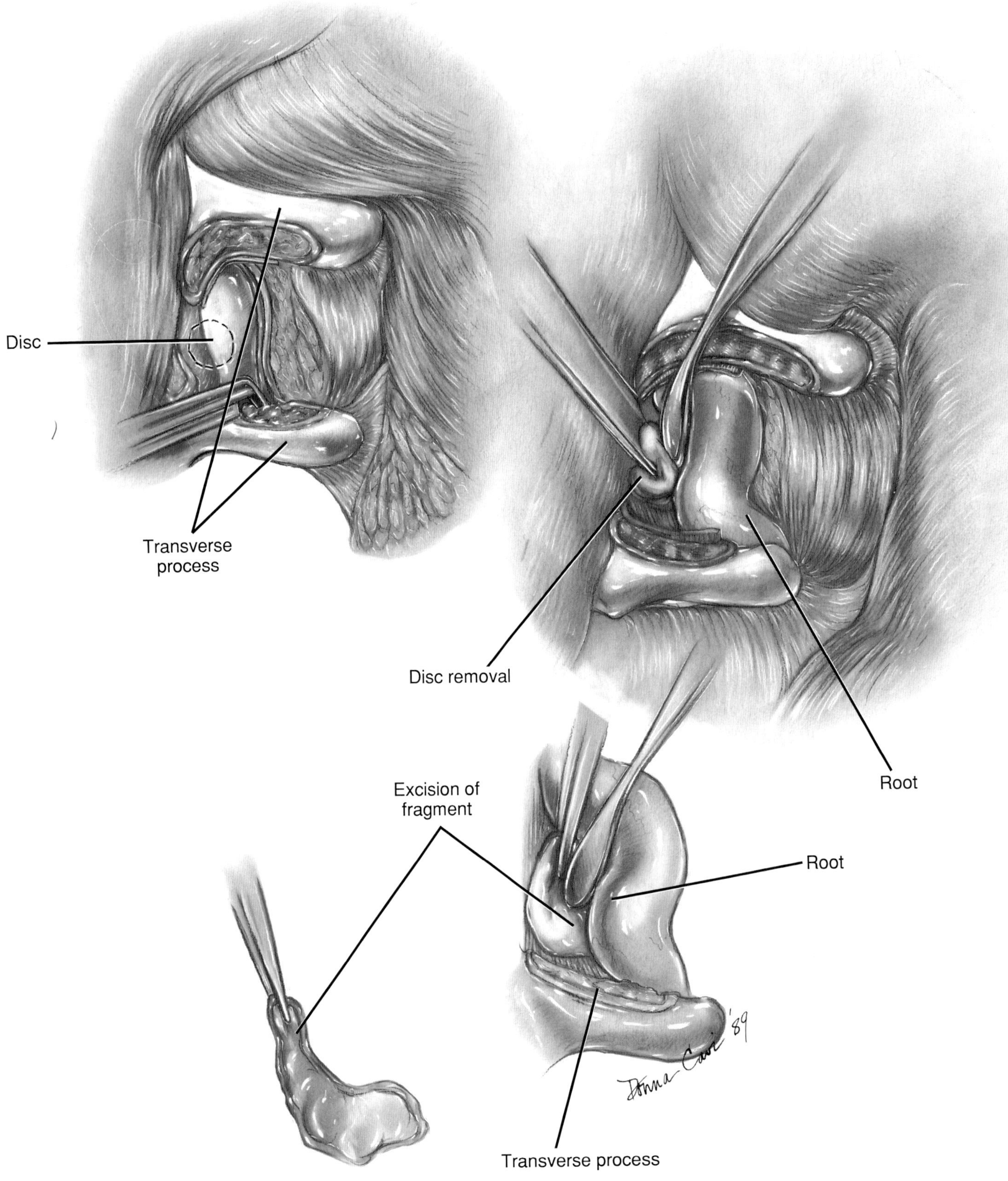
Disc
Transverse process
Disc removal
Root
Excision of fragment
Root
Transverse process

Figure 1.14.

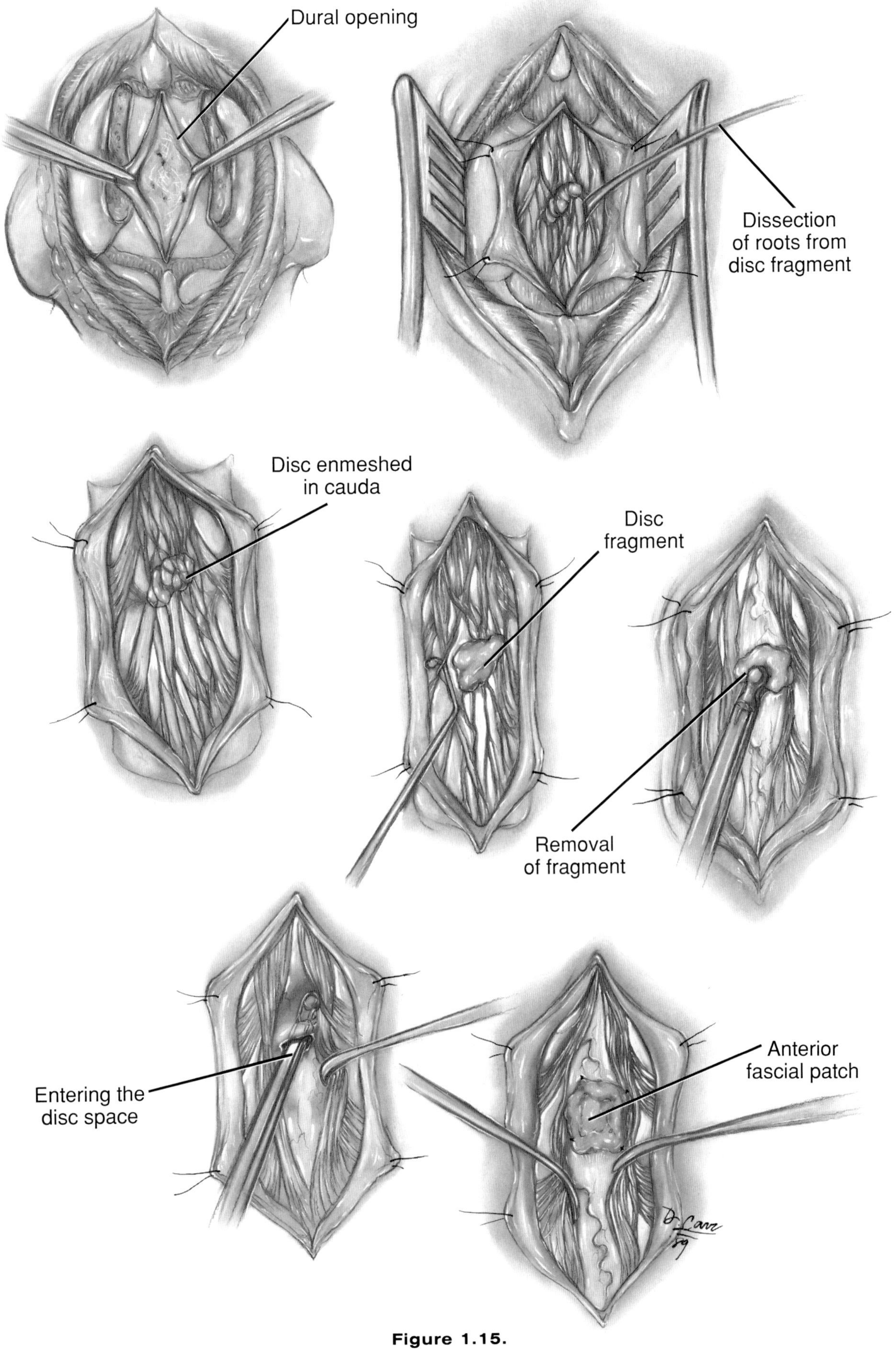
Dural opening
Dissection of roots from disc fragment
Disc enmeshed in cauda
Disc fragment
Removal of fragment
Entering the disc space
Anterior fascial patch

Figure 1.15.

be loose within the canal, but commonly the nerve roots are very adherent, and there is a localized arachnoiditis already beginning. The nerve roots must be identified under high magnification and dissected free from the disc fragment. The disc should not be removed until it is certain that every root is free. Then the disc fragment can be grasped with the disc rongeur and carefully withdrawn. Any root that is ventral to the disc and still adherent can be freed as it is carefully extracted. The hole in the dura and the posterior longitudinal ligament is usually easy to find. It commonly is immediately beneath the fragment. Sometimes, the disc fragment may have herniated a segment or more, and then it will not be possible to determine its origin. When the defect is visible, the roots should be carefully retracted, and the interspace entered through the defect (Fig. 1.16). The remainder of the degenerated material, which is easily removed with disc rongeurs, should be obtained. The anterior defect usually cannot be closed. Nevertheless, it provides a ready path for further disc herniation. If possible, fill the defect with a hemostatic agent, roughen the circumferential edges of the dura without causing epidural bleeding, and tack a small pledget of lumbar fascia over the defect to provide a solid scar (Fig. 1.15). This should be done only if these maneuvers are easy; under no circumstances should any risk be taken with the cauda equina in order to achieve a dural closure. It is much better simply to leave the defect if exposure is a problem. The posterior dura is closed in a watertight fashion. No further special considerations affect the closure.

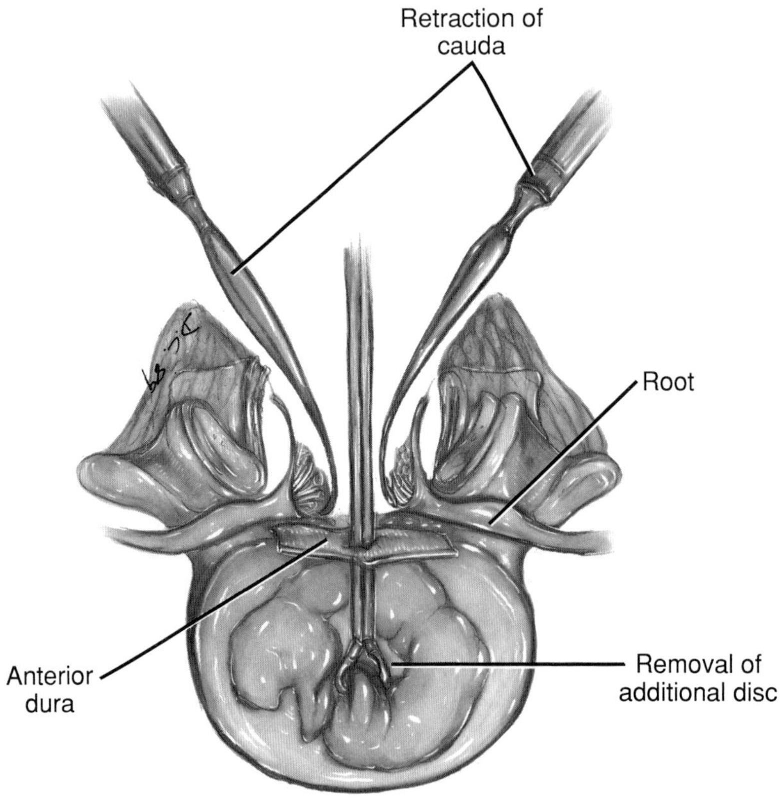

Figure 1.16.

2

Reoperation on Lumbar Spine

Reoperation for Herniated Lumbar Disc or Lateral Foraminal Stenosis

The operation is carried out with the patient under general anesthesia in a position similar to that which would be chosen for simple discectomy. The exposure of the interspace proceeds as for any first operation on the lumbar disc. When the interspace is exposed and the laminectomy retractors are in place, the surgeon is confronted with the previous laminectomy defect partially obscured by scar. This extraligamentous scar should be removed with a knife, exposing the bone circumferentially. The margins of the bone and the scar can be separated by a semisharp dissector such as the Adson periosteal elevator (Fig. 2.1). Then a few bites of bone on the laminae above and below will expose normal ligament or epidural fat and normal dura. A blunt dissector should then be used to free the remaining scar from bone, leaving a thin rim of scar attached to the dura. By exposing normal tissue above and below, the area of the root can be reached without cutting directly through the scar. The next step is to break down the adhesions that bind the scar and the root laterally to bone (Fig. 2.2). This is best done with a blunt or semisharp dissector such as the Olivecrona or the Adson periosteal elevator. It is quite common that a foraminotomy will have to be done if the root is be adequately mobilized because of the adhesions from previous surgery (see Fig. 2.11). Unless there is associated foraminal stenosis, it is likely that this can be done by using a 45° angled Kerrison-type laminectomy punch in the foramen, removing

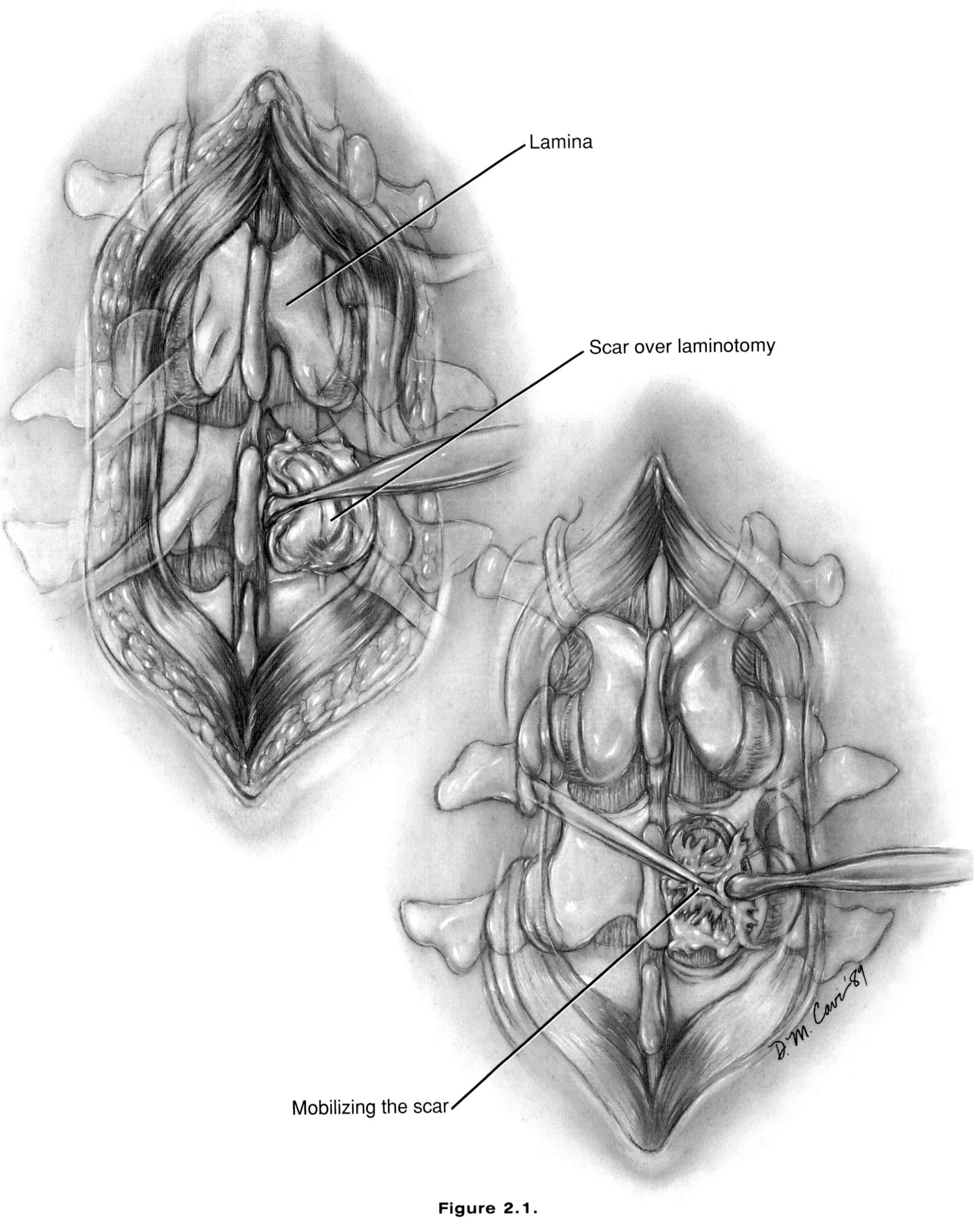

Figure 2.1.

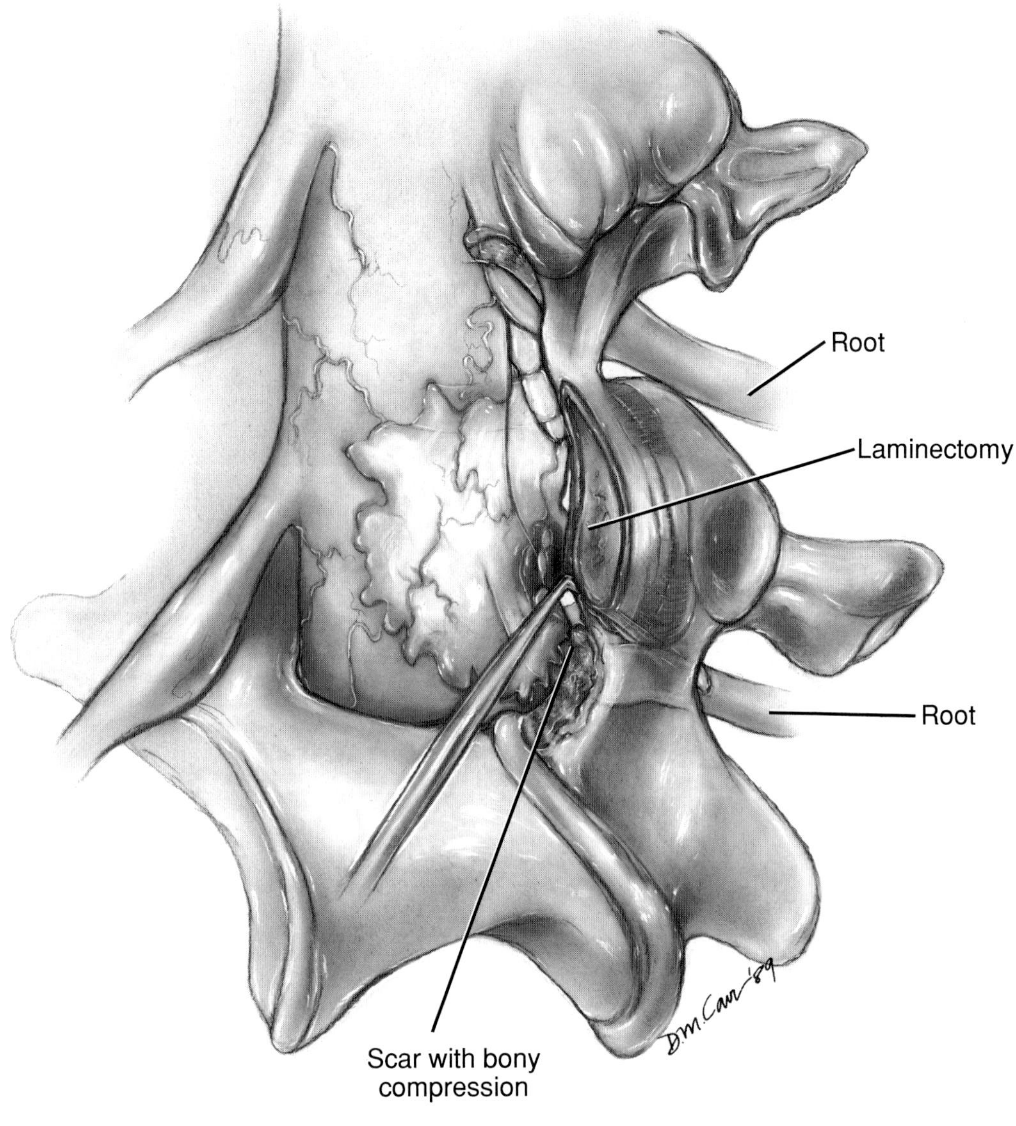

Figure 2.2.

the inferior portions of the superior articular process. Try to leave at least 50% of the joint. Commonly, the foraminotomy can be done without entering the joint at all. Collapse of the interspace often has occurred, and if there is true foraminal stenosis, it will be necessary to carry out a more extensive foraminotomy. In this situation, once the neural foramen has been opened with a punch, the pedicle should be chiseled or drilled away until the nerve is adequately decompressed and no longer distorted either by the pedicle or by the margins of the foramen.

When the foramen is tight, a chisel or a drill is more useful than a punch. The high-speed drill with a medial guard can be gradually inserted out the foramen, and the bone of the articular processes and the pedicle are removed until the nerve is free in the foramen. Small chisels can also be used to remove bone of both structures to accomplish the same purpose. If the problem is foraminal stenosis, then nothing further need be done once the foraminotomy is complete. If there is a recurrent disc fragment, however, or if the root is compressed by scar or ridge from beneath, more is necessary. Then the root should be gradually mobilized medially over the mass until the recurrent disc fragment is seen (see Fig. 2.4). As soon as it can be identified, the exposed fragment can be grasped with a disc rongeur and gradually teased out of its bed. This is better than an extensive dissection freeing the root over the disc over which it is often tightly stretched. If the disc fragment is not free in the canal, then it is necessary (1) to expose the root well out in the foramen so that it can be mobilized and (2) to expose the disc either in the axilla or laterally, as the situation requires. The root is then retracted either medially or laterally, exposing the ligament and the protruded disc beneath. The ligament should be incised in a cruciate fashion with a #15 knife, and the interspace entered with the disc rongeur to remove the disc fragment or fragments. If the disc simply is degenerated, the interspace should be thoroughly emptied of degenerated disc material with the rongeur. The technique does not differ from that described for primary disc herniation. The remaining disc material should be thoroughly curetted until all possible degenerated material is removed. The retractor is then removed, and the root checked again for the adequacy of the decompression. If the root remains under tension, it is necessary to relieve the tension by removing the offending structures whether this is a ridge beneath, more disc, or lateral bony compression in the foramen.

Reoperation for Epidural Scar

There is no evidence that removal of the generalized noncompressive scar, which sometimes complicates lumbar hemilaminectomy or laminectomy, is of lasting benefit. When there is local compression of the cauda equina or one or more nerve roots, however, removal of the offending mass has the same rationale as decompression for spondylosis, spondylolisthesis, or discectomy. The procedure varies according to the details of the original operation. Usually, it is helpful to know what the first surgeon did, but it is not always possible to obtain an accurate description of the operation. The newer imaging techniques give such a detailed view of the operative area that the details of previous operations are not as important as they once were. The operation itself must be planned to accomplish certain goals. There is no place for a hopeful exploration to see what is causing the pain. The procedure must be designed to correct the identified abnormalities that are presumed to be the cause of the problem.

Focal Epidural Scar with Root Compression

Focal epidural scar with root compression most commonly complicates a one- or two-level simple discectomy. Studies will show a mass of scar usually surrounding the root both anterior and posterior to it. There is usually a large dorsolateral mass pressing in, and the root is displaced medially. Computed tomography (CT) studies will also demonstrate foraminal stenosis if present. The differentiation of the mass from recurrent disc is frequently difficult, either by the imaging studies or even at surgery. This differentiation does not make a significant difference to the operative approach.

The first step simply is reopening the old incision if that incision is adequate. Reexploration requires more exposure than discectomy, and it is wise to have at least one interspace exposed in addition to those that have to be reexplored. The old skin scar should be excised if it is large, and the skin closed primarily with fresh edges. The original incision is carried down to the spinous processes in the midline, and the subperiosteal dissection is carried out as previously described. This is more difficult in the patient who has had a previous operation, but it is still important to make the dissection in the subperiosteal plane and disturb the muscle mass as little as possible with the osteotomes. Once the exposure of the interspace is complete, the effects of previous operations will be seen (Fig. 2.1). There usually will be densely adherent scar that obscures the margins of the site. The first step is to define the bone. This is done with a semisharp osteotome such as the Adson periosteal elevator, which is used to scrape the scar away until the margins of the previous hemilaminectomy are seen (Fig. 2.1). Excess scar can then be excised down to the bone margins if the CT myelogram has not shown any pseudomeningocele. Then the laminectomy needs to be extended slightly superiorly and inferiorly. Usually, it is difficult to extend it laterally at this point, but a few bites of bone taken above and below will expose relatively normal epidural space and usually expose the dura. Then, with the Adson periosteal elevator the scar is freed from bone laterally, leaving the remaining scar mass medially adherent to dura and nerve root (Fig. 2.2). A foraminotomy should then be done until adequate exposure is obtained. The foraminotomy is carried out beyond the epidural scar. The next step is to find the root and free it from scar. Usually, this is best done by dissecting laterally until the root is discovered in the foramen where it is less scarred. This maneuver isolates the scar from bone, leaving it on the root (Fig. 2.2). The actual dissection of the scar from the root may be done with a knife by experienced surgeons used to operating on such problems or with a sharp dissector such as a large Rosen knife or the Adson periosteal elevator. Which is used depends on the adherence of the scar to the dura. Less-sharp instruments are used if the scar will strip away from dura and root; the choice of instruments is determined by the amount of force required to strip the scar. If stripping is difficult, then a knife should be used to avoid undue traction on the root and possible injury. Usually, it is best to begin superiorly and medially, working the scar free along the root inferiorly and laterally. As the root is exposed, the massive scar is removed by the appropriate sharp and blunt dissection (Fig. 2.3). The scar is held with a toothed forceps such as a Cushing forceps rather than a heavier instrument that increases the risk of traction on the root. By these maneuvers it should be possible to remove the dorsolateral portion of the scar, exposing the nerve root beneath. The foraminotomy should be enlarged until the nerve root is free and not compressed. Then it is necessary to remove scarring that may be beneath the root. This is done very much like removal of a free disc fragment. With a blunt dissector or a sharp elevator such as the Adson, the root medially is mobilized. Massive scar often is as impressive in its compression as disc herniation. The mobilization of the root is usually best done from lateral to medial, but occasionally the scar mass will be more medially placed in the axilla, and then the root may be moved laterally (Fig. 2.4). The dissection of the root from the scar must be done gently and slowly until the root is mobilized and the scar can be removed. The scar will not come out easily the way the herniated disc does. Even when there is a recurrent disc, it is often densely adherent in the scar. The best approach is to cut the scar away with a knife, but this should be done only after the root is completely identified. A small sharp forceps such as the pituitary rongeurs can be used to remove the scar, but often the scar is too dense to be bitten away with such an instrument, and a knife is required for total removal. At the end of these maneuvers the nerve root should be free of scar and free of compression either by scar or by bone. Then the interspace can be checked to be certain there is no component of compression from a recurrent disc herniation. There is no reason to remove a degenerated disc unless nerve compression is present.

Closure requires some care. It is very important to have immaculate hemostasis. Application of hemostatic agents is important if there is significant bleeding. These scars are often very vascular, and great care should be taken to obtain perfect hemostasis. Gelfoam, Avitene, or any other substance that is used should be removed when hemostasis is obtained, if possible, though judicious packing with these agents is better than allowing a blood clot to form. As soon as hemostasis is adequate, a fat graft utilizing normal fat from the margins of the incision should be obtained. This free graft of fat need be only a few millimeters thick, but it should cover the entire operative exposure (Fig. 2.4). While there are no definitive studies proving its use, the suggestive evaluations that have been done indicate that it does reduce the chance of a new, heavy scar forming. Some surgeons have advocated always making a second incision to obtain the fat, but this is not necessary if normal fat can be obtained a few centimeters from the edge of the exposure by undercutting. The simplest way to remove the fat graft is simply to expose the subcutaneous layer by lifting the skin. The electric knife is then used to undercut 1 or 2 cm into the subcutaneous space, and then the same knife is used to fashion the fat graft of the appropriate size. Using electrocoagulation provides immediate hemostasis. The graft is carefully laid in place and tucked around the root. Then closure proceeds with a single layer in the lumbar fascia, closure of the subcutaneous space with obliteration of the fat graft site, and skin closure. If there is inadequate subcutaneous tissue available through the wound site, then a separate incision over

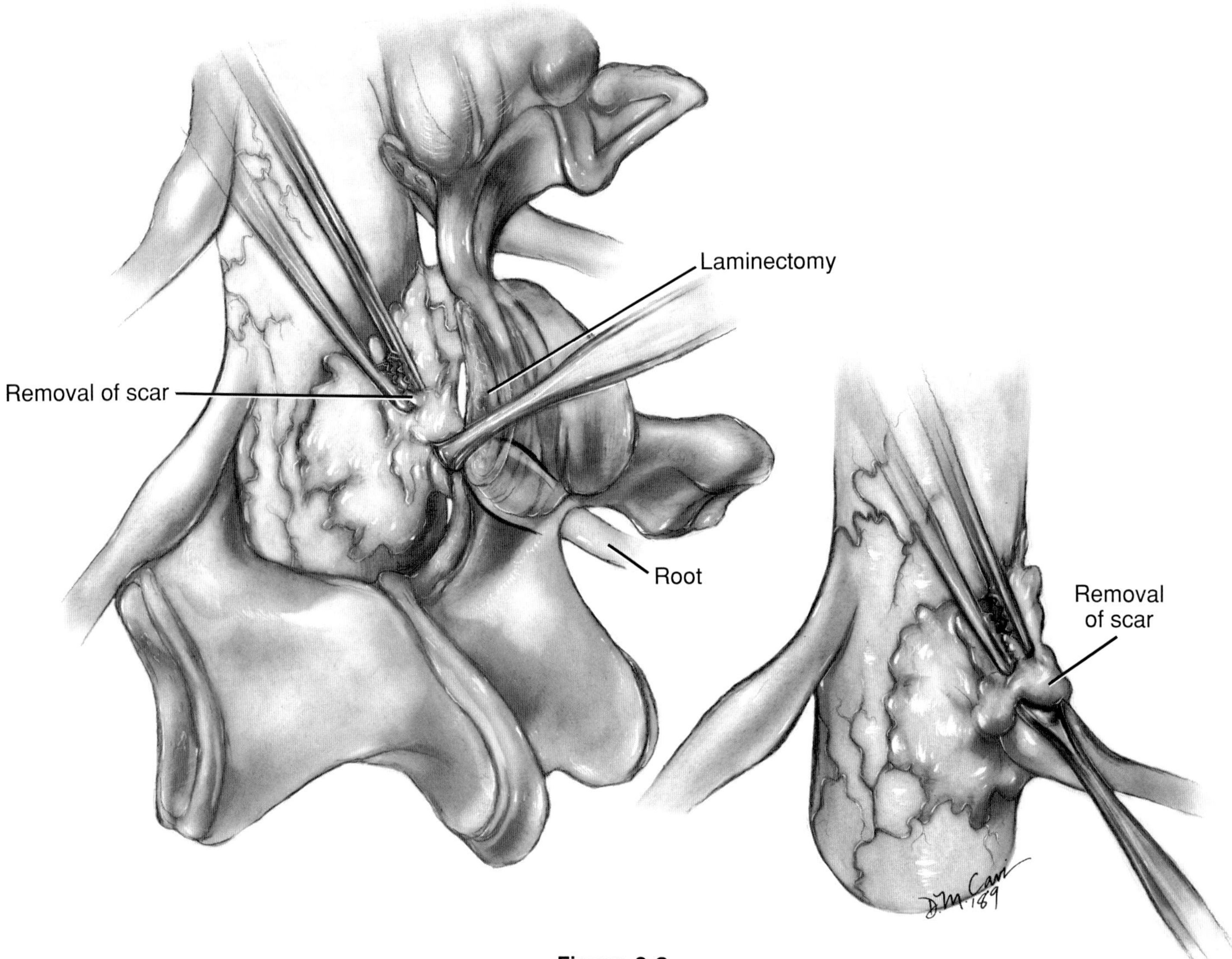

Figure 2.3.

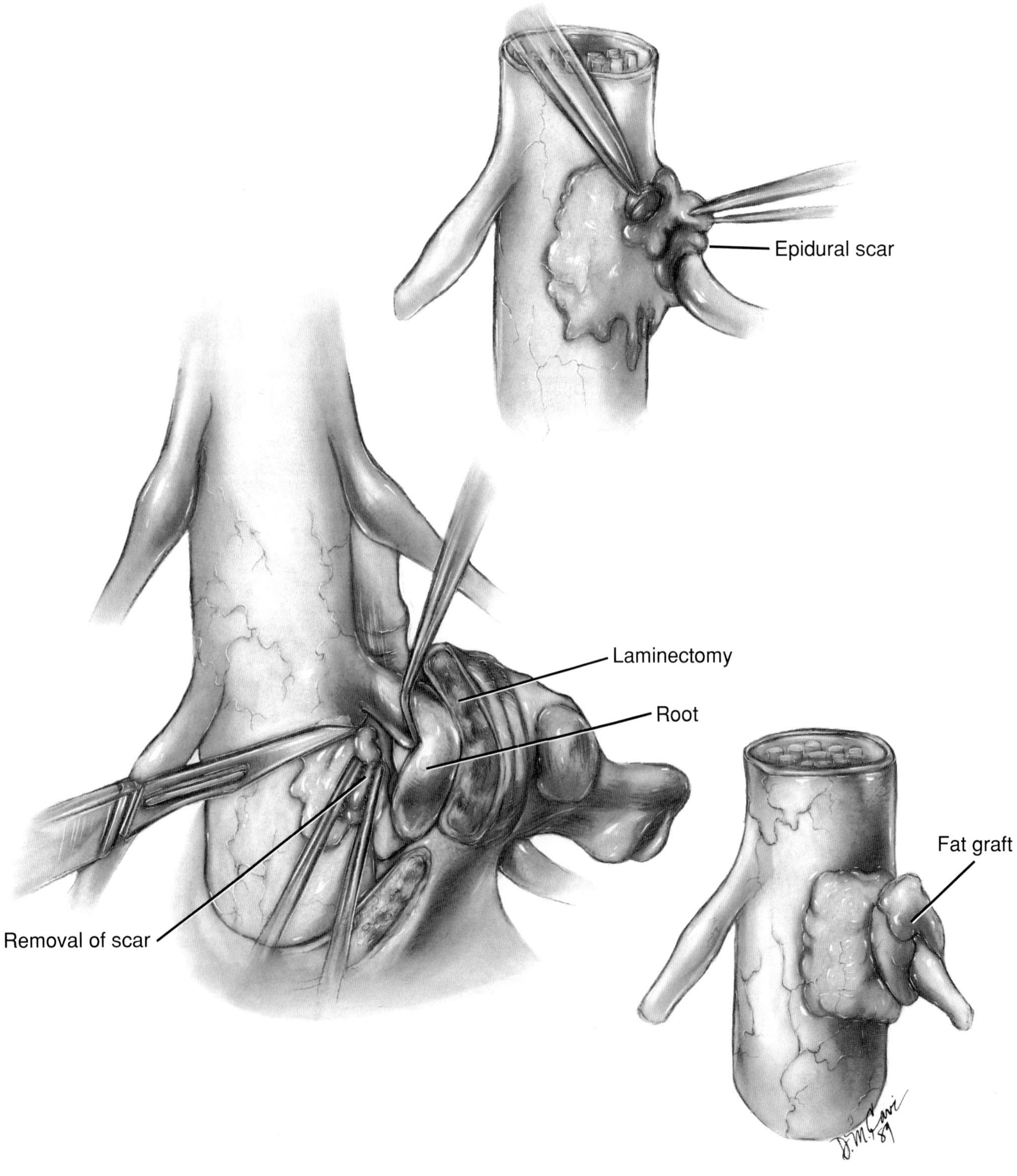

Figure 2.4.

the buttock, parallel to the cluneal nerves, can be utilized to obtain normal subcutaneous fat, which is usually present there.

General Cauda Equina Compression from Scar

When the patient has previously undergone a laminectomy, the scar presents a significantly different problem. Often, there is compression with virtually a total block from the posterior. The roots are enveloped with scar laterally. The removal of this kind of abnormality is a much greater problem than surgery for the circumscribed scar that affects only one root. It is very difficult to find the dura and roots through the scar. Therefore, the best way to obtain a plane between dura and scar is to look for the first normal level above, identify the dura, and then approach the decompression from that normal area.

The surgery is carried out by reopening the previous incision to the level of the first normal spinous process above. The incision should be planned so that one spinous process and the laminae above the previous surgical site are exposed (Fig. 2.5). The CT scan with intrathecal contrast will give the surgeon a reasonable estimate of the location of the dura. Be careful not to cut through the scar to such a depth that the dura is entered. If the incision through scar stops at the level of the base of the first normal spinous process, there should be no risk of injury to the dural contents. A subperiosteal dissection of the paravertebral muscle from that normal spinous process and laminae is then carried out. Once the level of the laminae is clearly identified, it is possible to split the scar down to that depth (Fig. 2.5). Remember that at L5-S1 the dura angles upward over the sacrum, and the incision through the scar should be similarly angled. Self-retaining retractors are put in place above and below. Sometimes, the scar is not so adherent to the dura, and a plane will be identified simply by spreading the retractors. More commonly, the scar is densely adherent, and a false plane must be created to facilitate the exposure. This is accomplished by undercutting the scar at the level of the laminae back to the zygapophyseal joints (Fig. 2.5). This will allow a wide exposure of the previous laminectomy site still covered by a few millimeters of scar and will greatly facilitate the scar removal. The interspinous ligament above the spinous process to be removed should be cut, and the spinous process removed with a bone cutting rongeur. The scar should be carefully dissected from the inferior margins of the normal laminae, and a laminectomy carried out, exposing normal extradural fat and dura (Fig. 2.6). The goal of this maneuver is to expose normal dura to allow the development of a plane between dura and scar. If possible, this can better be accomplished without a total laminectomy. Once the dura is seen, it is possible to begin to develop a plane between dura and scar in the midline (Fig. 2.6). This is best done by a sharp dissector such as the Adson periosteal elevator. A plane should be established, and a dissector carefully manipulated to free the dura in the midline. Leaving the dissector in place, a #15 knife is utilized to cut down onto the instrument. The flap of scar thus created can be grasped with forceps, and the dissection of the dural scar plane can be continued laterally to the margins of the laminectomy. The dural scar should then be removed with a knife, cutting it free from bone (Fig. 2.7). This maneuver is repeated throughout the length of the laminectomy until the dura is exposed to both extremities of the laminectomy and laterally to the margins of removed bone (Fig. 2.7). The next maneuver is to free the dura laterally underneath the retained bone and then down the pedicles into the foramen to expose the nerve roots. This should be done with a sharp periosteal dissector. The laminectomy may need to be widened with angled punches until it is complete and the foraminotomies can begin (Fig. 2.8). The most difficult part of this procedure consists of identification of the roots in the scar and the dissection of the lateral adhesions. Sometimes, a root is so encased that it is impossible to identify it without an actual knife removal of scar. In this situation, the location of the root must be identified, and the scar carefully removed in layers, until the dura of the root is seen (Fig. 2.9). This is a maneuver for the surgeon experienced in reoperation, and until it can be done with confidence, it is better to spend the time required for blunt dissection. If the dura is entered during any of these maneuvers, the laceration should be immediately repaired. Loss of a significant amount of cerebrospinal fluid (CSF) reduces the protection that the fluid-filled dural sac gives to the nerve roots during these dissections, and loss of tamponade also will increase extradural bleeding. To visualize the nerves adequately, particularly to allow removal of scar with a knife, it may be necessary to perform a foraminotomy. Once the root and scar are freed from

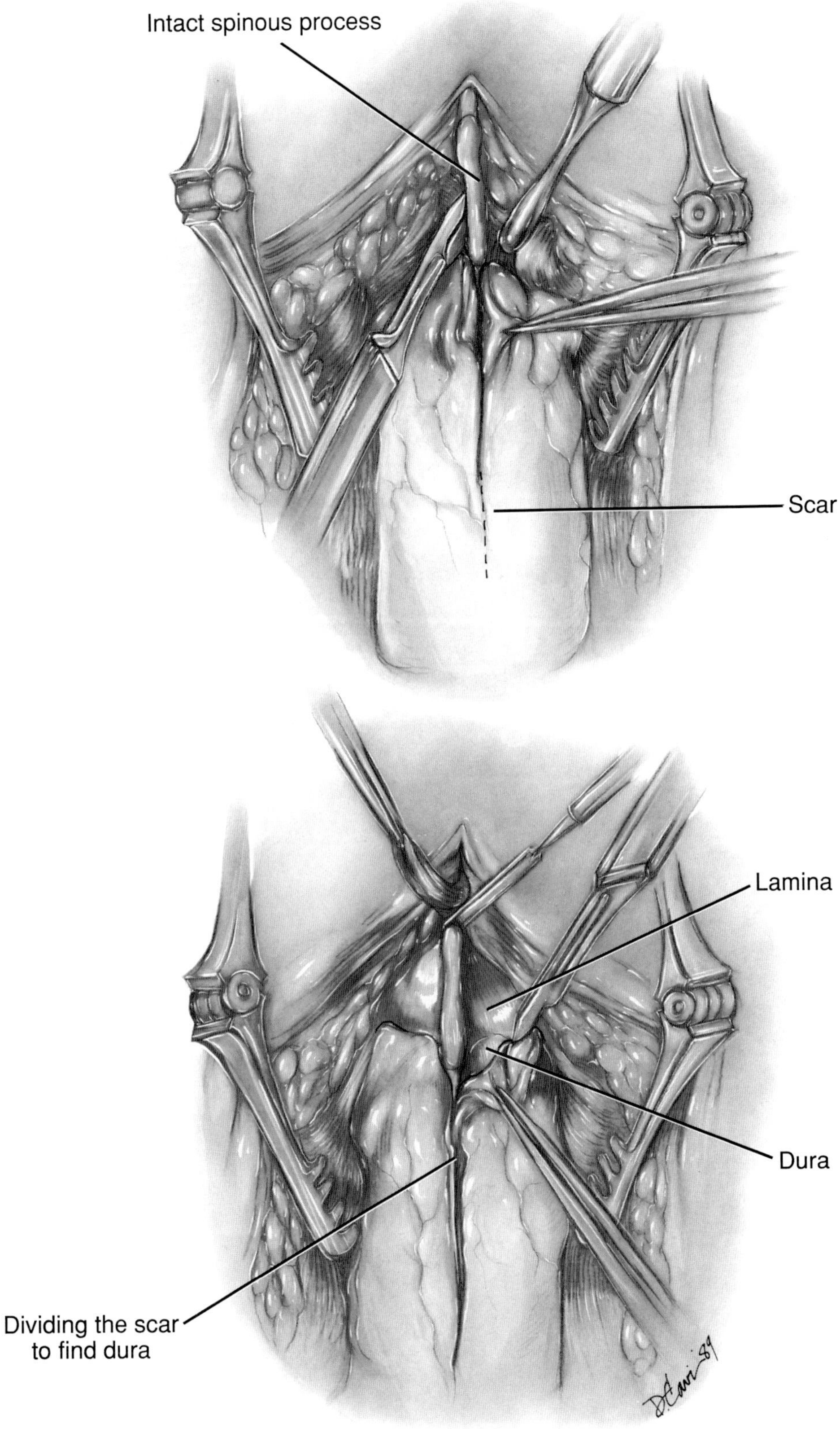
Intact spinous process
Scar
Lamina
Dura
Dividing the scar
to find dura

Figure 2.5.

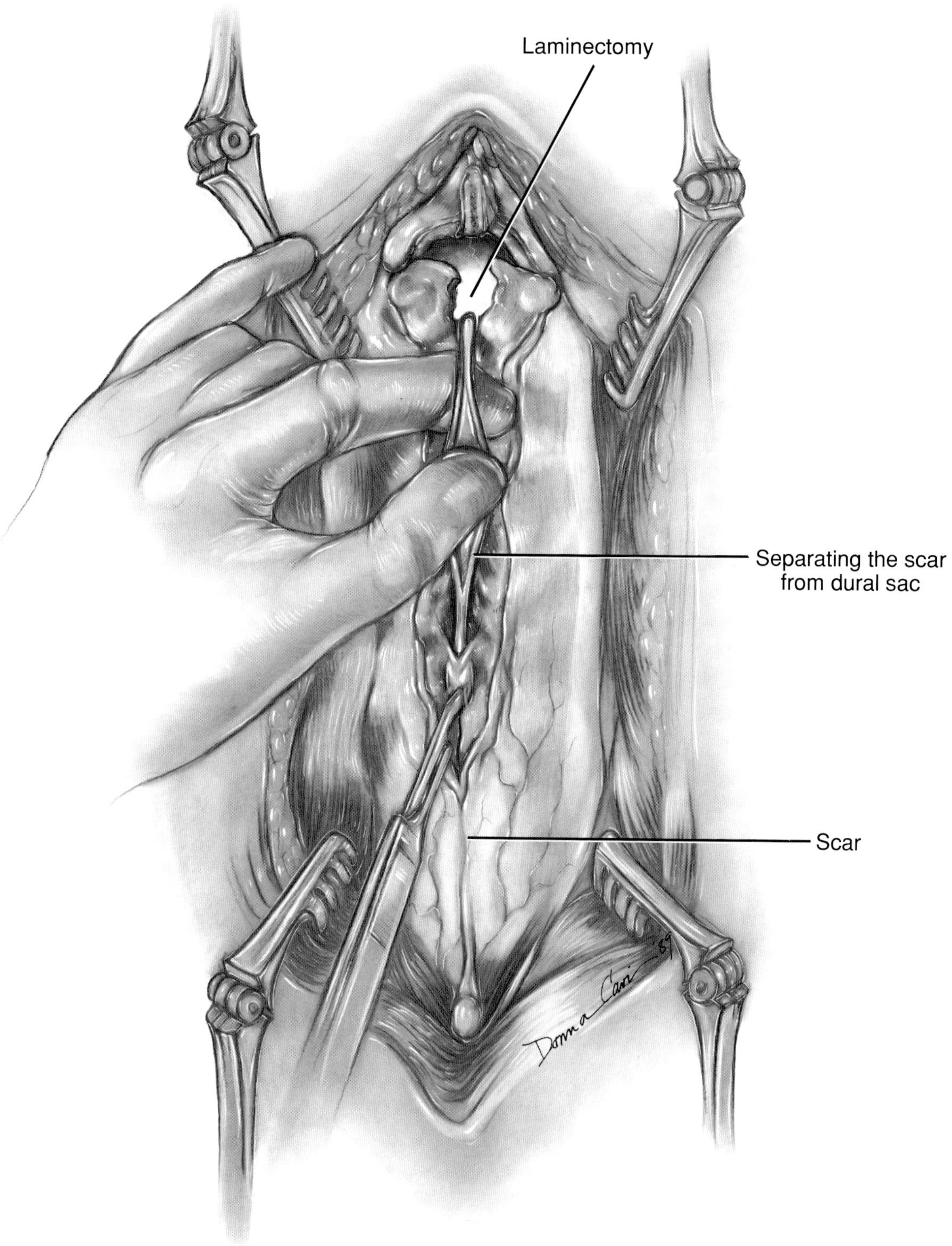

Figure 2.6.

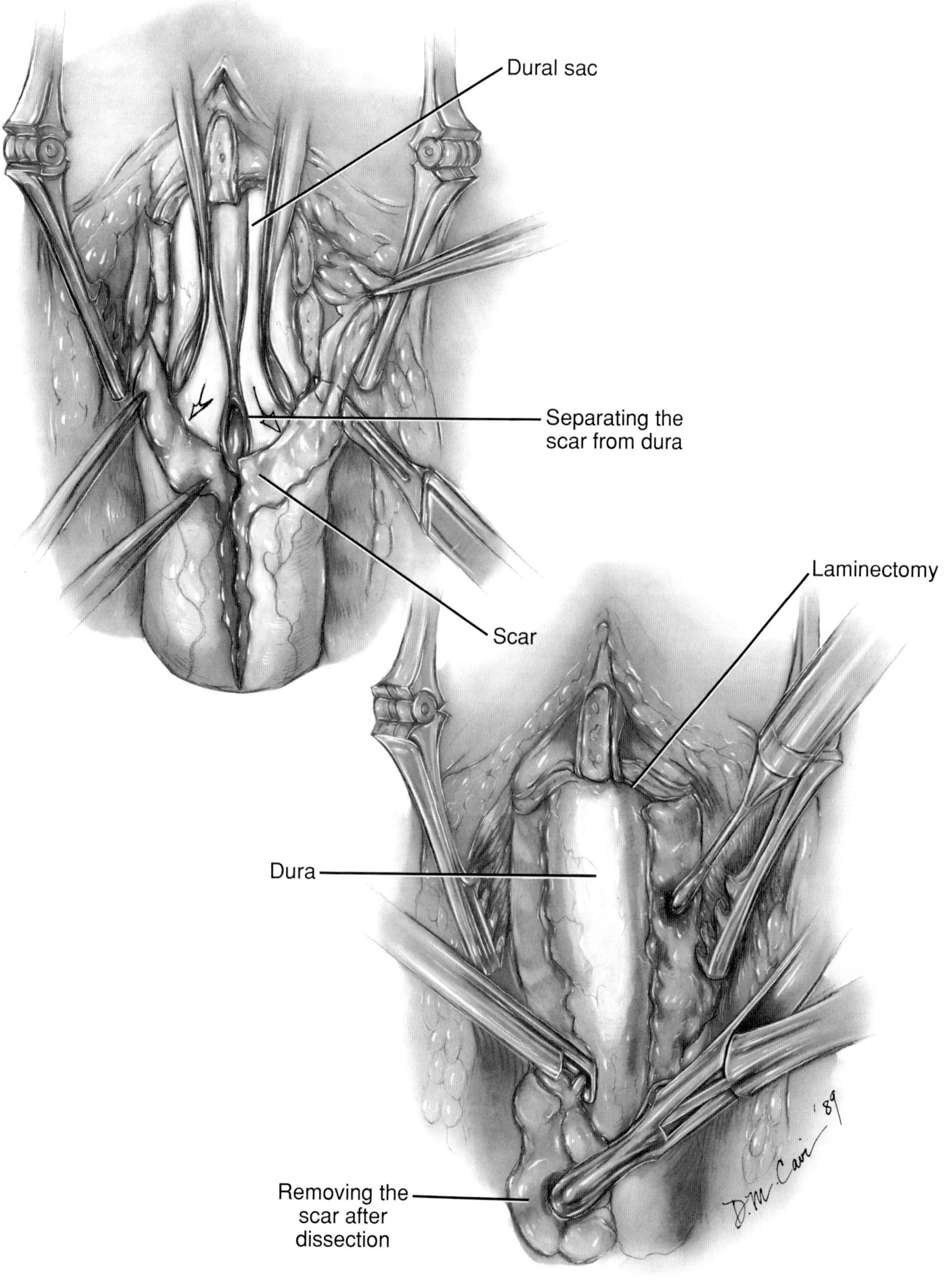
Dural sac
Separating the scar from dura
Scar
Laminectomy
Dura
Removing the scar after dissection
D.M. Cain '89

Figure 2.7.

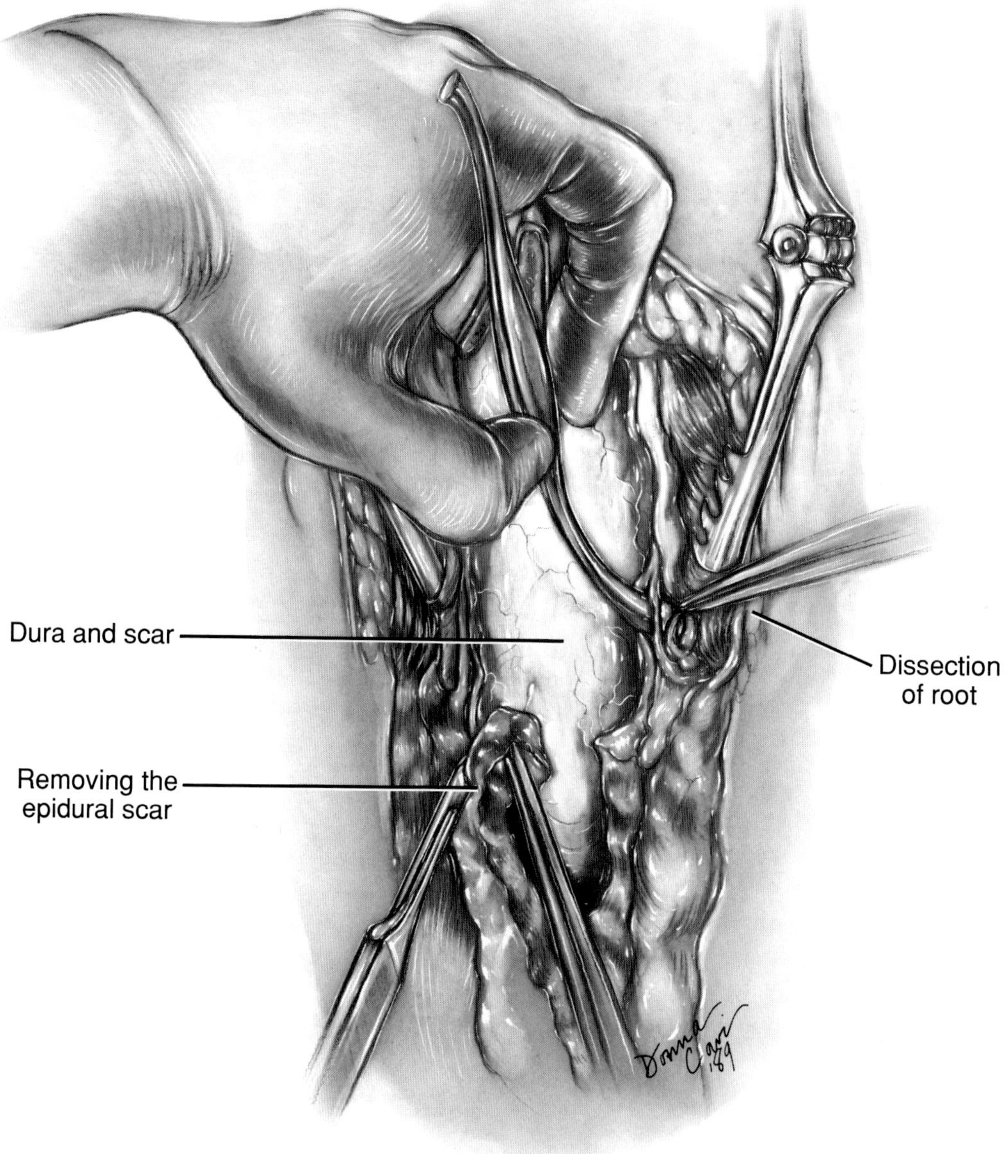
Dura and scar
Dissection of root
Removing the epidural scar

Figure 2.8.

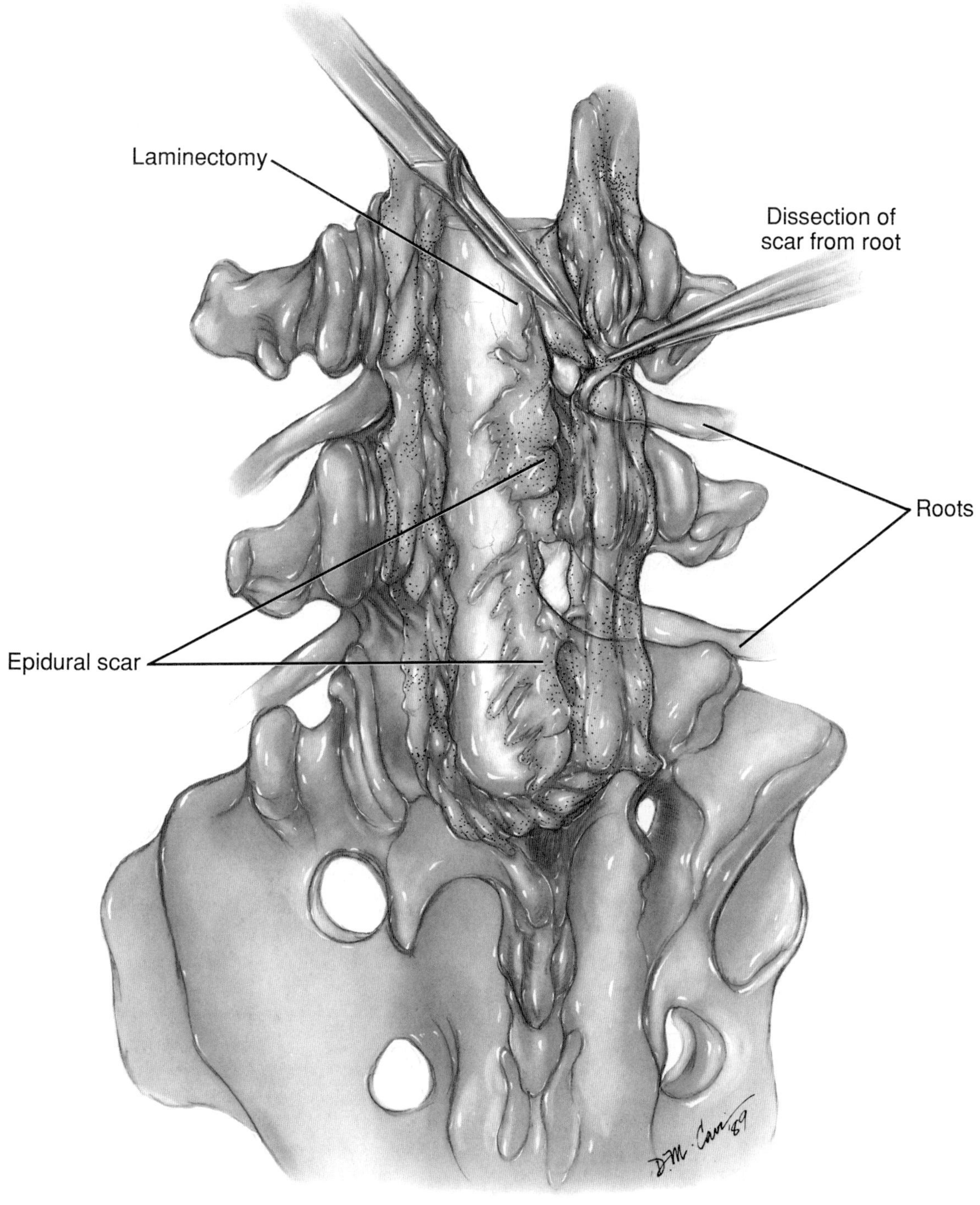
Laminectomy
Dissection of scar from root
Roots
Epidural scar
D.M. Carr '89

Figure 2.9.

bone laterally, the foramen can be identified with a blunt probe (Fig. 2.10). The removal of bone can be carried out with a high-speed drill, small chisel, or angled punches (Fig. 2.11). If the punches can be inserted into the foramen, they can be used to remove the lowermost portion of the superior articular process. Every effort should be made to avoid entering the joint space, but sometimes, in order to provide adequate decompression of the root, this is necessary. However, by angling the instruments beneath the joint itself, the size of the foramen can usually be increased by removing bone without entering the joint space. This is better than a right-angle bone removal in which bone from both the superior and the inferior articular process is removed. With such a maneuver the joint space must be entered. If the joint space is entered, try to leave at least 50% of it intact. If adequate root decompression requires removing the entire joint, this is what must be done. At the conclusion of the operation, stability of each motion segment should be carefully checked to determine if a fusion should be carried out. Most patients will not be unstable even with extensive bone removal at several segments if the anterior structures are intact. If severe degeneration has occurred or multiple discectomies have been carried out earlier, then the disruption of anterior integrity may lead to the need for fusion. A fusion should be performed only for demonstrated instability.

Use of a high-speed drill or chisels for the foraminotomy is important for any spine surgeon to learn (Fig. 2.11). The high-speed drills are made with guards that protect the dura, and these can be inserted in the foramen, drilling both pedicle and articular process bone and gradually enlarging the foramen out to the point where the root is no longer compressed. Small chisels can be used in the same way. It is important to remove the bone of the pedicle first with the chisels in order to make sure that there is free access to the foramen. Small shavings should be taken, and it is important to be certain that bone is removed down to the body so that no ridge is left to angulate the root. The chisels are then used to remove the inferior portion of the superior articular process, enlarging the foramen posteriorly. The foramen is large enough when a blunt probe can freely pass along the root on all sides and when the root can be moved easily in all directions (Fig. 2.11). The interspace should now be explored for recurrent disc or scar beneath the root. This requires mobilization of the root in all directions and exploration of the axilla (Fig. 2.12). If there is a large ridge beneath the root, it is best removed. The root is retracted medially in most instances, but the retraction should be in the direction that gives the best exposure, whatever that may be. Sharp pituitary rongeurs are usually enough to remove scar and thickened ligament. A small chisel is an effective way to remove a bony ridge. If the root is freely movable over the ridge, it is not necessary to remove the protuberant structures simply because they are present. The goal of the procedure is decompression of the root, and when this is accomplished, nothing further needs to be done. The procedure is repeated at each level required and bilaterally as necessary. When these maneuvers are all complete, the dural sac should be completely decompressed from posterior scar and bone. All of the involved nerve roots should have been explored and freed by lysis of scar and foraminotomy. The decision for or against fusion should have been made, and complete hemostasis obtained in the operative site. The dural sac should then be palpated to assess the extent of arachnoiditis and how much CSF has entered the decompressed sac. Occasionally, an intradural mass will be discovered when the contents of the dural sac have not been adequately visualized because of the block. These masses are usually arachnoiditis, and only under unusual circumstances does the dura need to be opened. The principal reason for opening the dura would be the discovery of a circumscribed mass.

Although there is no absolute evidence that it is beneficial, the experimental data on free fat grafting are such that this can be considered a surgical option. A strip of fat sufficient to cover the entire operative site can be obtained by undercutting the skin to normal fat. If no normal fat is available and the surgeon wishes to use a fat graft, it is better to make a separate incision over the buttock in order to obtain it. The graft needs only to be 3–5 mm thick, but it should be sufficient to cover the entire operative area completely. The data that suggest decrease in the ingrowth of scar indicate this will be a useful maneuver, but no clinical studies have appeared that prove its worth. The fat graft will also obliterate the dead space created by the original undercutting of the scar.

Closure requires simple reapproximation of the lumbar fascia. Deep stitches in the muscle will only lead to more scarring and fibrosis. If the paravertebral

Figure 2.10.

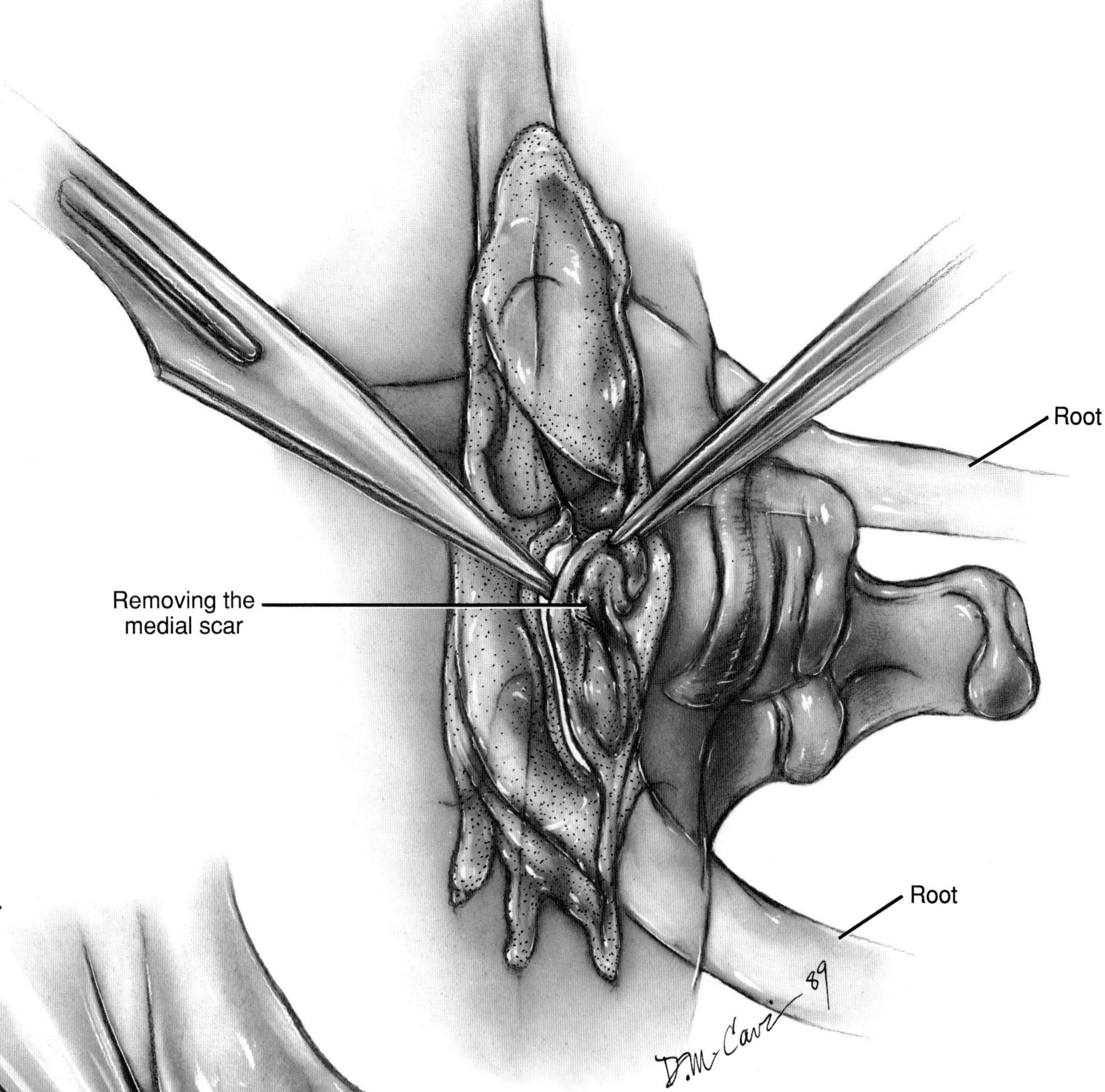

Figure 2.11.

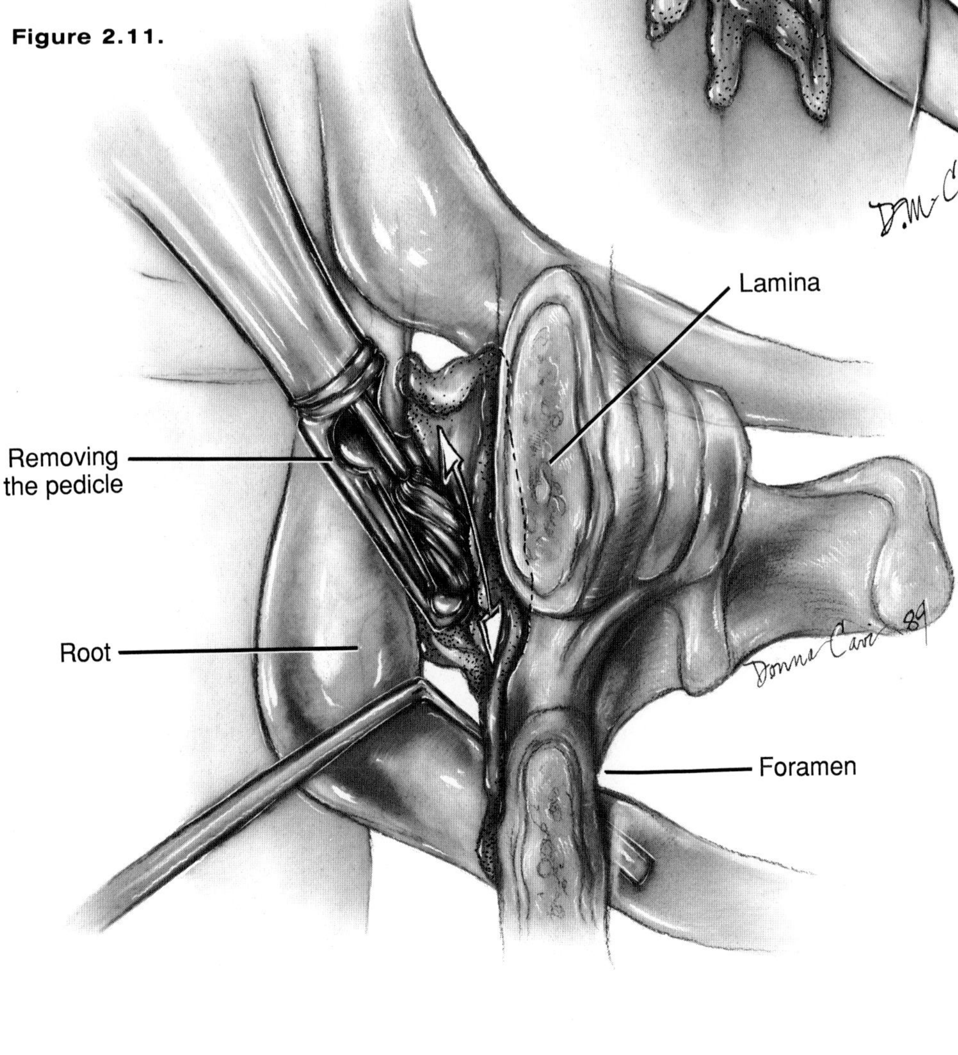

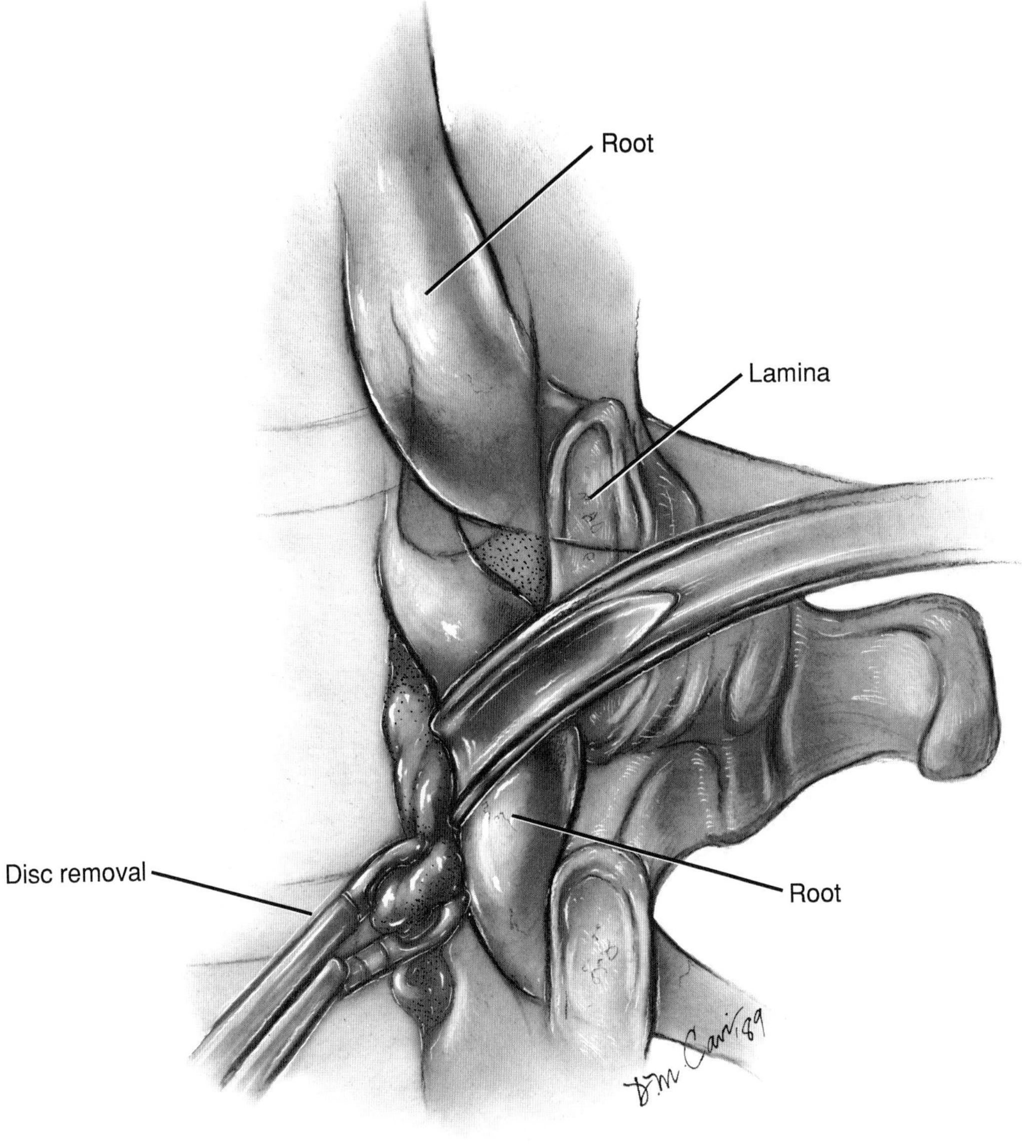

Figure 2.12.

muscles are badly scarred, it is worth considering transplantation of a lateral muscle mass. In this situation, the entire scarred muscle is excised throughout the length of the incision. The skin is undercut, and normal paravertebral muscles are found laterally. A relaxing incision is made in the lumbar fascia, and then a blunt finger dissection is utilized to isolate a portion of paravertebral muscle that can be brought to the midline and closed. This maneuver needs to be considered only when there is virtual replacement of the paravertebral muscle with scar medially. The subcutaneous tissue and skin are closed so that dead space from the fat graft is obliterated; no other special precautions need to be taken.

Fusion Removal

Sometimes, there is overgrowth of a posteriorly placed fusion that will lead to generalized spinal stenosis, or there is a significant focal overgrowth at the upper margin of a fusion with cauda equina compression (Fig. 2.13). Sometimes, a posterior fusion bony mass presents a pain problem because the skin is adherent over it and the mass itself is irritating to local structures. The relief of these problems requires removal of the fusion mass in order to provide adequate decompression.

Removal of Exuberant Posterior Fusion Mass

Sometimes, all that is required is to remove the great overgrowth of bone that has occurred posteriorly. The operation is done with the patient under general anesthesia and prone in an appropriate position for laminectomy. The old skin incision is opened and carried to the mass in the midline. The muscles and scars should be dissected free from the mass of bone via blunt dissection with Cobb elevators. The electric knife can also be used. The fusion mass should be exposed laterally to its margins and superiorly until a normal spine above is seen. It is not necessary to take down muscles from normal spine. The bone removal posteriorly can be done in many ways (Fig. 2.14). The easiest way is with a large chisel or gouge. The mass should be removed until it is near the level of the laminae but still strong. An excellent way is with the high-speed drill, used to shave the bone down to an acceptable level. It may be possible simply to close the skin and muscle mass over the bed of resected bone. Frequently, the medial muscle is so destroyed in the midline that there would be a large gap, so a midline closure is not satisfactory. In this case the skin should be undercut laterally, with the subcutaneous tissue remaining on the skin. The dissection is actually at the level of the lumbar fascia, which will not be identified in the midline but can usually be found a few centimeters from the midline. The dissection is carried out until the paravertebral muscle masses are exposed bilaterally. A relaxing incision is made in the fascia and the muscle laterally so that a sizable mass of muscle, preferably 4 or 5 cm in width, can be moved to the midline. This muscle mass is then closed to provide adequate coverage of the decompressed fusion mass. A single layer of sutures are placed in the fascia covering of the muscle medially, and no stitches should traverse the muscle itself. The skin and subcutaneous tissue are closed in the usual fashion.

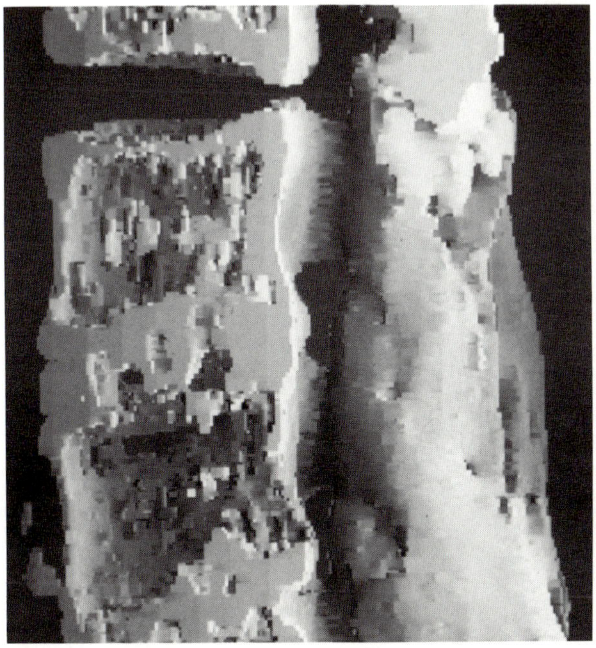

Figure 2.13. Three-dimensional reconstruction demonstrating severe foraminal stenosis beneath the fusion mass.

Removal of Fusion and Adjacent Laminae for Decompression of Spinal Canal

When there is actual compression of the cauda equina, it is more difficult to obtain an adequate removal of the fusion bone by working directly on the fusion. It is much easier to carry out a laminectomy one level above and then remove the fusion bone inferiorly. To do this, the original wound is reopened and carried down to the level of the fusion in the midline. The muscle and scar are scraped away from the bone with Cobb elevators or the electric knife. The fusion mass should be exposed from its upper extremity to its lower extremity and to its lateral margins. The incision must be long enough to allow the exposure of one segment above. The exposure described will allow a subperiosteal dissection of muscles from the spinous process and the laminae above the fusion. Self-retaining cerebellar-type retractors are put in place at this level, exposing these structures and the junction with

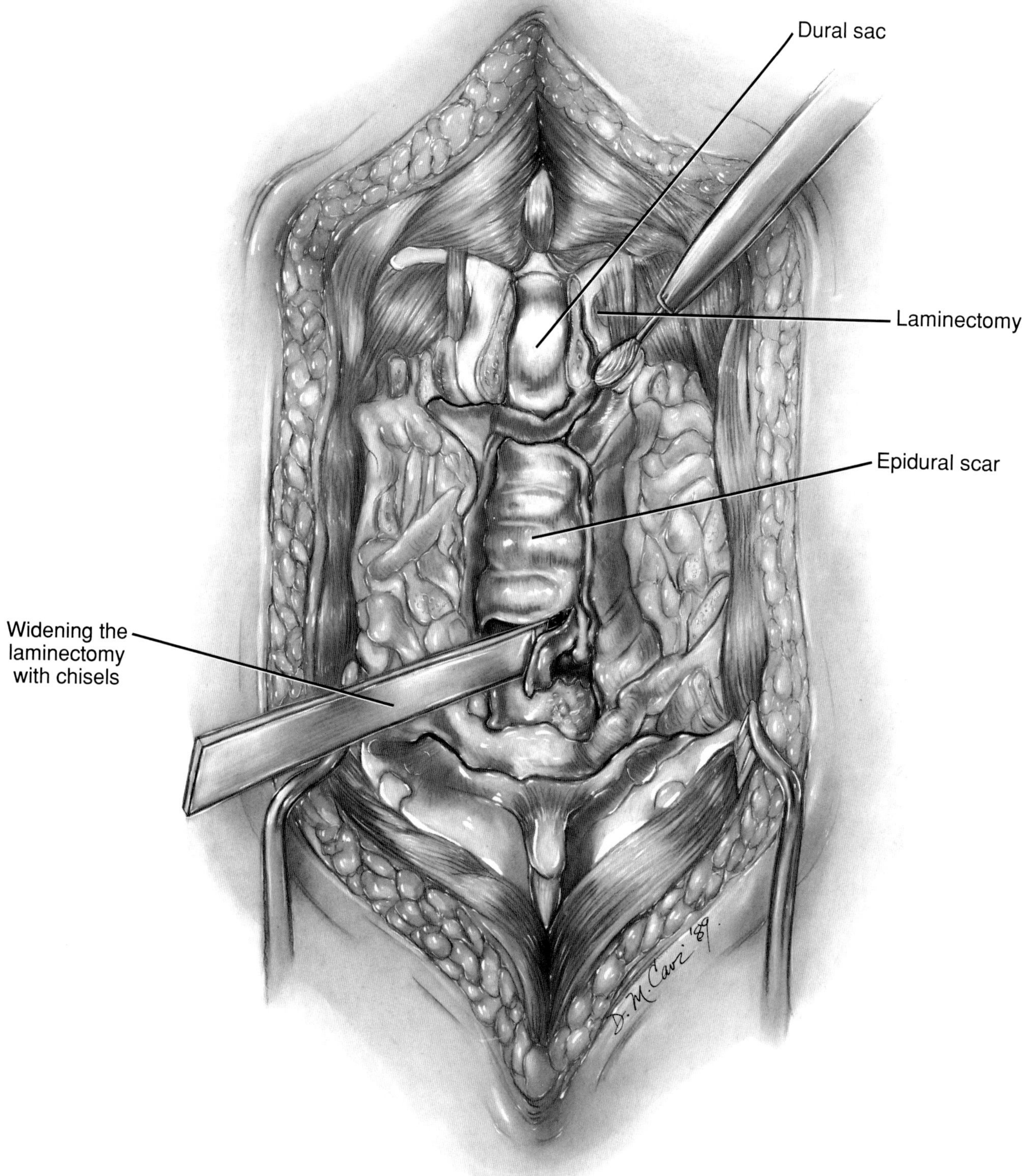
Dural sac
Laminectomy
Epidural scar
Widening the laminectomy with chisels
D. M. Cavi '89

Figure 2.14.

the posterior fusion. The spinous process should be removed, and a bilateral laminectomy carried out to expose the normal dura beneath. A complete laminectomy is not necessary if normal epidural space can be found without it, but usually a total laminectomy is required because there is nearly always some extension of scarring above the fusion. A dissector such as an Adson periosteal elevator or a Penfield #3 is then used to establish a plane between the dura and the fusion mass. Most of these exuberant fusion masses are too big to remove with laminectomy punches or rongeurs. It is necessary to reduce the bulk of the mass before the decompression can be carried out (Fig. 2.14). Everything is now fully exposed, so it is safe to use chisels or gouges or the high-speed drill. The high-speed drill is very accurate once the bulk of the bone has been removed with a chisel. Beginning above at the level of the laminectomy, use the drill to create a new spinal canal, skeletonizing the portion of the fusion next to the dura without drilling all the way through. When only a few millimeters of bone are left and the fusion is channeled from top to bottom to the full width of the laminectomy, then dura can successfully be freed from overlying remaining fusion bone and removed with an angled laminectomy punch (Fig. 2.15). If only decompression of the dural sac is required, the procedure can be terminated at this point. Frequently, there is lateral nerve root compression demonstrated on the CT scan. When this is the case, it is necessary to channel foraminotomies well out into the fusion. The location of the nerve roots can be estimated by identifying the nerve root at the first normal segment and then generally estimating the level of the next roots. With the high-speed drill or a rongeur, a potential channel is made laterally until the gutter is reached and the nerve root can actually be identified. Then the foraminotomy can be extended in the appropriate direction. The high-speed drill is an ideal way to do this, though rongeurs or chisels are also effective (Fig. 2.16). The fusion mass should be left intact laterally if at all possible, and the integrity of the fusion should be disrupted only if it is absolutely mandatory to obtain an adequate neural decompression.

It is quite common for there to be a marked reaction at the level above the fusion. The ligament is extremely thickened, and often bone also is thickened. The zygapophyseal joints may be relatively mobile. It may be difficult to expose the area because of the tremendous thickening of ligaments that is sometimes present. In general, a single-level laminectomy is adequate, and the ligaments can be removed piecemeal by a rongeur without difficulty. That the laminectomy be extended to a normal space above is important, since extending the laminectomy is better than trying to find the dura through the fusion or the markedly abnormal segment immediately above.

Closure is exactly the same as for any other lumbar procedure. The surgeon has the option of filling the defect in the fusion with a fat graft. Evidence that this is beneficial is not certain, but it has theoretical value. The muscle should be closed with a single layer, and muscle transplantation from the lateral can be carried out in the rare case where there has been severe destruction of paravertebral musculature. The skin and subcutaneous tissue are closed in routine fashion.

Surgery for Disc Space Epidural and Paravertebral Infection

Epidural Abscess

The patient with epidural abscess is usually identified because of systemic signs and symptoms indicating an infection. Such patients most commonly present with acute progressive neurological deficit suggesting the levels of spinal cord compression. As with epidural metastases, it is important to demonstrate the upper and lower boundaries of the infection so the surgical exposure can be judged. Remember that it is unwise to make a spinal puncture near an area where an epidural abscess may be found. If the symptoms are low thoracic or include the lumbar area, a C2 puncture is preferable. Since most of these are thoracic in location, it is unusual to require a cervical puncture, but it is extremely important to avoid puncturing the dura near an area of potential pus accumulation.

The treatment of epidural abscess that produces significant spinal cord compression and neurological deficit is surgical decompression and drainage. Operations are carried out under general anesthesia in the prone position. The laminectomy should be planned to uncover the most significant part of the accumulation of pus. The extent of the laminectomy should not be decided until the nature of the epidural mass is determined. Once it is certain that it is infection, then

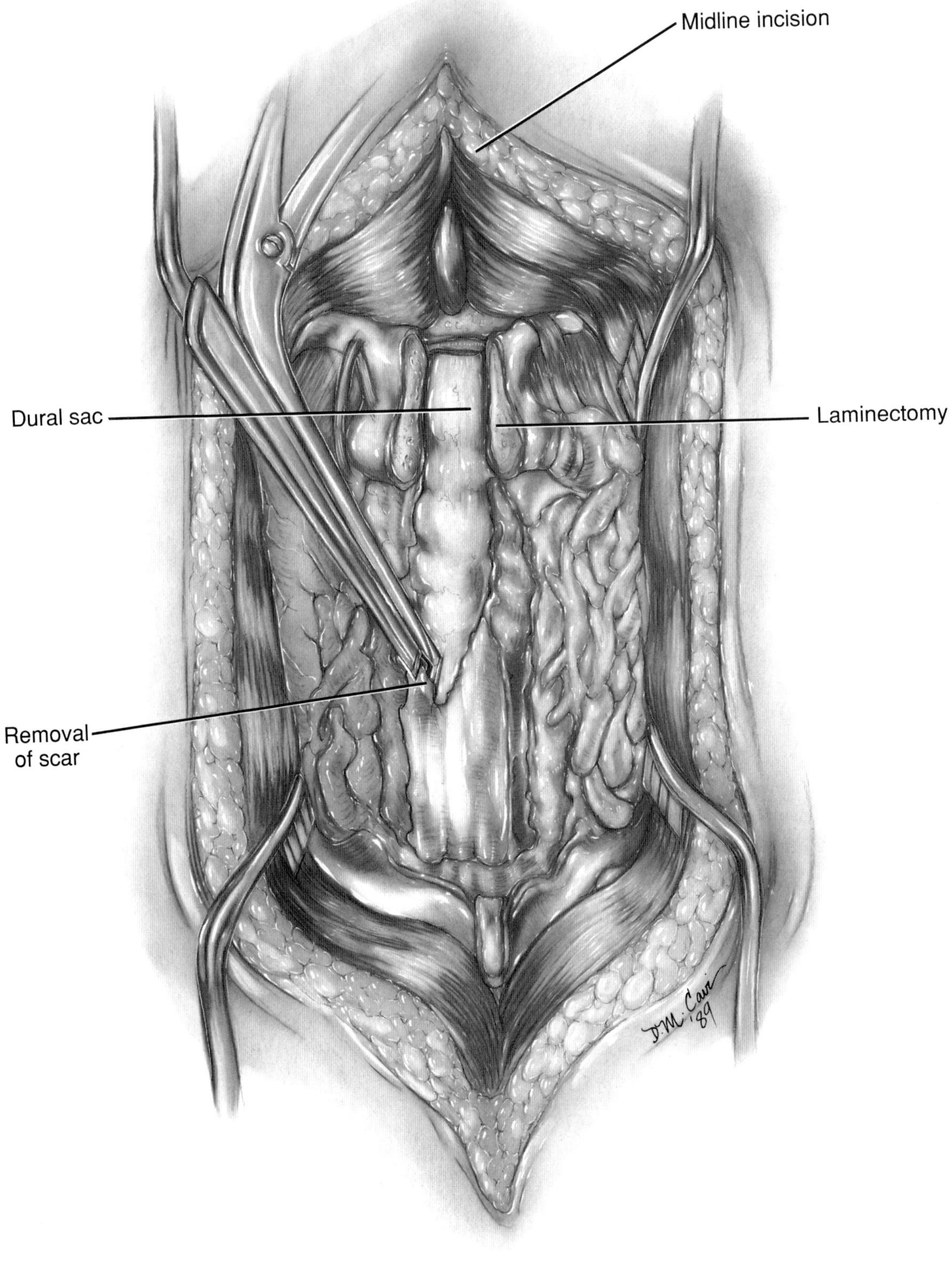
Midline incision
Dural sac
Laminectomy
Removal of scar
D.M. Carr '89

Figure 2.15.

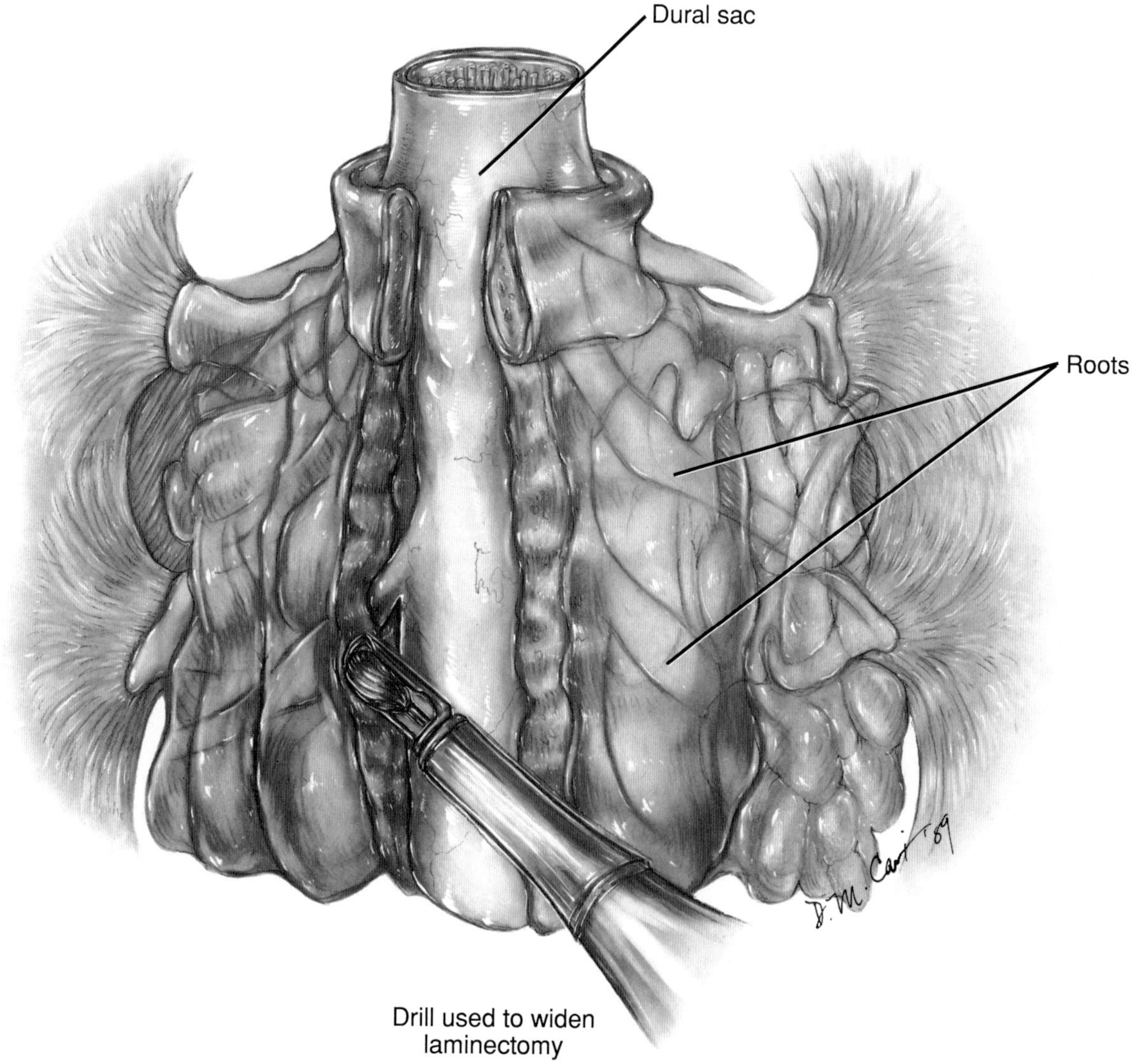

Figure 2.16.

the characteristics of the infected tissue determine what is done. The first step is to carry out routine laminectomy of one or two segments at the level of the major cord compression and neurological symptoms. At the same time, it is important to expose the patient so that an incision and bone removal can be performed beyond either extremity of the mass, if necessary. When the laminectomy is done, pus under pressure may be encountered. If the mass is liquid and expresses itself easily, the small laminectomy and decompression may be all that is required. A small, #8 red rubber catheter can be inserted into the epidural space, and the entire area irrigated thoroughly with antibiotic-bearing saline. An immediate Gram stain will give some idea of the nature of the problem, and cultures should be taken to cover all potential forms of infection. Then the irrigation proceeds until the epidural space is clean and there is no residual pus. It may be necessary to extend the laminectomy to obtain adequate decompression. Epidural suction drains should then be put in place to the upper and lower extremities of the lesion and brought out laterally through the skin. The closure requires no other special considerations.

Sometimes, the mass is not pus but is inflamed swollen tissue with thrombosed epidural veins. In such a situation the tumor mass must be removed as if it were neoplastic. This requires an extensive laminectomy that will expose the mass to allow complete removal. The granulating mass can be stripped from the dura by blunt dissection. Any bleeding points are coagulated, and adequate cultures and pathological specimens should be obtained. Although there does not appear to be pus, it is still wise to drain with epidural suction drains. The closure requires no special care otherwise.

There is an unusual situation in which this inflammatory thrombophlebitis process extends intradurally, causing thrombosis of intramedullary veins and venous infarction. Surgery will not benefit this condition, which is suspected when the myelogram shows an epidural mass that is noncompressive with systemic signs and symptoms of infection and relatively normal or swollen cord. The only reason for surgery is to obtain an appropriate culture. Epidural needle aspiration will usually suffice to obtain the culture, and surgery should be reserved for situations in which the nature of the problem is not clear.

Disc Space Infection

The disc space infection that requires surgery is relatively rare. When the diagnosis is made preoperatively, the approach should be retroperitoneal in the lumbar region, costotransverse in the thoracic area, and anterior in the cervical region. Most disc space infections can be treated effectively with antibiotics. The reasons for operation are limited: failure to obtain diagnosis on culture by any other means; drainage of a loculation of pus; and failure to eradicate the infection with antibiotics. The latter two problems will commonly be associated with intractable pain and progressive neurological deficits. With lumbar discitis, the development of pelvic thrombophlebitis is a dread complication that has both a high morbidity and mortality (Fig. 2.17).

Treatment of Inflammatory Discitis via Posterior Approach

Occasionally, the surgeon will operate on an apparent disc herniation only to find evidence of infection. This is most commonly the case with indolent infections of the disc, such as brucellosis or tuberculosis. Most commonly, the diagnosis will be made preoperatively because of the systemic signs and symptoms, and the retroperitoneal approach can be elected. If the surgeon finds the disc infection unexpectedly, however, special measures are required to deal with it.

The operation will have been carried out as for a disc removal or exploration. When the apparently herniated disc is entered, the extremely degenerated nature of the material removed should give the surgeon a clue that discitis is the appropriate diagnosis. Sometimes, frank pus will be obtained, but it is more likely that the disc material excised will simply be extremely degenerated, soft, and without its typical appearance. Some of the disc should be sent for Gram stain immediately, and some should be sent for culture, with all potential forms of possible infection covered. The interspace should then be thoroughly cleansed of all degenerative material with disc rongeurs and curettes. Remember that these maneuvers are much more dangerous in the face of infection because the protecting surrounding annulus is largely destroyed and the ligaments may be involved, so that it is easy to penetrate into the retroperitoneal space.

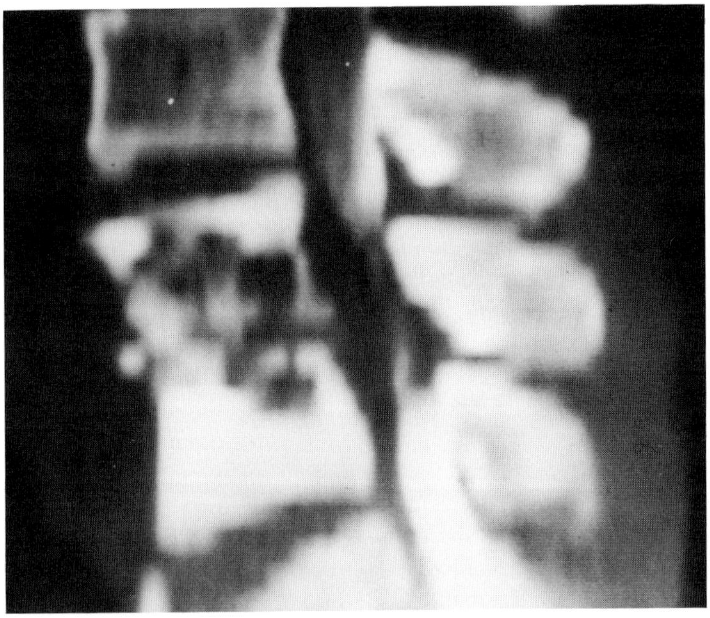

Figure 2.17. Typical picture of disc space infection with destruction beginning in the disc and spreading to the related body. The appropriate therapy will be radical resection because of the sizable epidural collection behind the infection that produced spinal cord compression.

The interspace should be carefully irrigated under pressure with a large quantity of saline until the return is clear and no more degenerated disc material can be obtained. A small suction drain should be placed through the hole in the posterior longitudinal ligament into the disc space and brought out through a separate stab wound several inches from the midline. The wound is then closed in the usual fashion, and the drain is left in place until the organism is identified and appropriate antibiotics are begun.

Retroperitoneal Approach to Lumbar Disc Infection

When the nature of the problem is identified in advance, a retroperitoneal approach is superior to the posterior approach. In such situations, the combination of imaging studies will have produced a probable diagnosis. The first step should be needle aspiration of the disc or paravertebral mass under fluoroscopic CT control. Saline can be irrigated through the needle and aspirated. Needle and saline cultures will frequently identify the appropriate organism. When patients do not have progressive neurological deficits or unusually septic conditions, a trial of eradications with antibiotics prior to surgery is worthwhile. Surgical exploration and debridement and drainage should be required in a minority of patients and reserved for those with serious sepsis, extreme pain or progressive neurological deficit, or progressive disease that does not respond to antibiotic therapy. A flank incision similar to incisions required for the anterior and anterolateral approaches for other disease is utilized. General anesthesia is mandatory because of the nature of the operation. The exposure is the same as required for fracture of a contemplated anterior fusion. The difference is that the infection in the paravertebral space has commonly created a large retroperitoneal cavity that may be filled with pus or granulation tissue. In one way this makes the dissection easier, but in another it adds to the risk because of the friability of the tissue. The vascular structures particularly are more easily injured. Once the offending interspace is exposed, any granulomatous material or pus in the retroperitoneal area should be gently washed away. Granulation tissue that does not easily come out with irrigation should be left. Adequate cultures should be taken as soon as the space is entered, and then the whole retroperitoneal area should be irrigated with large quantities of saline. If the organism is known, it may be feasible to use an antibiotic-containing solution for irrigation. If the organism is not known, saline is adequate. Irrigation will usually allow the disc space to be readily identified. When there is a significant paravertebral infectious process, the ligaments and annulus usually have been destroyed. In less serious paravertebral infections, these structures may still be intact. The ligaments and annulus are opened as necessary, and all of the infected material is removed from the disc space with suction. The Cavitron ultrasonic dissector is an excellent tool for this job. Infected discs should be entirely removed, and involved bone that is clearly infected should also be removed. All bone that is relatively normal should be left in place. The interspaces above and below the involved space should be inspected to be certain they are not involved, but unless there is strong evidence, intact ligaments and annulus should not be breached. It seems anachronistic, but grafting in the face of infection is almost always successful. The technique described in Chapter 7 is employed. Once the graft is seated, the whole area is irrigated with saline, and suction drains are put in place to drain both the disc space and the paravertebral retroperitoneal space. Two drains are usually required. These should be brought out through a separate flank stab wound; the drain should be left in place until there is no further drainage and adequate antibiotic coverage is instituted.

Costotransverse Approach to Thoracic Infection

When the infected disc is in the thoracic region, it is common for there to be a significant paravertebral mass. Tuberculosis is the most likely possibility in most parts of the world, but in the United States other organisms are seen at least as frequently. The principles of surgery for both are about the same. Whenever a thoracic paravertebral infection is found, it is wise to treat the patient and the surgery as if tuberculosis was the diagnosis.

The operation is carried out with the patient under general anesthesia and prepared for the costotransverse incision. The costotransverse approach is the same as described for a thoracic disc. The rib that allows best access to the involved discs should be chosen for the approach. When there is a significant paravertebral mass, the approach will immediately provide access to the mass. It is extremely important that the pleura not be entered in the face of a potential infection. Cultures should be obtained as soon as the paravertebral area is entered and the pus is encountered. The area should be thoroughly irrigated with saline, and the involved discs and destroyed bone should be excised. The Cavitron is an excellent tool for this excision. No sequestra should be left, but bony removal should be limited to clearly devascularized infected bone. These areas will heal well, and fusion usually occurs when the bony excision is not excessive and when the infection can be controlled. If extensive bony removal is necessary, interbody fusion (Chapter 7) can be employed.

Following bony removal, copious irrigation is utilized again. The wound should then be drained with soft suction drains, and the wound closed as for any other costotransverse approach.

Arachnoiditis

Surgery for adhesive arachnoiditis of the cauda equina is rarely indicated, but there are patients who have progressive neurological deficits or intractable pain that has failed every other method of relief for whom lysis of the adhesions has something to offer. Careful removal of the scar can result in predictable cessation of the progression of neurological deterioration, occasionally lead to some improvement, and has a 50/50 chance of making the pain better.

The operation for exposure of the dura is virtually always the same as for reoperation on the lumbar spine for removal of compressive epidural scar. The arachnoiditis has usually developed in the face of multiple operations, and the first portion of the operation, decompression of the dura, must be accomplished before the dura can be widely opened. Rarely, arachnoiditis will complicate trauma or myelography so that an uncomplicated laminectomy is all that is required. The bone should be removed at least one or two levels above the highest point of the expected scar. It is important to extend the laminectomy to normal structures in order to dissect the nerve roots free. A minimum of one vertebral segment above is required. The epidural scar is removed throughout the length of the exposure. Beginning in this normal location, the surgeon should then open the dura. The operating microscope is required even for opening the dura, for the adherence of nerve roots to the dural

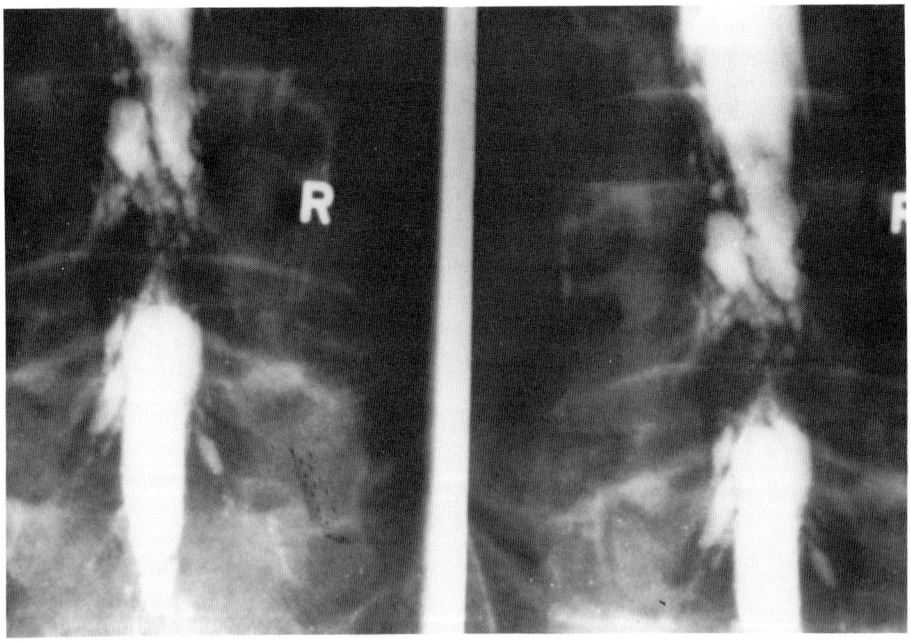

Figure 2.18. The myelogram demonstrates a focal (napkin-ring) block over the body of L4.

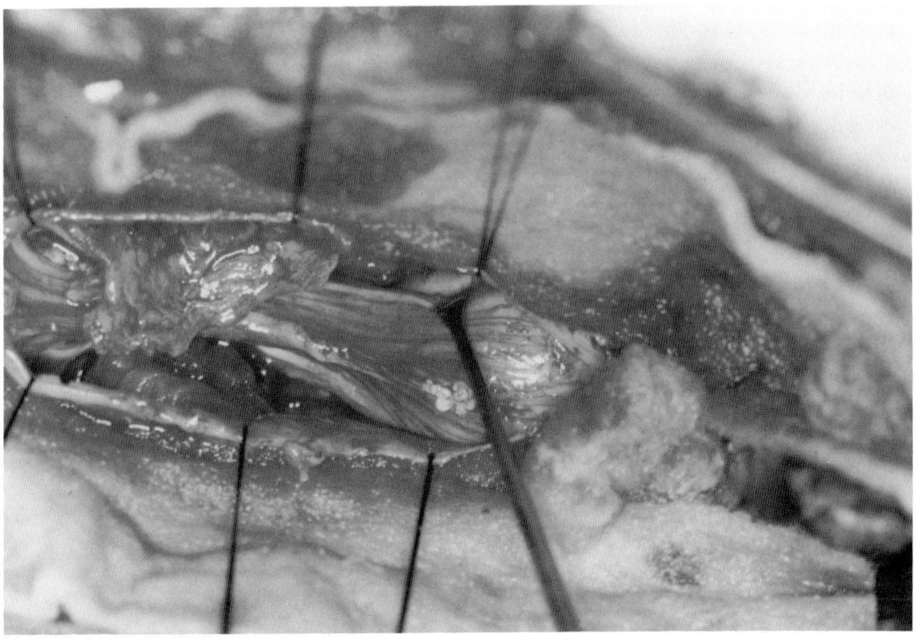

Figure 2.19. An operative photograph demonstrates the mass being dissected from the adherent roots of the cauda equina.

sac can be dense and it is very easy to injure roots when opening of the dura is attempted without magnification. As soon as the dura is opened, the thickened arachnoid will be seen (Fig. 2.20). This should be preserved and the dura dissected free from it. A small grooved director is a handy way to open the dura in the midline. The dissection should free the dura from the arachnoid laterally to the gutters; make sure that no roots are adherent to the dura under the incision. It is common for the roots to be circumferentially applied to the dura, and they can easily be injured by the opening knife, the lateral dissection, or dural retention sutures. Once the dura is opened throughout the length of the field, the edges of the dura must be freed from the arachnoid; this blunt dissection is carried laterally to the margins of the laminectomy and then down into the gutters. Dural retention sutures may then be placed to hold the dura out of the way. This will expose the mass of thickened arachnoid containing the nerve roots from normal subarachnoid space above to normal subarachnoid space below or to the sacrum (Fig. 2.21). The posterior roots are nearly always much more involved than the anterior roots, and when the process extends beyond the lumbar space and surrounds the cord, it is usually more serious posterior to rather than anterior to the dentate ligaments. The reasons for this predilection for the posterior space are unknown. The dissection should begin by opening the subarachnoid space at a normal level (Fig. 2.22). Individual nerve roots are then identified. It is easier to take the larger nerve roots first, for this will allow them to be moved out of the way for the more demanding dissection of the smaller roots. The arachnoid is removed from individual roots throughout the length of the incision. It is better to trace a single root the entire length of its course in the arachnoiditis than to work on multiple roots at the same level. It is not safe to hold the roots with any kind of retractor, but the adherent arachnoid makes a convenient handle. Divide the arachnoid throughout, leaving a small strip adherent to each root, and when the root is completely free, you can remove the last strip of adherent arachnoid. Occasionally, the arachnoiditis can be stripped via blunt dissection, but in such a situation there is always question whether the lysis needs to be done. More commonly, the arachnoid reaction is densely adherent to the roots and must be removed with microscissors. Arachnoid knives are a very handy way to strip long pieces of the arachnoid from the roots. Obviously, great care must be taken to avoid injury to the roots with a knife. Disposable right-angled blades are very convenient for this, since they are extremely sharp and have a point. The safest thing is to use the microscissors, but knives in experienced hands provide an increase in the speed with which the lysis of the adhesions can be done. The large roots do not present great technical problems, but it can be extremely difficult to tell the small sacral roots from arachnoid adhesions. If there is ever a question, it is better to leave any structure. The use of electrical stimulation for the identification of motor roots and those going to bladder and bowel can be employed, but it is not routine (Fig. 2.23). Once all the posterior roots are free, it is necessary to proceed anteriorly by cutting laterally around the mass of roots. It is very difficult to work through the scarred posterior roots. Fortunately, the motor roots are not nearly as involved as the sensory roots. They are larger, so division of the adhesions with a knife is less dangerous and there is usually much less scarring around them. The goal of the procedure is to eliminate all of the adherence between nerve roots and remove essentially all of the scar. Unfortunately, this is rarely realized, and the surgeon usually must compromise with total removal because of the fear of injury to nerve roots. The best guideline is that if injury to nerve appears likely, it is better to stop the procedure.

The most difficult of all the arachnoidal reactions that can be encountered is the true arachnoiditis calcificans. The removal of this densely adherent calcified material is virtually impossible with current microtechniques, and the surgeon should have a low threshold for stopping the procedure when it becomes evident that extricating the nerve roots from the calcified mass will probably be unsuccessful.

The decision to close the dura is an important one. If the dura can be closed, it is better to do so. If it cannot be closed, a patch is reasonable. Leaving the dura opened is an acceptable substitute but is less desirable. The closure then proceeds as described for any reoperation on the spine. If the dura has not been closed, a watertight muscle closure and a tight subcutaneous layer are important.

Dorsal Ganglionectomy

Dorsal ganglionectomy is occasionally indicated for patients with a serious injury to a lumbar root. Such

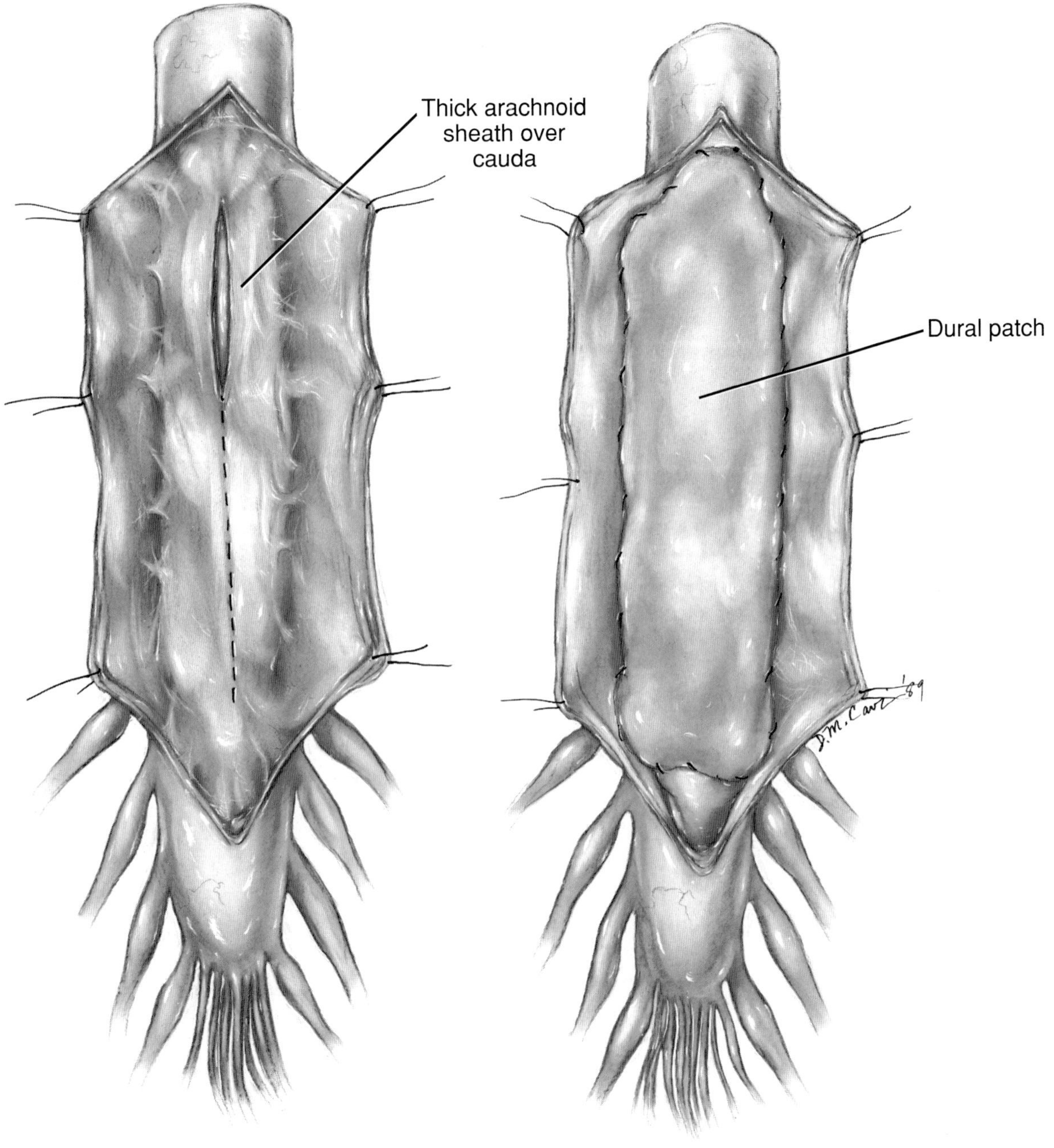

Figure 2.20.

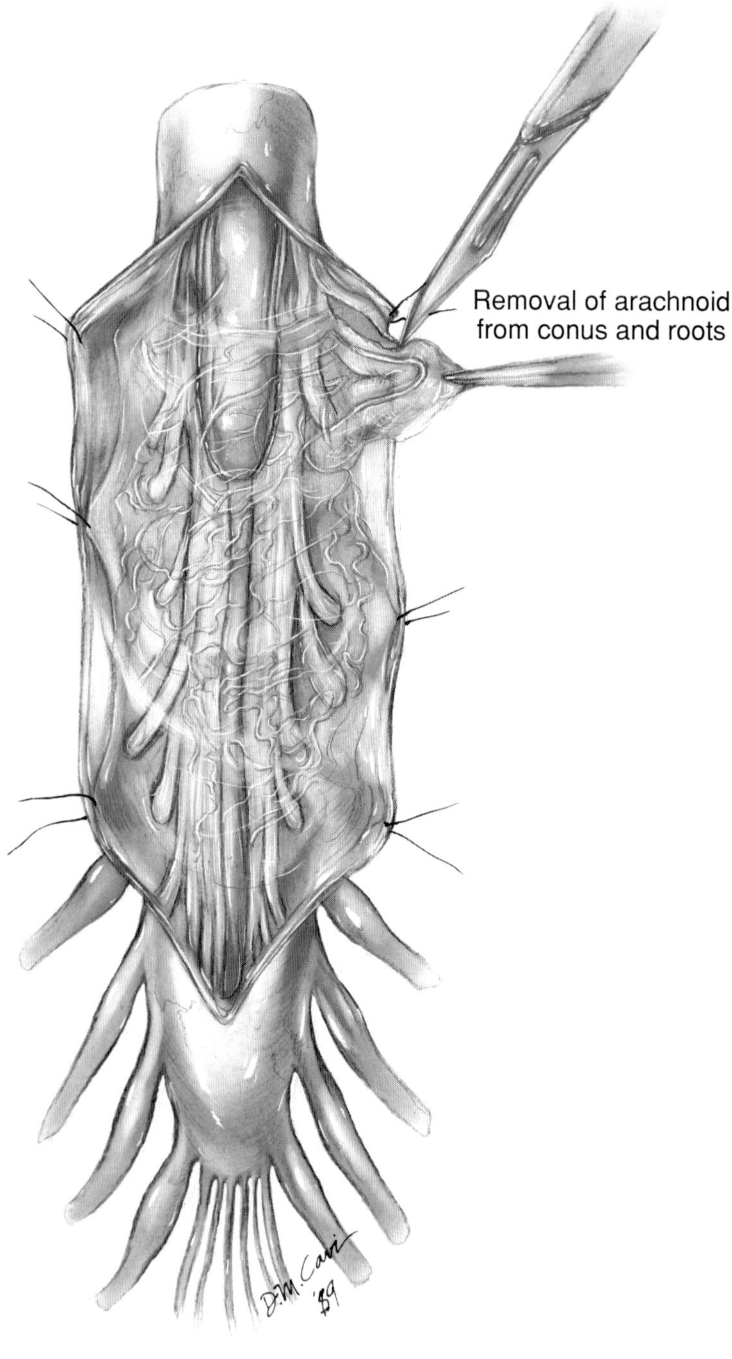

Figure 2.21.

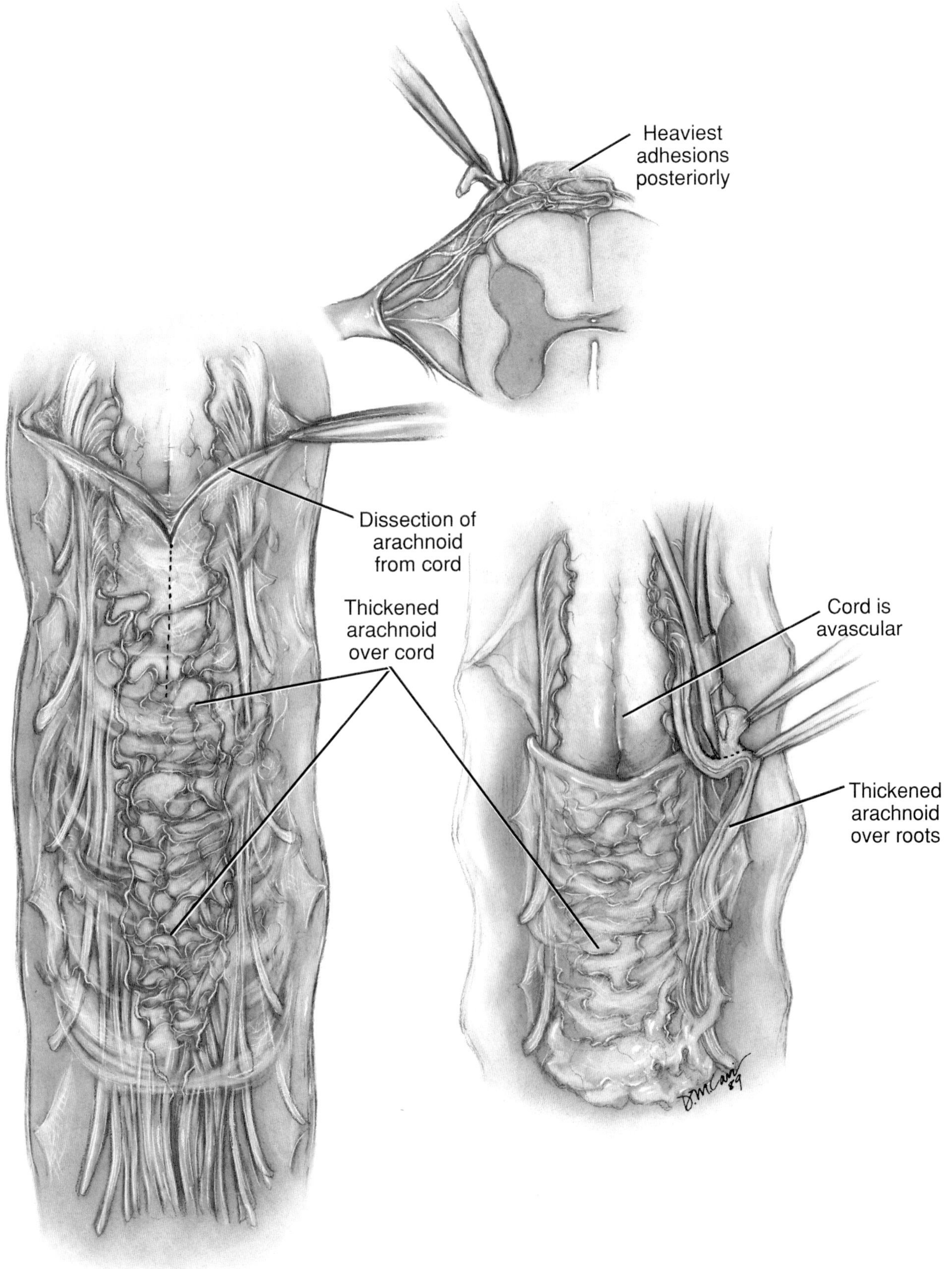
Heaviest
adhesions
posteriorly
Dissection of
arachnoid
from cord
Thickened
arachnoid
over cord
Cord is
avascular
Thickened
arachnoid
over roots

Figure 2.22.

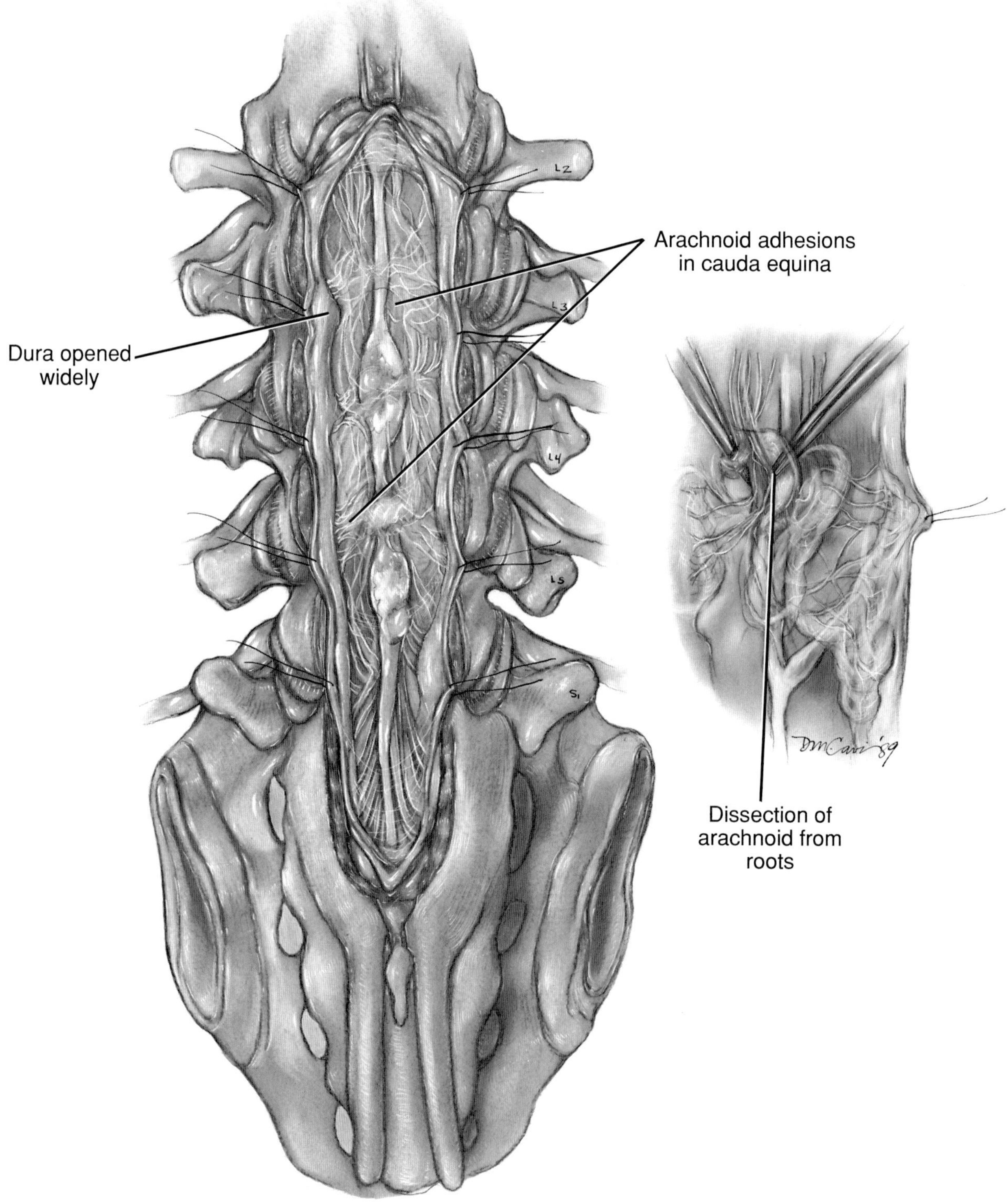
Arachnoid adhesions
in cauda equina
Dura opened
widely
Dissection of
arachnoid from
roots
L2
L3
L4
L5
S1

Figure 2.23.

patients have usually suffered root injury secondary to disc herniation or in the course of surgery for root compression. The typical patient has excruciating pain only in the distribution of the involved root. When selective root blocks relieve the pain, dorsal ganglionectomy may be indicated. This operation is chosen over posterior rhizotomy because it eliminates potential pain fibers entering the cord through the anterior roots. All such fibers have their origin in the dorsal root ganglion. These operations are carried out with the patient under general anesthesia in the prone position exactly as for excision of a lumbar disc. The goal of surgery is excision of the appropriate dorsal root ganglion without injury to the anterior root or entering the CSF.

When it is appropriately placed, the skin incision from the previous surgery simply can be reopened. If it will not allow access to the neural foramen, the incision must be modified so that a generous foraminotomy can be performed. Attention must be given preoperatively to stability, since a foraminotomy will be required and its extent cannot necessarily be judged in advance. Unless the zygapophyseal joint is disrupted on the other side, it is very unlikely that any instability will follow the unilateral foraminotomy. If it appears this will destabilize the spine, fusion must be considered.

Usually, the old skin incision is opened, and a dissection through the previous operative site is carried out to expose the foramen to be explored as well as the lamina above and the lamina below. The nature of the dissection will be determined by the configuration left by the previous surgery. The goal of the exposure is to be able to carry out a foraminotomy, and whatever is required to remove the postoperative scar to achieve this goal should be done. The general principles of exposure of an interspace for discectomy and foraminotomy apply. When the Williams retractor is put in place, the surfaces of the lamina above and the lamina below should be identified. The lateral dissection should be carried out to the lateral margin of the zygapophyseal joint so a generous foraminotomy is possible. The technique of gaining access to the foramen will also vary with the distortions of anatomy left by the previous surgery. In general, the principle of going from normal to abnormal should be followed (Fig. 2.24). Removal of a small portion of the lamina above or the lamina below, exposing dura, is easiest. The interface between the dura and the scar can then be developed to expose the foramen. If a significant foraminotomy has been done at an earlier surgery, it may only be necessary to remove the scar from the root. This is best done under magnification. As the epidural fibrosis is removed, the thickened, scarred root will come into view (Fig. 2.24). If a foraminotomy has not been accomplished, the foramen should now be enlarged until the medial and lateral extent of the dorsal root ganglion can be visualized. An alternative approach to removing lamina is to use a high-speed drill to remove the posterior wall of the foramen, i.e., about one half to two thirds of the zygapophyseal joint, to expose the root and ganglion. There is no need to extend the exposure medially except to find a normal plane. For ganglionectomy, the entire extent of the zygapophyseal joint and its relationships with epidural fibrosis medially in the area of previous surgery, the lamina above, and the lamina below must be seen. Then, with a large burr and a high-speed drill the foramen can be opened posteriorly. The bone in the foramen should be skeletonized to the point it is extremely thin, so that it can be easily removed with curettes or small rongeurs. The extent of the bony removal is related to the position of the dorsal root ganglion, and this must be judged by direct vision. Only the S1 ganglion is within the spinal canal. All others are extracanalicular in the foramen. At least half the joint, and frequently even more, must be removed to ensure adequate exposure (Fig. 2.25). The dorsal root ganglion is identified as a small mass bulging posteriorly on the root; it can be palpated as a firm rubbery mass in the much softer root. It is important to see the medial and lateral borders so the root is not opened excessively. The microdissection requires good hemostasis. These tend to ooze, and the liberal application of a hemostatic agent such as thrombin or Avitene is wise, so that the dissection can be carried out under direct vision without blood obscuring the field. When the exposure is adequate, a sharp small pointed knife, such as one with a #11 blade, is used to open the dural sheath in the midline from the medial to the lateral aspect of the ganglion (Fig. 2.25). The medial aspect is recognized because a few rootlets will come into view. Usually, no CSF is seen because of the extensive scarring among these posterior rootlets. Sometimes, a few drops of CSF will appear. This is of no consequence. The dissection is then carried laterally until a few rootlets entering the ganglion are seen. The

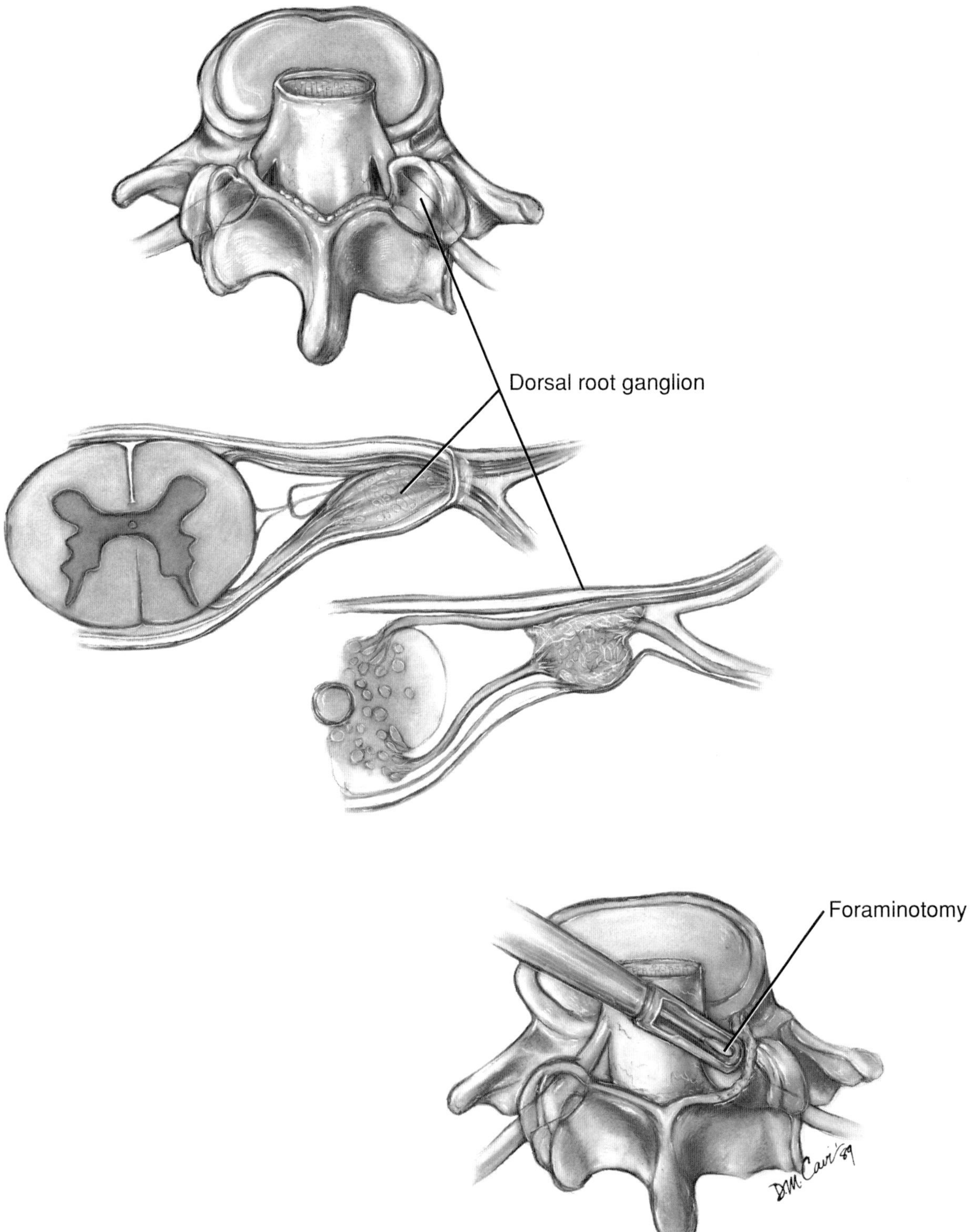

Figure 2.24.

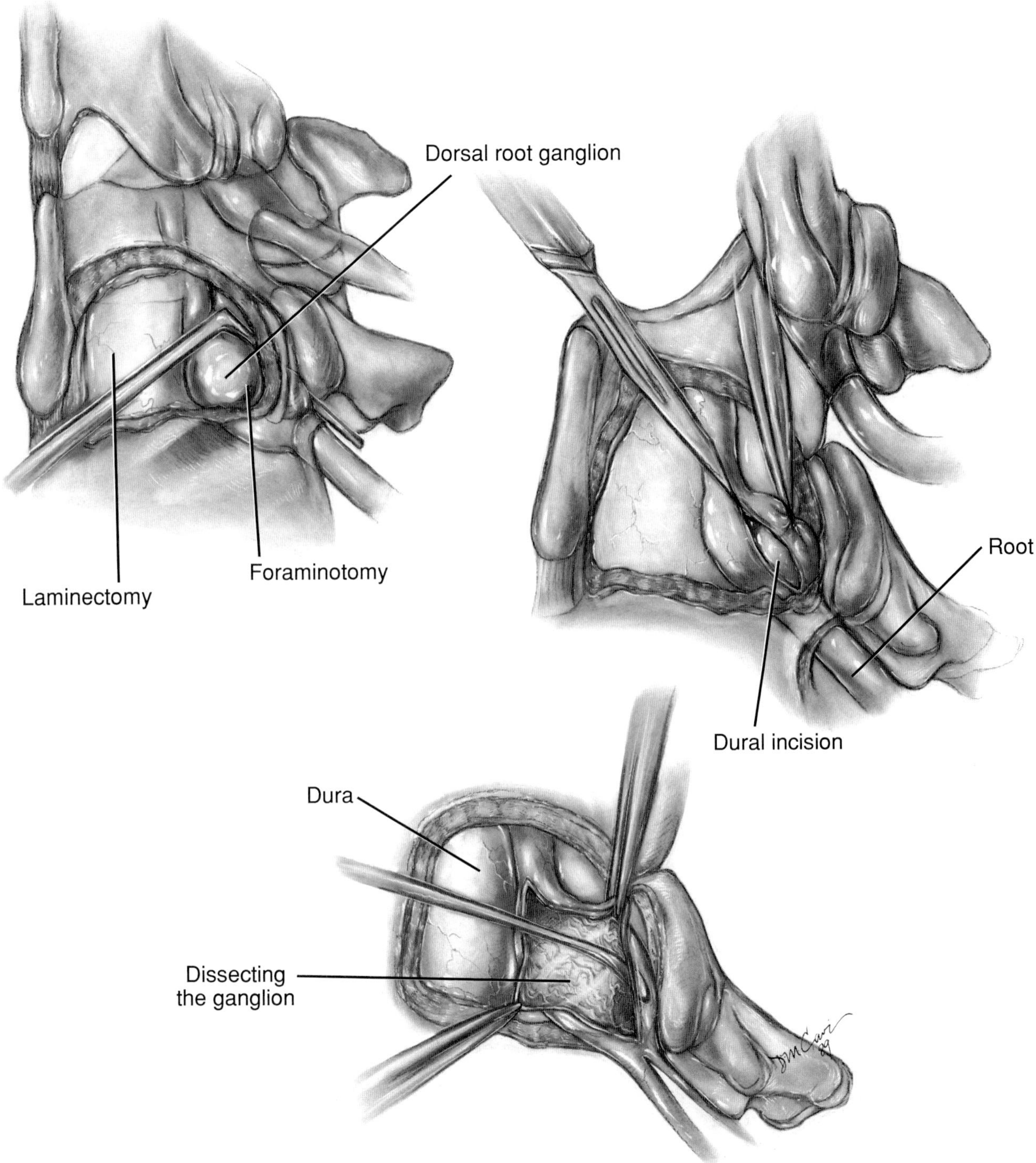
Dorsal root ganglion
Laminectomy
Foraminotomy
Root
Dural incision
Dura
Dissecting the ganglion

Figure 2.25.

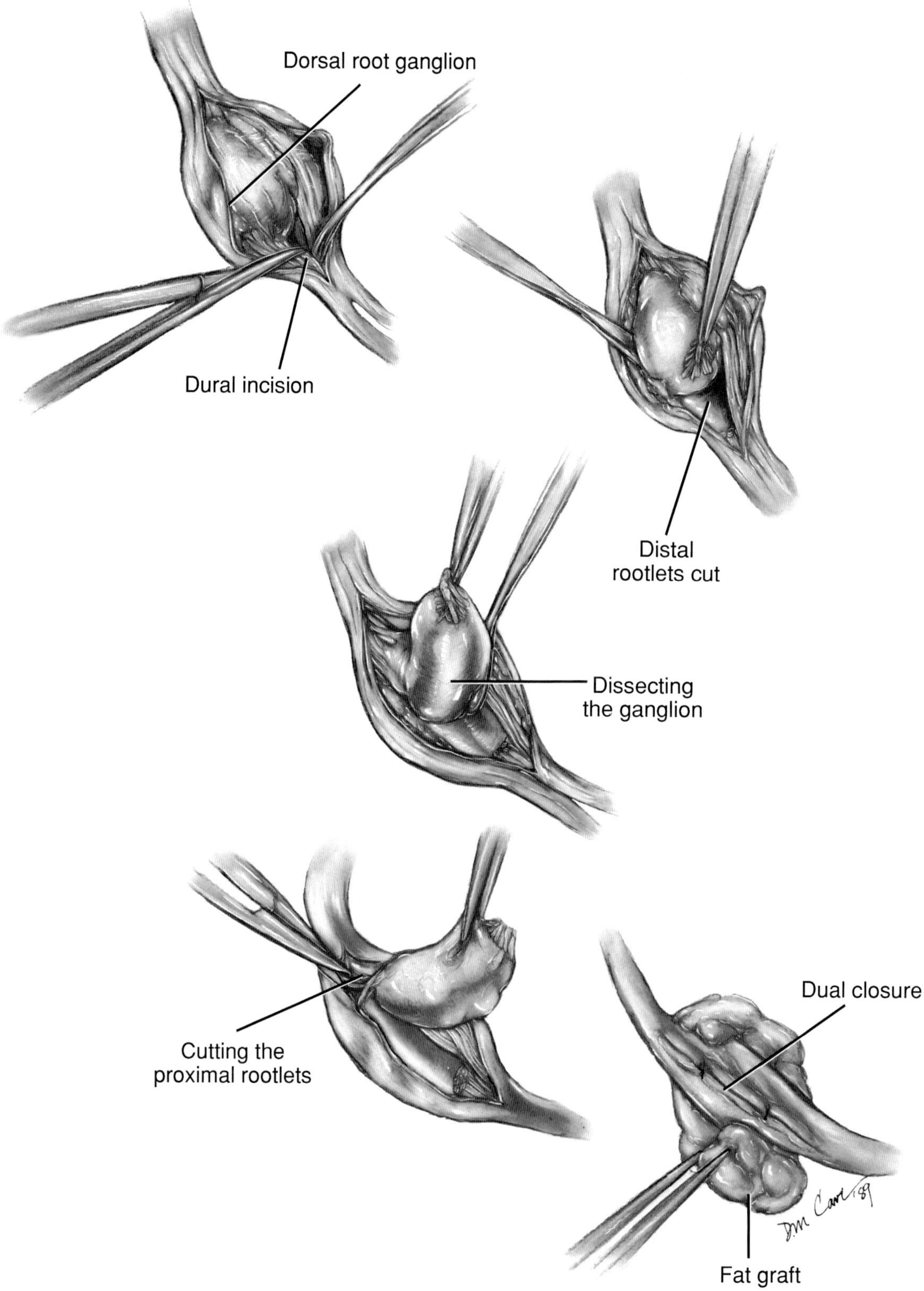
Dorsal root ganglion
Dural incision
Distal rootlets cut
Dissecting the ganglion
Cutting the proximal rootlets
Dual closure
Fat graft
DM Carr '89

Figure 2.26.

dural sheath should then be dissected free from the posterior ganglion circumferentially with a Rosen knife or other small sharp dissector. The ganglion will look like a small pea with rootlets on either side (Fig. 2.26). It is usually possible to dissect all the way around it without ever seeing ventral roots. Sometimes, because of scarring, it is not possible to proceed anteriorly until the posterior roots are cut. The posterior rootlets leaving the ganglion should be divided first, then the ganglion should be rolled from medial to lateral, dissecting it free from the anterior root. Once this is accomplished, the lateral rootlets next to the ganglion are divided. If CSF is not encountered, nothing more is necessary. If a CSF leak is present, the dural incision should be closed or the area tightly packed with fat. An assessment of the instability created by removal of zygapophyseal joint is necessary. Fusion should be required only if there is extensive disruption of the joints at other levels and on the opposite side. The lumbar fascia is closed in the midline; subcutaneous tissue and skin closure are routine.

3

Decompressive Lumbar Laminectomy

Lumbar Laminectomy for Spondylosis

Lumbar laminectomy for spondylosis is done with the patient under general anesthesia. The patient may be positioned prone or knee to chest (Fig. 3.2*A* and *B*). The lateral position is not as satisfactory for complete laminectomy. The patient should be positioned on rolls or a laminectomy frame that supports the lateral chest, abdomen, and pelvis from iliac crest to the shoulders. The skin incision should be planned to expose just the laminae to be removed. If there is any doubt, a film for localization should be taken before the skin incision is made. The incision should be made from the spine above the last level to be removed down to the sacrum or the spine below the last level to be removed. The incision is extended to the spinous processes in the midline, and self-retaining retractors are utilized to expose the entire area. Hemostasis should be obtained at each layer by electrocoagulation, but skin hemostasis is not required unless the bleeding is excessive.

The lumbar fascia should then be incised in the midline down to periosteum. Use of the cautery knife is a bloodless way to do this. The lumbar fascia is then undercut to the lateral margin of the spinous process, first on one side and then on the other. The interspinous attachments should be divided, leaving the muscle mass virtually undisturbed (Fig. 3.3). Square 1-inch periosteotomes are ideal for the subperiosteal

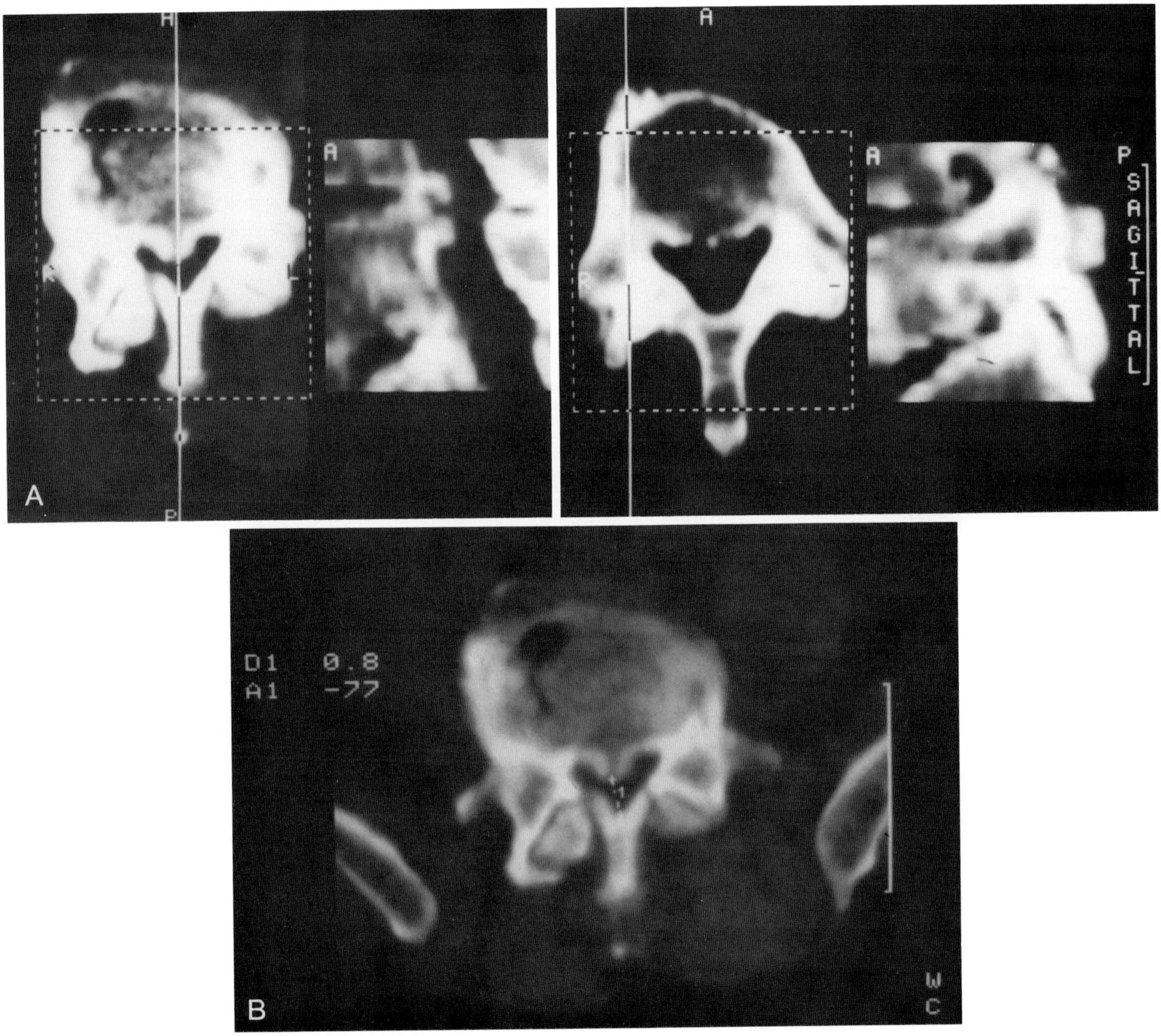

Figure 3.1. **A** *(left and right)*. Typical features of spinal stenosis are seen. The pedicles are shortened, the zygapophyseal joints are greatly overgrown, and the canal is further compromised by posterior spurring on the body. The triangular shape is typical. **B.** Severe spinal stenosis with calcification of posterior disc protrusion. Notice the short pedicles and overgrown facets that contribute to the problem.

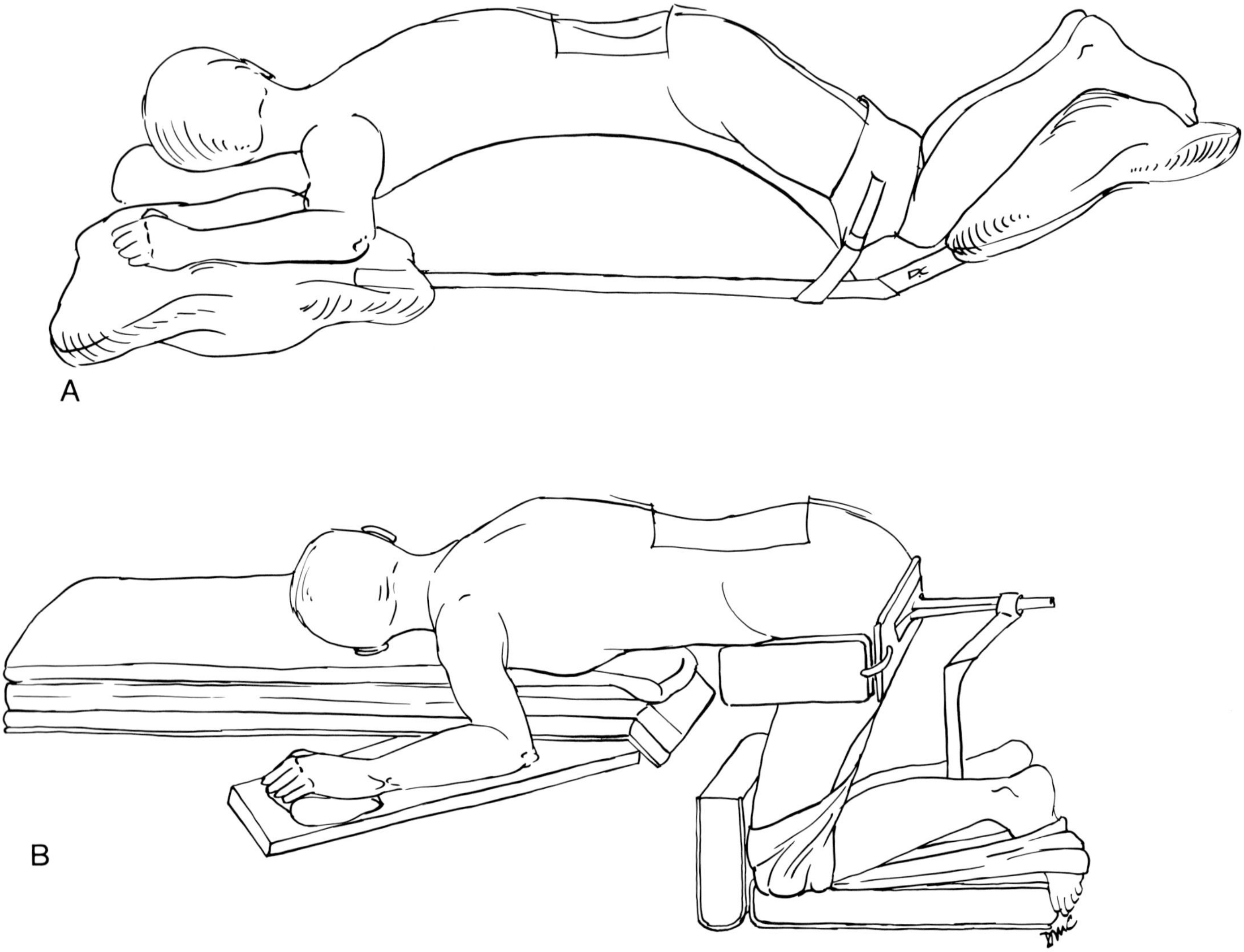

Figure 3.2. A. Patient on lumbar frame in optimum position. **B.** Proper position on the Andrews frame.

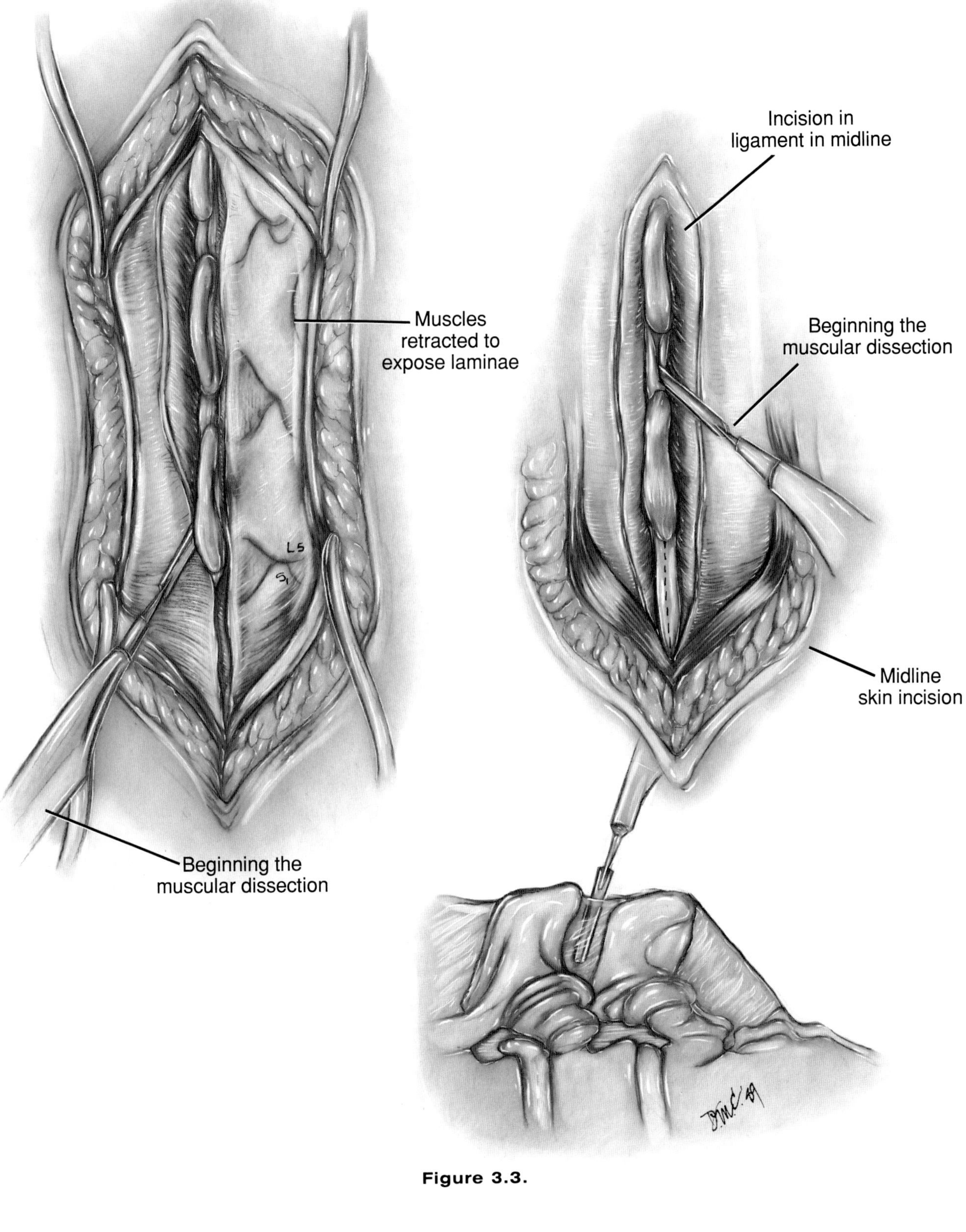
Muscles
retracted to
expose laminae
L5
S1
Beginning the
muscular dissection
Incision in
ligament in midline
Beginning the
muscular dissection
Midline
skin incision

Figure 3.3.

dissection of the muscles from the laminae. It is extremely important to be in a true subperiosteal plane. When this is accomplished, the muscle pseudocapsule is virtually undisturbed (Fig. 3.4). When a true subperiosteal dissection is not performed, the muscle mass will be entered, increasing scarring and postoperative pain as well as causing potential changes that will affect the biomechanics of the spine. The cuts with the osteotome are made in a sequential fashion so that the dissection can proceed with the least trauma and effort. The first cut is made directly down the spinous process, across the lamina, and out to expose at least the medial third of the zygapophyseal joint. Depending on which hand was used for the first subperiosteal incision, the next cut will expose either the inferior or the superior margin of the lamina. For a right-handed surgeon, the usual sequence is for the right-hand osteotome to be used to make the first spinous and laminar cut. Then, while the right-hand osteotome is used to maintain retraction, the left-hand osteotome is used to cut the superior space and the superior margin of the lamina and facet. Then the left-hand osteotome is used to maintain retraction while the right-hand osteotome is withdrawn and reinserted to cut the space below and the lower margin of the lamina out on to the facet (Fig. 3.5). The process is repeated in that sequence from either above or below, depending on where the original incision has been made. The sequence is carried out until all of the laminae are exposed, then this incision is packed with 4×4 sponges, and the procedure is repeated over the sponges to clean all bits of muscle and fat from the bone. The same procedure is done on the opposite side in reverse. The sponges are then removed, and angled cerebellar retractors or their equivalent is put in place. Place the lower one first, wherever it will be convenient for general exposure. Then place the upper retractor in exactly the position it should be left, and replace the lower in the most appropriate position. This means the entire exposure can be obtained by three retractor insertions. The levels exposed must be verified to be certain that the bony removal will be what is planned. If there is any doubt, an x-ray is the safest course.

There are two basic techniques for laminectomy. One is to remove spines and laminae as a single piece, and the other is piecemeal removal with rongeurs. The latter is the traditional technique. The first step is removal of the spinous processes (Fig. 3.6). A large flat bone-cutting rongeur is inserted to the base of the spinous process, and the spinous processes are sequentially cut from below upward. If the first process to be cut is grasped with a clamp, the spines and attaching ligaments can be lifted out of the way so that the spines that are already cut do not interfere with the next cut of the rongeur. If the ligaments are thick and well developed, it is better to divide the interspinous ligaments with a knife at the upper and lower extremities of the spine removal. Unless bleeding from the cut spinous processes is excessive, there is little reason to try to stop it at this point. The laminectomy is better done from below upward, since it is easier to cut under the lower margin of the laminae than it is to cut over the upper margin of the laminae. From the lowest level to be removed, an Adson or Leksell-type rongeur should be used to remove the laminae (Fig. 3.7). Usually, it is easier to begin in the midline, exposing the ligament by removing the lamina and the base of the spinous process. The ligamentum flavum runs from the upper margin of the lamina below to insert on the lower margin of the lamina above and extends underneath the lamina to approximately the midpoint. As the lamina is removed above the ligament, the epidural space will be entered. Once the epidural space is clearly seen, a Penfield #4 dissector or Adson periosteal elevator should be used to be certain that the dura and epidural fat are free from the ligament (Fig. 3.7). Then the rongeurs can be utilized to remove both ligament and bone in a single bite. In the lumbar region below L1, the rongeurs can be placed within the spinal canal with safety as long as the dural sac is intact. If the dura is opened and the tamponade of the cerebrospinal fluid is lost, then epidural bleeding and the danger of placing instruments within the canal will increase. If the dura is opened inadvertently, repair it immediately to prevent both of these annoying problems. The complete laminectomy should be done before the gutters are widened. Epidural bleeding is more likely to occur with the lateral decompression, and it is easier to remove the laminae throughout the length of the proposed incision before changing instruments. At each step be certain that there is no adherence between dura and overlying ligament or bone. Freeing any adhesions with the dissectors before removing the next lamina will ensure that the dura is not torn. When the appropriate number of laminae have been removed, the laminectomy should be widened until it is com-

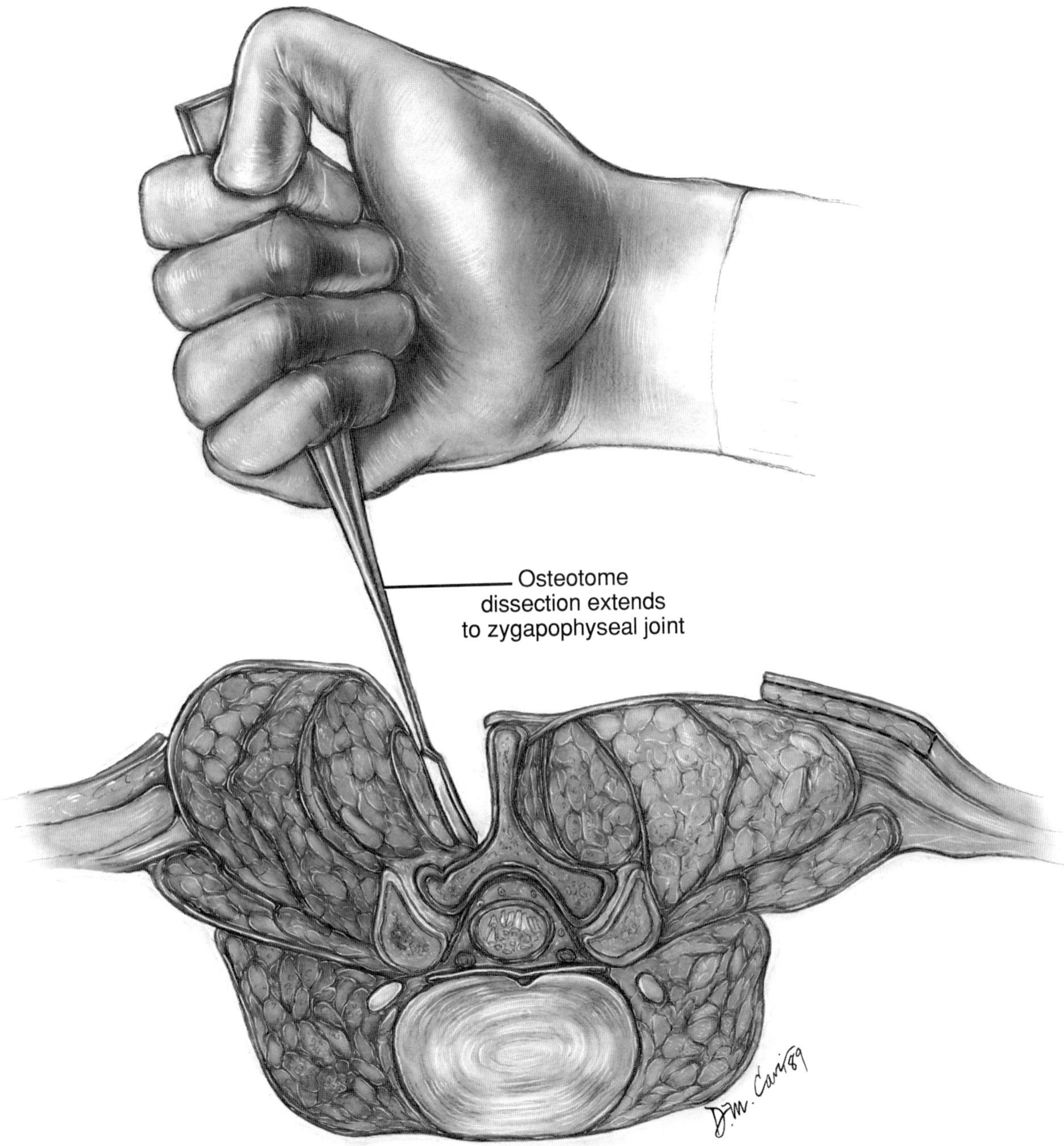

Figure 3.4.

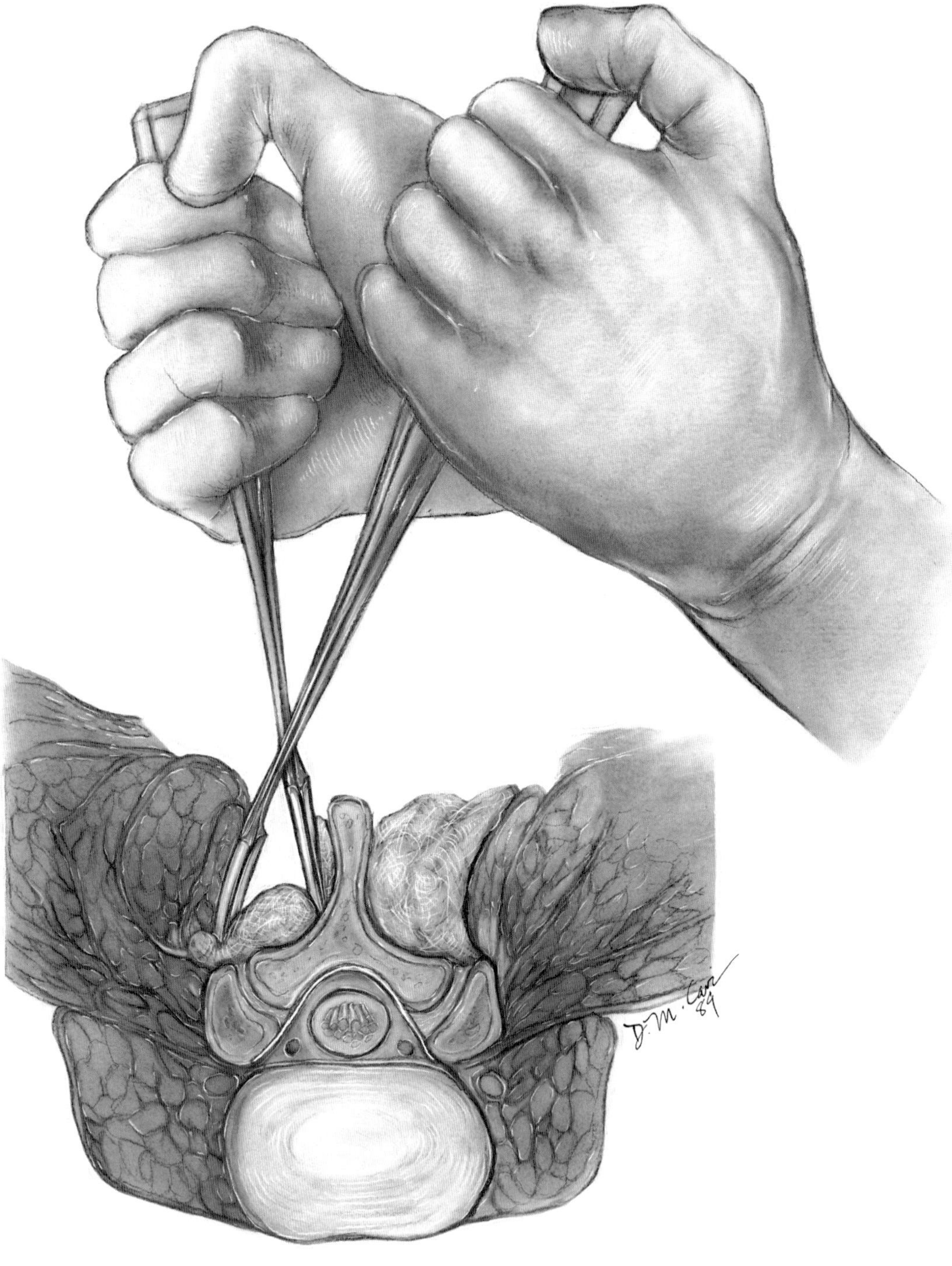

Subperiosteal dissection of paravertebral muscles from spines and laminae by use of osteotomes

Figure 3.5.

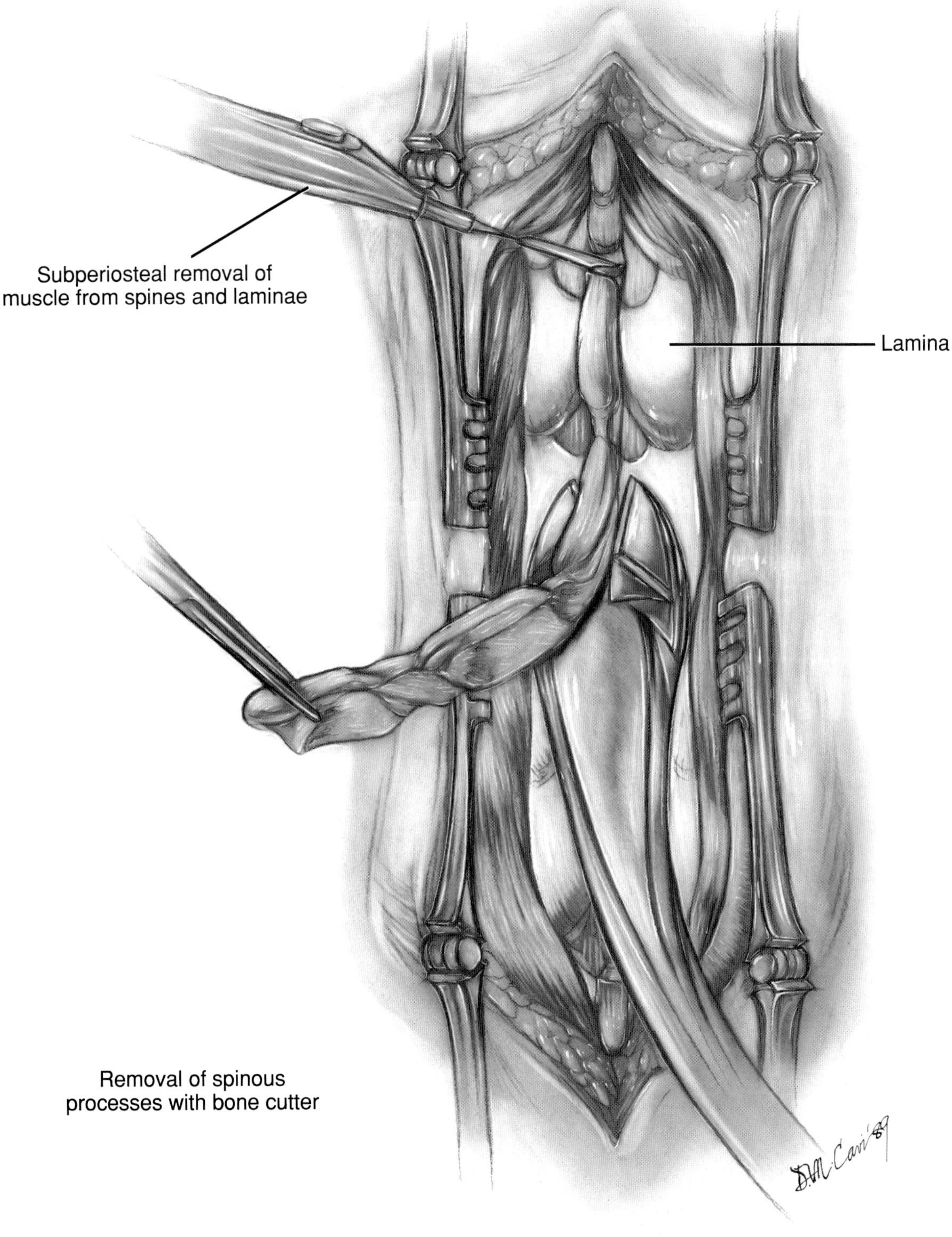
Subperiosteal removal of muscle from spines and laminae
Lamina
Removal of spinous processes with bone cutter
D.M. Cain '89

Figure 3.6.

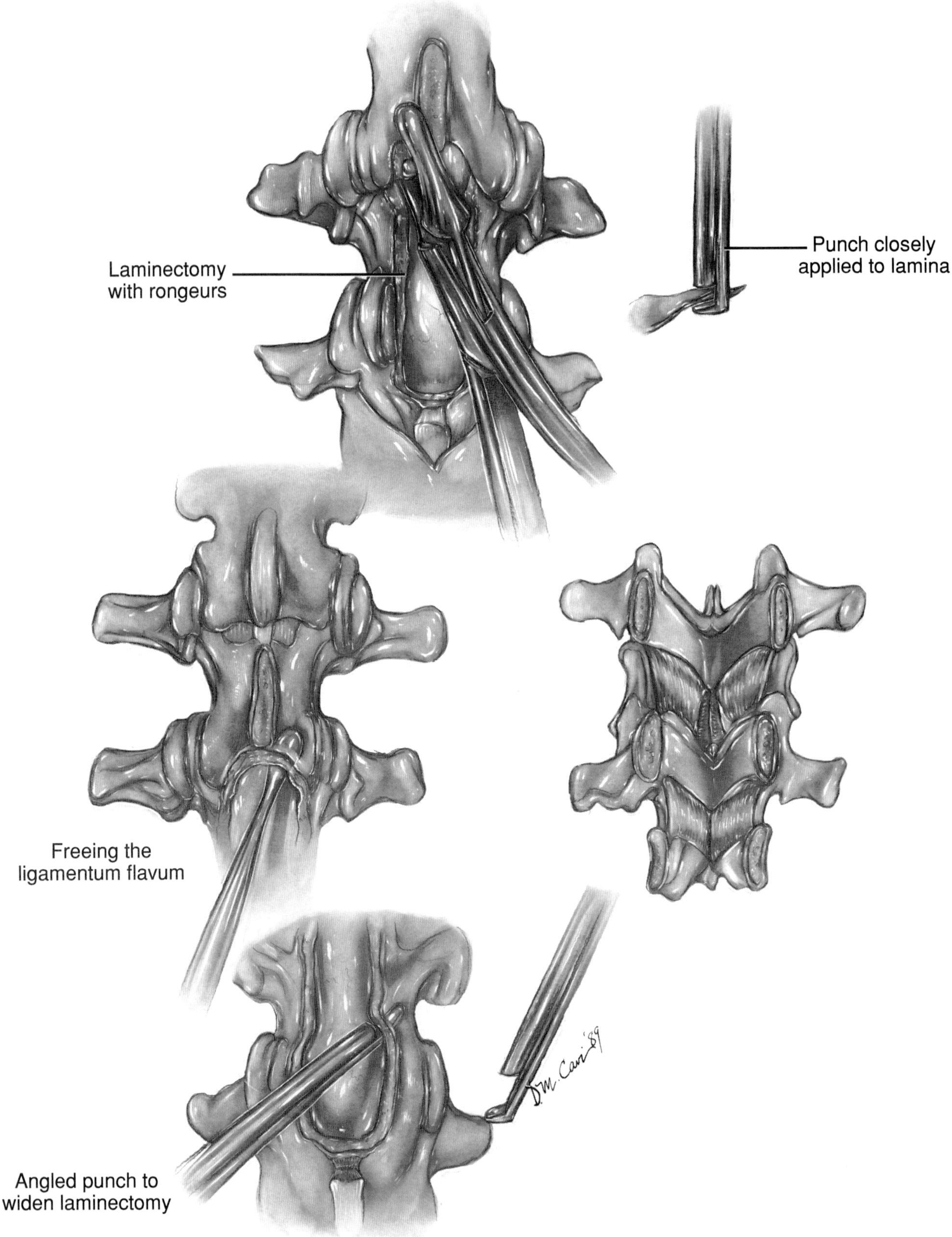
Laminectomy with rongeurs
Punch closely applied to lamina
Freeing the ligamentum flavum
Angled punch to widen laminectomy

Figure 3.7.

plete. This is better done with 45° angled Kerrison-type rongeurs (Fig. 3.7). Sometimes, the removal of the laminae themselves is difficult with the jawed rongeurs, and the Kerrison-type punch is superior. In the latter case, a 90° angled instrument is better. The 45° punches are then utilized to widen the laminectomy out to the margins of the articular processes and the pedicles until all of the lamina is removed. All that is required for decompression is that the articular processes and pedicles are not encroaching on the spinal canal. If there is any question about the adequacy of the decompression, it should be possible to slide a small catheter (6 or 8 French) up or down the spinal canal in the midline to be certain that the epidural space is adequate. The closure requires real care. Some investigators have advocated harvesting a graft of fat to fill the defect left by the lamina, in the hope of preventing ingrowth of fibrous tissue. There is no certain evidence that this improves results. If the patient has sufficient adipose tissue, the technique is simple. With an electric knife, a strip of fat approximately 0.5–1.0 cm thick and of appropriate width and length can be obtained from the subcutaneous tissue on one side of the incision. With reoperation, there is unlikely to be adequate fat, and a separate incision over the buttock to obtain the fat graft may be required. While the technique is currently popular, there is no proof yet that it is of value, and it must be considered the surgeon's preference rather than a mandatory part of these operations. With or without fat graft, the closure is important. No stitches should be placed in the muscle. It is sufficient to coapt the edges of the lumbar fascia with heavy sutures (Fig. 3.8). The subcutaneous space should be closed to the lumbar fascia in the midline. A subcuticular skin closure eliminates the need for later suture removal.

En Bloc Laminectomy

There are several ways in which the spines and laminae can be removed and replaced in order to provide a more or less intact posterior ring. There is no evidence yet that en bloc laminectomy is a superior

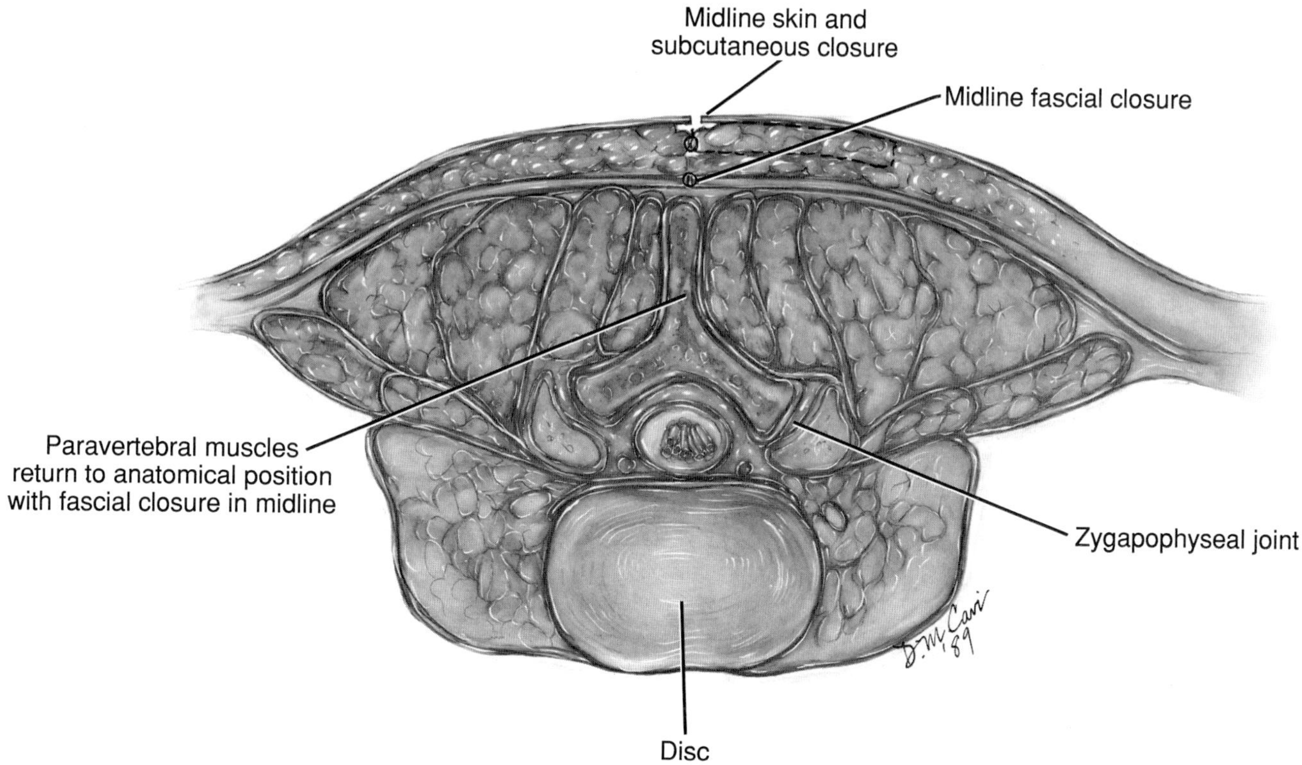

Figure 3.8.

technique, and it certainly is more difficult. However, changes in instrumentation make it increasingly possible to do this, and the technique is functionally appealing. The spines and laminae are exposed as for piecemeal laminectomy. There are now several high-speed drills with laminectomy attachments available. These are similar to the more commonly utilized craniotomes, in that they are a cutting saw with a "post" blade seated in a guide that deflects the dura (Fig. 3.9). The first step is to cut the interspinous ligament at the upper and lower margins of the incision. Then the drill footplate is inserted beneath the lamina as far laterally as possible, and the laminae are successively cut from the lower to the upper margin. If the lamina overlaps enough that it is not possible to obtain easy insertion, a small laminotomy may be required to gain access to the epidural space. Sometimes, it is difficult to remove the saw through a cut of several segments, and an alternative technique is used. This alternative technique consists of cutting both right and left sides of the same vertebra, then lifting that process lamina complex out of the way and cutting the next on each side. The technique has most merit for excision of intradural tumors. In the treatment of spondylosis where decompression is the aim, the ligaments and overgrown bone must be removed, refashioning the laminae to provide adequate room.

Once the intraspinal procedure is complete, the laminae are wired in place (Fig. 3.10). A right-angle drill is utilized to drill through the spinous process above and below, as well as those processes at the upper and lower margins of the removed segment. In addition, it is used to drill through the medialmost portion of the superior articular process at each level, and a hole is made in each laminae laterally. Wires are then passed to wire the bone securely in place at each level and through the transverse processes above and below (Fig. 3.11). The closure then proceeds as for any other procedure.

Foraminotomy

The technique of foraminotomy differs considerably when a complete laminectomy has been done. Bone has been removed to the medial margin of the foramen, so the identification of the exact location of the foramen is not difficult. The first step should be to identify the nerve root and determine whether it is compressed or not. If the nerve root is freely movable, then no foraminotomy is required. However, if there is compression, the goal of the foraminotomy should be elimination of the compressive elements (Fig. 3.12). The usual problem is pressure on the nerve root by pedicle and the undersurface of the superior articular process. The aim of surgery should be removal of the offending portions of the pedicle and joint. Usually, it is possible to do this without entering the zygapophyseal joint. When the compression is from a spur of bone arising from the lip of the interspace, it may be that this cannot be removed safely. Simply removing the roof of the foramen, i.e., the zygapophyseal joint, is a viable alternative. In this situation, it is probable that the joint itself will have to be entered and at least partially removed, but this is avoided when possible.

The foraminotomy can be accomplished in three ways. Traditionally, rongeurs are used. A small 45° angled punch is a very good way to remove the underportion of the superior articular process. The instrument is gradually advanced out the foramen, and the bones are bitten away, enlarging the foramen itself by removal of the underportion of the joint. Dramatic overgrowth of the articular processes accounts for the fact that a significant amount of bone can be removed without entering into the joint space itself or weakening the articulation. It is very difficult to remove a portion of the pedicle by this technique. Failed foraminotomy most commonly occurs because the component of compression by the pedicle is not recognized or relieved.

Foraminotomy can also be accomplished by means of small chisels or a high-speed drill. The chisels are easy to use and provide a handy way to reduce the pedicular component of the compression. With instruments ranging in size from a few millimeters to 1.5 cm and a lightweight hammer, small shavings of bone can be removed, with the foramen sculpted to its new dimensions. While doing this it is very important not to take too much bone, lest the joint be unnecessarily disrupted. The chisels provide an excellent way to shave the pedicle. Be careful not to turn down the chiseled piece of pedicle onto the nerve root or to leave a broken fragment of bone in the foramen. The nerve root should be visualized at all times during these maneuvers but does not require protection. The cuts with the chisel are precise, are controllable, and allow direct visualization of the nerve at all times.

The foraminotomy can also be carried out with a

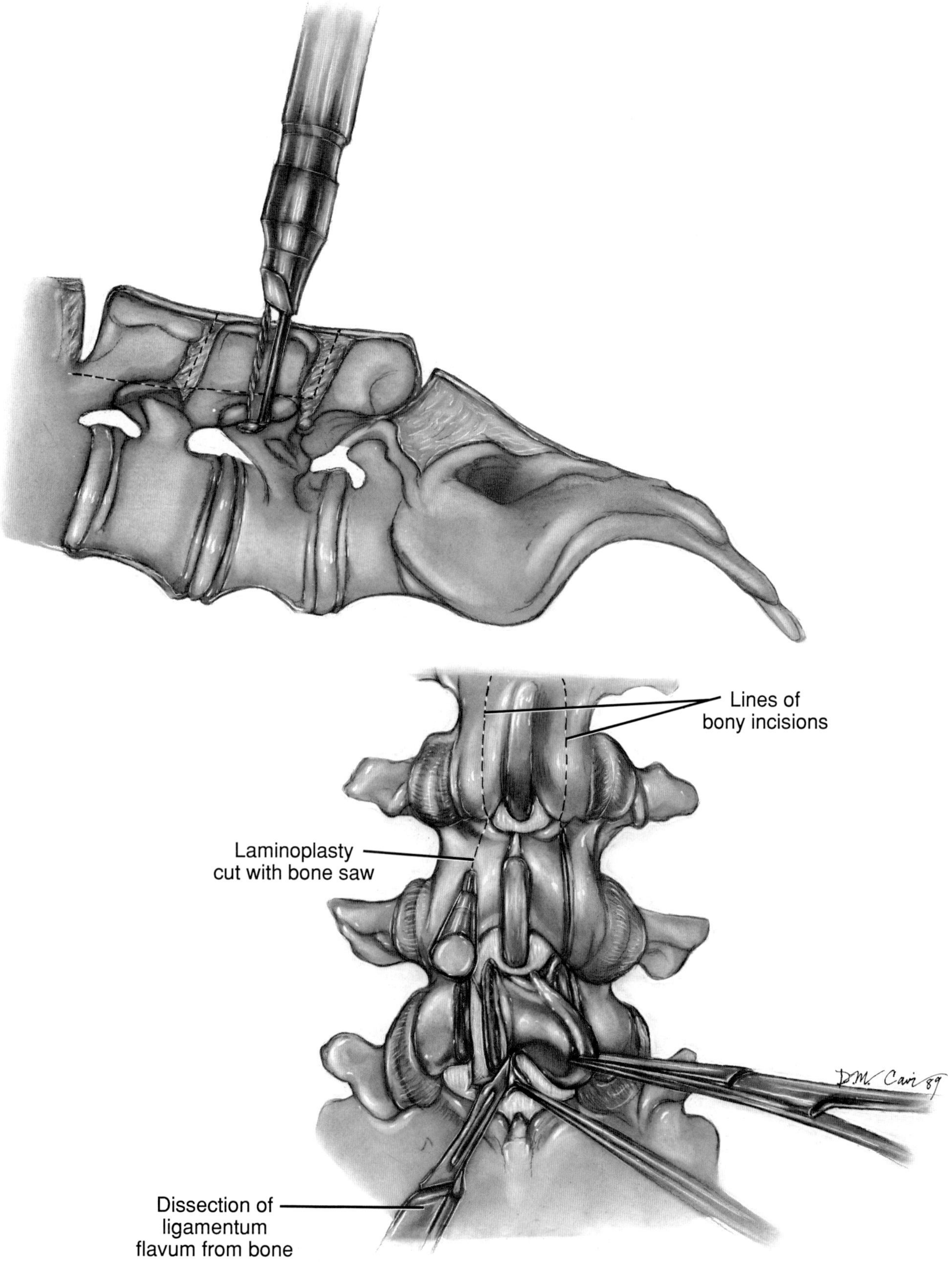
Lines of
bony incisions
Laminoplasty
cut with bone saw
Dissection of
ligamentum
flavum from bone

Figure 3.9.

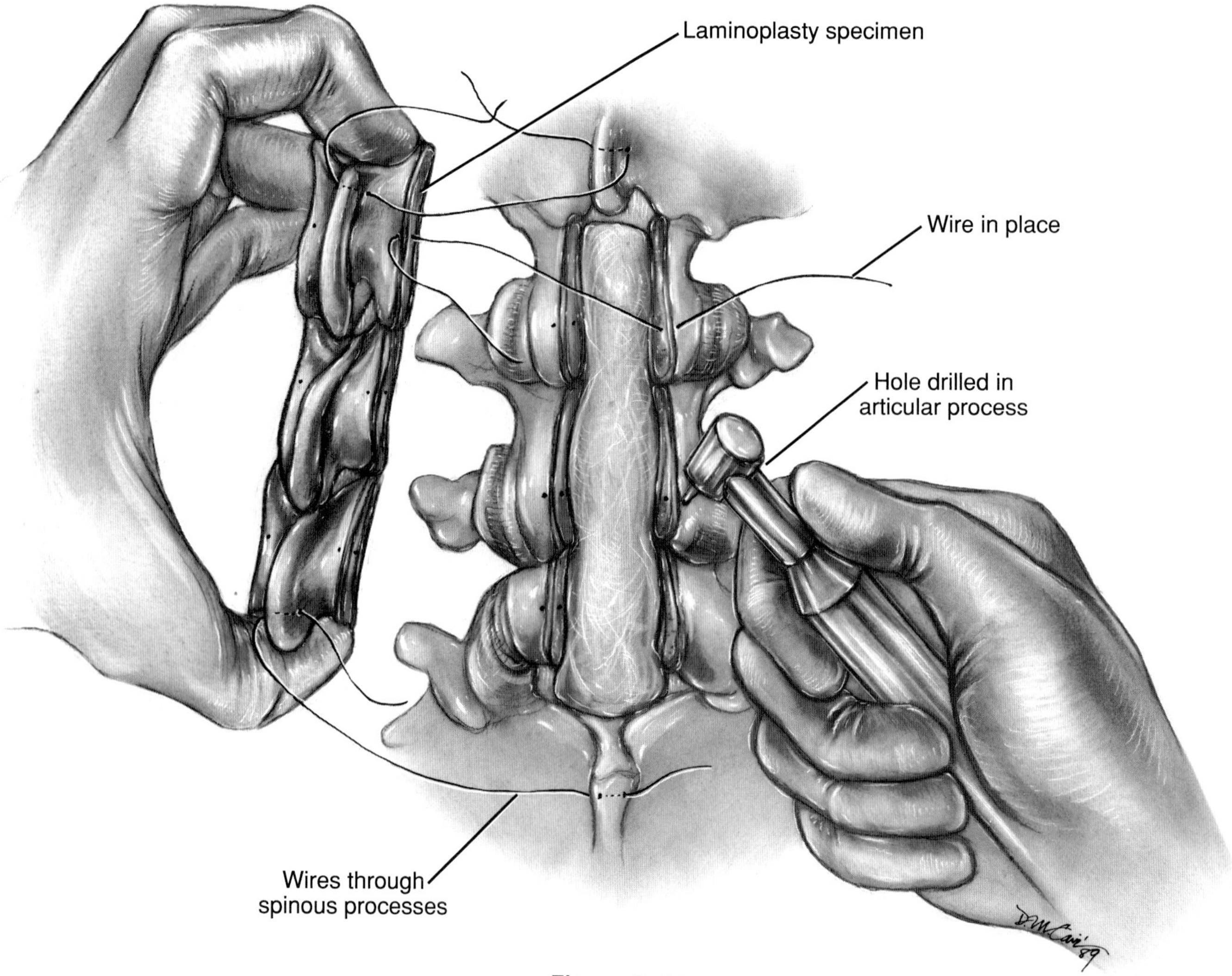
Laminoplasty specimen
Wire in place
Hole drilled in articular process
Wires through spinous processes

Figure 3.10.

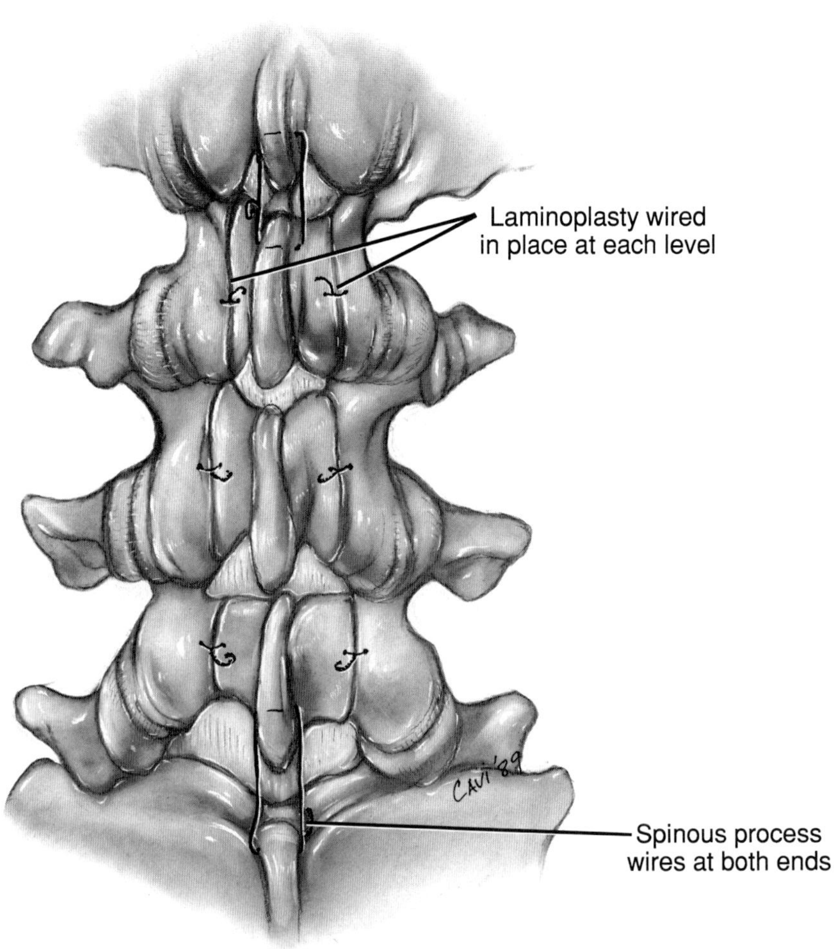

Figure 3.11.

high-speed drill. The best drills have a guard so that they only drill 180° of the circle. This is ideal for the foraminotomy, for it means that further protection of the nerve root is not necessary. By using one of the drills with the guard on and parallel to the nerve root, the drill can gradually be advanced, enlarging the foramen superiorly first by removing the inferior portion of the superior articular process and then, by angling the drill slightly, removing the lower half of the encroaching pedicle. Then the nerve root can be retracted, and the lower portion of the pedicle carefully drilled away. Drilling provides the fastest and most precise foraminotomy. However, the high-speed drill is a dangerous instrument and is not for the hands of the inexperienced. No one should use the drill in these tight quarters who is not thoroughly familiar with the intraoperative use of high-speed instruments and who has not prepared themselves, with both practice and a clear appreciation of the anatomy, for the actual foraminotomy. Nerve root decompression is adequate when the root is freely movable and a probe easily passes on all sides into the foramen.

Be sure not to thin the pars interarticularis too much. Later stress fracture can occur and is a worse problem than partial removal of a joint.

Fat Graft

Placing a free graft of fat over a laminectomy defect in an attempt to prevent adhesive scar formation is currently in vogue. There is no firm evidence that this is beneficial, but anecdotal observations from a

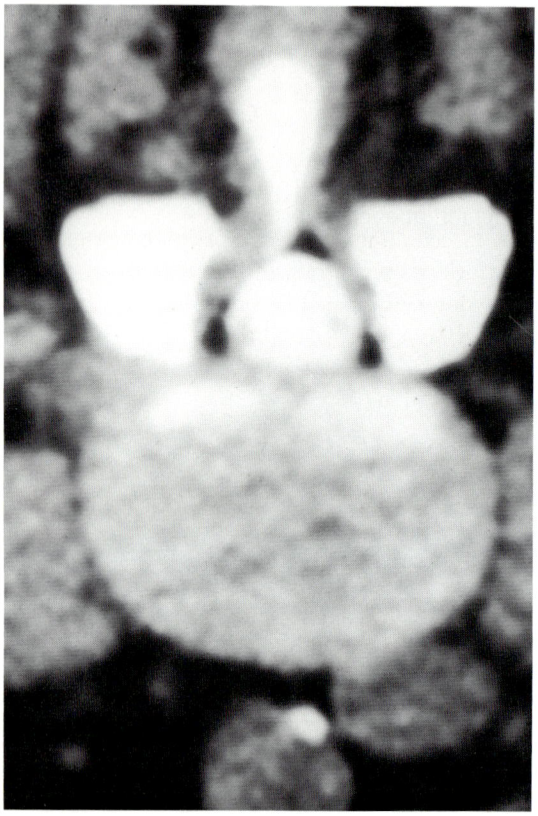

Figure 3.12. Lateral foraminal stenosis as seen by CT scan.

number of surgeons indicate that the amount of postoperative scarring does appear to be reduced. Since many now use the technique, it is worth describing, even though the efficacy of fat grafting in changing the outcome for significant numbers of patients remains unproven and probably never can be demonstrated. It adds little to the procedure and may be particularly suitable for the patient who has had a previous operation. To obtain a fat graft that is not densely scarred, the surgeon must take the graft from outside the operative area, unless the patient has had no earlier surgery. If fusion is contemplated, removing the fat from the bone graft incision is an alternative. A similar incision over the buttock specifically for the fat graft is possible. It is also feasible to undercut the incision out to the pad of fat, which is routinely found lateral to the psoas just above the iliac crest. The fat graft can be conveniently harvested with an electric knife, thus minimizing bleeding. The graft should be chosen to cover the defect in question with a thickness of approximately 0.5–1.0 cm.

The graft should be carefully shaped in size so that it fills the defect. Insofar as possible, it should be placed around nerve roots and over exposed dura. The principal goal is to reduce the adhesive scarring that occurs. This is best done if the graft is interposed between dura and surrounding structures. An appropriate insulation may require considerable shaping and cutting, but this actually adds little time to the procedure. Once the graft is put in position, be careful not to suck it out again. The wound can then be closed without further precaution.

Decompression for Paget's Disease and Other Lesions

Paget's disease of the spine is notoriously painful, yet surgery is of little value for most widespread disease. There is, however, the rare patient who suffers root compression from foraminal narrowing or cauda equina compression from accelerated stenosis who will be benefited by surgical decompression. Neither operation requires special surgical technique. Cauda equina compression is treated by lumbar laminectomy done as for any other spondylotic disease. The only difference is that bone involved with Paget's disease can be extremely vascular. Liberal application of bone wax may be necessary to keep blood loss at an acceptable level. Often the technique required is one bite with the rongeur, followed by bone wax, followed by another rongeur bite. This technique, though somewhat tedious, does minimize blood loss.

Decompression for Paget's Disease

Occasionally, Paget's disease involving lamina, pedicle, and articular processes will progress to the point that there is significant foraminal compression and neuropathy. The differences between this surgery and that required for spondylitic foraminotomy are not many, but there are some that are different enough to require separate description. These principally relate to the different character of the Paget's diseased bone. The Paget's diseased bone may be very soft when the process is in its vascular phase. Thus in the late burned-out phase, the bone may be exceptionally sclerotic.

The positions and the approach are the same as for any other foraminal compression. The subperiosteal dissection described for lumbar hemilaminectomy should be carried out but is modified in that most of the dissection around the involved bone is done sharply with a knife under direct vision with care taken so that the large, sharp osteotomes do not tear the soft bone or plunge through it. The area to be removed is exposed with self-retaining retractors. A hemilaminectomy is not necessary. The goal of the procedure is foraminotomy (Chapter 1). Only enough lamina should be removed to expose the root. The procedure is begun by isolating the bone to be removed by using a sharp dissector to free ligamentous attachments and expose the zygapophyseal joint. Bone removal then begins immediately medial to the facet with a few bites of laminae sometimes being necessary to gain adequate access. The ligamentum flavum is excised and removed, exposing the lateralmost aspect of the epidural space. The pedicle is identified, the zygapophyseal joint is appreciated, and the course of the nerve is anticipated. Bone removal should then begin. If the process is sclerotic, the high-speed drill is an ideal way to remove bone. Entrance into the zygapophyseal joint should be avoided, and bone removal should include pedicle and the undersurfaces of the two articular processes until the root is free. The Paget's process may continue well out into the foramen, and it may be necessary to undercut for a significant distance or even remove some or all of the zygapophyseal joint to obtain an adequate decompression. This should not stop until blunt dissectors can be passed into the extravertebral space along the nerve roots in all directions. Small chisels may also be used to remove pedicle and the underportions of the processes. They are particularly useful in removing the compressive portions of the pedicle down to the level of the vertebral body, thus creating a new channel for the nerve. When the bone is extremely vascular, use of the high-speed drill is difficult. Then, chisels or rongeurs are better. The soft bone often breaks, and it is not as easy to tailor the removal, sparing the joint. In this situation it is much more likely that decompression will be carried out by removing all bone including the joint, which often cannot even be identified because of the bony abnormalities. Bony removal should continue until the nerve root is free in the lateral recess, around the pedicle, and in the foramen. Hemostasis is best obtained by the liberal use of bone wax, but packing with hemostatic agents may also be necessary. Closure requires no special care in either instance.

Aneurysmal Bone Cyst

The surgical management of the aneurysmal bone cyst remains a frustrating exercise. A number of techniques have been recommended, but none are entirely satisfactory. Now, with appropriate imaging, the diagnosis is virtually always made in advance and is based on scanning for a complaint of pain. Patients also occasionally present with mass lesions complicating the bony abnormality and rarely with infarction secondary to a steal phenomenon.

Embolization

The first step following the diagnosis on computed tomography scanning or magnetic resonance imaging is to carry out a spinal angiogram to identify feeding vessels, if there are any. These can be immobilized at the same time. In the rare patient who has undergone cord infarction from steal phenomenon, there usually are sizable vessels, and in the patients with the so-called capillary type of aneurysmal bone cyst (which is probably better termed capillary angioma), there may also be significant feeding vessels. Definitive surgery should proceed within a few days.

Anterior Approach

Both the retroperitoneal approach and a transcavitary approach are equally satisfactory. The involved body should be exposed. When there is no soft tissue mass, the goal of surgery is to obliterate the bone cyst of the body involved by making a hole in the anterior surface and then rapidly curetting the cancellous portion of the bone and the bone cyst in order to disrupt the trabeculations. Bleeding will be dramatic. It cannot be controlled until the entire cyst is broken down. A heavy angled curette is the best way to break down the trabeculations completely. Once a unitary cavity is achieved, the bleeding can be controlled by packing the cavity with Avitene or thrombin-soaked Gelfoam. Pressure over the hemostatic agent will stop the bleeding. As much of the hemostatics as possible should be removed, and the area packed with bone fragments obtained from the ileum.

When the body is more involved, a collapse has occurred, or a collape is considered a risk, radical surgery is required. In such a situation, the discs above and below should be excised, and then the involved collapsed body should be rapidly removed with rongeurs. Bleeding will be brisk, and the trick of the operation is to proceed as rapidly as possible, since the bleeding cannot be controlled until the cyst is completely obliterated. As soon as the body is removed, the operative resection can be packed with hemostatics. Then an anterior fusion as described in Chapter 7 is performed. The excised body must be replaced and a block fusion is required.

Some of these tumors are associated with a significant soft tissue mass within the spinal canal. These masses most commonly occur in front of dura at the level of the body. The diagnosis is suspected when a significant neurological deficit occurs in conjunction with a typical x-ray appearance of an aneurysmal bone cyst. It is extremely difficult to manage these lesions by the posterior approach. They are very vascular, and bleeding can be difficult to control if the soft tissue mass is entered posteriorly. When such a mass is found unexpectedly, it is usually better simply to carry out adequate decompressive laminectomy and then return for a definitive anterior excision.

These operations are also done with the patient under general anesthesia by the lateral or anterior approach described. The principal goal of surgery is excision of the mass for decompression of the cord. Stabilization follows as a secondary procedure. In most instances, with a large intraspinal mass, there is such destruction of the body that a complete excision and fusion are necessary. The disc above and the disc below the involved body should be completely excised, and then the body rapidly removed. This will expose the posteriorly placed soft tissue mass. The Cavitron is an ideal tool for removing this mass. The goal is speed, since bleeding can be impressive. Since the neural elements are involved, the surgeon is faced with the twin requirement of rapid tumor removal and protection of the cord or cauda. The Cavitron is ideal because of the speed with which it removes tumor and because of the preciseness of the control. Often, because of the volume of the blood loss, two large suctions are required until the tumor is out. Once the dura is decompressed, the area should be packed with hemostatic agents, which are then gradually removed. As soon as the tumor is out, hemostasis can be obtained. Fusion then proceeds as described.

None of these operations require special closure.

4

Decompressive Laminectomy for Congenital Anomalies

Two techniques of surgery are necessary to treat the neural compression syndromes of achondroplasia. The most common problem is spinal cord or cauda equina compression by the progressive spondylotic change. Another problem present in young children is medullary compression at the foramen magnum or under C1.

Decompression of Spinal Cord and Cauda Equina

Irrespective of the level of compression, decompression of the spinal cord and decompression of the cauda equina are done in the same way, and the same concerns apply. The operations are carried out with the patient under general anesthesia in the prone position. When cervical decompression is planned, immobilization of the patient with tongs or a head holder during surgery is a useful precaution. Remember both children and adults can be extremely difficult to intubate and great care must be taken during intubation not to compromise the cervical spinal cord. If there is any major difficulty, a nasal intubation may be necessary. The incision should be planned so that the entire area of block can be decompressed. This means that at the time of myelography, it is usually

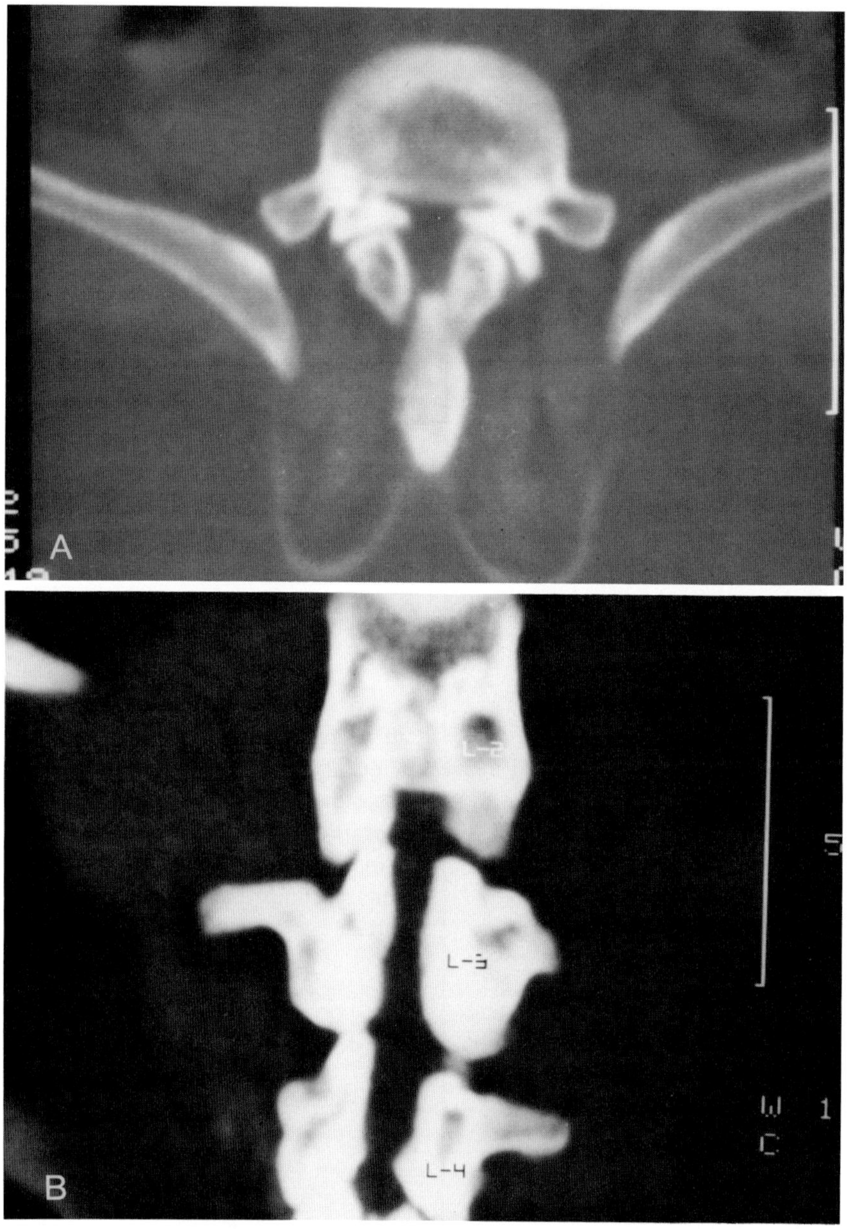

Figure 4.1. The typical spinal cord changes of achondroplasia are demonstrated. Note the short pedicles, the overgrown facets, and the compromise of the spinal canal in all directions, particularly in the lateral recess.

necessary to instill dye both above and below the block to see the extent of compression. When the problem is in the lumbar region, it may be impossible to demonstrate the lower level, but in other locations it is usually feasible to place dye in both the cervical and the lumbar subarachnoid space to define the length of the compression. The surgery should then be planned to carry the decompression above and below the demonstrated abnormality. Monitoring cord function is an important safeguard.

A skin incision is made appropriately, and the original incision is taken to the spinous processes in the midline. Remember to make the incision so that the subcutaneous portion and the skin incision are of the same length. The typical canoe-shaped incision may result in the original bony decompression being inadequate. A subperiosteal dissection of the muscles from the spines and laminae is then carried out. This is difficult to do because of the trough-like nature of the laminae and overhanging zygapophyseal joints. The smooth removal of the paravertebral mass of muscles from spine and laminae that is possible with normal anatomy cannot be carried out as easily. Because the laminectomy is likely to be extensive, it is necessary to expose the zygapophyseal joints over at least half their width, preferably to the outer extremity. Self-retaining laminectomy retractors are then put in place, exposing the laminae throughout the length to be removed and at least one normal space above and below. The spinous processes can be removed with a bone-cutting rongeur defining the length of the laminectomy. The laminectomy should begin below the lower extremity of the block and proceed upward until the compression is relieved. It is difficult to overestimate how dangerous this laminectomy is to cord function. The techniques that suffice for normal bony anatomy can lead to catastrophic results in the achondroplastic patient. The bone may be extremely hard and very difficult to remove. There is no room in the spinal canal, and instruments cannot be inserted underneath the laminae. The ligaments are extremely thick and can be densely adherent to the dura. The dura may also be adherent to the periosteum where the ligaments are thin. The zygapophyseal joints are overhanging and may virtually meet in the midline with little laminae present at all. The pedicles are short, and as the laminectomy extends laterally, the dura will balloon out of the defect, which makes it easy to enter the dura and difficult to continue the laminectomy without doing so.

Several techniques are available to help avoid these pitfalls. Piecemeal removal of the bone with large blunt rongeurs is the most commonly employed technique. The laminectomy should be carried out with the jaws of the rongeur perpendicular to the laminae, and the instruments should never be inserted into the spinal canal. Once the laminectomy is complete, the canal opening may be widened by the use of angled laminectomy punches, but again great care must be taken not to insert the footplate underneath the bone except where the neural elements are clearly visible and compression will not occur. The original laminectomy should be continued until the entire decompression is complete. Bone removal should be wide enough at this state that herniation of the dura through a narrow channel cannot compress the spinal cord. The laminectomy can then be widened by using laminectomy punches. The high-speed drill with a large cutting burr is an excellent way to perform the laminectomy. It may be necessary to enter the zygapophyseal joints, and this is appropriate if required for adequate neural decompression. Try to leave at least half the joint, but the goal of this operation is decompression of the neural elements, and instability has never occurred in our series no matter how radical the bone removal. Using the drill throughout the laminectomy procedure is feasible but requires an experienced hand. Drilling in the achondroplastic spine is not a place to learn to use this equipment. Nevertheless, when appropriately done, the removal of the laminae with the drill can be carried out more quickly than with a hand rongeur and with greater safety. The drill is particularly useful when the laminae are fused into what is virtually a single bony mass. This is not unusual in the older achondroplastic patient. The drill is the fastest way to channel the bone in this circumstance. A third technique is the use of a sharp osteotome or chisel to remove the lateral masses of bone after the midline removal is complete. When these instruments are used, it is important that the technique be to shave small pieces of bone from the lateral aspects of the laminae. Sections of bone 3–4 mm in width can be removed with a few judicious blows at each level, and then the whole process can be repeated if the canal needs to be widened further. It is important to make certain that the overgrown facets are free of muscle and that the chisel or osteotome be angled slightly medially so the section of bone that is freed will break easily at the limit of the laminectomy. A sharp chisel can be even faster than the high-speed drill or rongeur, and this is a technique that any spinal surgeon should master.

In cervical and thoracic areas, rarely is there a radicular component to the compression. In the lumbar region, however, there may be foraminal stenosis, and compression of roots as well as of cauda equina occurs. When this is the case, foraminotomies must be carried out. The area of the foramen can be very difficult to identify because of the changes in the zygapophyseal joints, which mask the normal relationships. After the laminectomy is complete, the roots should be identified by exploration in the epidural space, and the region of the foramen thus identified also. It is virtually impossible to carry out the foraminotomies with rongeurs. There simply is not enough room to insert any instrument into the foramen. The high-speed drill or chisels are ideal. The drill is particularly valuable here because the channel can be made to conform to the nerve root exactly, and unnecessary bone is not removed. The chisel may be a more effective way to remove the pedicle. A drill with a guard should be employed as the foramen is enlarged and the pedicle is removed. The chiseling is done judiciously, with shavings of 1 or 2 mm in thickness removed with each chisel placement. Each foramen should be enlarged until the root is clearly decompressed along the length of the foramen. Usually, it is the short pedicle that is the major compressive force, and this must be removed partially in order to allow the root free access to the foramen. In the achondroplastic patient, the dura of the root may be tightly adherent to the bone in the foramen, and it is necessary to be extremely careful in bone removal. Usually, there is such bony overgrowth that the foraminotomy that removes the inferior portion of the pedicle and the inferior portion of the superior articular process does not even enter the joint space. Even if the joints are excised, instability is a rarity. These are long operations that are difficult to do, and the risk to the patient is considerable. Careful and continuous attention to detail is required if the operation is to be done safely. Physiological monitoring of both potentials is an important adjunct for the protection of the roots and spinal cord.

Decompression of Cervicomedullary Junction

For a group of children who present with sleep apnea, decompression of the cervicomedullary junction is important treatment. There is compression at the cervicomedullary junction from the posterior rim of the foramen magnum and the posterior rim of the foramen magnum and the posterior elements of C1. There may be a true Chiari malformation, but this is not necessarily the rule. The bony compression is easily demonstrated by magnetic resonance imaging or sagittal reconstruction of computed tomography (CT) scans. Dilute intrathecal contrast in conjunction with the CT scan provides a graphic demonstration of the compression but is not mandatory to the diagnosis. Since the compression is nearly always from the posterior elements, then posterior decompressing is usually the procedure of choice. The operation is done with the patient under general anesthesia, with skeletal fixation used. Skeletal traction is also satisfactory (Figs. 4.2 and 4.3). These children are vulnerable during intubation, and the intubation itself may be difficult because of the laryngeal anatomy. Measurement of spinal evoked potentials during intubation provides a measure of safety. The patient is then placed in the prone position, and evoked potentials are monitored throughout positioning. It is not unusual to compromise these potentials by the position of the patient; be certain that this has not occurred before the incision is made. A midline skin incision is made from the inion to the midcervical area, and the original incision is extended to the spinous processes of C2 and C3 and the occipital bone (Fig. 4.4). Self-retaining retractors should be put in place at this point, and a sub-

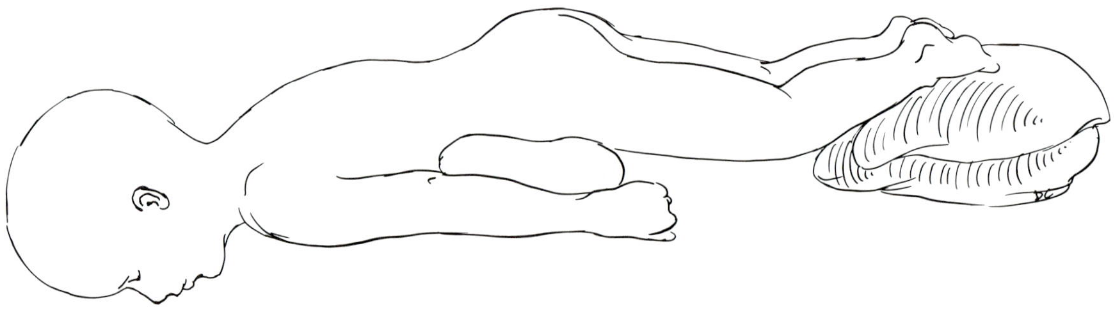

Figure 4.2. Child in proper position for posterior cervical surgery.

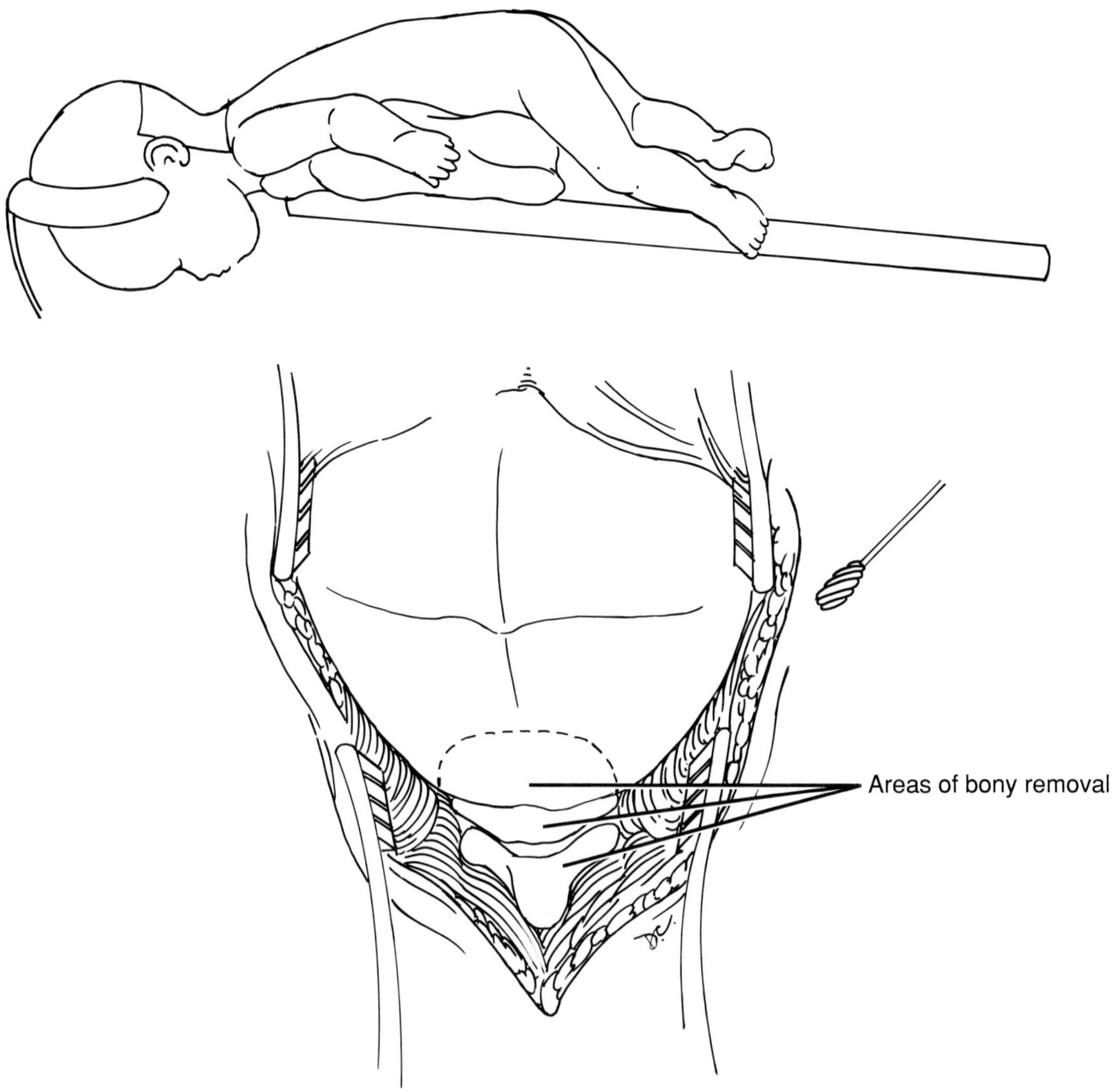

Figure 4.3. Achondroplastic child in head rest.

periosteal dissection of the cervical musculature from C1, C2, and C3 carried out. Do this dissection with a knife blade rather than with osteotomes. There is little margin for safety in dealing with these compressed cords, and the bones of these young children are often soft. Posterior defects in C1 in the midline are not uncommon. The dissection should be carried laterally with a knife until the entire width of the spinal canal is seen. This is usually best judged by the location of the C1-C2 articulation. It is also important to remember that for reasons that are not known, the vertebral artery may have an unusually medial course in achondroplastic children and can easily be entered by the knife dissecting on or above C1 (Fig. 4.5) Once the bony dissection is complete, the area between muscle and bone should be packed with sponges, and the periosteal elevator used to lift periosteum and muscle from the occipital bone. Around the foramen magnum this may be difficult, and it is better to cut these attachments with a knife rather than run any risk of

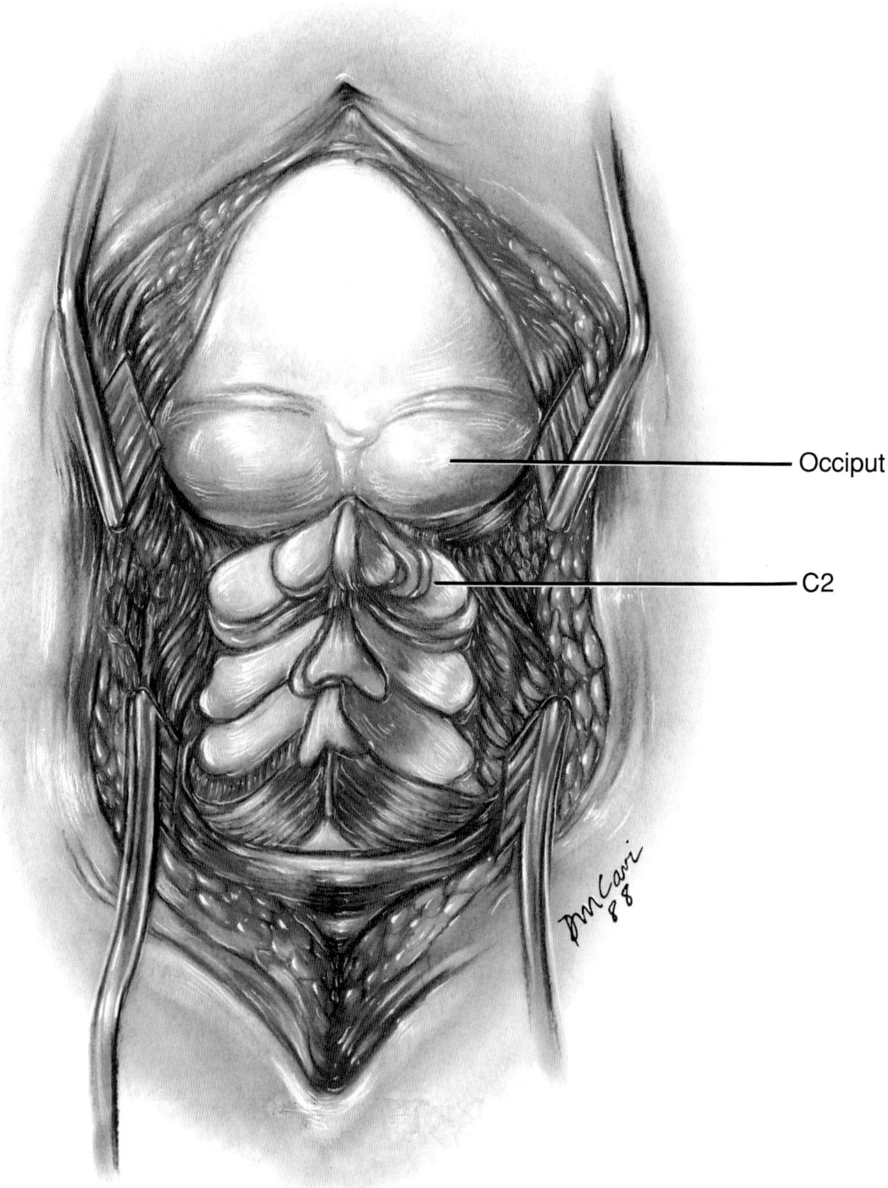

Figure 4.4. C1 cannot be seen.

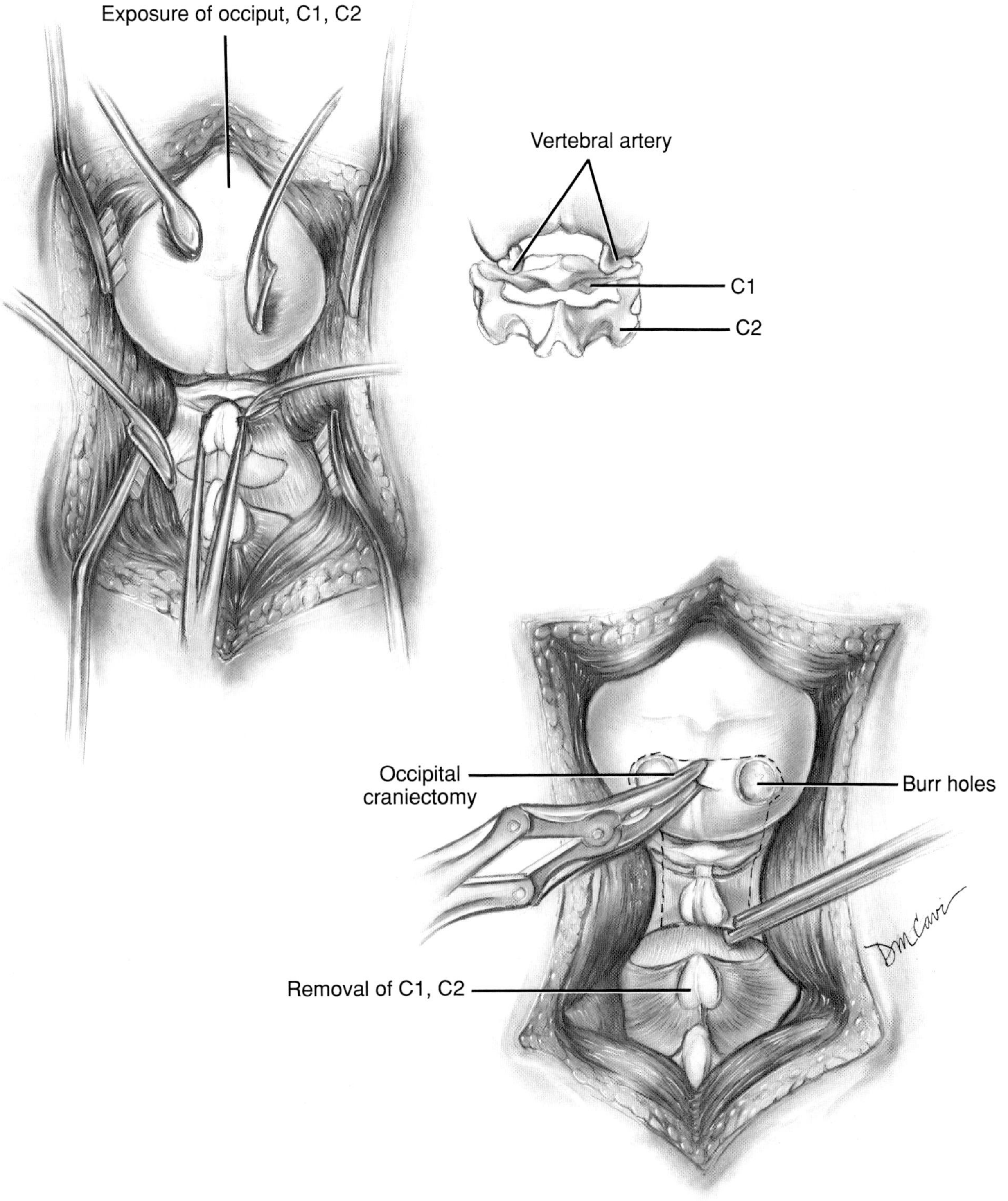

Exposure of occiput, C1, C2
Vertebral artery
C1
C2
Occipital craniectomy
Burr holes
Removal of C1, C2

Figure 4.5.

spinal cord compression because of movement from an attempted blunt dissection. Next, the bony configuration must be seen (Fig. 4.6). It is not uncommon for the arch of C1 to be virtually hidden beneath the laminae and spinous process of C2, and the foramen magnum rim may be tucked under the arch of C1. The order of bone removal depends on what is seen, but it is usually easier to remove C2 first (Fig. 4.7). The spinous process can be removed piecemeal, and then the laminae can be removed by utilizing the blunt rongeurs perpendicular to the dura. Do not put the rongeurs beneath the laminae. It is reasonable to use laminectomy punches laterally, but only after the canal has been widely opened and the cord decompressed. When C1 becomes visible, it is removed. The periosteum of C1 and the dura will be intimately fused, and it may be difficult to remove the bone without tearing the dura. It is particularly important not to try to place even a periosteal elevator beneath the bone. It is better to remove all the soft tissue from the margins of C1 sharply. Blunt instruments must be used with great care. The bone is removed by directing the rongeurs perpendicular to the spinal canal. The high-speed drill is an ideal way to remove C1, but the unusual locations of the vertebral artery may complicate these procedures. The occipital bone and the rim of the foramen magnum are then removed (Figs. 4.6 and 4.8). One technique is to drill bilateral holes on either side of the midline in the most available flat portion of the occipital bone and then to remove the occipital bone with rongeurs. This can be safely done with either jaw rongeurs or punches down to the margin of the foramen magnum, which is removed by using the perpendicularly angled rongeurs. The high-speed drill also is conveniently used in the posterior fossa craniectomy. This reduces the temptation to place the rongeurs beneath the bone near the margin of the foramen magnum (Fig. 4.9). Once the laminectomy and craniectomy have been extended laterally beyond the limits of the spinal cord and brain stem, the dura is opened. The dura covering the cervical cord should be opened in the midline (Fig. 4.10). A thickened band of dura beneath the rim of the foramen magnum always stretches transversely, compressing the cervicomedullary junction. Unless this band is divided, decompression of the junction is not possible. Ideally, the dura is opened just beyond this band, and then the superior arms of a Y-shaped incision are extended from this point laterally toward the upper outer margins of the craniectomy. This provides an excellent decompression when closed with a patch. There is a very real danger in this maneuver. Venous anomalies of the posterior fossa are not at all unusual. The band may contain a sizable circular sinus. This sinus may be unusually large, extending upward for several centimeters. Sometimes, the posterior fossa dura can virtually be a lake of blood, and both excessive blood loss and air embolism are very real risks. When blood is encountered at this level or at the level of the band, it is very important to use clips to obliterate the sinus and then open the dura between the clips. The venous pressure is such that coagulation usually will not suffice, and if the dura is widely opened in the face of inadequate control of the sinus, catastrophic blood loss may ensue. Once the dura is widely opened, the cervicomedullary junction should be carefully inspected. The compressive marks of bone and dura are usually obvious. There may be a true Chiari malformation, but this is not always present. Extensive exploration, lysis of adhesions, or removal of tissue is nearly always unnecessary in these children. The dura should be closed with a triangular or quadrangular patch (Fig. 4.11). A watertight closure is desirable. The muscles should be closed superficially so that compression from a tight muscular closure cannot occur. The closure does not require special care otherwise. Rarely, one of these children is or will become hydrocephalic, and the possibility of increased intracranial pressure must be kept in mind, during the postoperative care of these children. The sleep apnea does not always relent immediately but may improve over weeks or months. For this reason, these children should be monitored carefully in the postoperative period. Respiratory problems following extubation are not at all uncommon, and the tube should be left in place until the child is awake and breathing well after surgery. Apnea monitoring can be a useful adjunct.

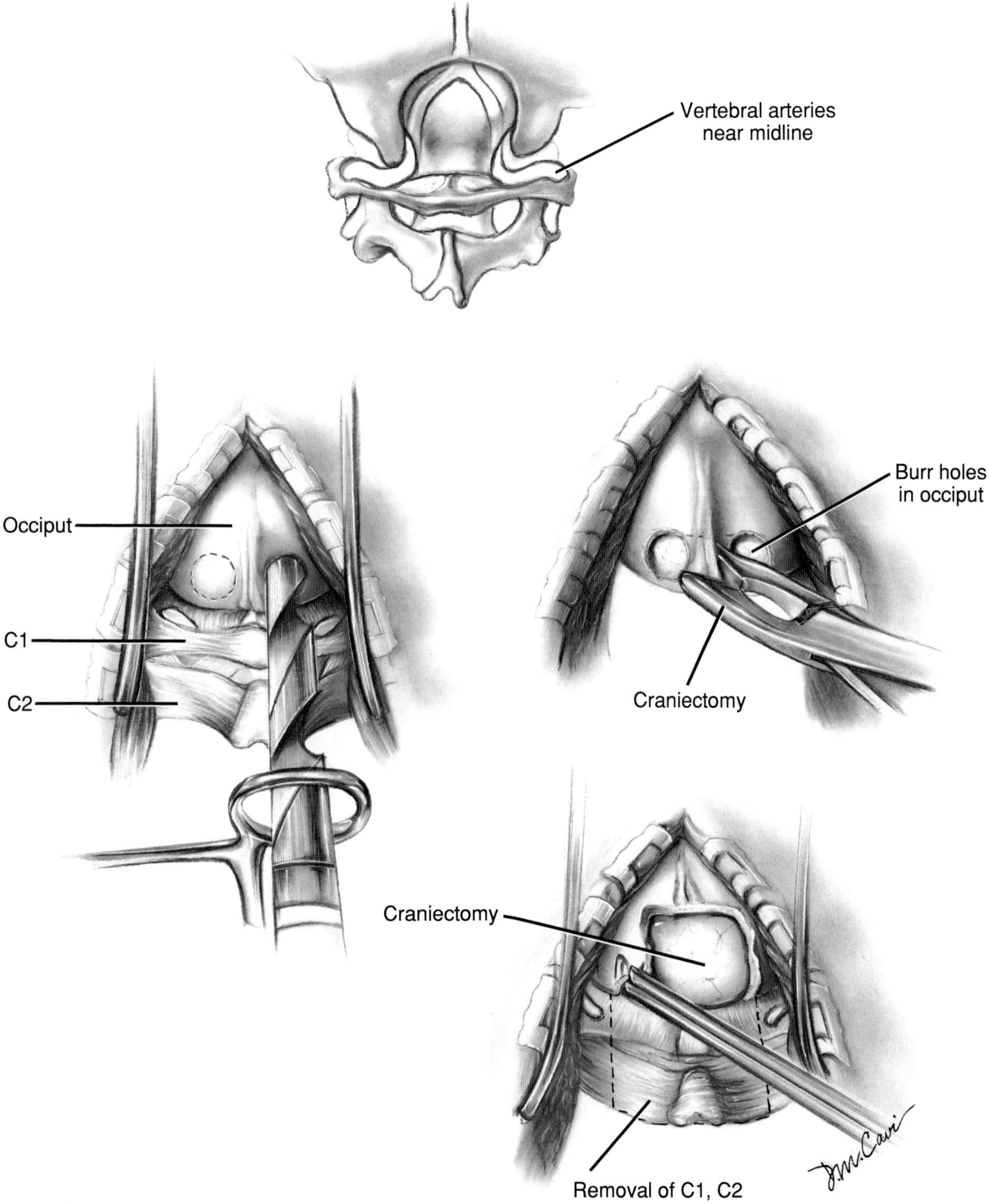
Vertebral arteries
near midline
Occiput
C1
C2
Burr holes
in occiput
Craniectomy
Craniectomy
Removal of C1, C2

Figure 4.6.

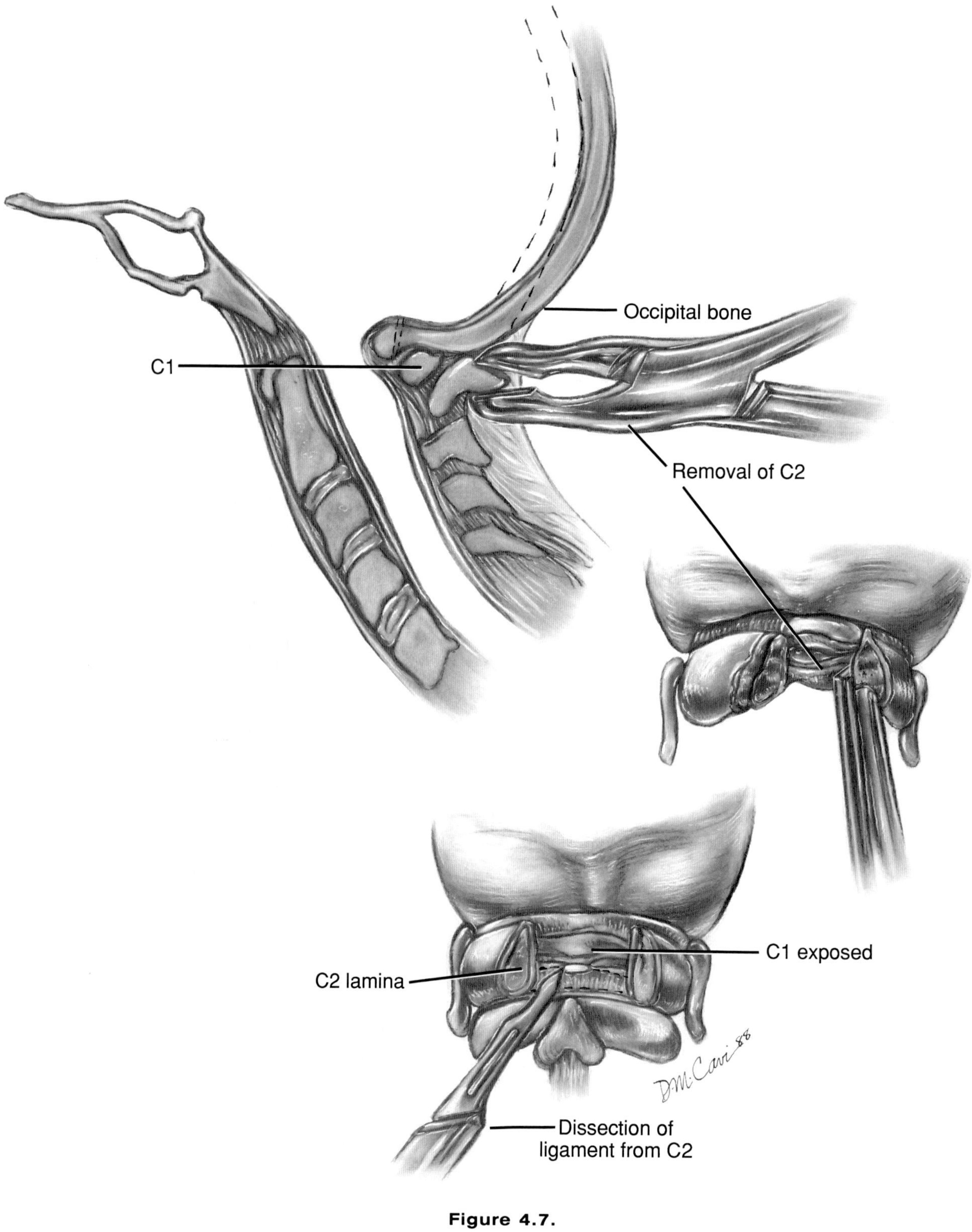
Occipital bone
C1
Removal of C2
C1 exposed
C2 lamina
D.M. Cavi 88
Dissection of ligament from C2

Figure 4.7.

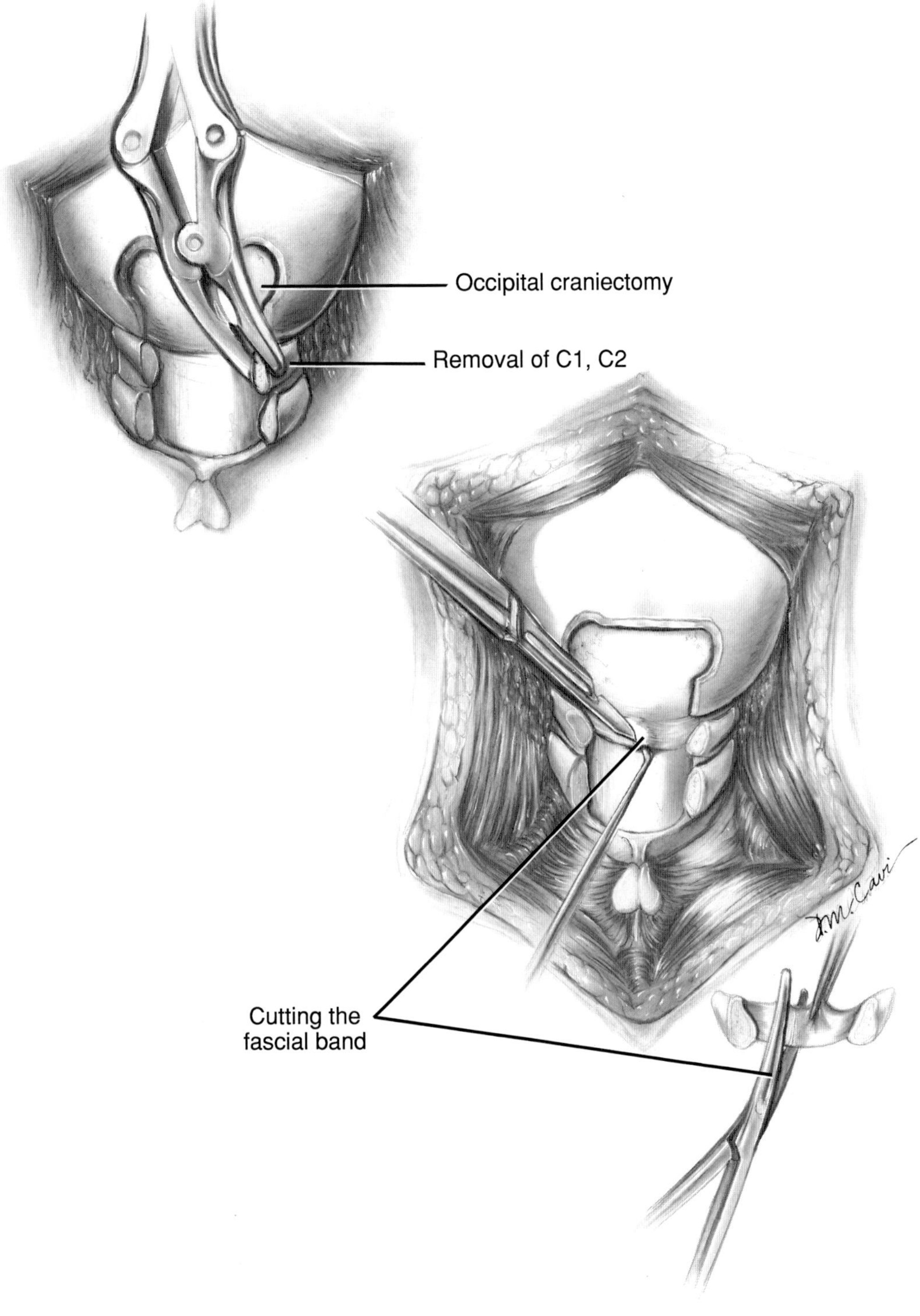
Occipital craniectomy
Removal of C1, C2
Cutting the fascial band

Figure 4.8.

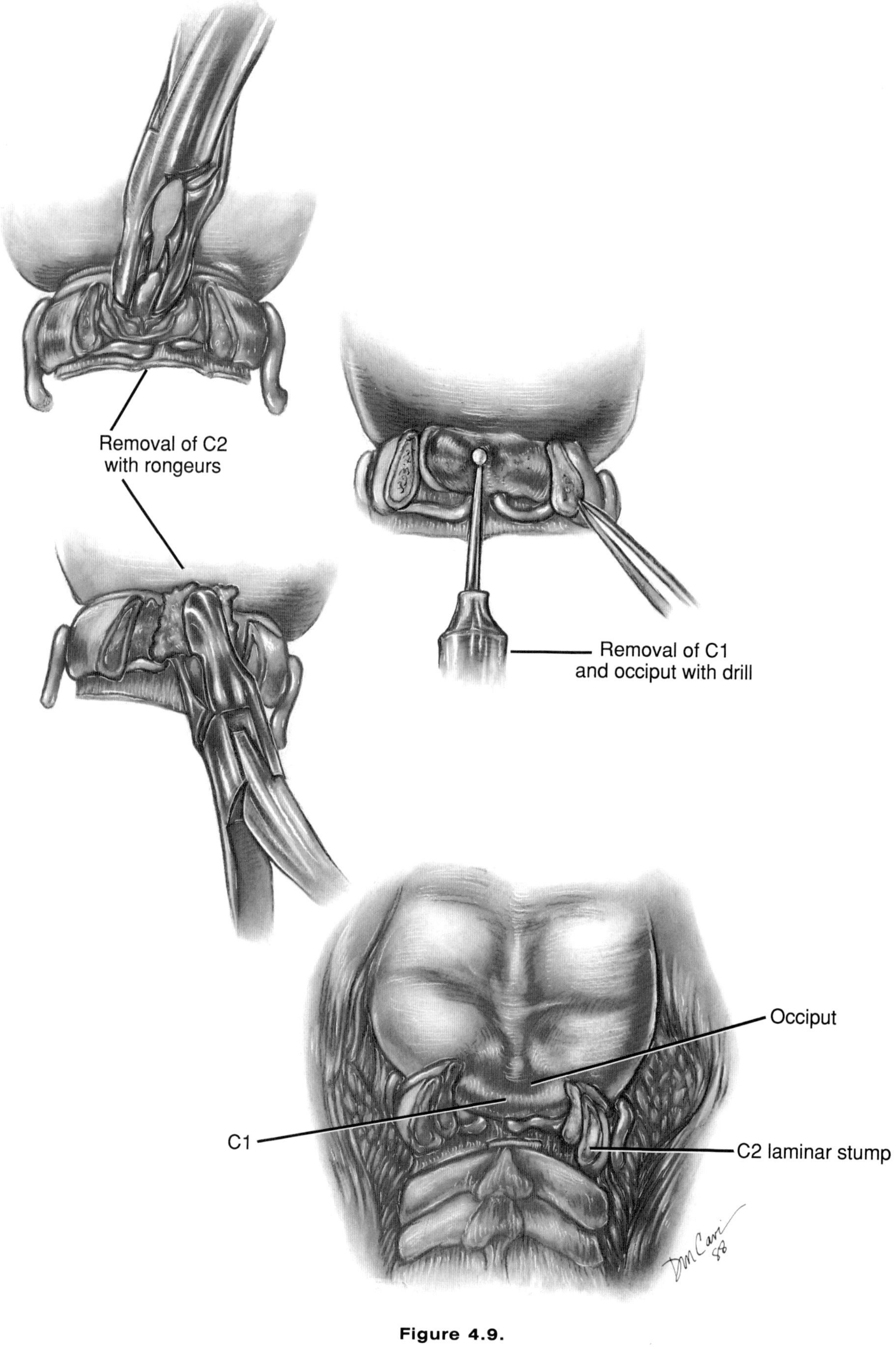
Removal of C2
with rongeurs
Removal of C1
and occiput with drill
Occiput
C1
C2 laminar stump

Figure 4.9.

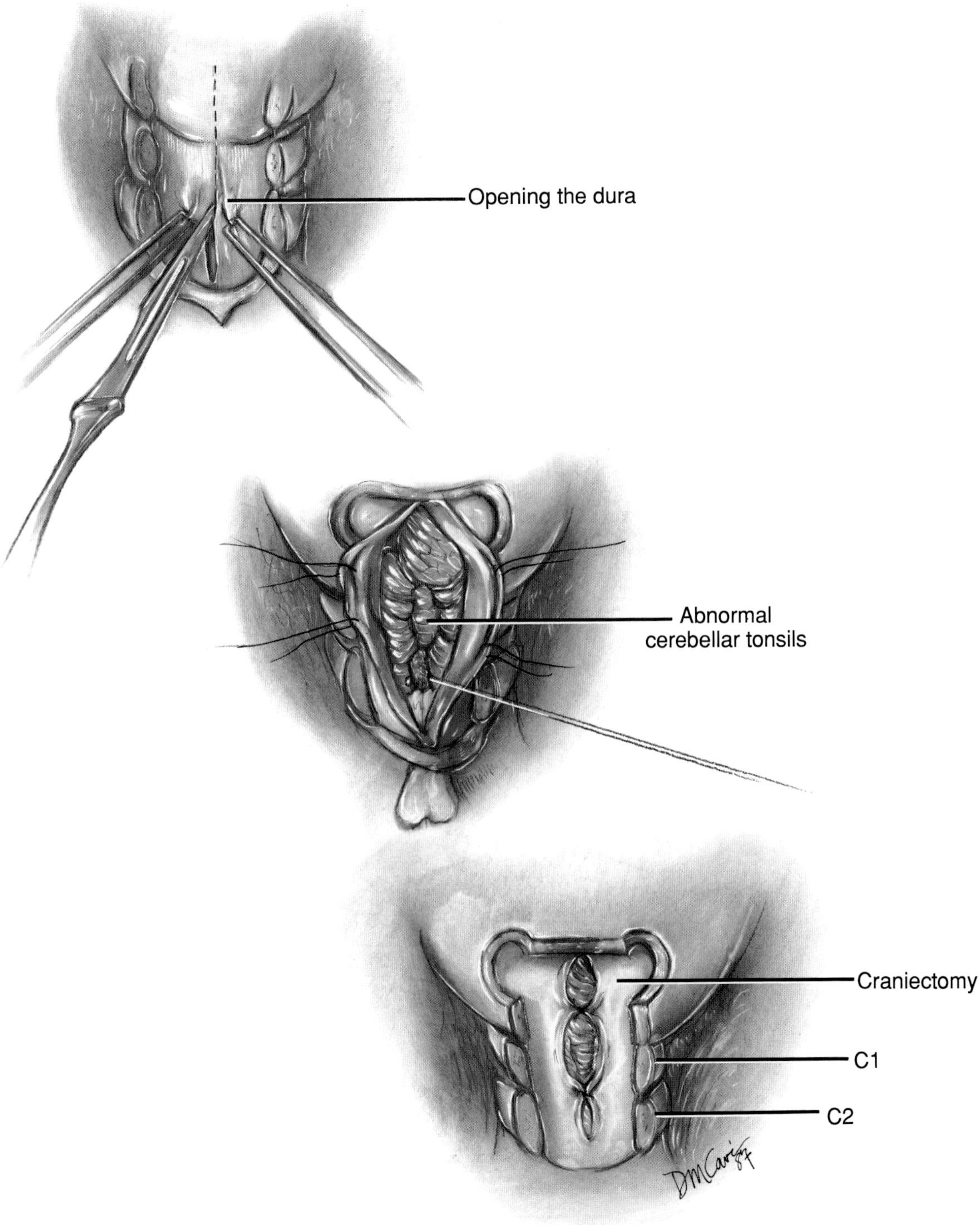
Opening the dura
Abnormal cerebellar tonsils
Craniectomy
C1
C2

Figure 4.10.

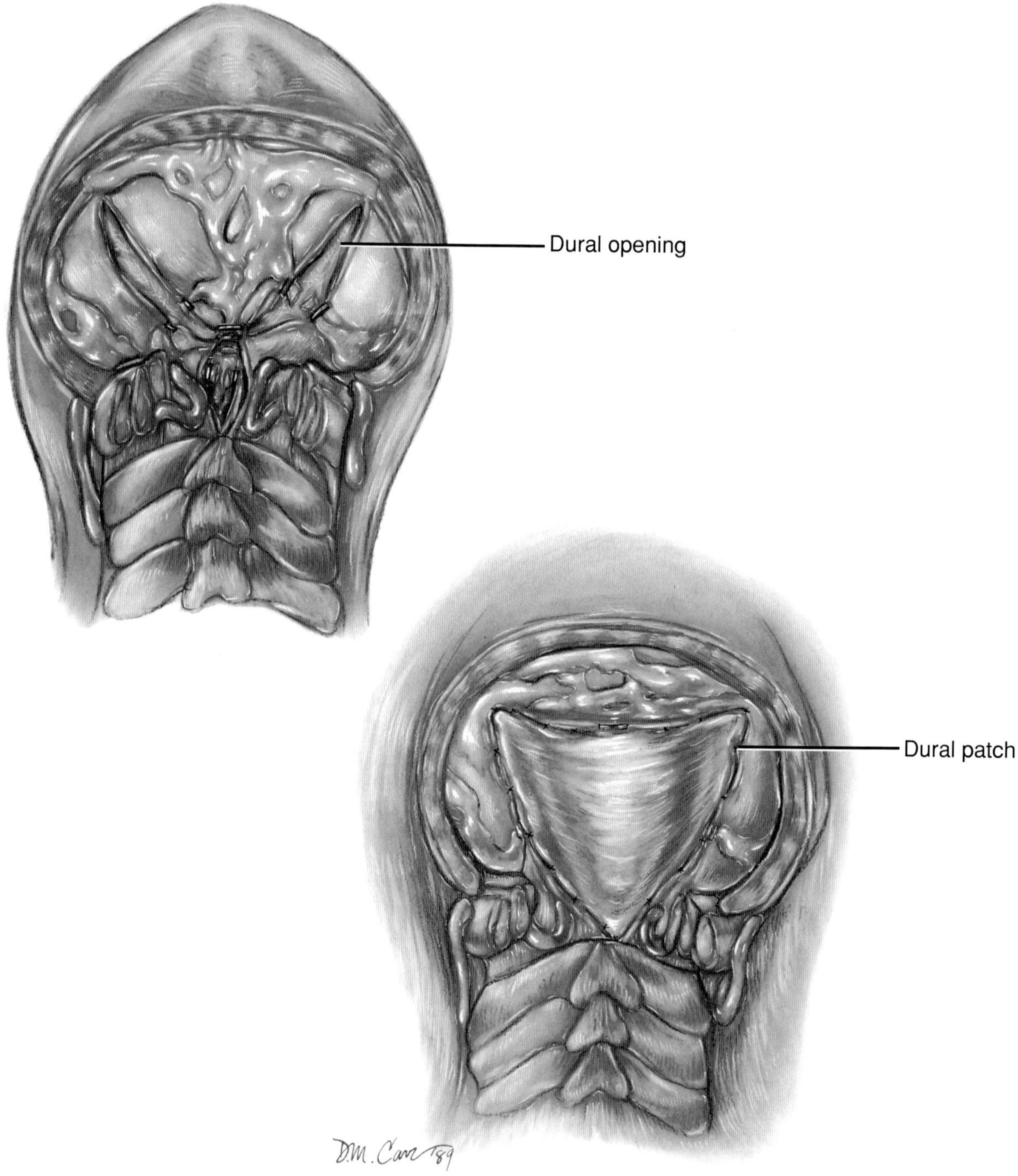

Figure 4.11.

SECTION 2

Lumbar Fusion

5 Lumbar Pedicle Screw Fixation and Fusion

Cotrel-Dubousset Instrumentation in Spondylolisthesis

Posterolateral spinal fusion with iliac crest bone graft is considered the standard treatment for symptomatic spondylolysis and spondylolisthesis. Pseudoarthrosis rates of up to 60% have been reported in the literature, however, and techniques of improving the fusion rate are being sought. Internal fixation in selected cases of spondylolisthesis is gaining acceptance in the armamentarium of spine surgeons as one means of achieving this goal.

Various means of achieving a stable fusion through the use of internal fixation have been and are currently being developed. One such method is the innovative instrumentation system developed by Yves Cotrel and Jean Dubousset. This system was originally designed for the correction and stabilization of scoliosis. Because of its versatility, however, it can be used for the treatment of a variety of spinal disorders, including spondylolisthesis. A two-level stabilization of most grades of spondylolisthesis can be achieved with the use of a short Cotrel-Dubousset rod and pedicle screws. In addition to a potentially higher fusion rate, this system has the advantage of preserving the adjacent motion segments, thus minimizing loss of flexibility of the lumbosacral spine and secondary degenerative changes at unfused motion seg-

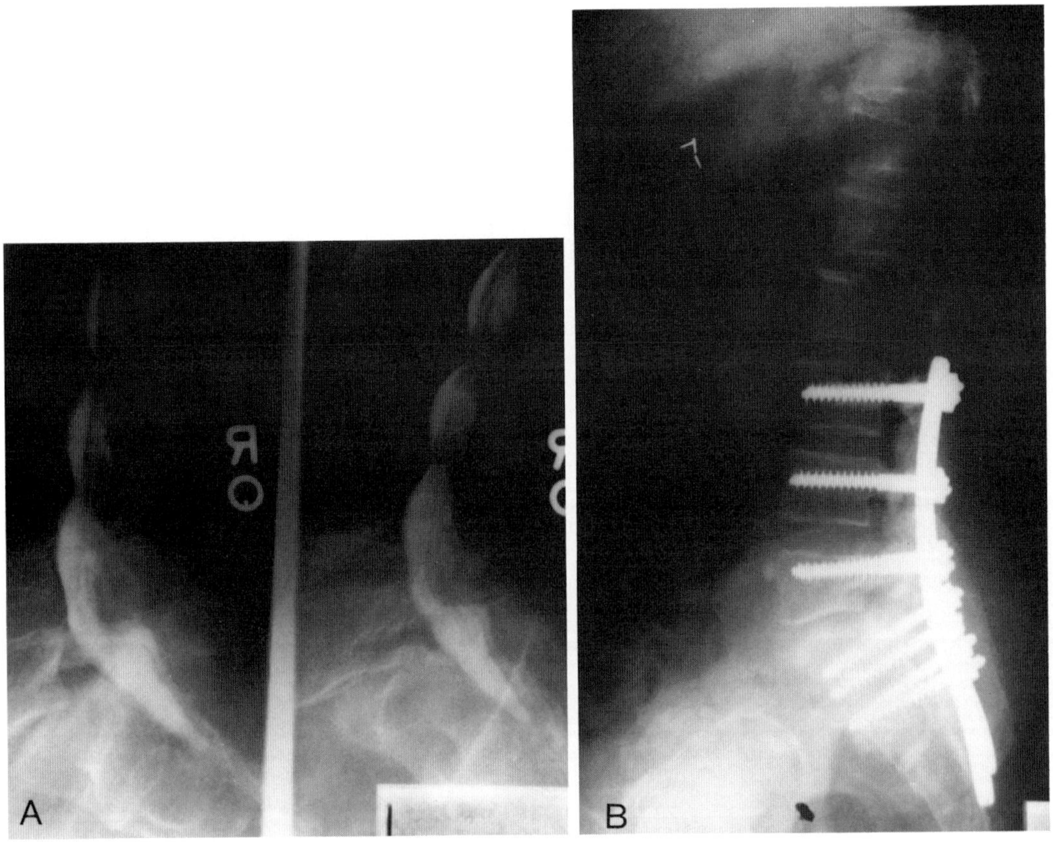

Figure 5.1. A. The patient has an L5-S1 spondylolisthesis congenital in origin. **B.** The problem has been corrected by the use of Steffee system with screws in the sacrum and the pedicles of L5, L4, and L3. The correction is excellent and stabilization was complete.

ments. Another advantage of this system is that the need for postoperative external support is minimized.

Although the long-term efficacy of this system is yet to be established, the placement of pedicle screws appears to be safe when the technique as described below is carefully followed. Fixation is readily achieved with the insertion of a short knurled rod within the heads of the pedicle screws. Reduction can be attempted, but we prefer to use this instrumentation as a neutralization device to facilitate in situ fusion. If *reduction* of spondylolisthesis is desired, then Steffee variable screw placement (VSP) instrumentation should be utilized. The technique described below is that used in patients with a grade I or II isthmic L5-S1 spondylolisthesis.

Technique

The use of a spinal frame that allows the patient's abdomen to hang free, thus minimizing bleeding, is highly recommended. We prefer to place our patients in the knee-chest position on the Andrews frame. After preparing and draping the patient in standard fashion for a posterior lumbosacral approach, the spine is exposed from L4 to the sacrum in standard fashion. The dissection should proceed laterally so as to expose the ala of the sacrum and the transverse process of L5. Laminectomy of L5 and L5-S1 foraminotomies (Gill procedure) are then performed in most cases.

The entry point for the placement of the L5 pedicle screws is next selected. This entry point is defined by

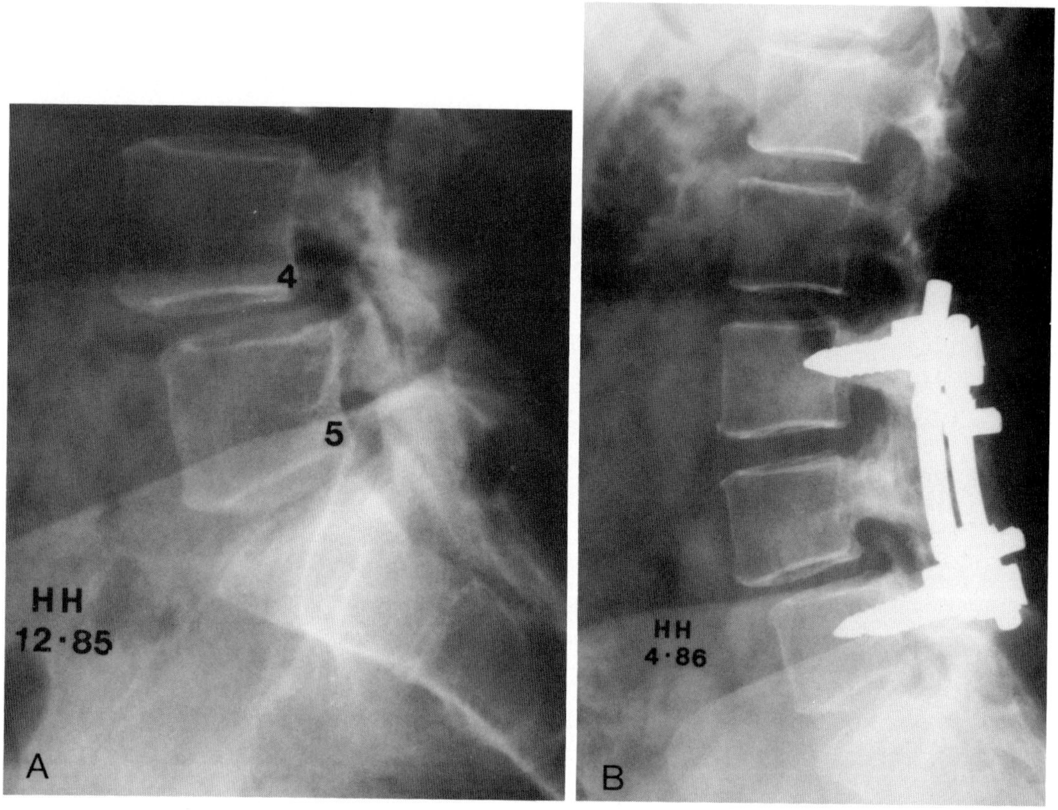

Figure 5.2. The patient has an L4-L5 degenerative spondylolisthesis **(A)** corrected by a Steffee plate with pedicle screws **(B)**.

the intersection of a horizontal line bisecting the base of the transverse process and a vertical line through the lateral aspect of the superior articular process of L5 (Fig. 5.1). After careful selection of the entry point, a Leksell rongeur is used to decorticate 2 mm of bone at this point. Care should be taken to minimize destruction of the L4-L5 facet joint capsule so as to avoid spontaneous extension of the fusion to L4.

A 000 curette is used to carefully probe the intended path of the screw. The tip of the curette should be angled 15° medially from the entry point in order to follow the center of the pedicle into the vertebral body (Fig. 5.2). If the curette (or subsequently the screw) is angled less than 15°, there is the danger of exiting the lateral wall of the pedicle and missing the vertebral body altogether. If angled more than 15°, the medial wall of the pedicle may be exited and the spinal canal violated (Fig. 5.3). The use of radiographic control is recommended to confirm the intrapedicular position of the curette, especially when this technique is used for the first time. (C-arm fluoroscopy can be used if desired.) After experience is gained with this technique, a "feel" for the walls of the pedicle can be appreciated with the probe. The use of a power drill, even with variable speed, is not recommended as a substitute for manual probing, since this eliminates the tactile feedback of manual probing of the pedicle. A 45-mm closed pedicle screw is selected and carefully placed into the pedicle by using the Cotrel-Dubousset pedicle screwdriver. The opposite L5 pedicle screw is placed in similar fashion.

The entry point for the sacral pedicle screws is selected in a somewhat different manner, since there is no transverse process to serve as an anatomic landmark. The entry point for the sacral screw lies on the vertical line that bisects the articular process just caudal to its most caudal extent (Fig. 5.4). A Leksell rongeur is used to decorticate the entry point, and a 000 curette is used to probe the path of the screw, with the tip of the curette angled again 15° medially but also 30° distally from the entry point so that the screw path will be parallel to (and thus will not pen-

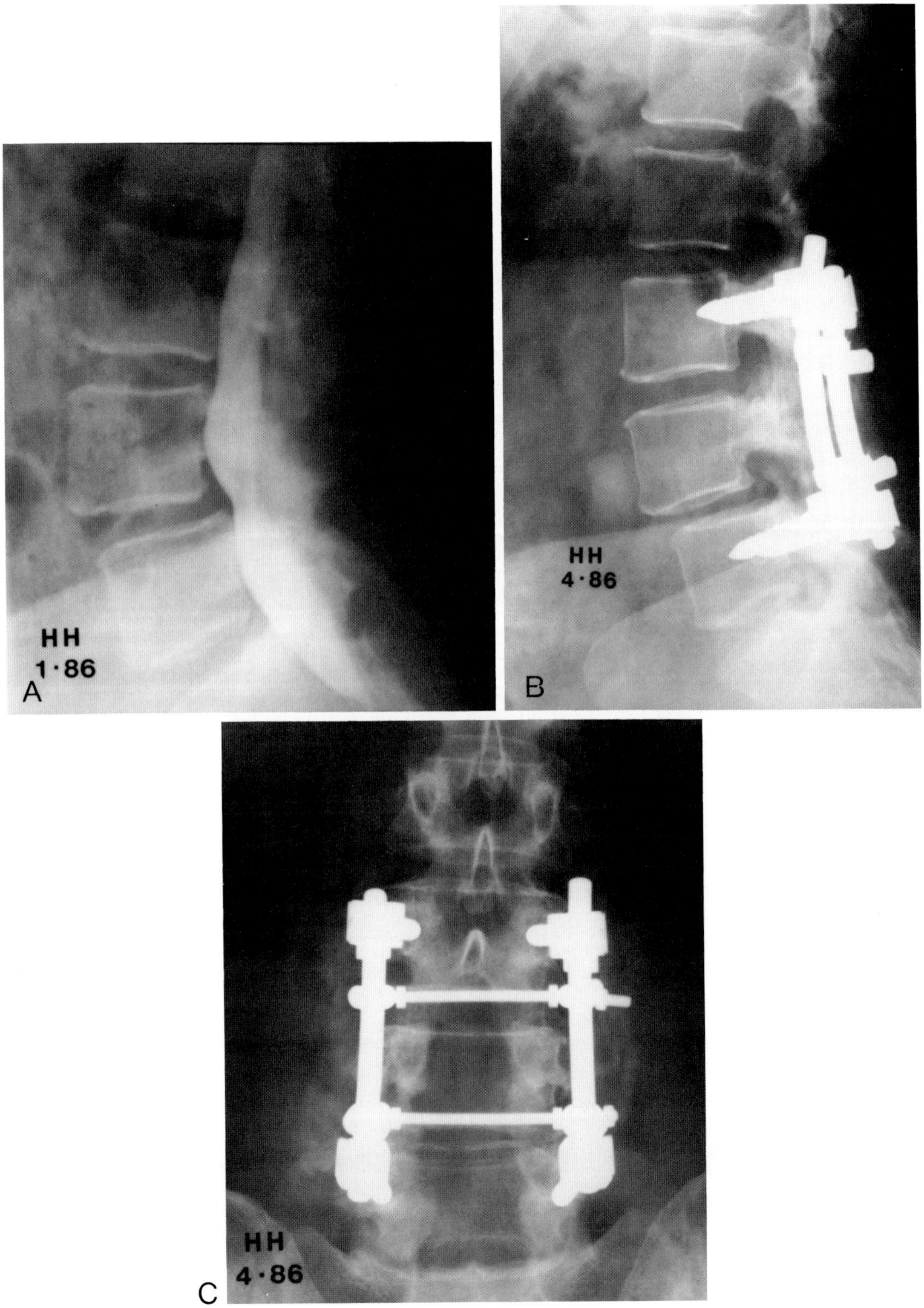

Figure 5.3.

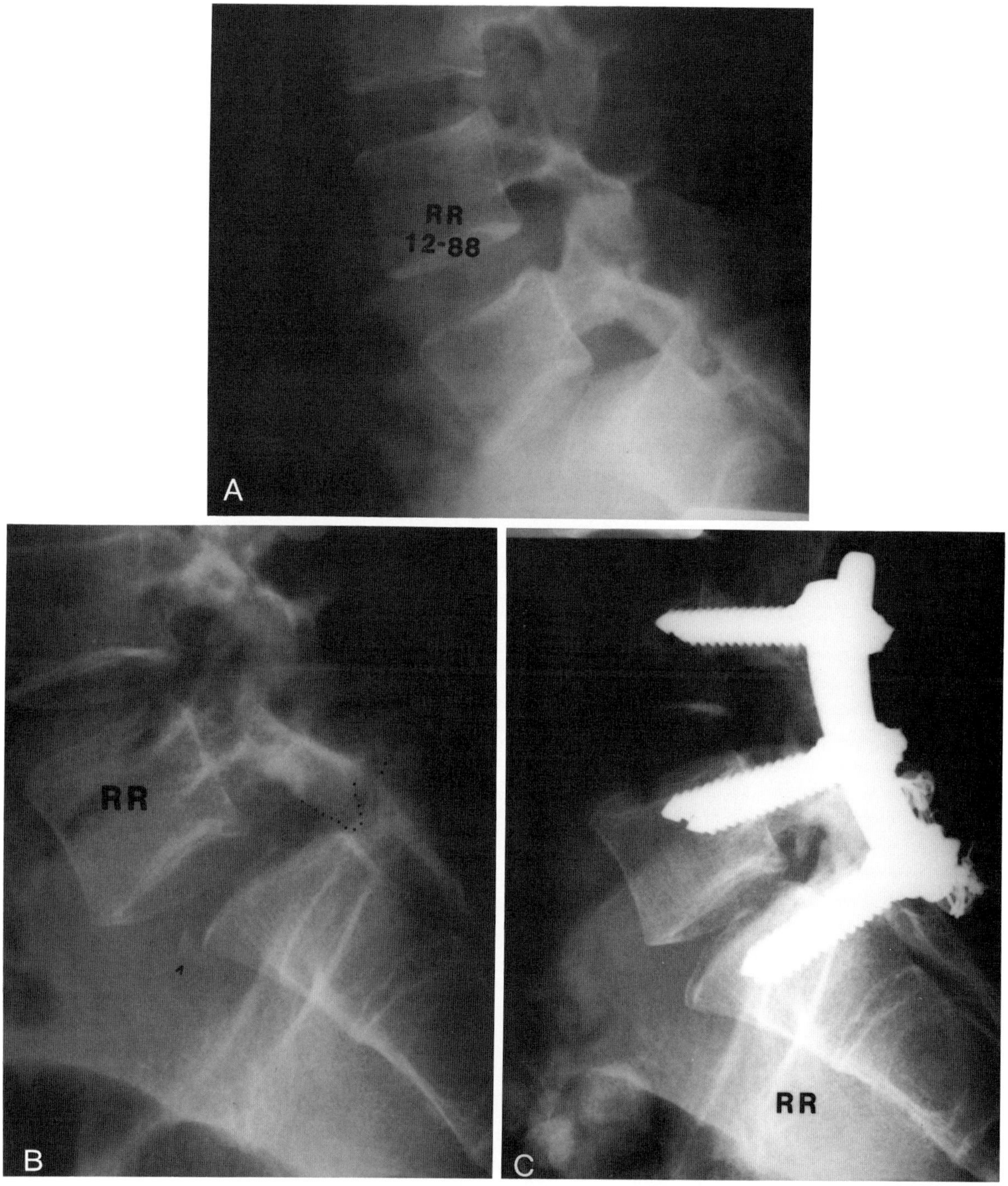

Figure 5.4.

etrate) the superior end plate of S1. This angle is quite variable and should correspond to the angle of sacral inclination as seen on the lateral preoperative radiograph. A 30-mm pedicle screw is then selected and carefully placed with the pedicle screwdriver. The anterior cortex of the body of the sacrum may be felt while driving the screw. If this occurs, the pressure on the screwdriver should be *slightly* increased in order to penetrate this cortex, and the screwdriver should be turned no more than two 360° turns to avoid injury to the S1 nerve root.

Once all four screws are in place, the appropriate length Cotrel-Dubousset rod is selected (and cut if necessary) and secured into place with the set screws. The rods should be bent into slight lordosis prior to securing them to the pedicle screws. Distraction between the pedicle screws should be avoided in order to preserve L5-S1 lordosis. A confirmatory lateral radiograph is obtained to evaluate the technique, the set screws are overtightened with the T-wrench, and the set screw heads are broken off. Corticocancellous and cancellous bone graft is harvested from the posterior iliac crest through the same skin incision but a separate fascial incision. The transverse processes of L5 and the ala of the sacrum are decorticated (with the use of an osteotome, a gouge, and/or a high-speed burr), and the bone graft is packed into place laterally. Care is taken to avoid placement of the bone graft medial to the instrumentation in order to avoid the development of a secondary spinal stenosis.

Large suction drains are placed into both wounds, and the wounds are closed in layers. Care should be taken to eliminate the dead space over the iliac crest fascial incision by suturing the subcutaneous layer to the fascia in this area.

Postoperatively, radiographs are obtained and the patient is mobilized without a brace. The patient should be followed with serial radiographs until a solid fusion is documented. Fusion is usually achieved within 6 months. Rarely does this instrumentation require removal. If this is necessary, the rods can be cut between the pedicle screws, and the screws removed with the screwdriver or hook holder.

Steffee Transpedicular Instrumentation

Steffee transpedicular instrumentation is also called the variable screw placement (VSP) bone plate and bone screw system, which can be used by surgeons to address a number of different clinical situations. The basic background for Steffee instrumentation depends on the concept of the pedicle being the "force nucleus" of the normal vertebra. The "force nucleus" of the normal vertebra is located at the junction of the ridge on the superior articular process, the ridge on the pars interarticularis, and the ridge of the transverse process. These three ridges converge at the direct posterior landmark corresponding to the correct placement of the transpedicular screw. The "force nucleus" serves as a window into the intramedullary canal of the pedicle. The primary indications for Steffee transpedicular instrumentation are: spinal trauma, degenerative spondylolisthesis, isthmic spondylolisthesis, degenerative disc disease, adult-onset scoliosis, fixation following posterior vertebral osteotomies, and postlaminectomy instability. There are several definite absolute contraindications to transpedicular instrumentation: a history of infection and dysplastic pedicles preventing safe screw fixation; and morbid obesity, severe osteopenia, and open wounds contraindicating the use of transpedicular screw instrumentation with posterior plates. In addition, patients having a history of metal allergy are not candidates for Steffee instrumentation. The instrumentation is made of a high-grade stainless steel known as 22 chromium-13 nickel-5 molybdenum. The VSP bone plates are fabricated from 316 LVM implant-grade stainless steel. Patients with a history of allergy to jewelry can have a plate taped to their skin for several days to determine if redness develops in reaction to the plate. Several devices augment and increase the stability of Steffee transpedicular instrumentation. There are, for example, washers or plate spacer wedges used behind the integral nut of the screw that increase the rigidity of the instrumentation system by increasing the congruence of fit between the screws and the plates.

Surgical Technique

The patient is placed under general anesthesia on an Andrews spinal frame or similar frame that keeps the abdomen free (Fig. 5.5). Currently, there is an Andrews operative table manufactured that allows anteroposterior and lateral fluoroscopic views to be performed during pedicle screw fixation. Surgeons first developing familiarity with the technique of pedicle fixation may find that continuous monitoring using

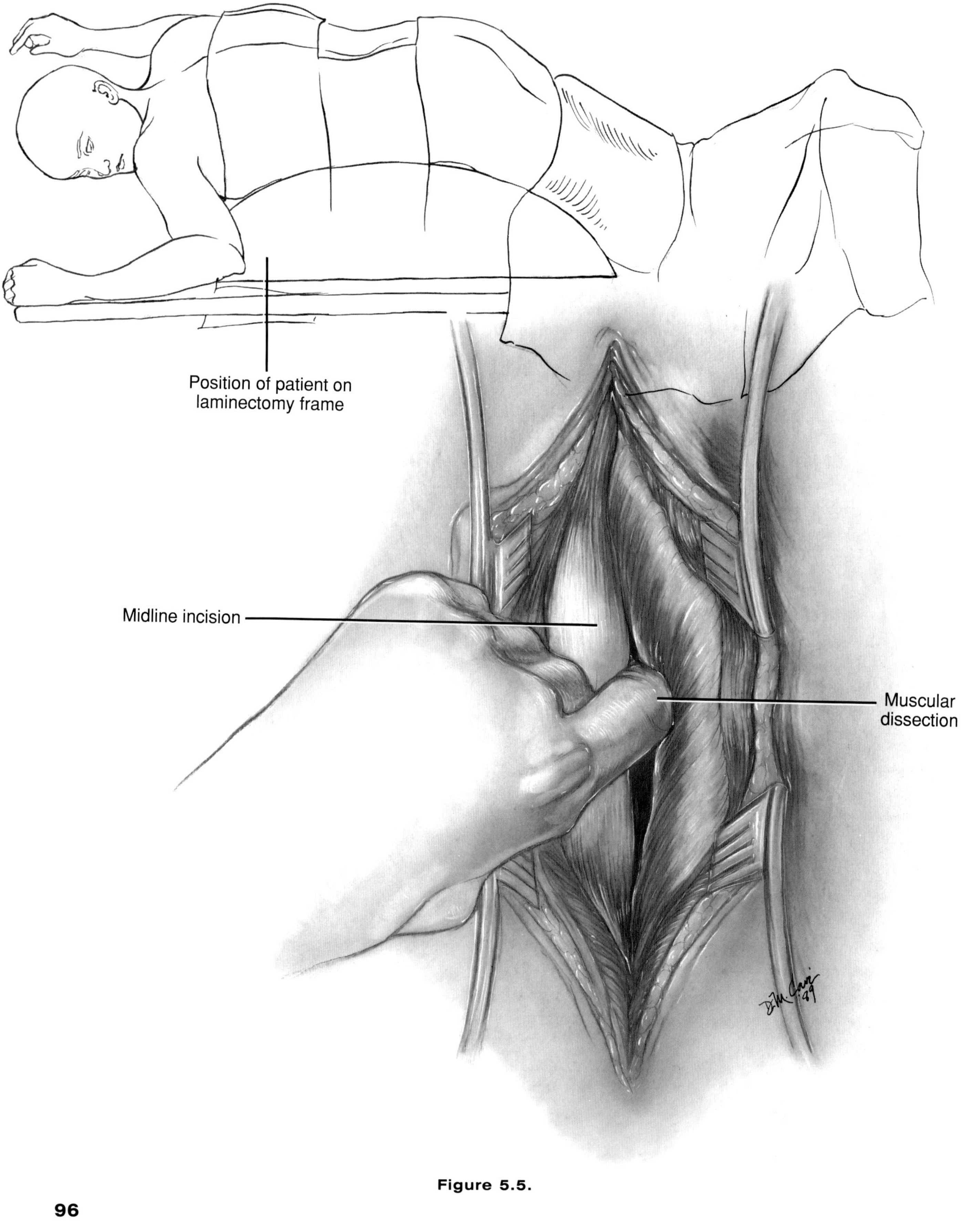
Position of patient on
laminectomy frame
Midline incision
Muscular
dissection

Figure 5.5.

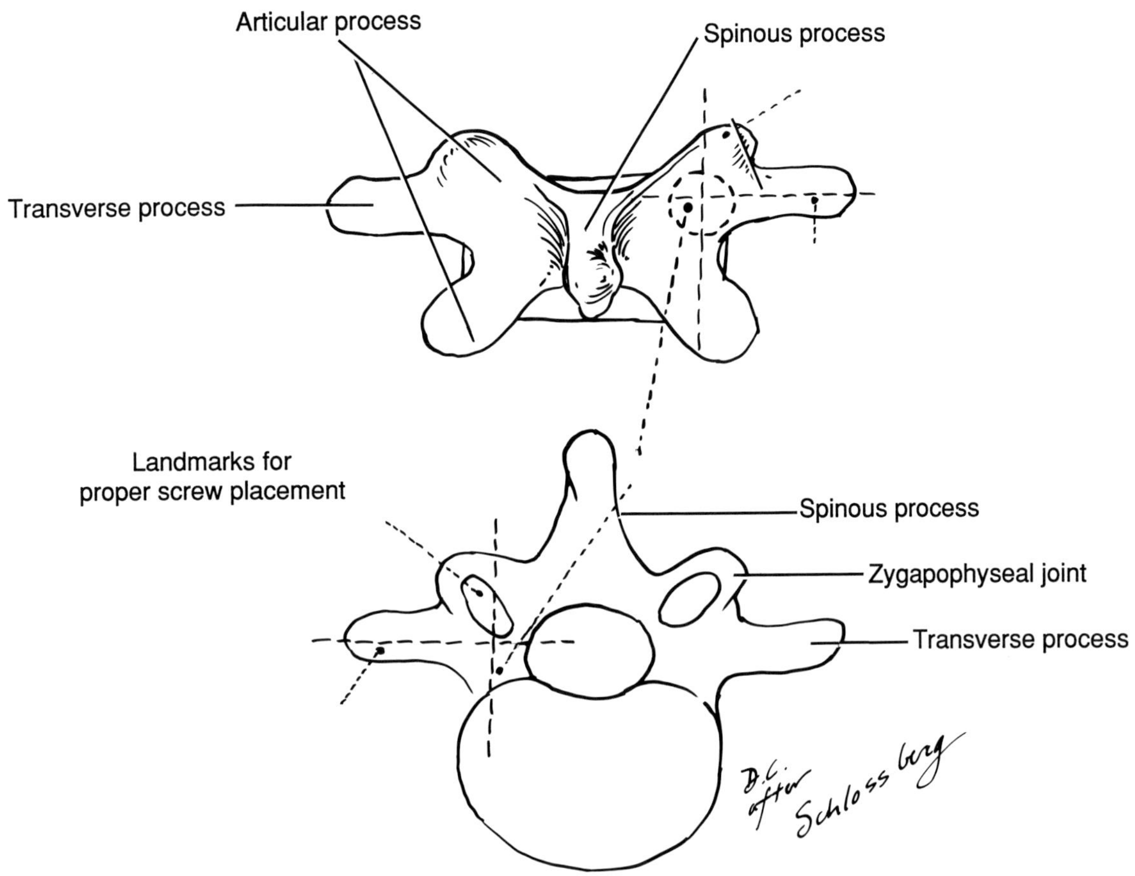

Figure 5.6.

anteroposterior and lateral and oblique fluoroscopy will increase the safety of transpedicular instrumentation. The use of posterior implanted plates and screws requires a working knowledge of anatomic subtleties in order to identify correct pedicular placement. If the specific lumbar vertebra in question has a mamillary process, this area can be decorticated with a rongeur, and a Steffee pedicle probe can be inserted directly at this location. If the vertebra does not have a mamillary process, then a transverse plane should be formed at the midportion of the transverse processes. The sagittal plane can be determined by the midportion of the superior articular processes. Where the parasagittal and transverse lines intersect is the correct position for insertion of pedicular instrumentation. After stripping the paraspinal muscles and transverse processes of the vertebrae to be fused, a small burr is used to decorticate the posterior ridge of the pedicle. A ridge exists on the top of the transverse process, the superior articular process, and the pars interarticularis. The point of convergence of these three ridges represents the correct entry point for all types of intramedullary fixation (Fig. 5.6). The Steffee pedicle probe is particularly well suited for gaining entrance into the pedicle because its taper prevents overpenetration of the vertebra and thereby prevents penetration of the anterior great vessels. With experience the surgeon can develop the "correct feel" of entering the intramedullary canal of the pedicle. This is described as a unique and identifiable sensation by Dr. Arthur Steffee. After the pedicle probe is withdrawn, a 6.5-mm tap is used to cut threads within the pedicle in the vertebral body. A pedicle sound can be inserted to document that no walls of the pedicle have

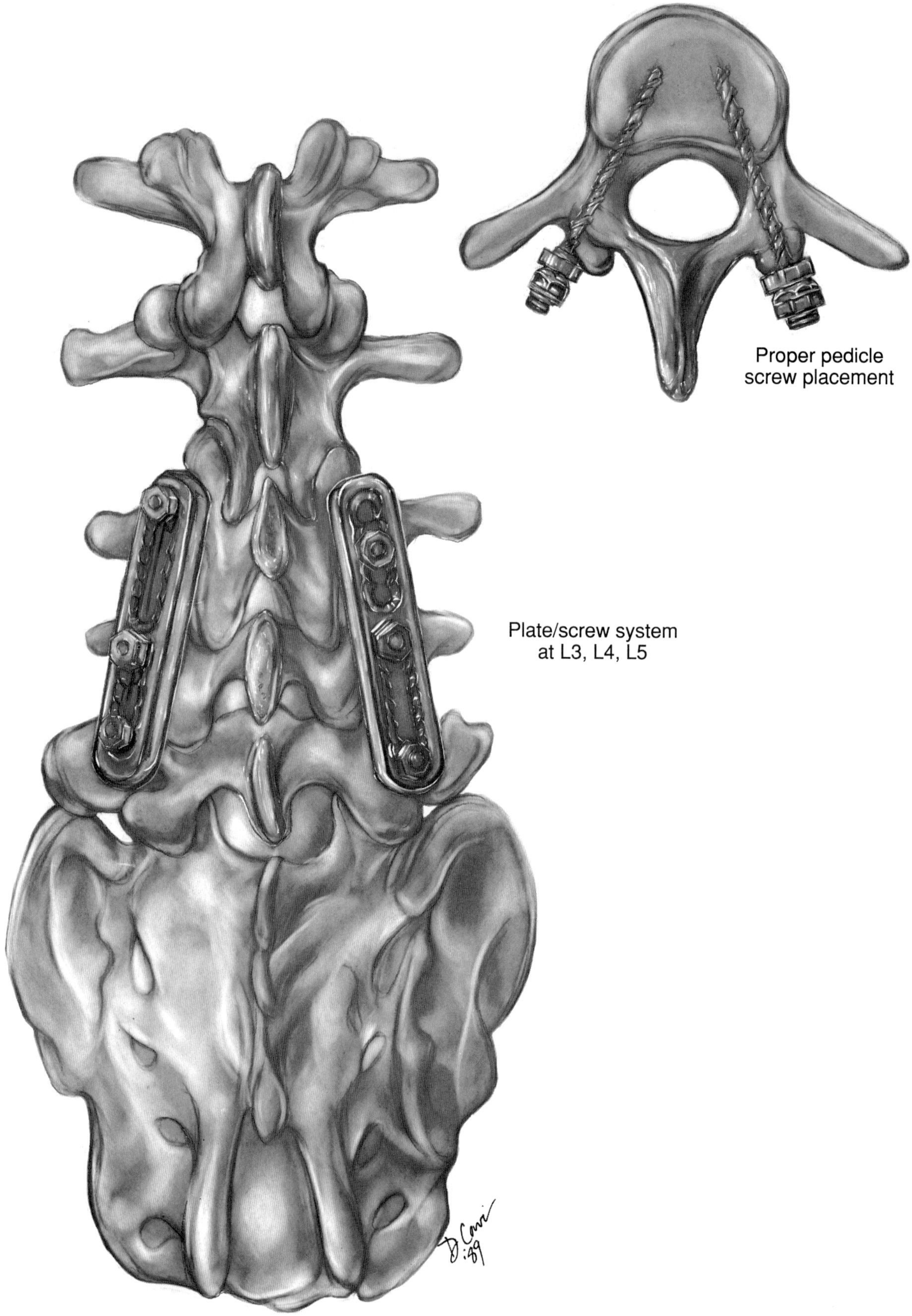
Proper pedicle
screw placement
Plate/screw system
at L3, L4, L5

Figure 5.7.

been violated. It is recommended for osteopenic bone to insert methyl methacrylate cement to increase the purchase power of a pedicle screw. We would recommend that methyl methacrylate should not be used. Several studies have been conducted that document that methyl methacrylate, when placed under pressure, will extrude for the pedicle and can actually form a mass within the spinal canal. After threads for the pedicle screws are cut, various size Steffee pedicle screws can be inserted. The current generation of screws utilizes an integral nut, which means that a hexagonal nut has been milled within the pedicle screw, which prevents anterior penetration of the tip of the screw. The correct plate is then contoured to the patient's desired lumbar lordosis. The plate is then inserted with its slotted holes over two to four vertebral levels. The plate is then locked in place over the pedicle screws by utilizing a double-nut locking system. The holding power of the plates and screws is determined by a spiral lock nut thread that is of space age design and offers superior holding ability compared with that of conventional machine threads. A machine nut is then inserted over the second conical locking nut. When this is maximally tightened, excellent stability and fixation are obtained (Fig. 5.7).

A specific point should be mentioned with regard to fixation to the sacrum. The Steffee transpedicular system is the best and most stable means of securing fixation to the sacrum because bicortical purchase of the sacrum can be achieved. The screws penetrate the anterior cortex of the sacrum. This can be accomplished safely because the common iliac vessels bifurcate at L4, and the promontory of the sacrum typically has no overlying major vascular or visceral structures as long as the screws at the S1 pedicle are directed toward the midline. The most important aspect of the Steffee transpedicular instrumentation is to decorticate the transverse processes and facet joints before applying the plates. The plates are extremely bulky and wide and may interfere with the amount of bone that the surgeon can place in performance of the spinal arthrodesis. Therefore, it is recommended that the posterior elements and facet joints be decorticated and the cancellous posterolateral bone graft be inserted after inserting the pedicle screws but before applying the posterior longitudinal plates.

Posterior Lumbar Interbody Fusion

Posterior lumbar interbody fusion can be performed with the reamers and broaches of the AcroMed system in a more standardized and safer manner than was done previously. Several broaches can be used to apply bone grafts measuring $11 \times 11 \times 30$ mm. The use of broaches and reamers allows for posterior lumbar interbody fusion to be performed in conjunction with posterior transpedicular instrumentation and plate fixation. This allows the surgeon to perform a circumferential arthrodesis of the spine in conjunction with posterior instrumentation. Transpedicular instrumentation allows the surgeon to achieve fixation along all three longitudinal columns of spinal stability, the anterior column, the middle column, and the posterior column. Postoperative immobilization with a Boston overlap brace or a custom-molded thoracolumbar orthosis is recommended.

6

L4-S1 Lumbar Transverse Process-Iliac Crest Fusion

The patient is anesthetized in the supine position. Following the completion of satisfactory general anesthesia, the patient is turned prone onto the operating frame. The frame is specifically positioned such that the abdomen is free of all extrinsic pressure to reduce epidural venous stasis and pressure. In females, particular attention is paid to the positioning of the breasts to make sure that the areolae are free from pressure from the frame (Fig. 6.1). The back is prepared and draped with the drapes extending slightly out more to the side of the iliac crest that will be used for the graft. The initial portion of the procedure involves a standard approach through skin, down to the lumbodorsal fascia. A meticulous subperiosteal exposure is performed with the aid of the cautery to minimize bleeding out to but not beyond the zygapophyseal joints (Fig. 6.2). Further dissection at this point will create unnecessary bleeding and should be delayed until any necessary neural decompression is completed. At the completion of the decompression, the standard laminectomy retractors are removed, since they often inhibit the ability to obtain a wide lateral exposure to the very tips of the transverse processes. The exposure is best accomplished with the use of a Meyerding retractor held by the assistant on the op-

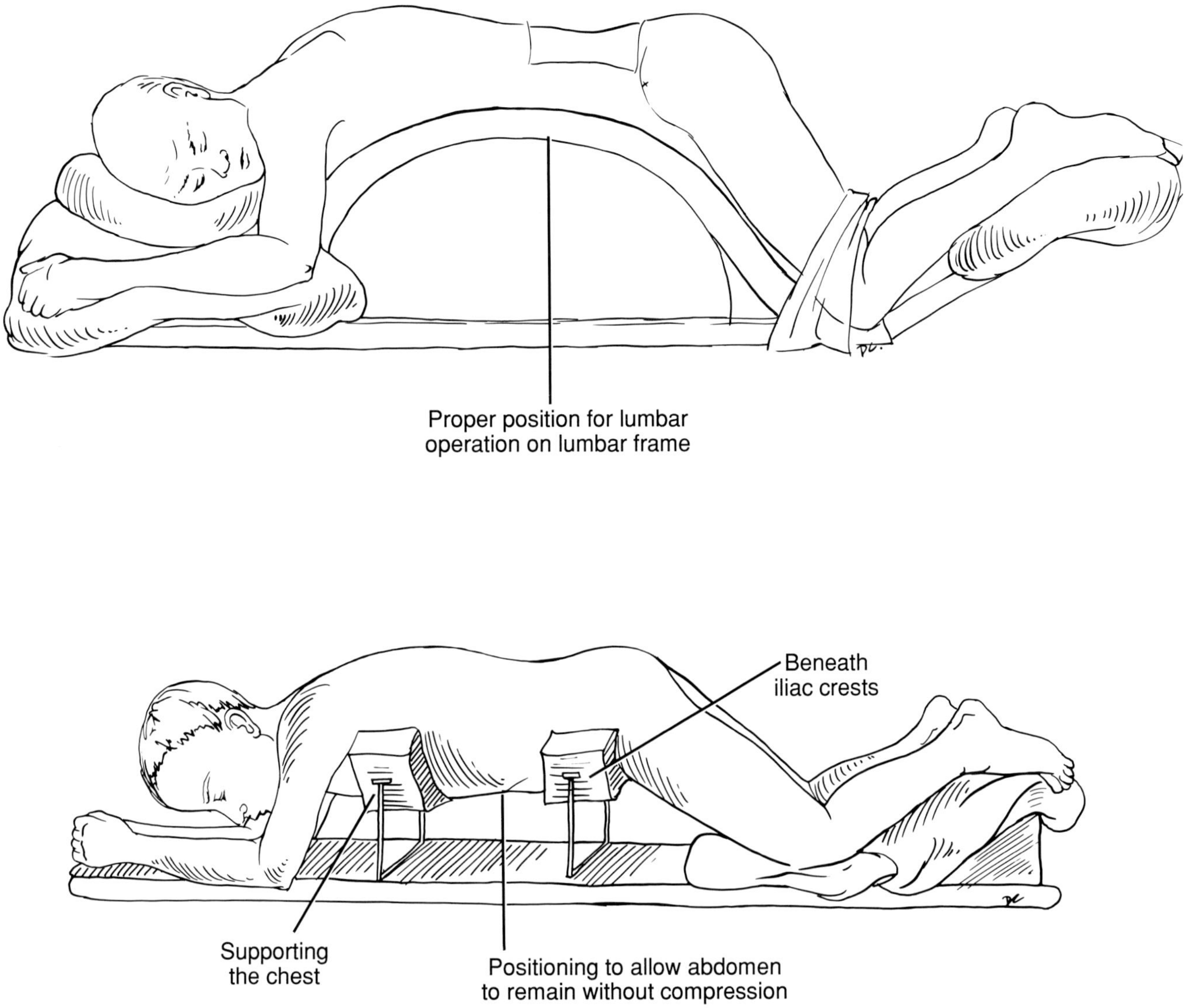

Figure 6.1.

posite side of the table. Any of several large self-retaining retractors are satisfactory also. Headlight visualization facilitates the visualization of the transverse process and dissection. At the superior part of the wound, the cautery is used to elevate the multifidus and erector spinae lateral to the L3-L4 facet (Fig. 6.3). Particular attention is paid to not damaging the capsule of this joint, since it will not be incorporated in the fusion. However, it is important to remember that the L4 transverse process is directly lateral to the L3-L4 facet and that it is important to visualize completely and expose this facet to facilitate exposure of that process. Once the L4 transverse process is adequately visualized, its surface is cleaned with a combination of the cautery and a #2 curved curette that is able to remove soft tissue over the process and, more importantly, in the lateral gutter extending up onto the lateral surface of the superior facet of L4 (Fig. 6.3). This affords maximum surface area for later lateral fusion. Once this is completed,

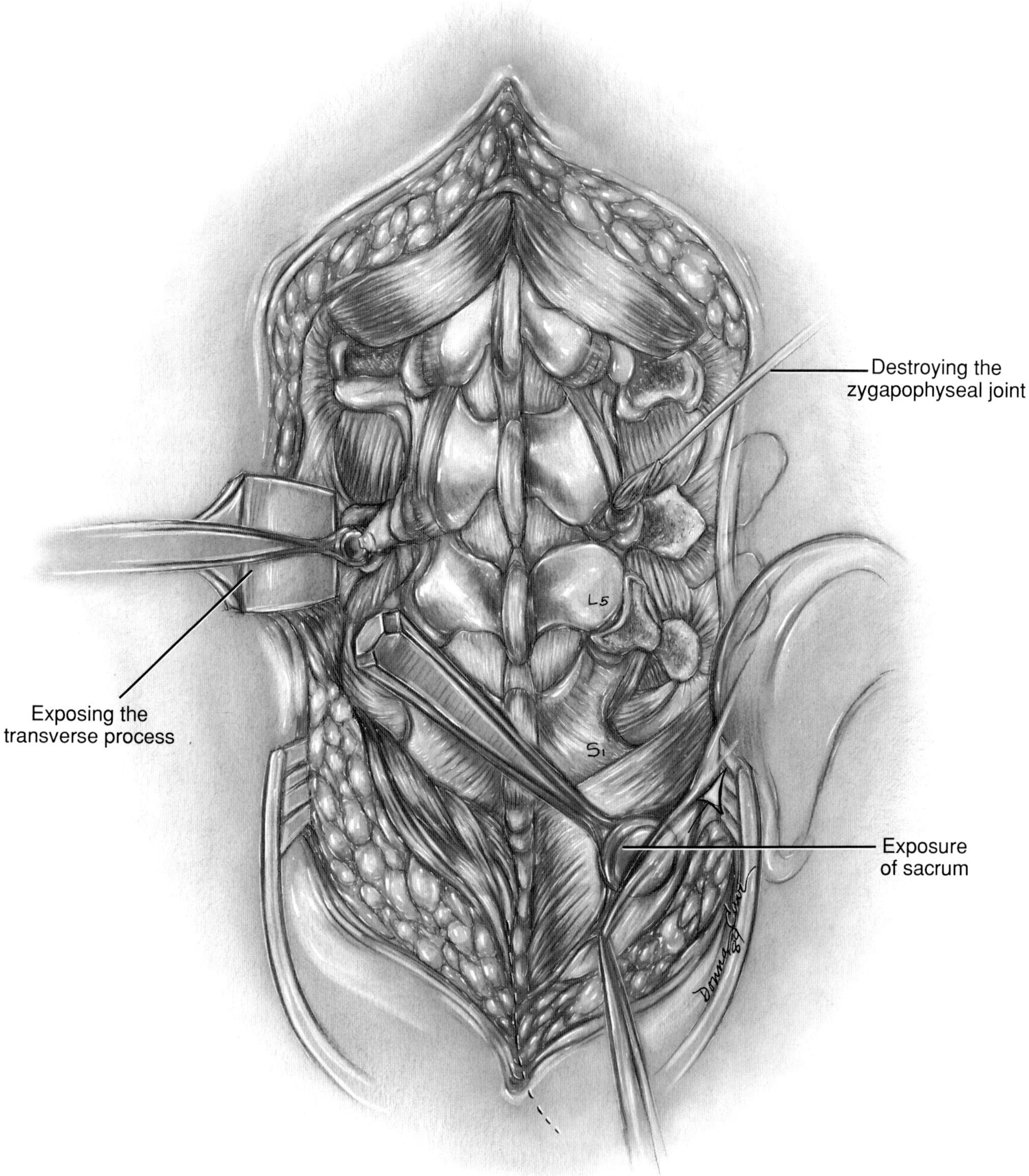
Destroying the zygapophyseal joint
Exposing the transverse process
L5
S1
Exposure of sacrum

Figure 6.2.

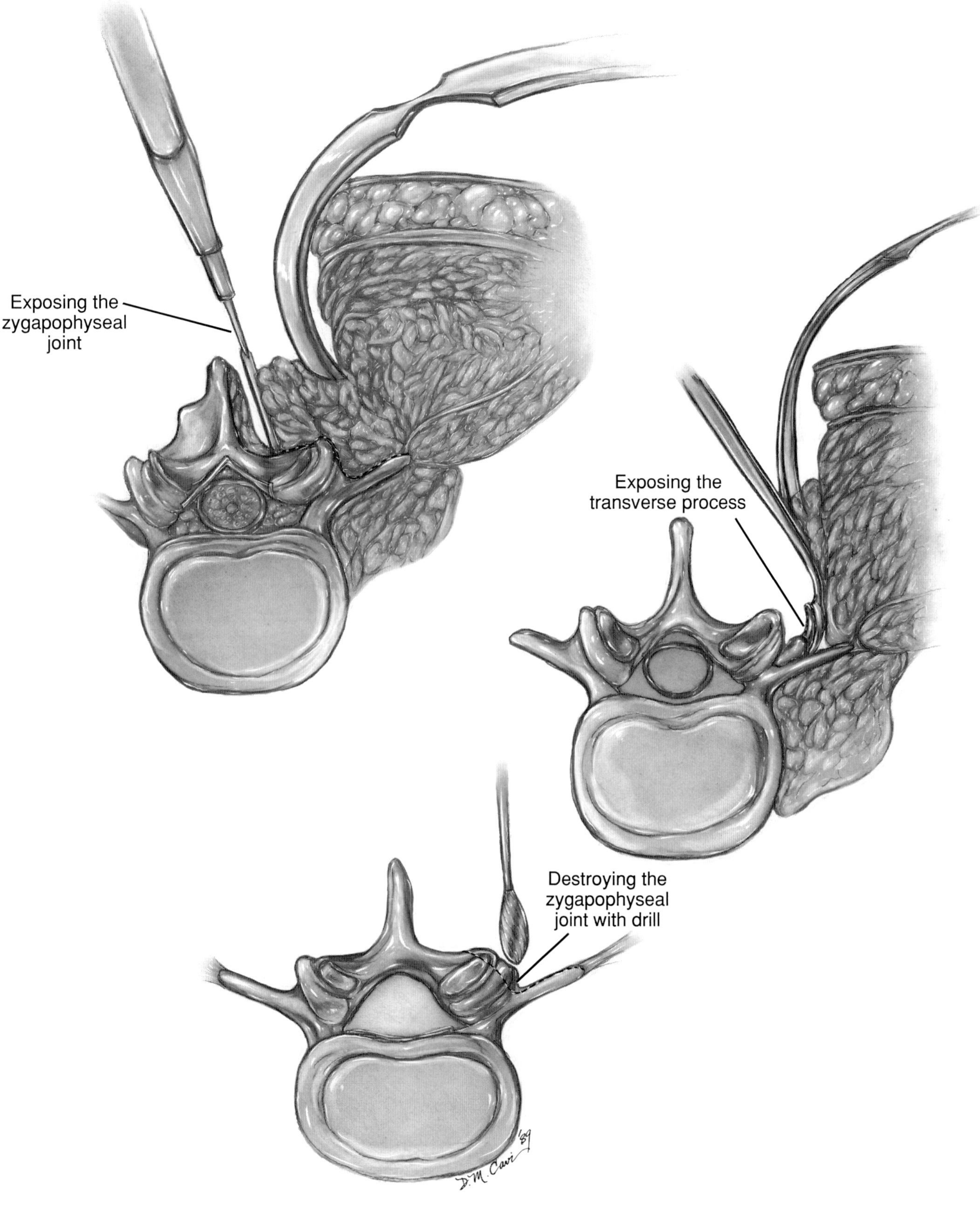
Exposing the zygapophyseal joint
Exposing the transverse process
Destroying the zygapophyseal joint with drill
D.M. Cavi '89

Figure 6.3.

the retractor can be moved one space caudally where a similar procedure is performed over the L5 transverse process. Finally, attention is directed at the sacral ala, with the Meyerding retractor holding the musculature laterally. The soft tissues are cleaned from the sacral ala, exposing an area of bone approximately 1 cm laterally and approximately 2 cm superiorly and inferiorly. Once this is completed, a motorized high-speed burr is used to decorticate the surfaces of bone in this lateral gutter, including the transverse processes and the lateral side of the superior facets of the involved vertebrae (Fig. 6.3). Finally, the vertically oriented facet joints of L4-L5 and L5-S1 are identified. Motion at these joints is able to be visualized by the pressure of a Cobb elevator. The facet capsule of these joints is stripped with a combination of a #3 straight curette and cautery. Once these facets are completely identified, the facet surfaces and the articular cartilage are destroyed with the high-speed burr. It is important to include these facets in the decortication process, since they are important in the later stabilization of the fusion. A failure to include them results in a higher pseudarthrosis rate. A similar process is then performed on the opposite side.

The iliac crest bone graft is taken through the same skin incision. A second incision approximately 3 cm in length is made on the selected crest, and a flap over the lumbodorsal fascia is raised (Fig. 6.4). The top of the iliac crest is identified and the fascia is divided, exposing the iliac crest beneath the subperiosteum. Dissection is continued out laterally and over the side of the iliac crest with the use of a Cobb dissector. Attention is particularly paid to hemostasis and to stripping the musculature subperiosteally to minimize bleeding. A Taylor retractor is then placed carefully over the lateral aspect of the iliac crest. The point should be carefully placed to avoid displacement and slippage into the sciatic notch that could damage the sciatic nerve or the superior gluteal artery. A ½-inch osteotome is used initially to create vertical strips in the iliac crest, and then a 1½-inch curved osteotome is used to scarify the inferior surface so that the grafts can be removed in toto without splintering of the lower aspect of the iliac crest (Fig. 6.5). Each graft is approximately ¼ inch wide, 1½ inches long, and ⅜ inch thick. Smith-Peterson gouges are used to obtain strips of cancellous bone. At the completion of bone removal, the iliac crest site is thoroughly irrigated and packed, awaiting completion of the fusion prior to closure. The primary wound is then reopened, and cortical strips of bone are laid directly on the transverse process with the cancellous side facing the decorticated transverse processes. These are packed out as far laterally as possible and laid from transverse process to transverse process (Fig. 6.6). Following this, the large amounts of cancellous bone are laid into the overlying gutter and decorticated facet joints, completing the fusion (Fig. 6.7). A watertight closure is effected over the iliac crest graft site by using a vacuum drain. A standard wound closure of the posterior lumbar region is finally performed.

The patient is nursed recumbent until lessening of pain enables the patient to be mobilized in a polypropylene body jacket. Use of the jacket usually extends for approximately 3 months until x-rays show consolidation of the fusion mass.

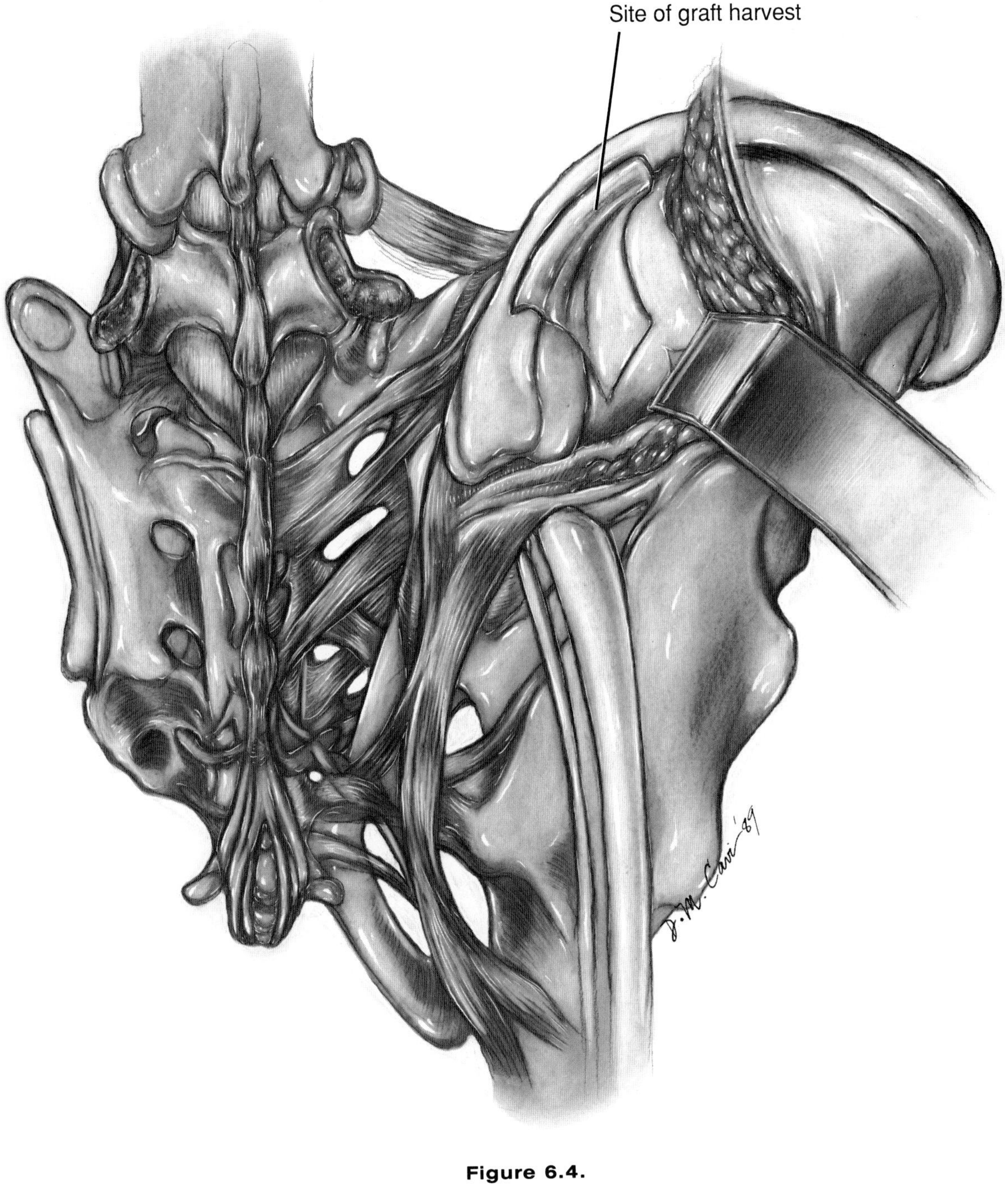

Figure 6.4.

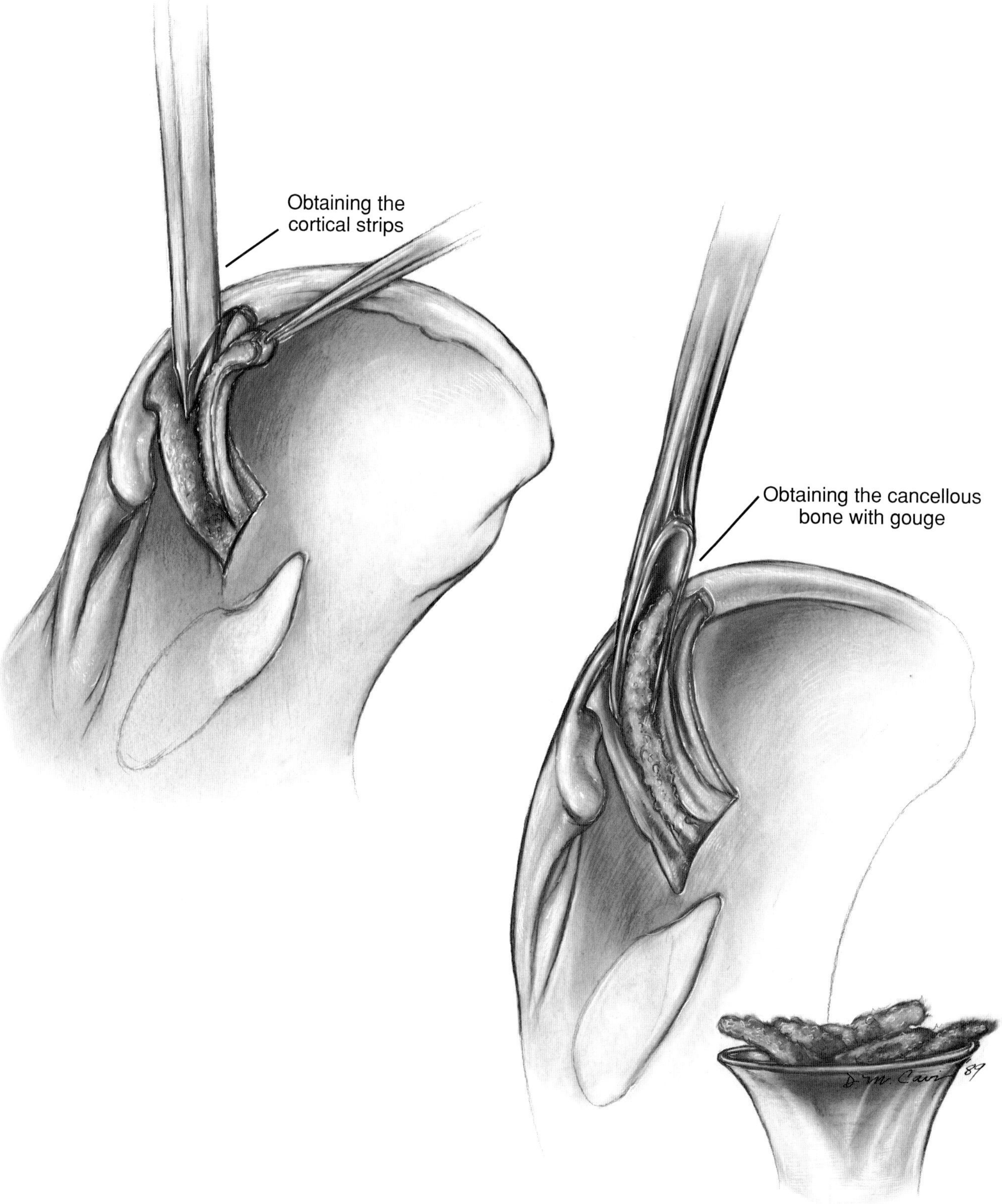
Obtaining the
cortical strips
Obtaining the cancellous
bone with gouge

Figure 6.5.

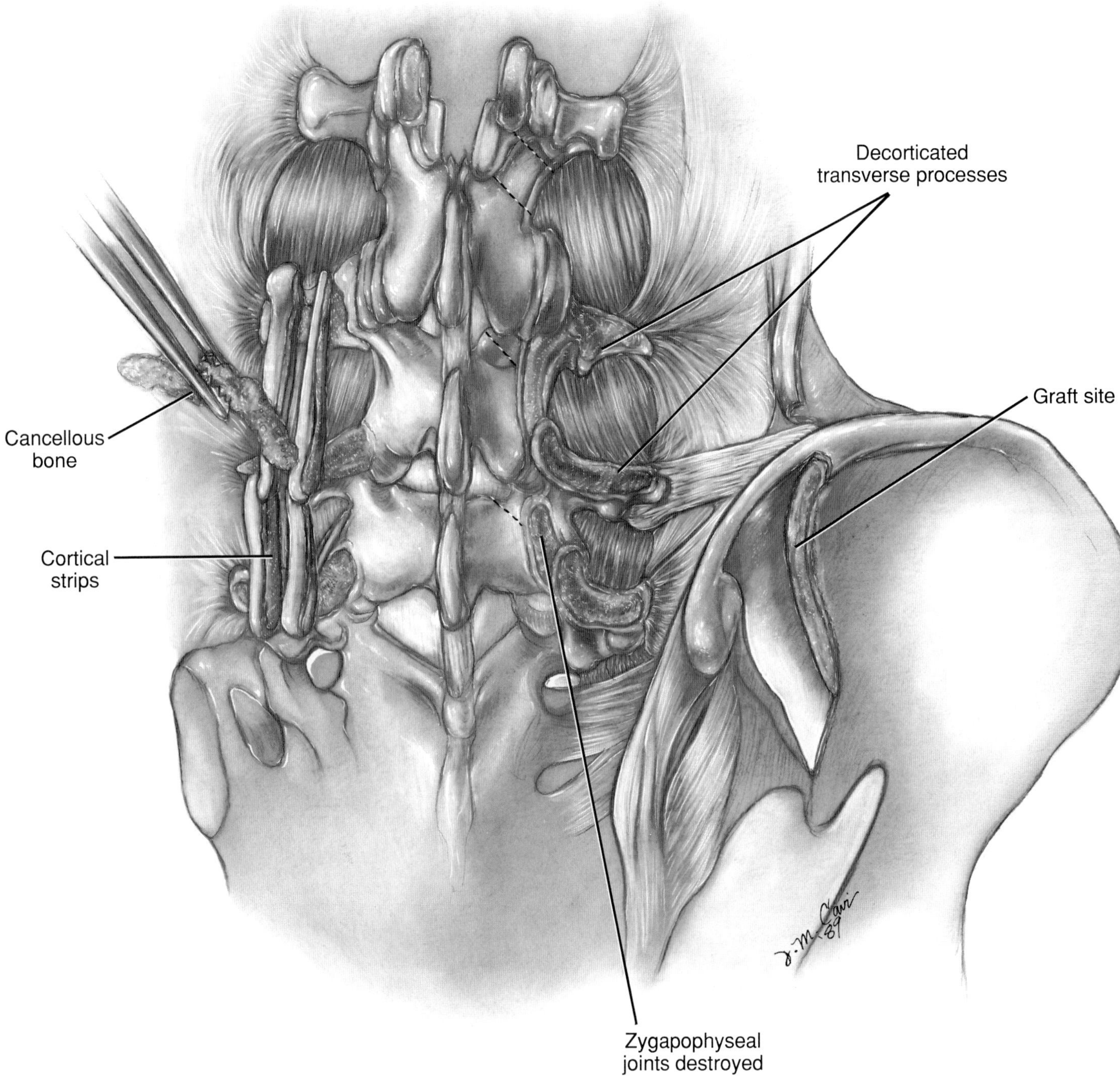
Decorticated
transverse processes
Graft site
Cancellous
bone
Cortical
strips
Zygapophyseal
joints destroyed

Figure 6.6.

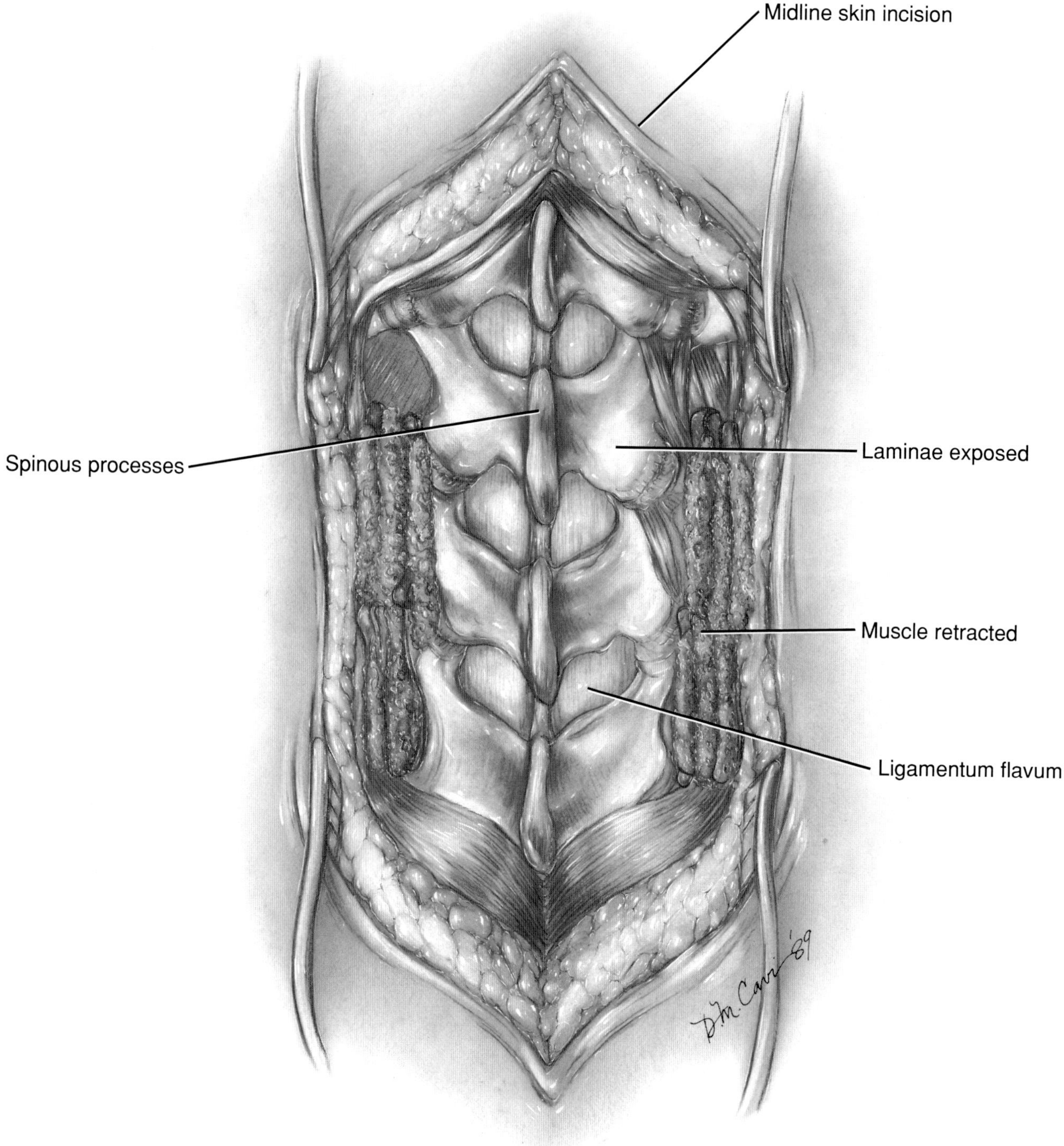
Midline skin incision
Spinous processes
Laminae exposed
Muscle retracted
Ligamentum flavum
D.M. Cavi '89

Figure 6.7.

7

Anterior Operations on Lumbar Spine

Transperitoneal Approach to Lumbosacral Junction Anterior L5-S1 Fusion for Spondylolisthesis and Instability

The transperitoneal approach to lumbosacral junction anterior L5-S1 fusion for spondylolisthesis and instability has enjoyed a reputation for technical difficulty and is held to be associated with unusual postoperative complications—especially retrograde ejaculation and functional sterility in males from disruption of the presacral sympathetic plexus by subperiosteal dissection anterior to L5-S1. Because the superior hypogastric plexus is situated directly anterior to the fifth lumbar vertebral body and intervertebral disc space, it is susceptible to injury in midline exposures of the lumbosacral spine from the front. However, a review of the literature and an informal poll of leading spinal surgeons yielded only 16 patients of many hundreds of procedures with documented sterility. Sterility has been overrated as a complication and is quite uncommon. Impotence is no more common after anterior spine fusion operations than after other procedures on the back.

Excessive bleeding from the retroperitoneal vessels can be avoided if the surgeon is aware of the anatomic variability of the lumbar retroperitoneal venous system. The incidence of variation from the accepted anterior relation of the great retroperitoneal veins to the two lower lumbar vertebrae is estimated, by cadaveric and in vitro study, to range between 50% and 32%.

Indications

Anterior approach and fusion of L5-S1 are indicated for (1) failed posterior fusion for spondylolisthesis, (2) a previously infected posterior approach, (3) L5-S1 instability evidenced by greater than 4-mm translational motion on flexion-extension radiographs, (4) L5-S1 instability with severe spina bifida or radical laminectomy with no lumbosacral posterior elements, and (5) greater than Meyerding grade II spondylolisthesis.

Technique

The patient is placed in the supine position on the operating table (Fig. 7.1). The patient should be placed with the crest of the ilium even with the flexion crease of the table, which allows for hyperextension of the lumbar spine to gain greater exposure.

The abdominal incision is a midline vertical incision that is paraumbilical (curving to the left), extending just proximal to the pubis to permit full exposure of the sacral promontory. A transverse abdominal incision is advocated by some as having a more cosmetic resultant scar; however, this incision requires transection of the rectus abdominis muscles.

For the midline approach, an incision is carried through the skin, subcutaneous fat, and tissue and through the relatively avascular linea alba of the rectus sheath. The bodies of the rectus abdominis muscle are bluntly separated by fingertip to expose the anterior peritoneum.

If a transverse incision is employed, the initial skin incision should run horizontally in a gently curving fashion between the anterior superior iliac spines, ending approximately 1 cm superior and 5 cm medial to each anterior superior iliac spine. The anterior portion of the rectus sheath is identified and then is opened transversely. The body of the rectus abdominis muscle is elevated and transected by using a diathermy technique. The posterior rectus sheath, fascia transversalis, and the peritoneum are conjoined posterior to the rectus muscle. The posterior rectus sheath and fascia are carefully dissected down to but not through the peritoneum.

The peritoneum is carefully elevated and opened the length of the incision, with care taken not to damage the intestinal viscera. A Foley catheter is mandatory to decompress the bladder, as the bladder is usually at the inferior extent of the peritoneal incision. The balloon of the Foley catheter can be palpated for orientation. The operating table is then placed on slight Trendelenburg position, and the peritoneal contents are then packed away.

The sacral promontory is palpated and the posterior peritoneum is identified, as well as the aortic bifurcation. The location of the L5-S1 intervertebral disc is usually 2–4 cm inferior to the aortic bifurcation. The retroperitoneum is infiltrated with normal saline and epinephrine solution to elevate the peritoneum off the important vascular structures. Bipolar cauterization of vessels is utilized. This helps prevent retrograde ejaculation, as the nerves and vessels supplying the hypogastric plexus can be preserved. The posterior peritoneum is incised along the left common iliac artery to its bifurcation and then parallel and medial to the left ureter.

Although there may be some hemorrhage encountered in this area, the use of electrocautery should be avoided anterior to L5-S1 to avoid damage to the sympathetic plexus. Any small vessels encountered may be ligated individually. An important point is to pass Silastic vessel loops around the aorta, iliac arteries and veins, and vena cava. This permits elevation of the great vessels and provides control of the vessels in the advent of an inadvertent tear—avoiding catastrophic hemorrhage.

At this point, the left common iliac vein is identified coursing underneath the aortic bifurcation crossing the anterior surface of the L5-S1 disc. By using gentle blunt dissection of the posterior peritoneum, the peritoneum is elevated from left to right across the left iliac vein and anterior surface of the L5-S1 intravertebral disc. The middle sacral artery and vein are now encountered and should be ligated and divided without tying off any branches of the hypogastric plexus. If cautery is to be used, bipolar is preferred to unipolar because of the greater control of the area of soft tissue affected by the spark gap.

Cobb elevators are used to dissect off any residual soft tissue remaining on the anterior surface of the disc, and four Steinmann pins can be inserted into the bodies of L5 and S1 for soft tissue retraction. Alternatively, Deaver-type retractors may be positioned for soft tissue retraction.

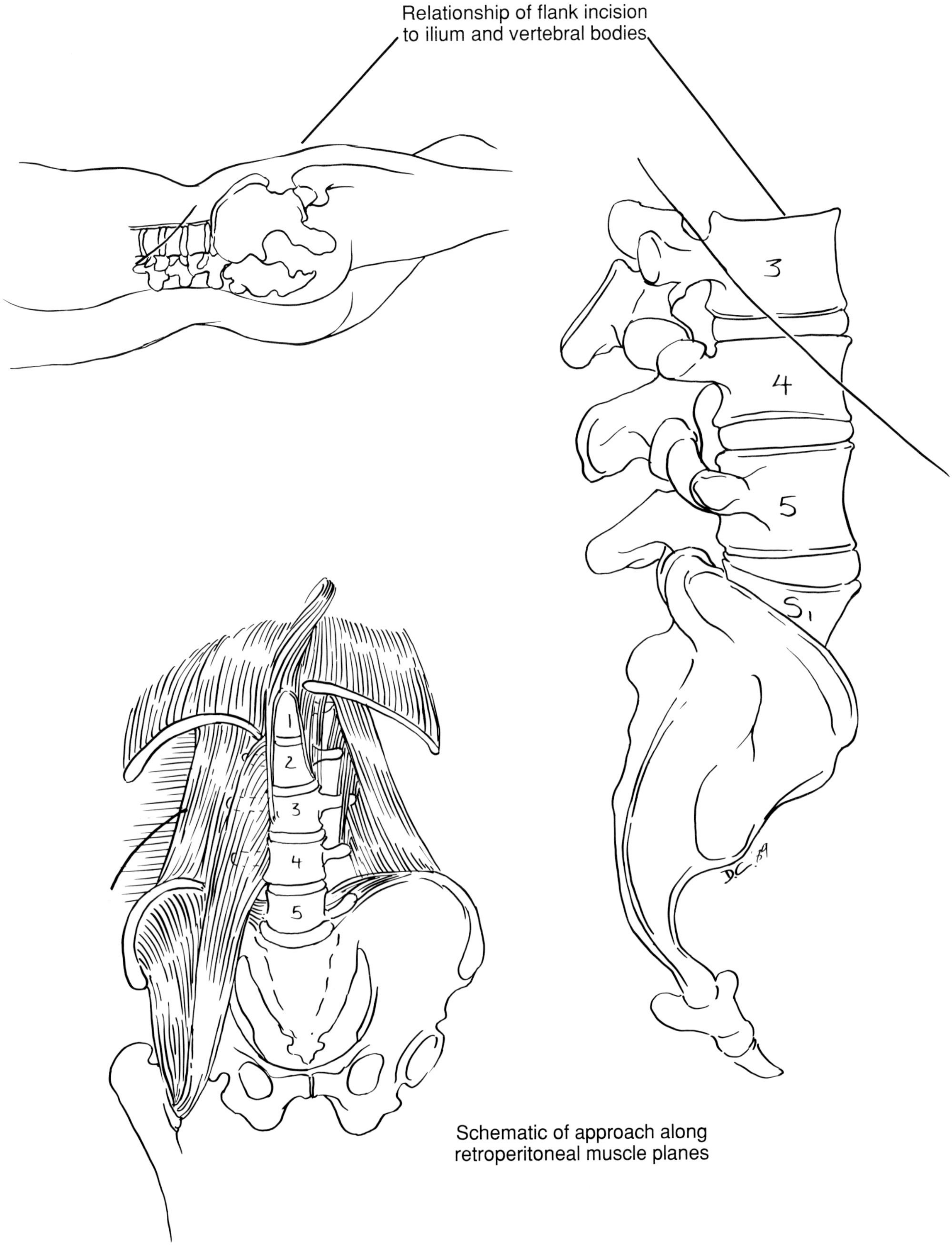
Relationship of flank incision
to ilium and vertebral bodies
3
4
5
S1
1
2
3
4
5
Schematic of approach along
retroperitoneal muscle planes

Figure 7.1.

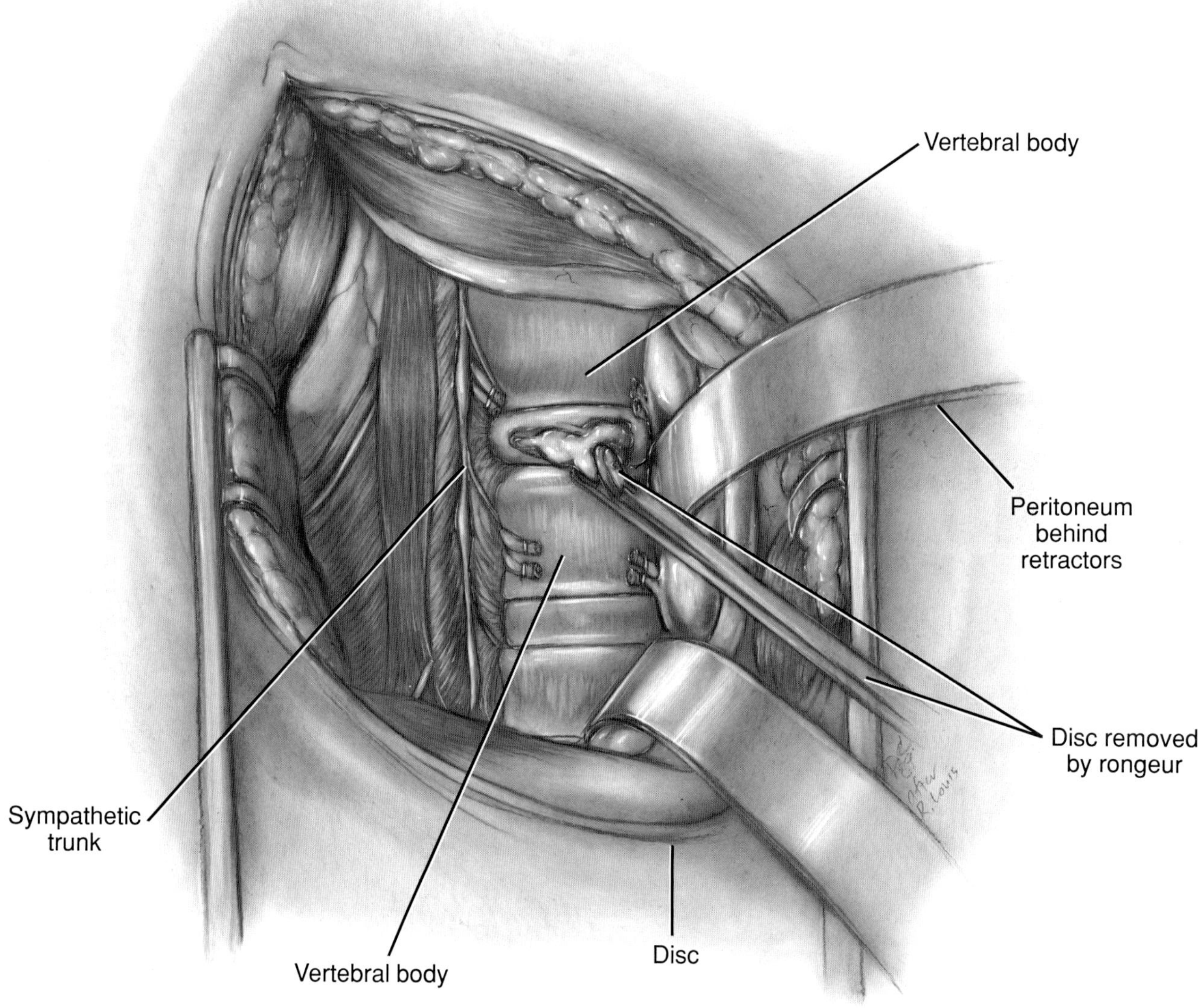

Figure 7.2. Lateral retroperitoneal exposure of vertebral column.

The disc level should be confirmed at this point by utilizing either intraoperative x-rays with a metallic marker or discography with a radiopaque dye.

The disc is excised with a #15 blade through a H-shaped incision in the annulus fibrosus. Anterior grafting or stabilization procedures can then be performed. Two segments of the tricortical iliac crest graft are harvested by using a powered oscillating saw. A malleable probe is fashioned to determine the appropriate height and depth of the graft.

For the average 75-kg man, these grafts measure 10–14 mm in height and 20–25 mm in depth. A horseshoe-shaped bone tamp is used to countersink each of the two grafts in place. The flaps of the H-shaped incision in the annulus fibrosus can be sutured with the grafts locked in place with heavy absorbable figure-of-8 stitches. A cross-table radiograph is taken at this point to document the position of the grafts. Any extension of the lumbar spine or operating table is corrected, which also helps to lock the grafts into position.

If additional exposure is required superiorly to reach the L4-L5 disc space, the level of the aortic bifurcation and any anatomic variation of the iliac veins will determine how the vessels can be retracted. This requires ligation of the left iliolumbar vein as it passes posterolaterally around the L4 vertebral body. The exposure is a fairly deep hole, and failure to ligate the left iliolumbar vein before retracting the left iliac vein has been reported to cause fatal hemorrhage.

The wound is closed in a layer-by-layer fashion, with care taken to reapproximate the posterior and the anterior peritoneum, the overlying anterior abdominal fascia, the subcutaneous tissue, and the skin.

Anterior Retroperitoneal Approach to Thoracolumbar Junction

The anterior retroperitoneal operative approach as described was originally developed to provide enhanced exposure of the kidney. It evolved from a costotransversectomy procedure in order to give better exposure with less tissue damage. This exposure provides an extraperitoneal approach to the anterior thoracolumbar junction and, as such, is useful for anterior decompression, tumor resection, anterior bone grafting, or anterior instrumentation from T11 to L4, although its major utility is for exposure of the upper lumbar spine (L1-L2). The lateral two thirds of the twelfth rib is resected subperiosteally; with the pleural cavity avoided, the anteriolateral abdominal musculature is divided. The major dissection takes advantage of the potential space behind the kidney between the renal fascia (Gerota's fascia) and the quadratus lumbar and psoas muscles. Retraction in this interval provides exposure of most of the lumbar vertebral bodies and sufficient working space for extension excision grafting and instrumentation.

One of the major complications of the retroperitoneal approach through the periosteal envelope of the twelfth rib is damage to the parietal pleura and inadvertent vilation of the thoracic cavity. The twelfth rib varies in length from 1.5 to 14 cm, with the average being most frequently between 11 and 14 cm. The pleura attaches to the undersurface of the posterior 6 cm of the rib and then extends anteriorly over the T11–T12 interspace for a distance of 10–11 cm from the midline. If a shorter twelfth rib is encountered, it should be considered to be covered with pleura for its entire length. There are two tricks to help prevent perforation of the pleura: studying maximum inspiration chest x-rays to locate the lowest extent of the pleura, and making longitudinal incision in the periosteum and inner aspects of the last rib sufficiently far out to be below the pleural reflection.

Technique

The patient is placed in the right lateral decubitus position with the left side up. The patient's twelfth rib is positioned over the break in the table, which can then be "jacknifed" and the table extended to provide increased working space between the thorax and the left iliac crest.

The skin is incised along the twelfth rib from the costotransverse junction to within 1 cm of the tip of the twelfth rib. The dissection is then carried through the subcutaneous tissue and the intervening muscle layers (latissimus dorsi and serratus) superficial to the rib. Care should be taken to keep the skin incision and subsequent deeper dissection directly in line with the curve of the rib. The dissection is then carried down through the periosteum. Care should be taken to avoid sliding off of the rib inferiorly and damaging the subcostal neurovascular bundle. The rib is dissected subperiosteally. The rib is disarticulated from its costotransverse attachment with a Cobb periosteal elevator and is cut at the costotransverse junction. Elevate the rib with a bone clamp, and dissect the rib free from the rib bed from posterior to anterior. Remember that the diaphragm is attached to the superior edge of the twelfth rib. The tissue at the tip is then gently split while the rib is being elevated and then dissected free, again with care taken to avoid violating the parietal pleura or diaphragm.

In the periosteal bed from which the rib has been dissected, note the transverse abdominal musculature inferiorly and the diaphragmatic insertion superiorly. Gently retract the diaphragmatic insertion cephalad and the abdominal musculature cauda. A thin layer of the retroperitoneal spare fat should be identified. This is carefully opened with Metzenbaum scissors in a gentle cutting and spreading fashion until the peritoneum is noted. Bluntly dissect the peritoneum from the undersurface of the abdominal wall.

The incision is extended through the external oblique and internal oblique muscular layers by using electrocautery. At this point, identify the transverse abdominal musculature. This muscle layer is gently spread to expose the transversalis fascia. The peritoneum is retracted anteriorly, and the retroperitoneal space is revealed. The transversalis fascia is then bluntly dissected from the left psoas muscle. The posterior renal fascia, perinephric fat, left kidney, and peritoneal contents are retracted anteriorly with a large abdominal pad. This maneuver exposes the left crus of the diaphragm and the origin of the left psoas muscle and facilitates ligation of the segmental vertebral vessels. With the kidney retracted forward, identify the ureter on the undersurface of the peritoneum. The ureter needs to be dissected out and is retracted with the peritoneum. A Finochietto rib retractor is placed between the eleventh rib and the iliac crest.

Palpate the spine to find the soft prominent disc spaces. The overlying retroperitoneal soft tissue over the intravertebral disc is bluntly spread. Excess bleeding is avoided by staying on the surface of the disc and not on the vertebral body where the intercostal vessels are located. The aorta can be mobilized anteriorly and protected with a malleable retractor. Then, by using meticulous subperiosteal dissection, the crus of the diaphragm superiorly and the psoas muscle inferiorly can be elevated off, exposing the first lumbar vertebral body. If the vertebral body must be removed, it is advisable to remove the T12-L1 and L1-L2 intervertebral discs first—to clearly establish the limits of the dissection—and then remove the vertebral body in piecemeal fashion. The graft is applied as described in Chapter 6. The wound is closed by reapproximating the rib bed and then closing each abdominal muscle layer in turn.

Anterior Approach for Metastatic Spinal Disease

Exposures for the treatment of metastatic spinal disease are the same as those required for fracture. The goals are the same, and the only difference is in the way the bony injury is treated. Once the mass is identified and circumscribed, it should be removed as expeditiously as possible with the technique that ensures the best hemostasis. The ultrasonic dissector is an excellent way to remove metastatic tumor. En bloc resection often is not possible and rarely is curative. It is important to achieve a gross total removal so that local recurrence is not as likely and adequate spinal cord decompression is ensured. Many tumors can be removed by suction. Piecemeal excision is also feasible. A Cavitron allows precise tumor removal with considerable control. Tumor should be removed until all of the involved bone is gone and there are adequate surfaces for purchase in all directions where the graft or prosthesis will be placed. The neural structures must be completely decompressed. This usually means seeing the dura throughout the length of the bony resection. Only rarely is the dura actually involved with tumor. Hemostasis is obtained by the application of hemostatics until it is dry enough that the graft can be placed. Then the graft or prosthesis is fitted in the same manner described for fracture.

8

Operative Technique for Luque Segmental Spinal Instrumentation for Neuromuscular Scoliosis

Neuromuscular scoliosis presents a great challenge to the spine surgeon. Neuromuscular curves, long and sweeping, usually involve more levels than idiopathic curves. Pelvic obliquity is often an associated problem. Bracing is usually inadequate and surgery is often required. This involves long fusions in osteoporotic bone with often-uncooperative patients. Respiratory compromise, mental retardation, seizure disorders, and the need for prolonged immobilization contribute to these difficulties. Blood loss and complication rates have generally been higher with neuromuscular spinal deformity. Rigid internal fixation and fusion using segmental spinal instrumentation with Luque rods provide a solution to many of these problems. Biomechanical studies have shown segmental spinal instrumentation, with its multiple fixation points, to have a clear mechanical advantage over traditional instrumentation in providing and maintaining correction in the three-dimensional deformities of scoliosis.

The goals of surgery in neuromuscular scoliosis are stability and balance; these are accomplished by achieving a level pelvis with a well-balanced spine above it. With segmental spinal instrumentation this maximum safe correction can be obtained and held while arthrodesis takes place. The instrumented portion of the spine is secured by sublaminar wires at each vertebral level to smooth rods that lie at the base of the spinous process on either side of the spine. The spine will fracture above or below the area of Luque segmental instrumentation before the implant will fail. This strength allows immediate mobility without casting, which results in improved balance, pulmonary toilet, and bowel and bladder habits and facilitates postoperative care. Indicative for segmental instrumentation is progressive deformity secondary to a neuromuscular disorder with osteopenic bone, seizure disorder, and lack of patient compliance. This group has a high risk of traditional instrumentation failure.

The principles used in selecting the length of spinal fusion in Harrington instrumentation are applicable to segmental instrumentation. In general, fusion should extend from neutral vertebra to neutral vertebra and include the pelvis when obliquity is a problem. Patients without moderate spine flexibility should not be considered for posterior surgery alone. Preoperative evaluation should include forced bending and bending radiographs—when a residual curve persists, no attempt is made to gain a full correction. Prior to surgery a template to the corrected curves is fashioned with a malleable rod and via both anteroposterior and lateral radiographs. Pulmonary preparation including pulmonary function studies, arterial blood gases, and incentive spirometry instruction is important.

Following satisfactory endotracheal anesthesia, the patient is placed in the prone position on the Hall frame, with the anterior abdominal wall allowed to clear the table. Careful padding and inspection of anterior soft tissue and bony prominences are carried out (Fig. 8.1). A straight midline incision is used, and dissection is carried out to the spinous processes with the electrocautery, staying in the avascular fibrous intermuscular tissue. If present, the spinous process apophyses are split longitudinally and dissected to either side. Subperiosteal dissection using the Cobb elevator is performed to remove the paraspinal muscles. Electrocautery is used for meticulous control of bleeding. Self-retaining retractors are used to keep the wound open as dissection is carried out subperiosteally onto the laminae and laterally to the facet joints. All soft tissue is removed with curettes and rongeurs (Fig. 8.2). Tendinous attachments of the short rotators to the laminae are detached with the electrocautery. There are many methods of identifying spinal levels; most investigators believe an intraoperative radiograph should be used in each case. During the first pass of dissection, which is carried out distally to proximally on one side at a time (surgeon with Cobb elevator, assistant with cautery), stripping subperiosteally is carried only to the facet joints to reduce blood loss. Following instrumentation, dissection is continued to the tips of the transverse processes. The facet joints are cleared with curettes and rongeurs—all ligamentous and capsular attachments should be removed (Fig. 8.2). Sponge packing to control bleeding is used as the spine is progressively cleared.

The ligamentum flavum is then excised in the following manner: (1) the midline cleavage is exposed, (2) the ligamentum is freed from tissues within the canal, and (3) the ligamentum is finally excised (Fig. 8.3). A rongeur is used to excise the tissue between the spinous processes and expose the midline cleavage of the ligamentum. In the thoracic spine, some bone must be cut due to the inferior slant of the spinous processes. This is done with the rongeur held perpendicular over the interlaminar space, with as much bone as possible preserved. At this point, a Penfield dissector is inserted in the midline and passed deep to the ligamentum, freeing it from tissues within the neural canal. A gentle touch is required. While this maneuver is performed at one level, the rongeur should be used by the assistant to expose the ligament at the next level. Once all the levels are cleared, each surgeon uses a Kerrison punch or Leksell rongeur to excise the ligament level by level. Following completion of excision at each level, Gelfoam is placed to protect neural structures and to control bleeding. The ligamentum must be removed quickly and carefully at each level of fusion.

Once this exposure is completed, the 16-gauge sublaminar wires can be passed by the the surgeon and first assistant while a second surgeon prepares the 3/16

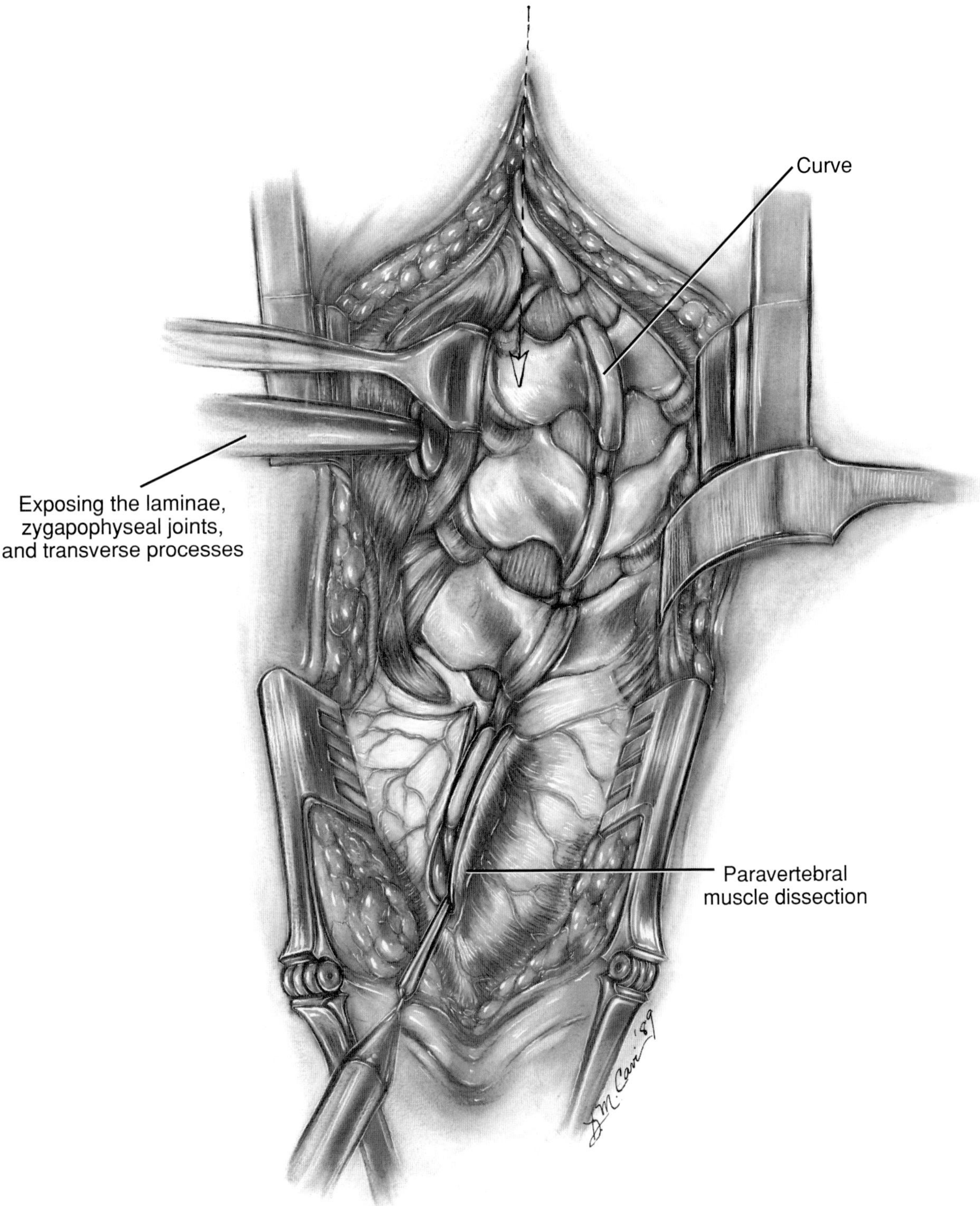
Curve
Exposing the laminae,
zygapophyseal joints,
and transverse processes
Paravertebral
muscle dissection
D.M. Corri '89

Figure 8.1.

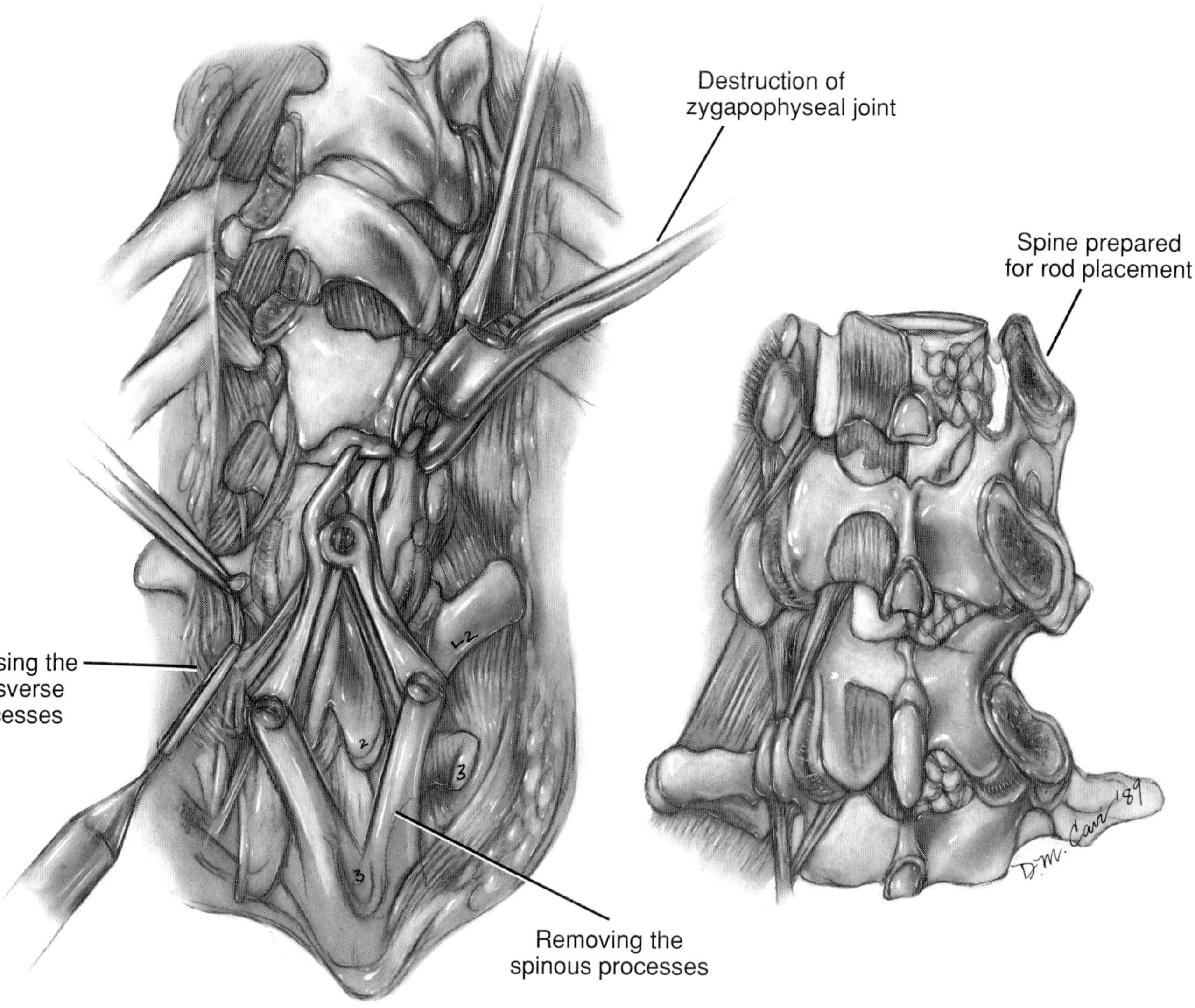

Figure 8.2.

rod (or ¼-inch rods in larger patients), using rod benders and the template that was prepared preoperatively (Fig. 8.4).

The 16-gauge wire should be cut in 50-cm lengths and folded in half—the area at the hairpin bend should be left open slightly to permit grasping with a clamp and should be shaped into an "S" configuration with smooth curves. The wires are inserted level by level from cephalad to caudad in the following manner (Fig. 8.5). The tip is placed into the removal canal at the inferior edge of the lamina in the midline and is advanced cephalad 5–7 mm, so that it clears the sublaminar origin of the ligamentum flavum. The curve then allows the wire to be rolled with a needle holder so that the tip emerges above the lamina. Tension must be kept on the tails to keep the wires pressed against the underside of the lamina. The assistant then places a clamp through the emerging hairpin loop, and the wire can be pulled through halfway, again with tension maintained to avoid push-

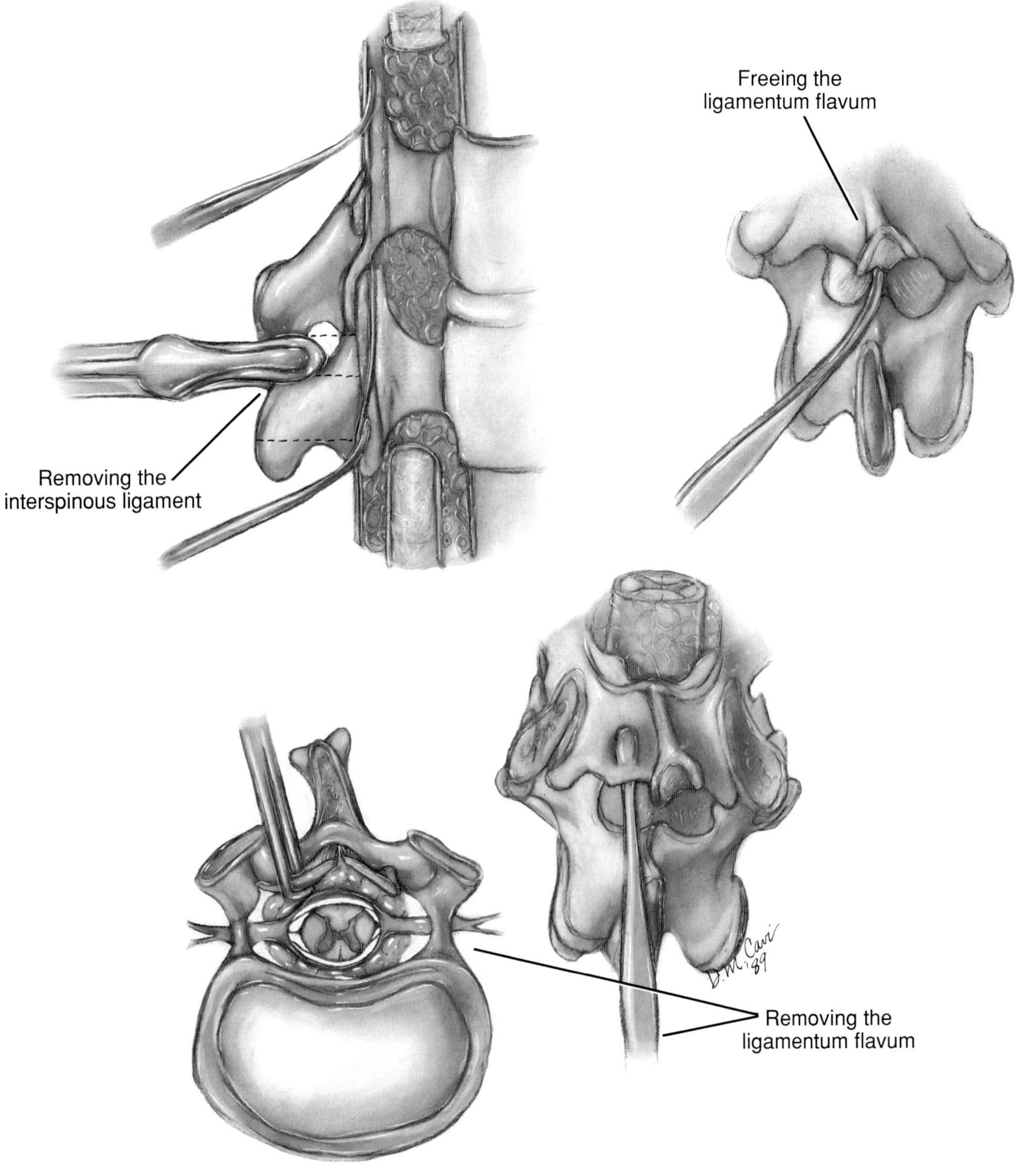
Freeing the
ligamentum flavum
Removing the
interspinous ligament
Removing the
ligamentum flavum

Figure 8.3.

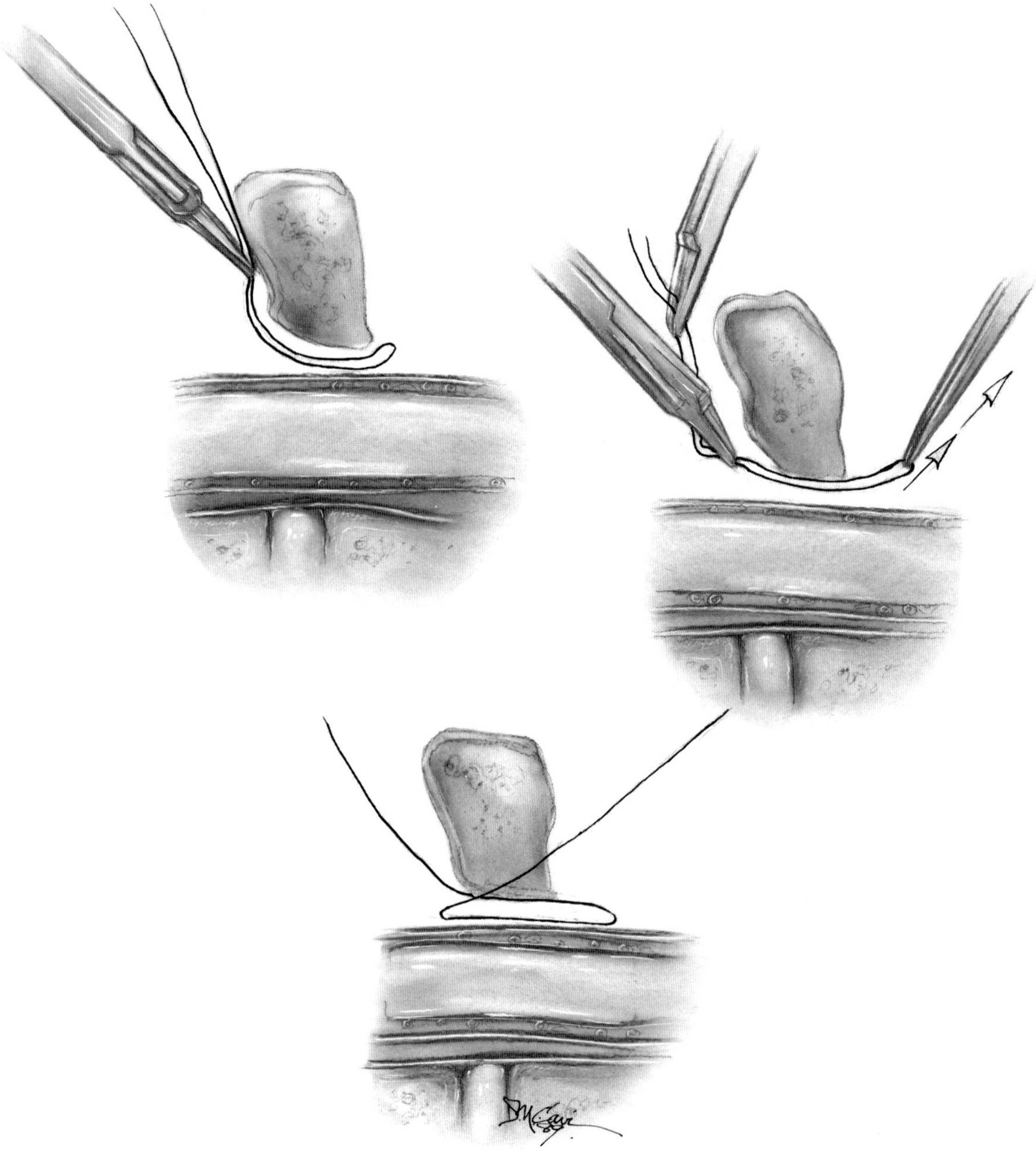

Figure 8.4. Passing the sublaminar wires.

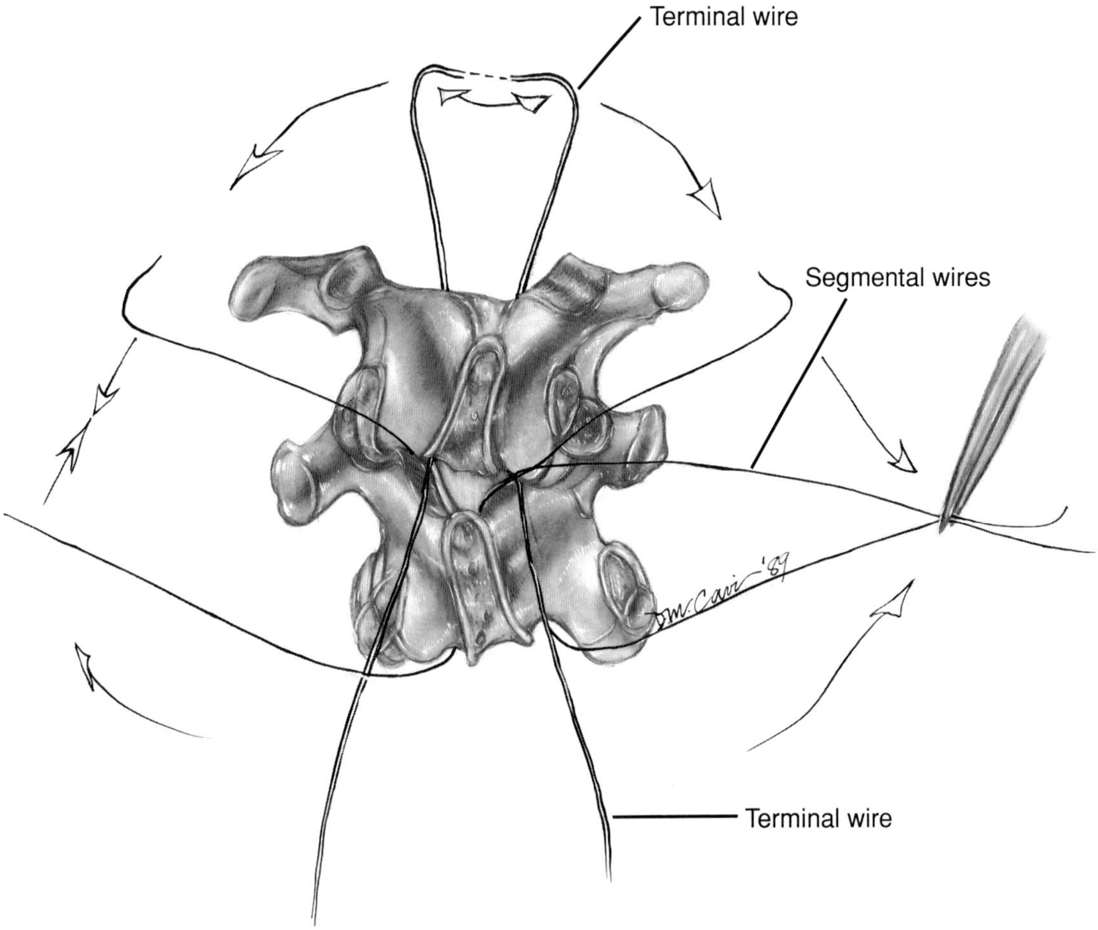

Figure 8.5. Wire placement.

ing the wires into the canal. Crimping the wires superiorly and inferiorly over the posterior portion of each lamina prevents their exerting pressure on the neural canal. All the wires are passed before they are attached to the rods, so great care must be taken not to push or dislodge the wires anteriorly. As the wires are placed, they are secured by hemostats shod with rubber tubing. These hemostats are then joined with a long clamp placed through their handles.

While the wires are being placed, the smooth 3⁄16 rods can be bent to fit the template that was prepared preoperatively (Fig. 8.6). Remember to incorporate the secondary spinal contours into these rods and include lumbar lordosis and thoracic kyphosis where indicated. The planes of these contours must be kept the same and should be orthogonal to the scoliotic contours. To add these contours, add torsional stress to the rods, and this stress will tend to rotate the short "L" limb of the rod. This rotational force should be kept in a posterior direction so that the short "L" limb will not rotate into the neural canal. This can be accomplished in two ways. First, it should be noted that the long limb of the rod will tend to rotate into the curve of the spinal column, so that less lateral correction is obtained. Second, if the long limb of one rod overlies the short "L" limb of the other rod, any posterior rotational force of the short "L" limb can be shared by the long limb of the other rod. Therefore, by offsetting the secondary contours approximately 20–30° away from the concave side of the scoliotic

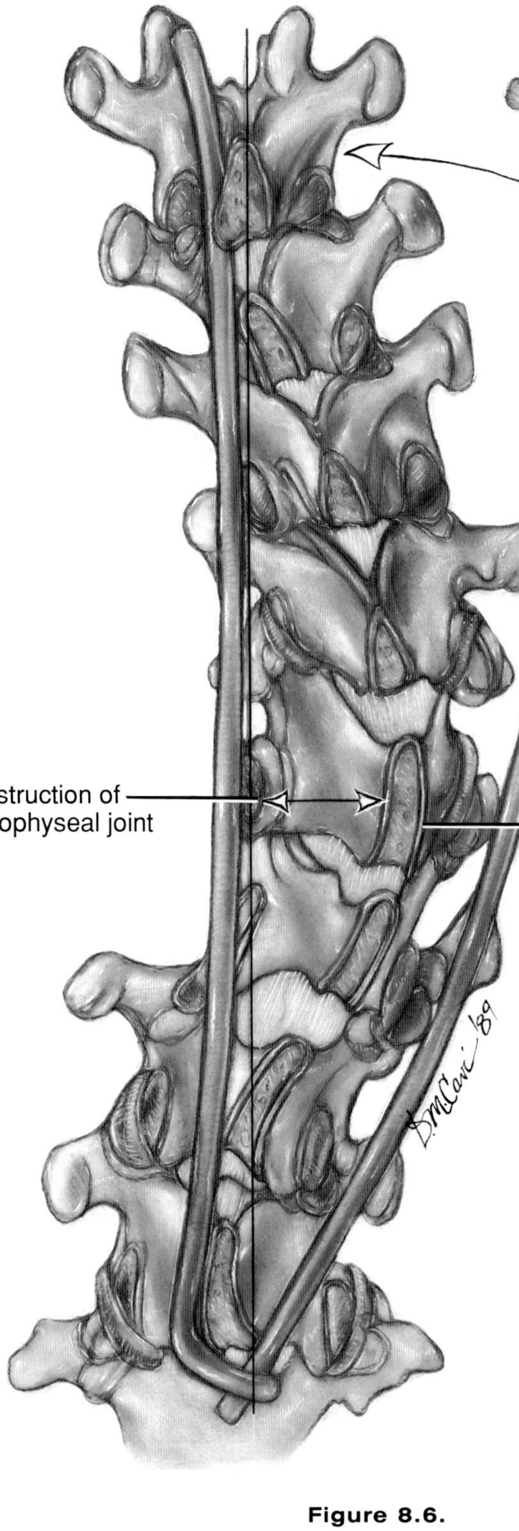
Rods are bent
to conform to curve
Destruction of
zygapophyseal joint
Removal of
spinous process

Figure 8.6.

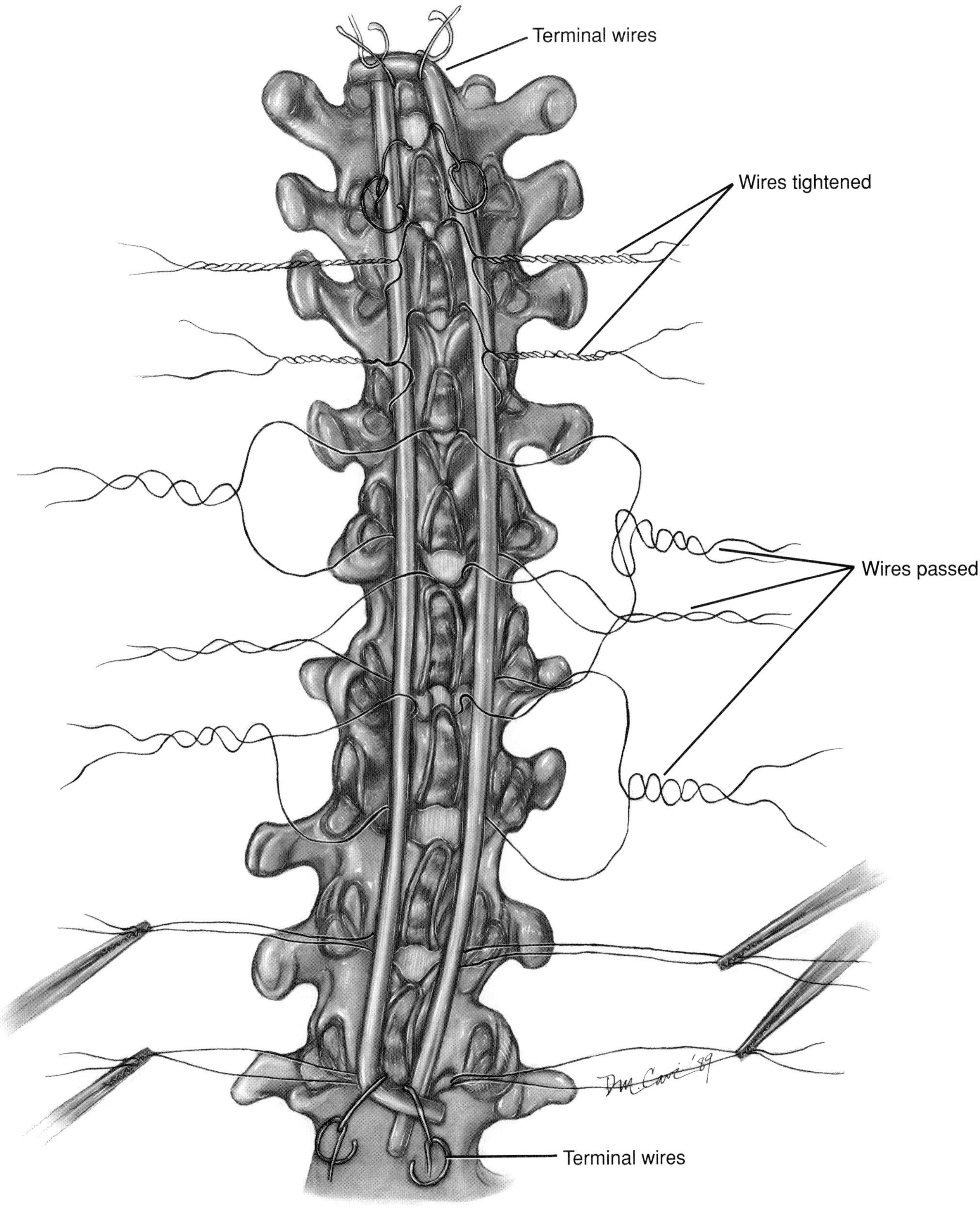
Terminal wires
Wires tightened
Wires passed
Terminal wires

Figure 8.7.

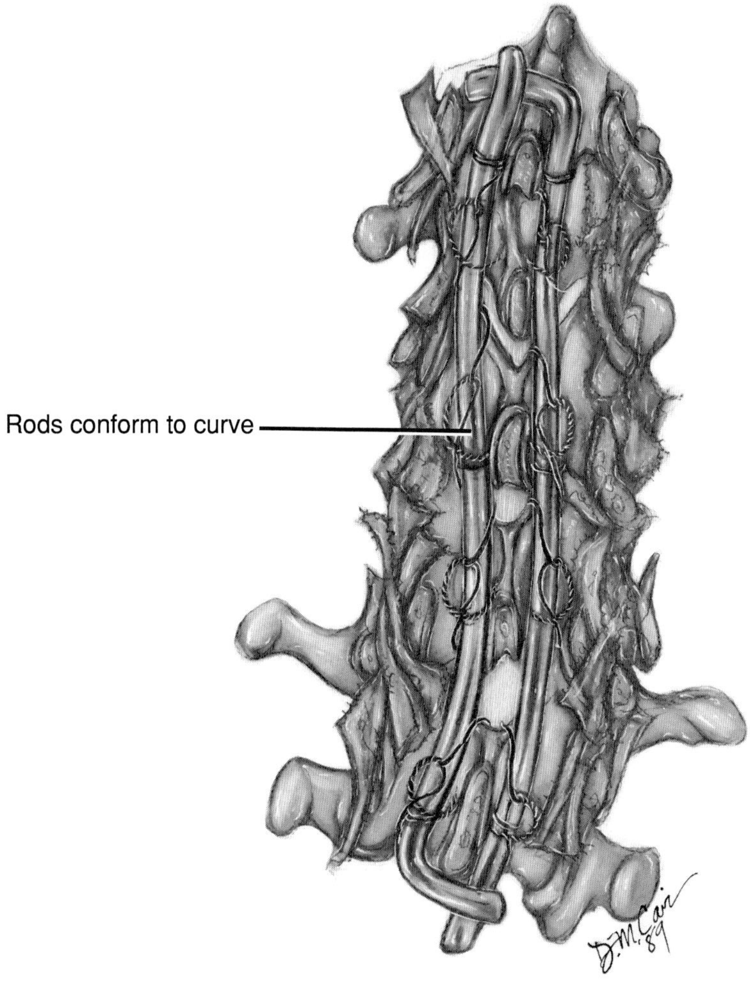

Figure 8.8. Luque system in place.

curve and by making sure that the long limb of one rod overlies the short limb of the other, torsional stress can be distributed over the entire construction.

Once the wires are placed, the rods are prebent, and complete facetectomies are performed, rod insertion can begin (Fig. 8.7). The hairpin bend is cut from each sublaminar wire, and the two wires are separated—one to the right side and one to the left side of each lamina. For thoracic curves the initial rod is placed on the convex side of the curve, and for lumbar curves the initial rod is placed on the concave side of the curve. In the thoracic spine, the short "L" limb is placed superiorly for the initially inserted rod. The wires are tightened sequentially with a jet wire tightener as the rod is levered to the spine. In the lumbar spine, the initial rod is placed with the short "L" limb below the spinous process of the lowermost vertebra to be instrumented. When the rod is to be fused to the pelvis for obliquity, the intraosseous pelvic portion of the rod is placed first. Wires are sequentially tightened while an assistant effects manual correction. Counterforces should approximate the rod and the spine so that the wires only maintain correction and are not fatigued by being used to achieve correction. In lumbar curves, to prevent rod rotation, the short "L" limb may need to be temporarily secured on the convex side of the deformity (with a single wire), especially if lumbar lordosis is prebent into the rods.

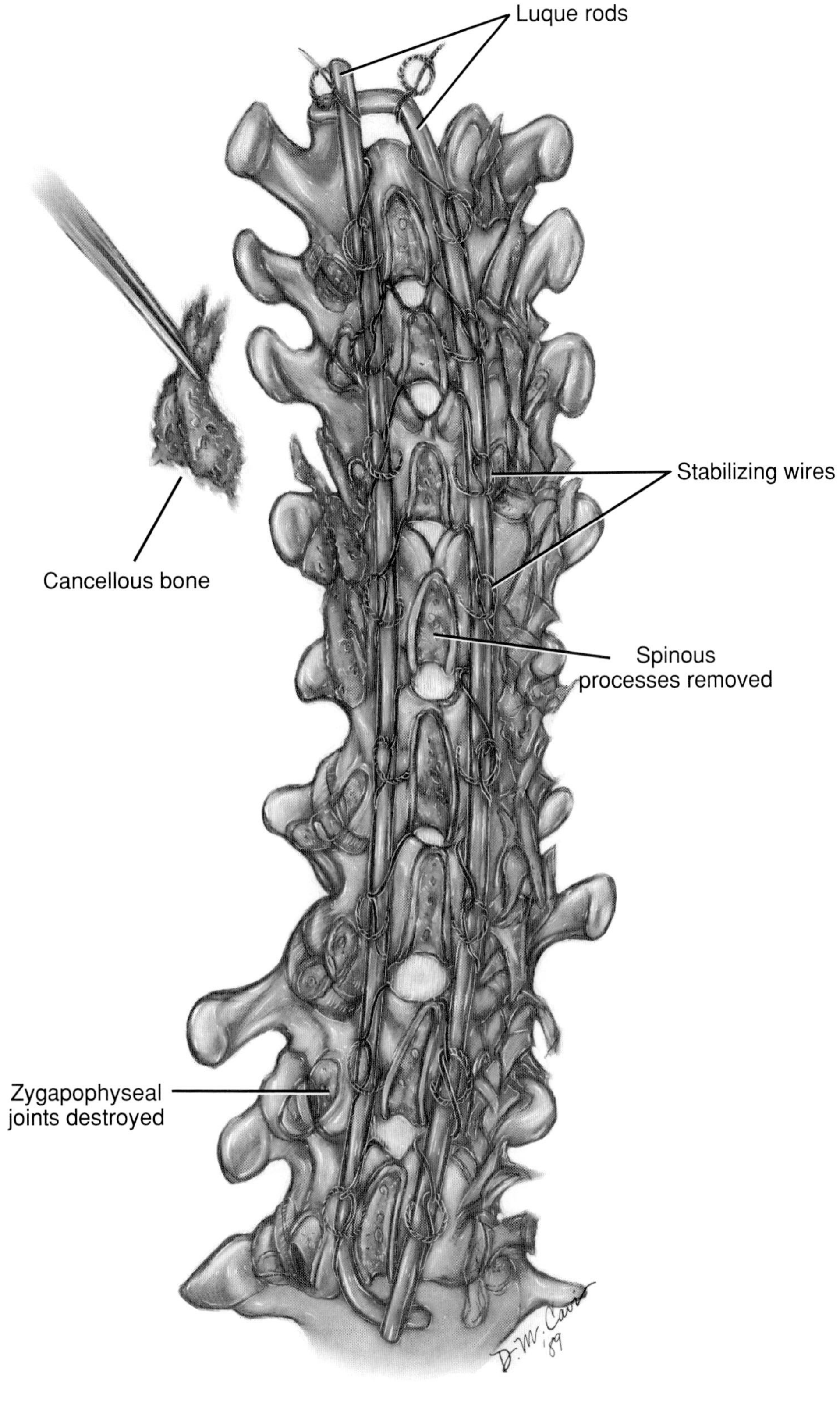
Luque rods
Stabilizing wires
Cancellous bone
Spinous
processes removed
Zygapophyseal
joints destroyed
D.M. Cain '89

Figure 8.9.

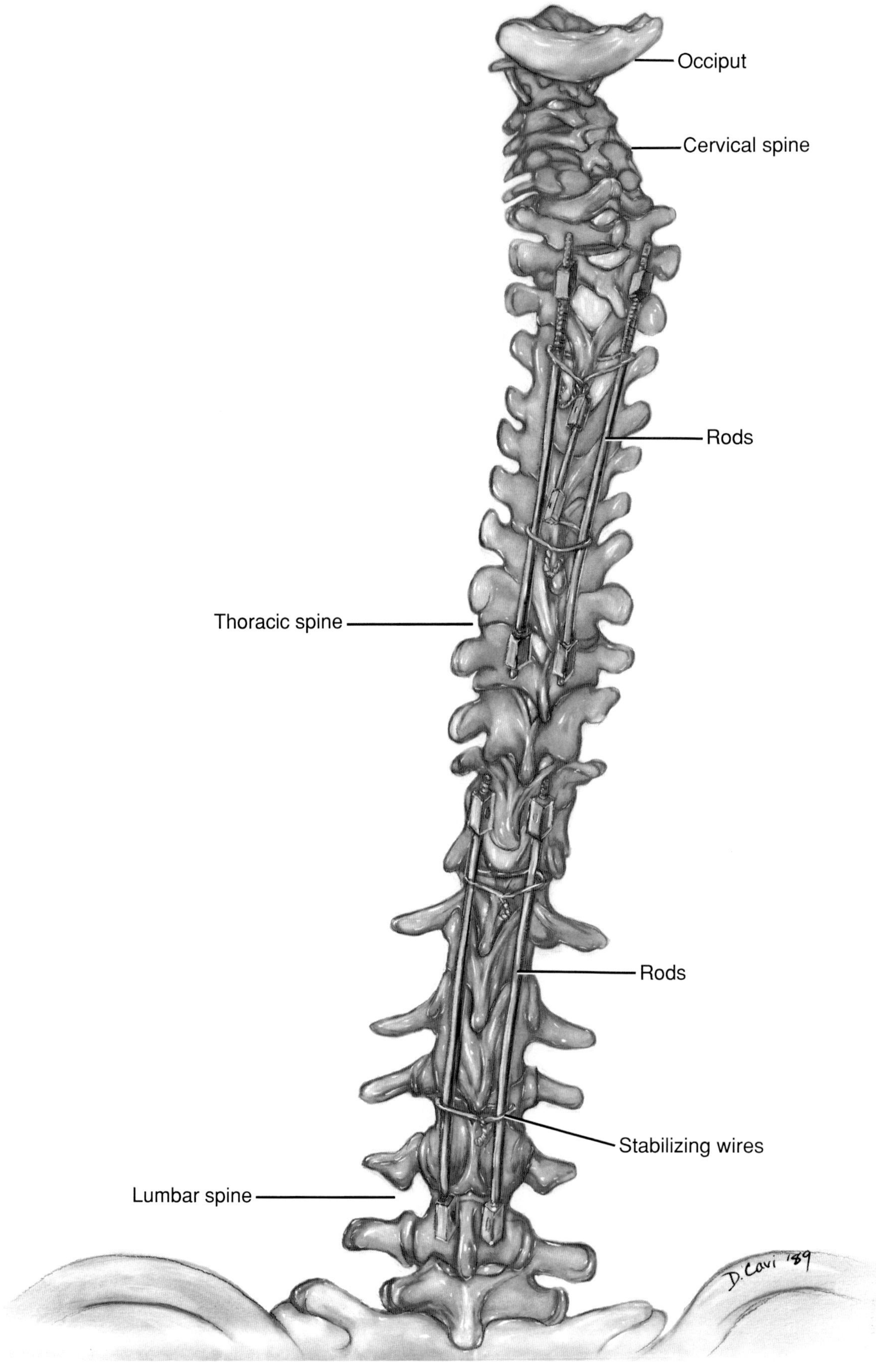
Occiput
Cervical spine
Rods
Thoracic spine
Rods
Stabilizing wires
Lumbar spine
D. Cavi '89

Figure 8.10.

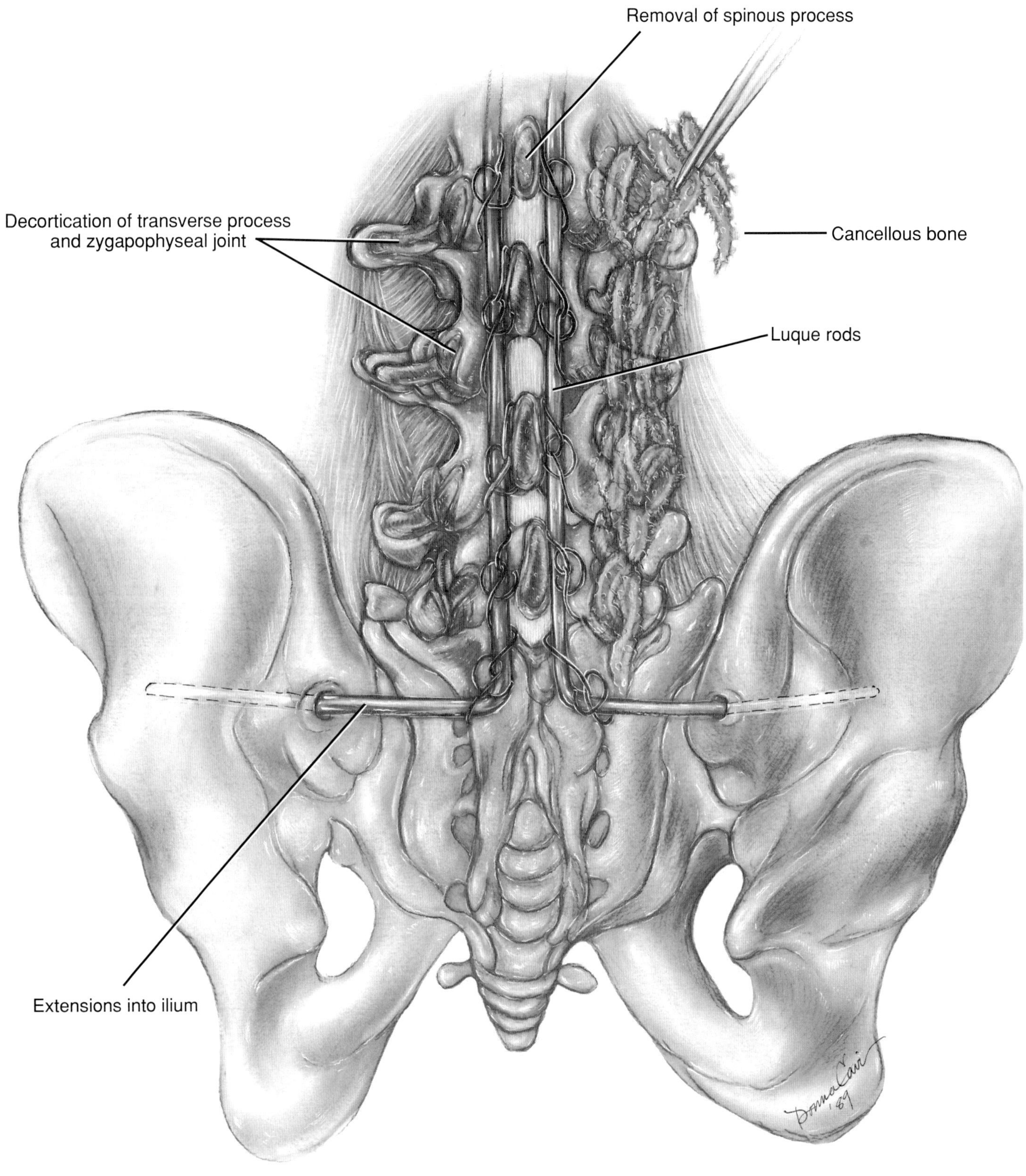
Removal of spinous process
Decortication of transverse process
and zygapophyseal joint
Cancellous bone
Luque rods
Extensions into ilium

Figure 8.11.

The wires should be tightened with their superior portion passing medial to the rod and their inferior portion passing lateral to the rod. If the inferior portion of the wire is passed medial at a point where part of the spinous process is removed during the exposure, it could lay up against cancellous bone and cut through during tightening. Supramedially and inferolaterally the wires are kept over good edges of cortical bone. However, this arrangement is reversed for the double wires at the "L" limbs of the rods both cephalad and caudad, to gain a more secure fixation of the rods.

After rods are placed and secured on both sides of the spine, coupling wires are placed between the two rods in each third of their length (Fig. 8.8). When these are tightened, they will approximate the rods to the midline at the base of the spinous processes. This position ensures maximum rigidity. Following this, the wires are retightened at each level and cut to a 1-cm length. They are then bent toward the midline and caudally to keep them away from the area of fusion. The end wires that are under more stress will tend to stick straight out from the rods, becoming more prominent and irritating. To avoid this, they may be cut long, bent longitudinally to overlie the rods, and incorporated underneath the above-mentioned interrod wires. This will secure them to the rods (Figs. 8.9 and 8.10).

Pelvic fixation is necessary when there is obliquity, and this can be obtained by placing the "L" ends of the rods into each ilium in the following manner. The best position is intraosseously along the transverse bar of the ilium (Fig. 8.11). This allows a long lever arm and permits harvesting of posterior iliac crest bone graft in the usual manner. Both iliac crests are exposed from the midline, and the gluteal musculature must be elevated to access the sciatic notches. The sacrum must also be cleared by elevating the musculature subperiosteally from the midline. The entrance point for the rod is identified just posterior to the sacroiliac joint at the level of the posterior superior iliac spine. A pin the same size as the rod is placed at this point and advanced slowly with a mallet. The surgeon keeps one finger in the sciatic notch and guides the pin superior to the notch and intracortical in the ilium. The pin should advance 6–9 cm and is left in place to be used as a guide in bending the rod. Two bends need to be made—one at the point where the rod will exit the bone (to approximate the rod to the surface of the sacrum) and a second at the point where it reaches the sacral spinous process at the midline and runs up the spinal column. It is easier to make the second bend first, and this is made after measuring the distance from the midline to the bone entry point and adding it to the intracortical length. The bend is made this distance from the end of the rod. The other bend is then made to allow the rod to be parallel to the posterior sacrum where it emerges from the ilium. No short "L" limbs are needed at the cephalad end of the instrumentation when pelvic fixation is used, as rotational forces will be taken up by the intrapelvic portion of the rods. Spinal contours and lateral deviations are bent into the rods. The rods are inserted first into the ilium, and then segmental wires are tightened in caudad to cephalad progression. The rods are secured and the wires are cut as described above (Fig. 8.9).

The remaining lateral gutter and transverse processes are then decorticated, and after copious irrigation, iliac crest bone graft is applied. Closure is performed in the standard fashion. Spinal cord monitoring is used intraoperatively.

Postoperatively, routine medical care is performed with the patients at bedrest. Pulmonary toilet is stressed. The patients may gradually advance activity and begin sitting and/or walking at approximately 1 week postoperatively. No cast or orthosis is necessary, but patients are restricted from heavy activity for 8–12 months. Follow-up care is otherwise similar to that for other types of spinal instrumentation.

SECTION 3

Cervical Disc and Related Problems

9

Cervical Hemilaminectomy and Foraminotomy for Spondylosis and Herniated Disc

The posterior approach to the cervical disc or spur is useful for patients with radicular symptoms or for spondylotic myeloradiculopathy. The operations may be carried out with the patient in the prone or the sitting position. Single-level foraminotomy can be performed with the patient under local anesthesia, but a general anesthetic is preferred by most surgeons. The critical factor in the cervical region is identification of the appropriate interspace. The most reliable landmark is the large posterior process of C2, so that when this is exposed in decompressive laminectomy, there is no question about the level of the bone removal. When only a single space is to be exposed, the skin incision is too small to allow C2 to be identified. Then, the most reliable anatomical guide is the x-ray appearance of the cervical spine. The first bifid spine can be identified on the anteroposterior x-ray and utilized to identify the appropriate interspace. If there is any question at the time of operation, a lateral spine film may be obtained to verify localization.

Posterior Operation for Cervical Disc

A skin incision 1–2 inches in length is made at the appropriate location in the midline and carried to the spinous processes. The approach must be exactly in the midline, and if it is, very little bleeding will ensue and the muscles will not be disturbed except in anatomical planes. Self-retaining retractors are put in place, exposing the spinous processes, and the appropriate level is defined. With a #15 knife or a small electric knife, the cervical musculature and ligamentous attachments are cut away from the spinous processes above and below the space to be exposed. Square cervical osteotomes are then utilized to perform the subperiosteal dissection of muscles from the spines and laminae. The ligamentous attachments to the bifid spines are such that the smooth subperiosteal removal possible in the lumbar and thoracic regions is not as possible here. As soon as the dissection down the spine is begun, a clearly defined plane of areolar tissue should be found, and the remainder of the muscular dissection should be bloodless. Staying in the proper muscular plane will greatly reduce postoperative pain for the patient. The interspace is exposed by a self-retaining retractor placed immediately adjacent to the zygapophyseal joint. The retractors with a single post, to be placed between the spinous processes, and a broad flat-toothed blade, to retract the paravertebral muscles, are excellent. With the retractor in place, the interspace should be identified to the lateral margins of the zygapophyseal joint. With a small rongeur, a partial hemilaminectomy of the laminae above the space to be explored should be carried out. The hemilaminectomy is quite small and, medially, need not be beyond the exit of the dural sheath around the root. A few millimeters of medial dura are all that needs to be exposed. An equally small hemilaminectomy is carried out below until the dura is exposed medial to just above and just below the exit of the root sheath. The procedure is then carried laterally, removing laminae until the root is clearly identified. If the foramen is not completely filled with herniated disc material, small angled cervical punches are satisfactory. If the root is tight at all, a high-speed drill is preferable. A curette is also a reasonable alternative. Be careful not to allow the footplate of the curette to be tilted down onto the root during the curettage. The curetting should be carried out on the upper and lower margins from medial to lateral so that any slip is out and away from the cord. The size of the foraminotomy is dependent on the tightness of the root. If the problem is a hard spur and no soft free fragment disc is likely to be present, then a generous foraminotomy is all that is required. This should be carried out over at least half the zygapophyseal joint. The lateral distance of the foraminotomy can be judged by the computed tomography (CT) appearance of the spur. Decompression of the root and the adequacy of the foraminotomy can be judged by inserting a fine probe out, to be certain there is room for the root in the remaining foramen. Some surgeons prefer to leave the ligament intact, further reducing the risk of nerve injury during foraminotomy. It also is reasonable to remove the ligament to allow thorough exploration of the root. Before CT imaging, when it was sometimes difficult to differentiate a herniated disc from a bony spur, exploration of the root was an important part of the procedure. Now that the difference can be virtually certain, further exposure of the root can be halted. The foraminotomy should be generous enough to be certain that it is beyond the margins of the root above and below and far enough lateral to allow free mobility of the root between the edge of the foraminotomy and the spur.

Cervical Disc Herniation

If a disc fragment is expected, then a slightly different technique is employed. The procedure including the foraminotomy is the same, but the disc fragment must be excised. When the foraminotomy is complete, the ligamentum flavum is incised over the existing root sheath parallel to it and removed. This allows the upper and lower margins of the root and the junction of the root sheath with the dural sac to be identified. The root should then be carefully palpated to determine the location of the mass. The approach to the disc fragment should be from the direction where mobilization of the root is least traumatic. Remember that anterior and posterior roots are often in what are virtually separate dural sheaths and it is easy to retract the upper root, see a glistening white structure beneath, assume it is the bulging posterior ligament, and incise it only to find that the anterior root has been cut. Be certain that the entire root is mobilized adequately before any incision is made. If possible, approach the root from the superior surface, since the

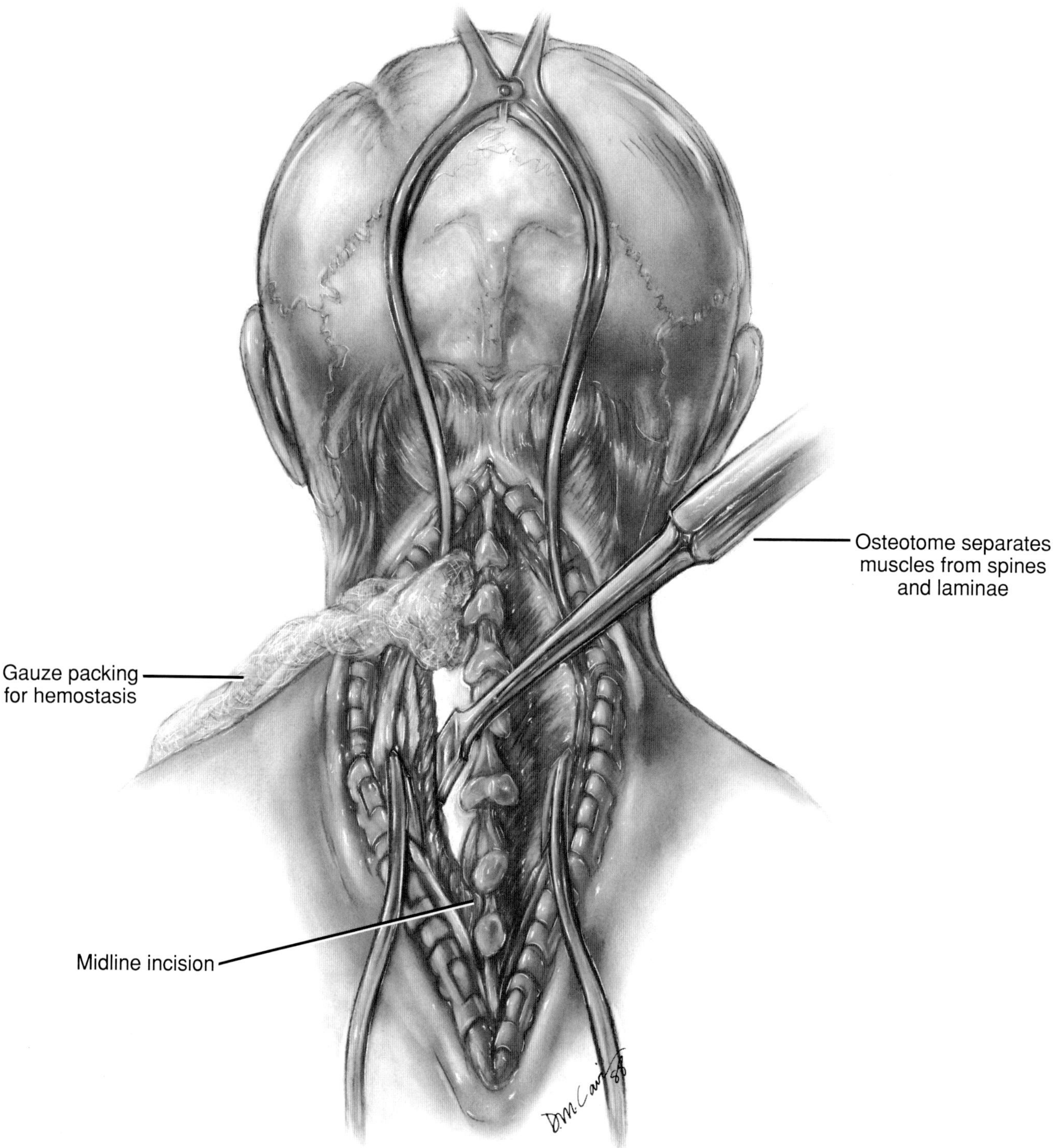

Figure 9.1. The patient may be positioned either sitting or prone for extensive cervical laminectomy.

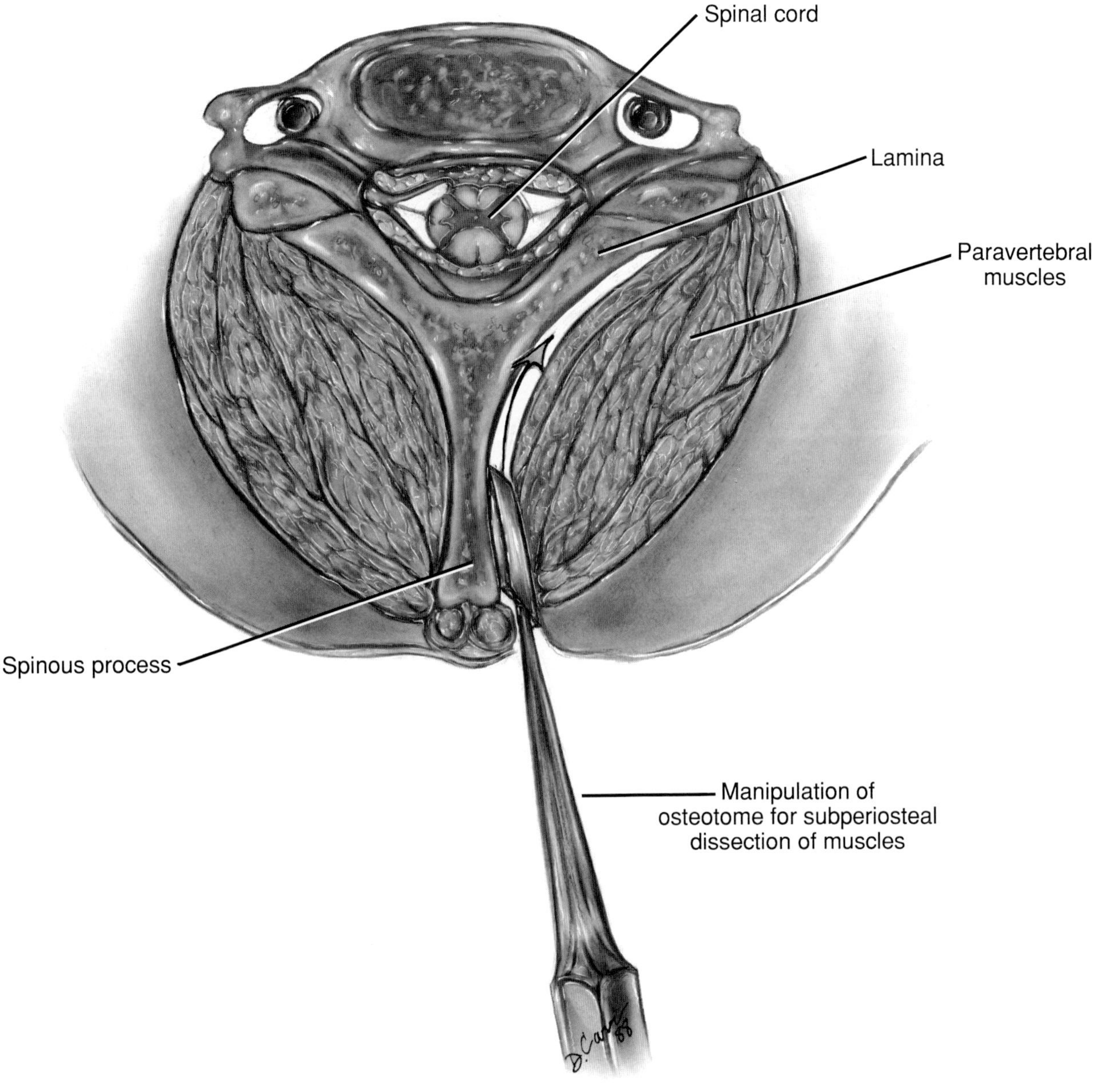
Spinal cord
Lamina
Paravertebral muscles
Spinous process
Manipulation of osteotome for subperiosteal dissection of muscles

Figure 9.2.

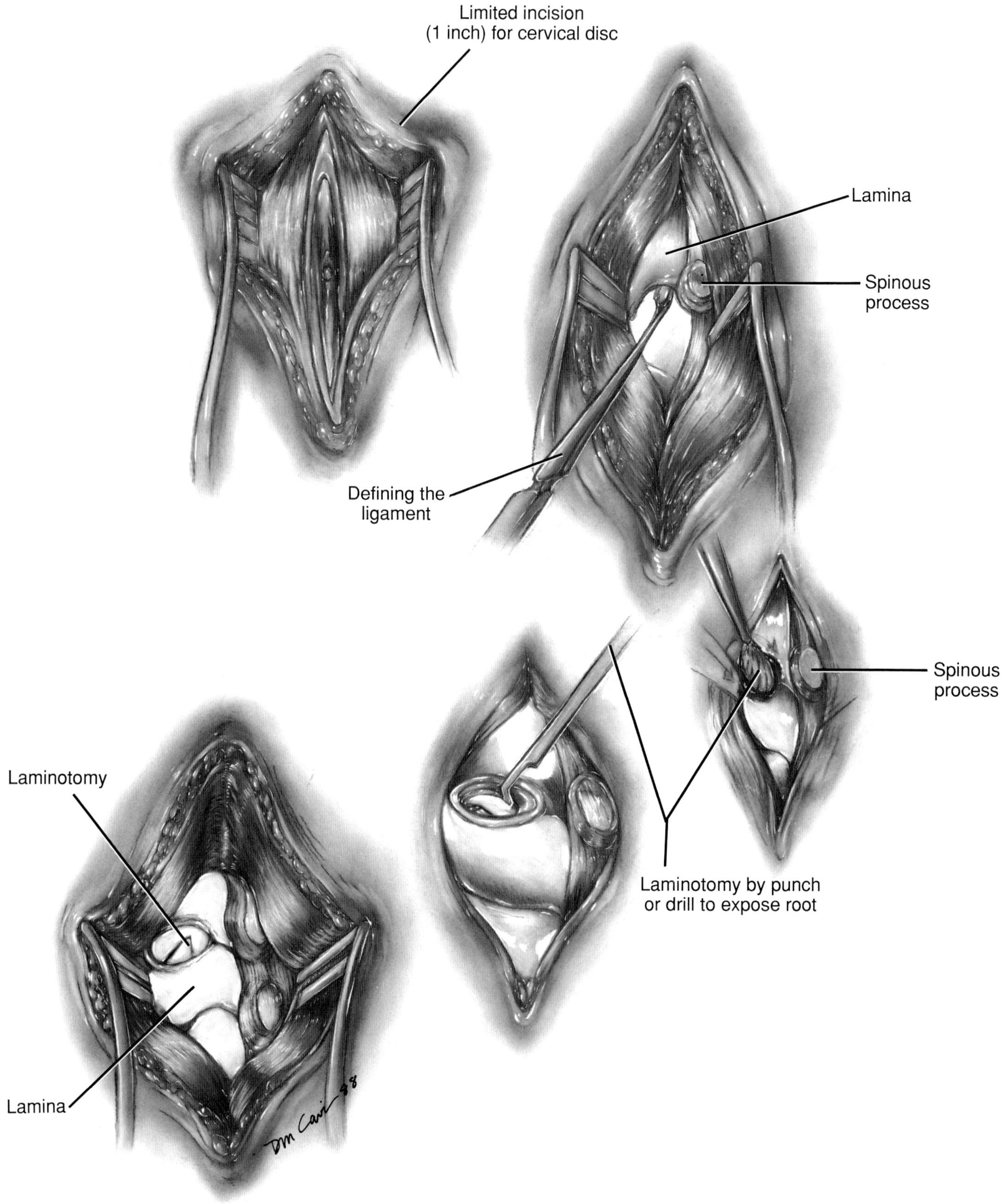
Limited incision
(1 inch) for cervical disc
Lamina
Spinous
process
Defining the
ligament
Spinous
process
Laminotomy by punch
or drill to expose root
Laminotomy
Lamina

Figure 9.3.

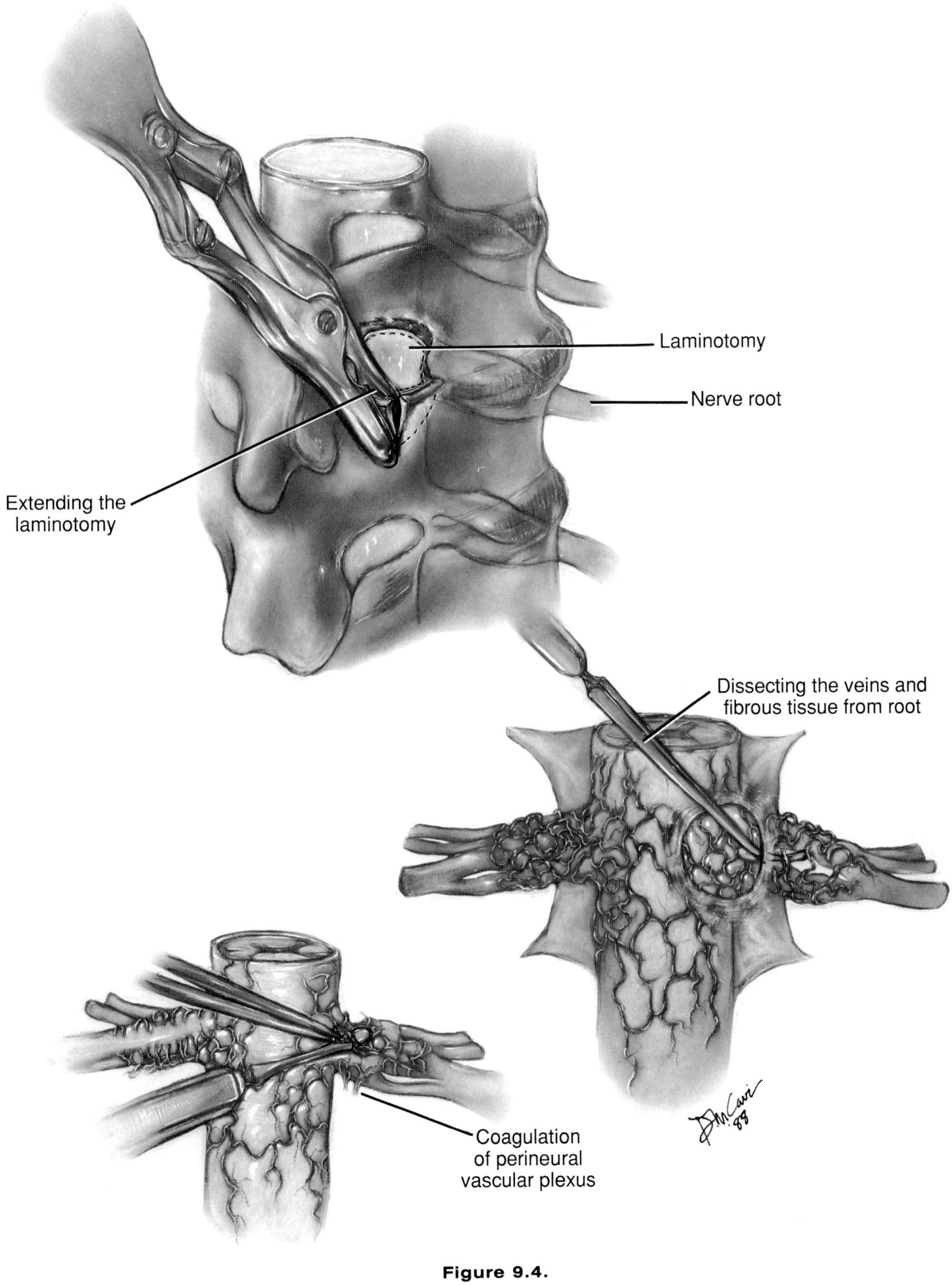
Laminotomy
Nerve root
Extending the laminotomy
Dissecting the veins and fibrous tissue from root
Coagulation of perineural vascular plexus

Figure 9.4.

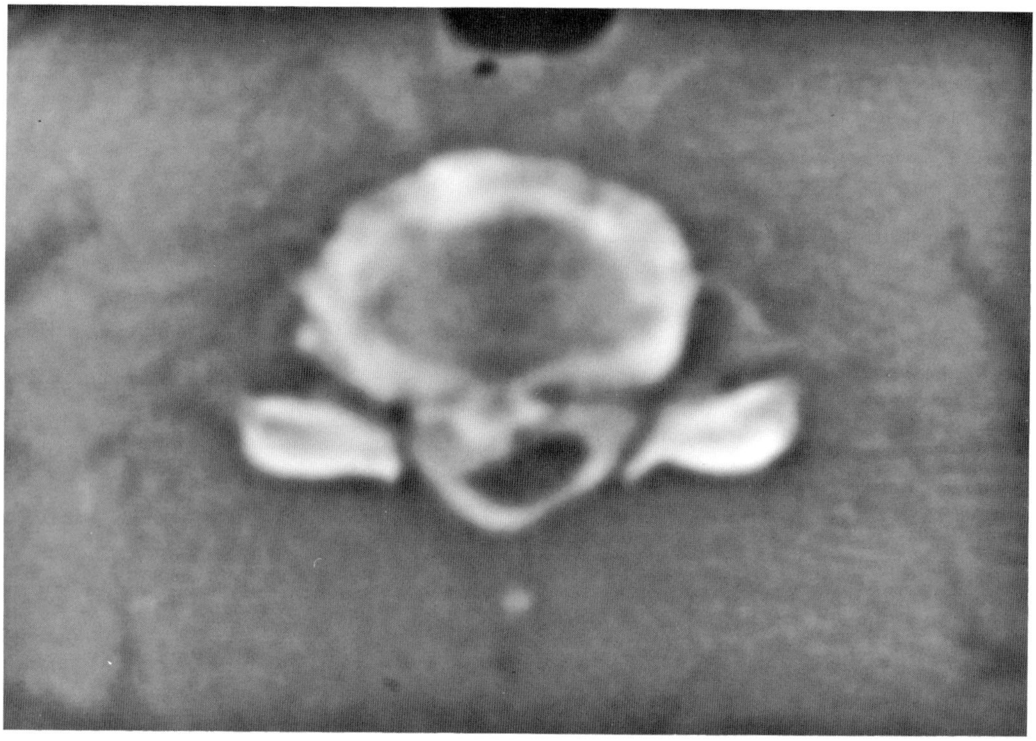

Figure 9.5. Cervical CT myelogram demonstrates a large posterior osteophyte displacing the spinal cord and impinging on the nerve root.

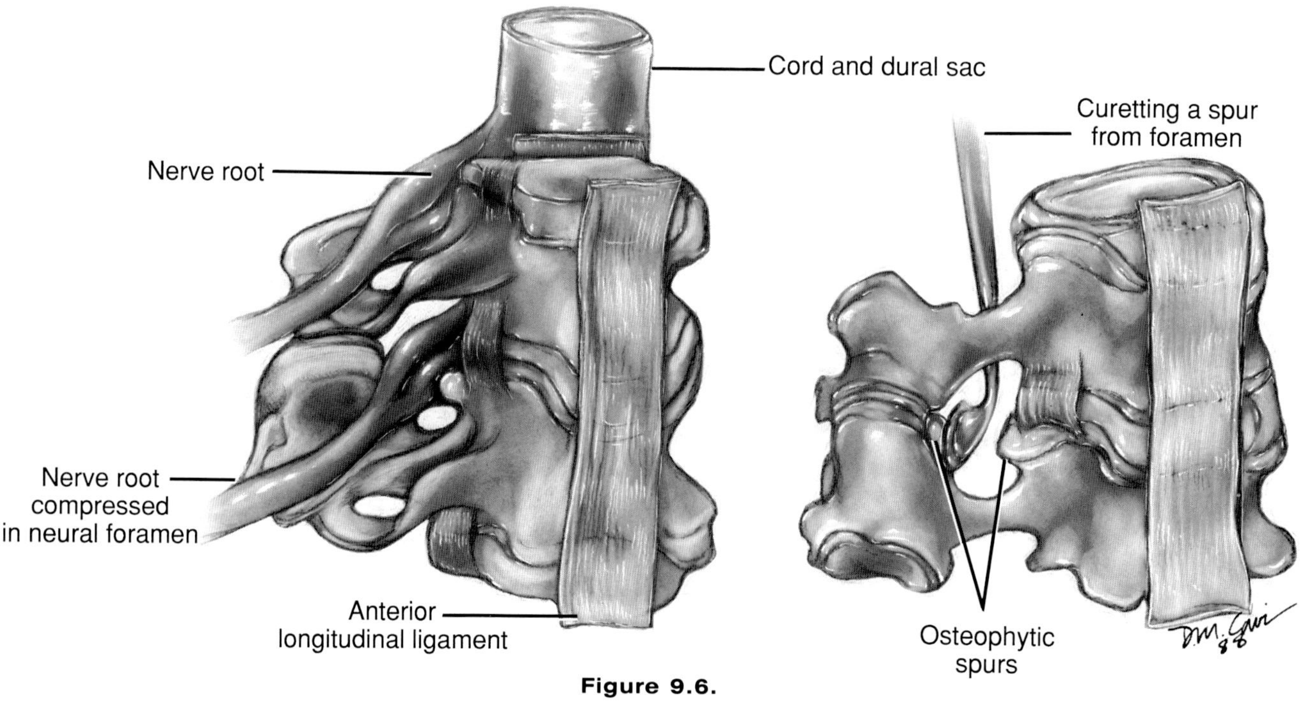

Figure 9.6.

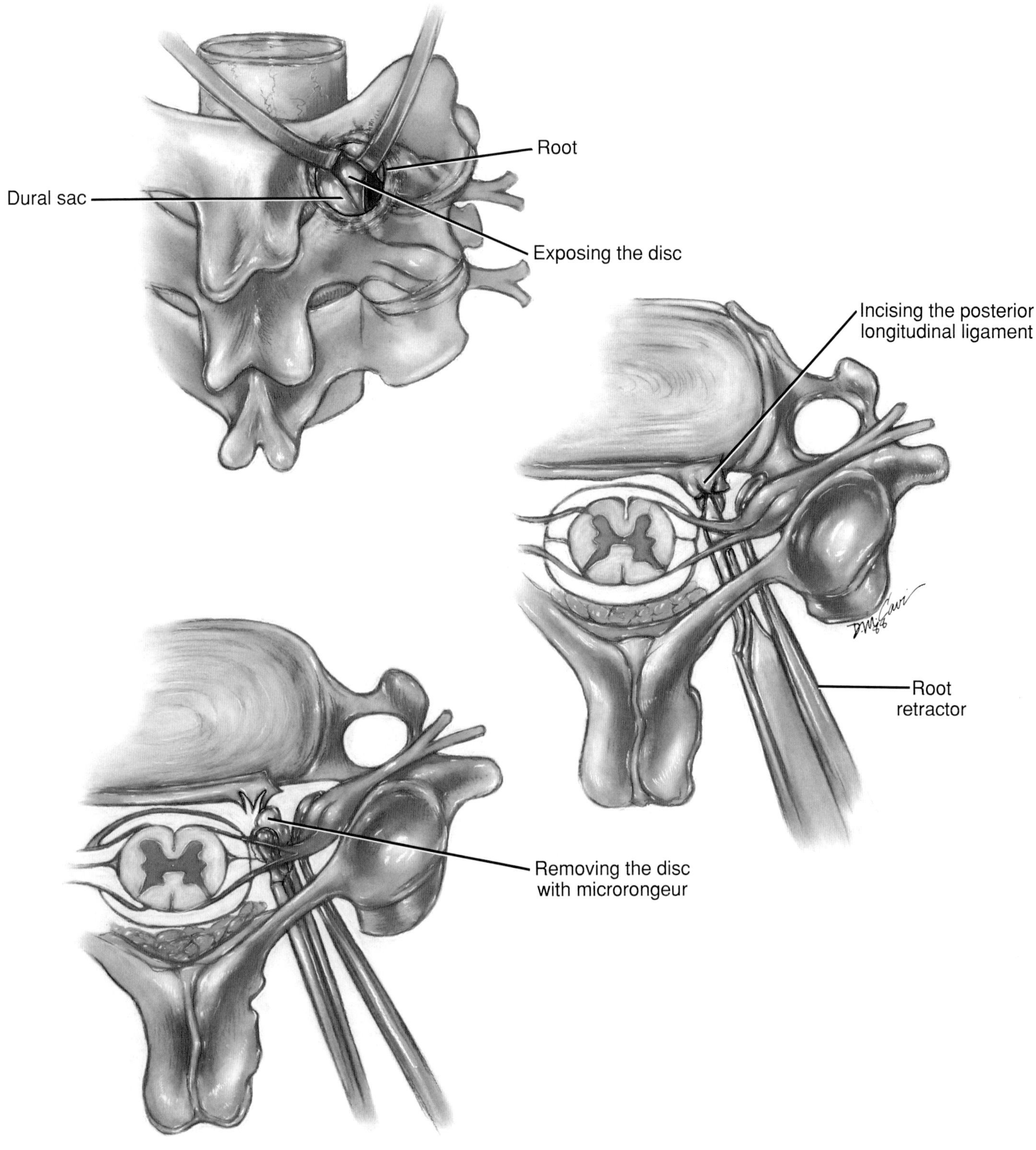
Root
Dural sac
Exposing the disc
Incising the posterior longitudinal ligament
Root retractor
Removing the disc with microrongeur

Figure 9.7.

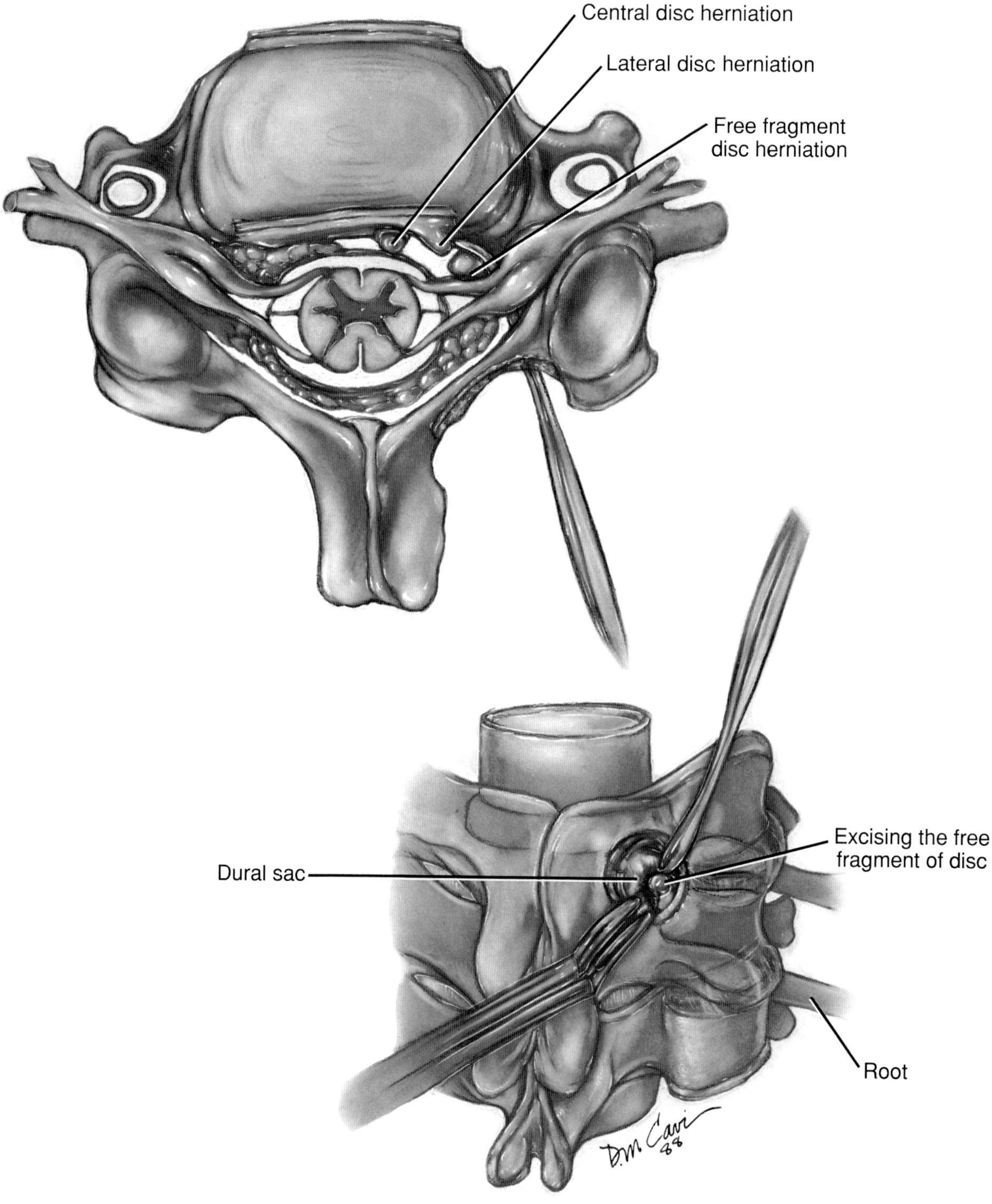
Central disc herniation
Lateral disc herniation
Free fragment
disc herniation
Excising the free
fragment of disc
Dural sac
Root

Figure 9.8.

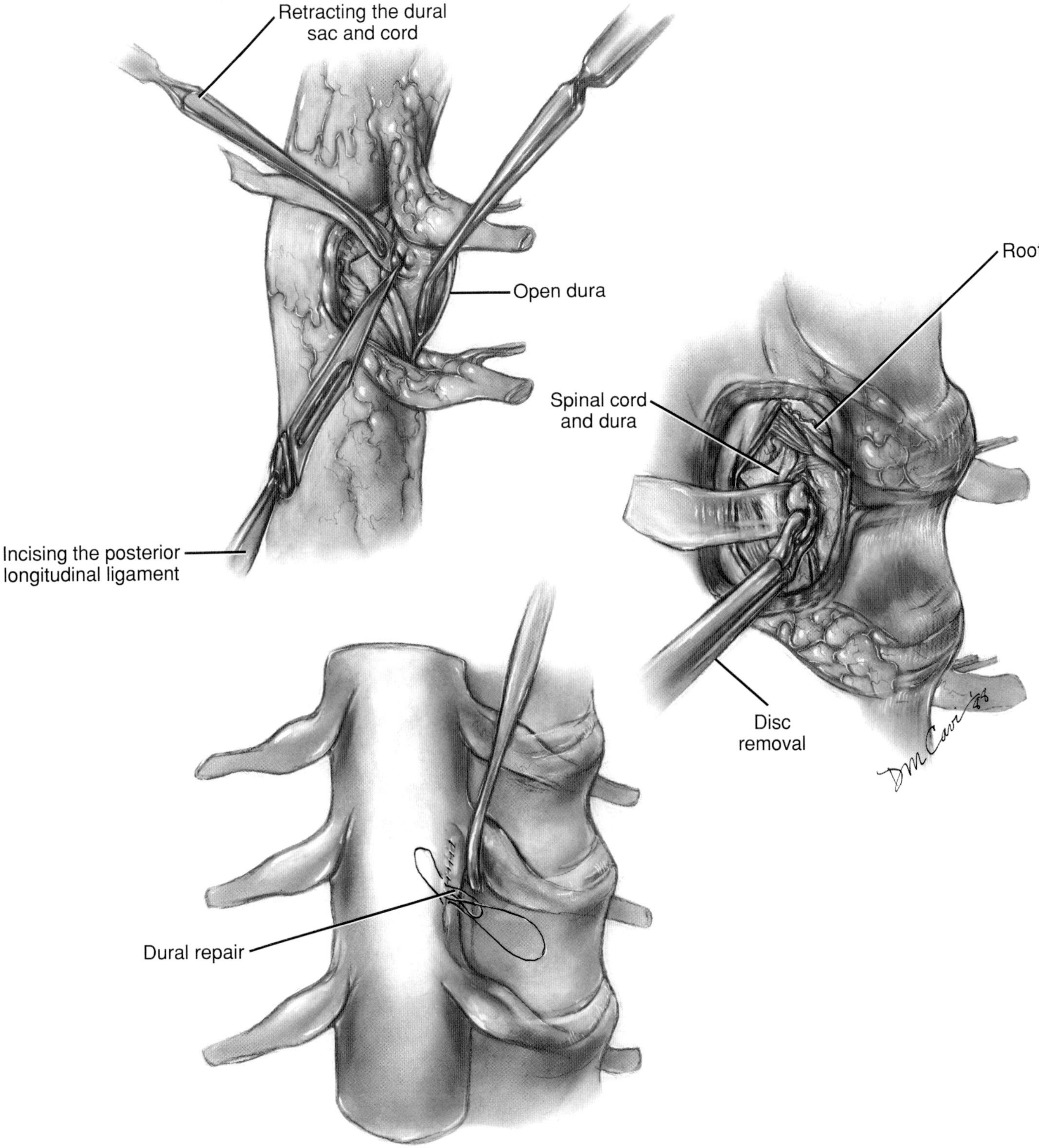
Retracting the dural sac and cord
Open dura
Incising the posterior longitudinal ligament
Root
Spinal cord and dura
Disc removal
Dural repair

Figure 9.9.

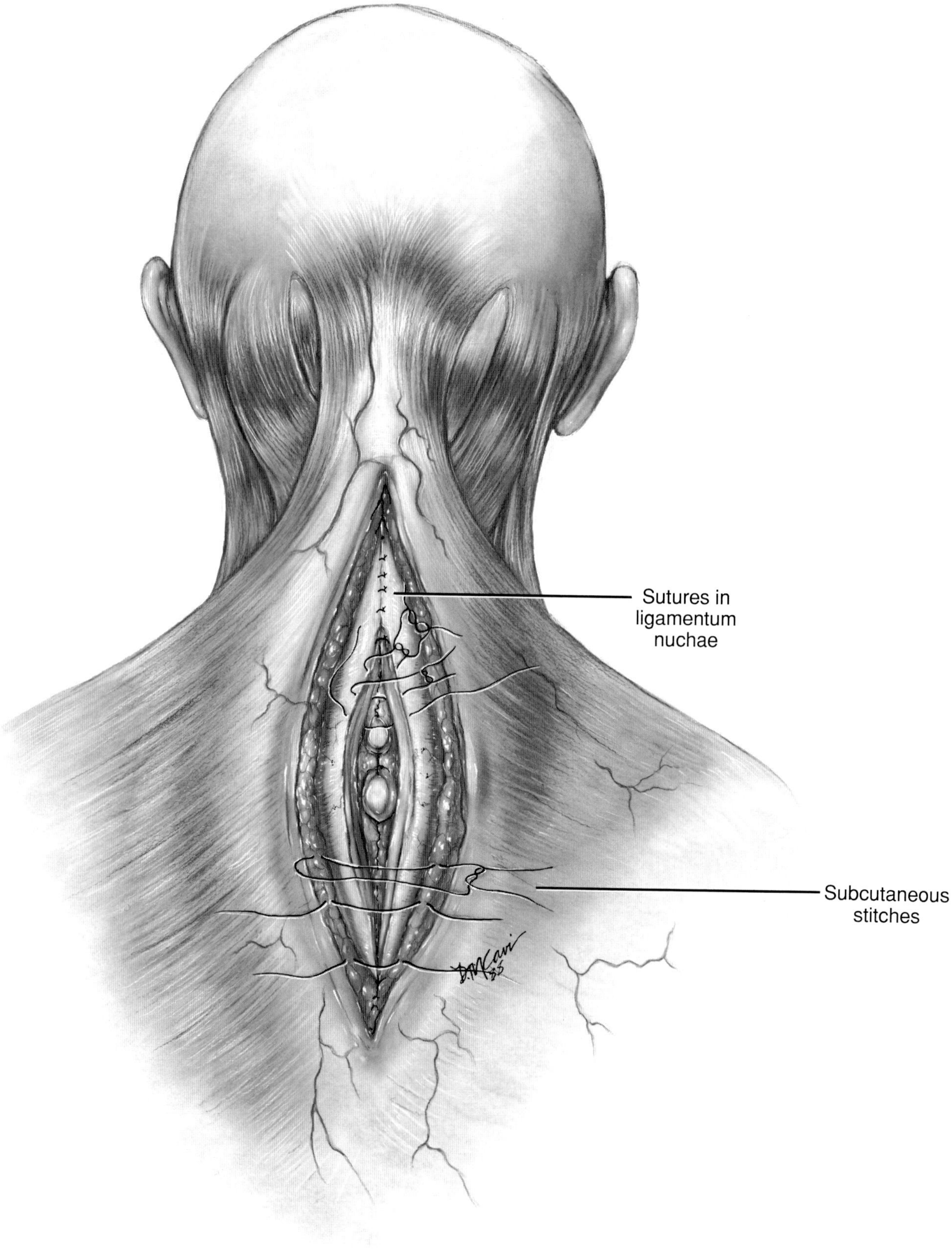

Figure 9.10.

anterior root is more inferiorly and anteriorly placed. If the disc herniation is a true free fragment, then gentle manipulation of the root usually allows a corner of the fragment to pop into view. This is grasped with a small pituitary-type disc rongeur, and the fragment is teased out of its location. Rhoton microrongeurs are ideal for the tight spaces often present in cervical disc herniation. If the disc cannot be easily seen with gentle root retraction, then a small blunt hook swept under the root may snag the fragment, which can gradually be eased into the operative field and removed. If the disc is still contained by posterior ligaments, no fragment will be seen; rather, the glistening dome of ligament over the fragment will be visualized. With the root carefully protected, the ligament can be incised with a #15 knife. Usually, a single puncture or a small cruciate incision will suffice. The disc immediately extrudes into the field where it can be grasped with the disc rongeurs and removed. All of these maneuvers require immaculate hemostasis. If any bleeding occurs from epidural veins, they should be packed with small amounts of hemostatic agent or small cottonoids so that everything can be done under direct vision. Magnification is helpful but not mandatory. Once the fragment is removed, a blunt hook should be swept medially under the dura and laterally under the root to be certain that no additional fragments are present. The sweep should be such that any disc material caught by the hook is brought into the field rather than pushed away from it.

Transdural Removal of Cervical Disc

Occasionally, the cervical disc is located so far medially that it cannot be exposed by retraction of the root. Then, a transdural excision is necessary. Such discs are virtually always located in the axilla and quite near the midline. The anterior approach is preferable for the removal, but in the situation in which they are encountered by the posterior approach, they can be removed quite easily by a transdural route. The dura is opened laterally in the axilla of the nerve root approximately at the level of the junction of the root with the spinal cord. A small dural opening no more than 1 or 2 cm is required. The roots should be gently retracted up, and the arachnoid opened, exposing the anterior dura. A small blunt dissector can be utilized to identify the disc fragment, and a #15 knife used to make a small linear incision through the anterior dura and ligament into the disc. The free fragment will immediately extrude into the incision. A small disc rongeur is utilized to grasp it and remove it. Again, the margins should be palpated thoroughly to be certain that there is no further fragment. The anterior dural sac does not need to be closed. The posterior dura should be closed in a watertight fashion.

The closure of all of these approaches is the same. The cervical muscle is not sutured, but the ligamentum nuchae is sutured in the midline. Subcutaneous and skin stitches are required, and the patients need no special postoperative care.

10

Anterior Operations on Cervical Disc

Smith-Robinson Fusion

Smith-Robinson fusion is done with the patient under general anesthesia and supine. The approach may be either from the left or from the right. Dr. Robert Robinson, the originator of one of the major approaches, believes that if the exposure is done from the left side, there is less danger to the recurrent laryngeal nerve, and extensive experience with his operation indicates that this is correct. The patient should be placed in a halter traction, and about 5 pounds utilized immediately to hold the head completely straight. The placement of the skin incision can usually be judged by comparison with the plain lateral x-ray. The transverse process of C6 can usually be palpated once the patient is asleep. Then the skin incision can be judged so that it lies exactly over the interspace to be entered (Fig. 10.2). If a two-level fusion is planned, then the incision should be halfway between the two levels. The opposite iliac crest is exposed if a bone graft is going to be used. The skin incision should be made from just off the midline laterally to just beyond the medial border of the sternocleidomastoid muscle. A convenient skin fold can usually be found for this transverse incision. The incision itself is quite small; 1 inch is usually sufficient, and 2 inches are more than adequate. The platysma is next isolated and divided, also in a transverse fashion (Fig. 10.3). This will expose the anterior bor-

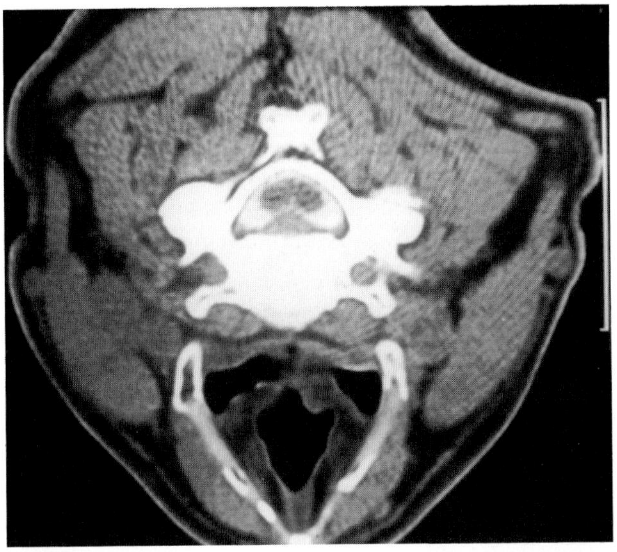

Figure 10.1. Computed tomography myelographic demonstration of a midline cervical disc protrusion best treated by anterior cervical discectomy.

der of the sternomastoid and the medial structures with their fascial coverings. The incision is now changed from transverse to vertical and carried along the anterior border of the sternocleidomastoid in the fascial plane that is avascular. It should be carried up and down far enough that exposure of at least three interspaces will be easy to accomplish. The dissection is then carried down to the carotid sheath. The dissection then proceeds medially, so that the carotid sheath and all it contains are lateral with the esophagus, larynx, and trachea medially (Fig. 10.4). The omohyoid muscle will usually be in the way of the exposure. It should be divided and does not need to be approximated on closure. If it is not obstructing the surgeon's view of the prevertebral space, then it can be left and retracted out of the way. The dissection is done with a pair of scissors and should be in a completely avascular plane. It is taken to the prevertebral fascia and musculature. The dissection should be carried superiorly and inferiorly enough so that three spaces could be easily exposed if necessary. The dissection behind the esophagus in the prevertebral space is better done bluntly with a Kutner dissector or with the surgeon's finger (Fig. 10.5). A single thyroid retractor is then utilized to expose the operative site, by retracting all of the medial structures, esophagus, larynx, and trachea to expose the midline. This will normally uncover at least two disc spaces. The next step is the absolute identification of the space. Take an x-ray to be certain. An 18-gauge spinal needle with beads soldered on at 1 cm so there is no possibility the needle can be driven through the interspace into the spinal canal by a heavy instrument or drape is a nice marker and allows discography if desired (Fig. 10.6). Two are placed in the adjacent discs, and a lateral x-ray is taken. As soon as the interspaces are identified, the self-retaining retractors are put in place. This is done by reinserting the thyroid retractor and again retracting the medial structures to expose the midline and the needles. Leave the needles where they are at this juncture. The Cloward retractor or a similar instrument designed for this purpose is utilized to provide exposure of the interspaces. Appropriate lengths for the blades of this retractor are chosen by the depth of the neck incision. The smooth blade without teeth is placed medially exactly opposite the interspace to be entered. A similar-sized tooth blade is inserted into the paravertebral musculature at the same level, and the retractor is assembled and spread. This provides excellent exposure medially and laterally and frees the surgeon and the surgical assistants from the necessity of retractor holding. A similar smaller retractor designed for the superior-inferior exposure is used; toothed blades are not utilized on this instrument. Be careful of the carotid artery. The retractor teeth should be firmly embedded in paravertebral muscle; it is wise to palpate the carotid sheath above the retractor to be certain that the carotid is not injured. The unnecessary needle can be removed, but the interspace to be opened is marked by incising the anterior longitudinal ligaments around the needle before the needle is taken out. This guarantees that no error in placement will occur. The disc incision is made at the junction of disc and bone, above and below, and taken laterally to the margins of the vertebral body (Fig. 10.7). The disc is removed piecemeal with rongeurs. Magnification is helpful but not necessary. The microscope or magnifying loupes make the removal of the disc more controlled. The cartilage plates are carefully curetted away with small curved curettes designed for this operation. It is not necessary to remove the posterior rim of the interspace. In fact, the small ridges that commonly are there in spondylitic patients help prevent the bone plug from being

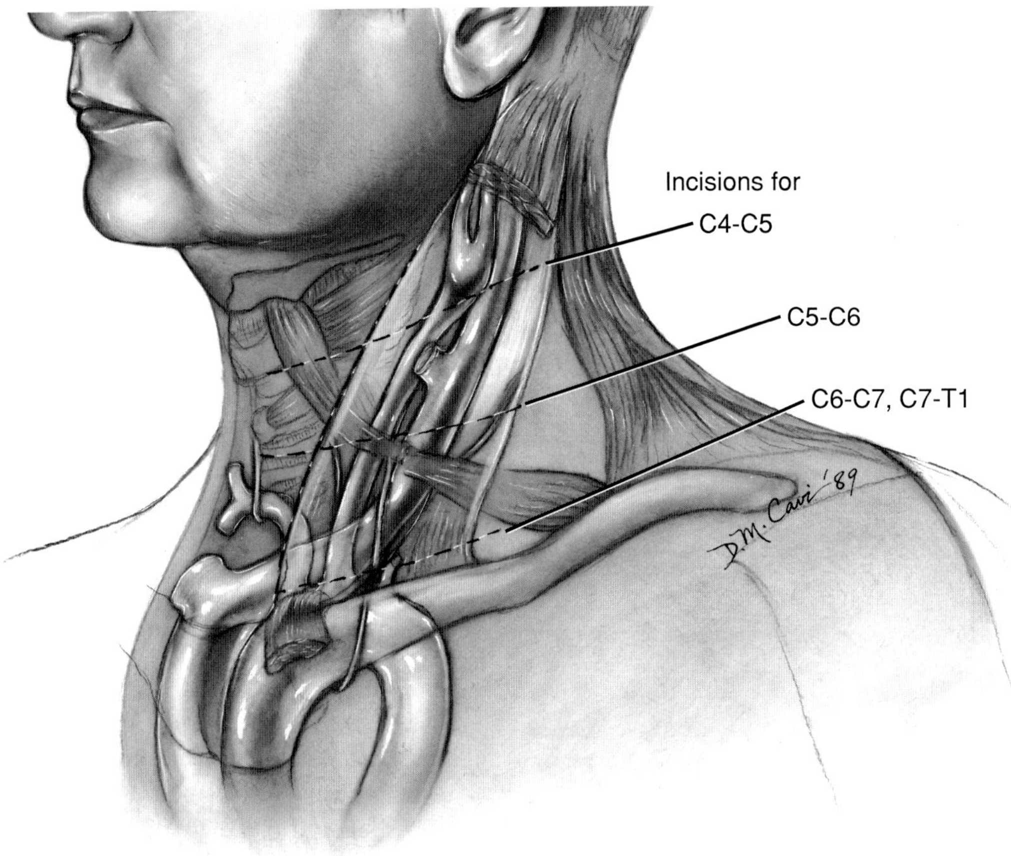

Figure 10.2.

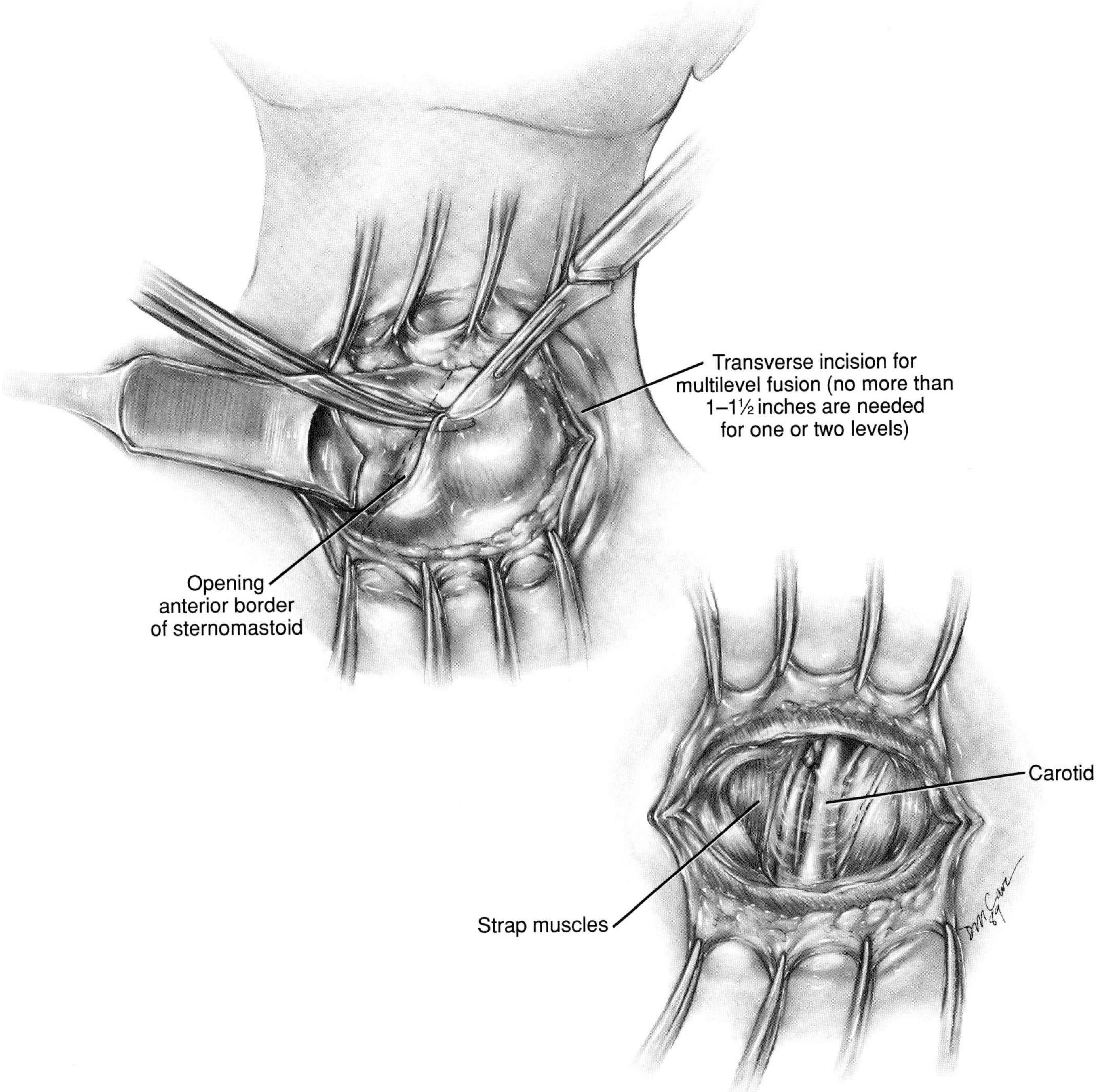
Transverse incision for multilevel fusion (no more than 1–1½ inches are needed for one or two levels)
Opening anterior border of sternomastoid
Carotid
Strap muscles

Figure 10.3.

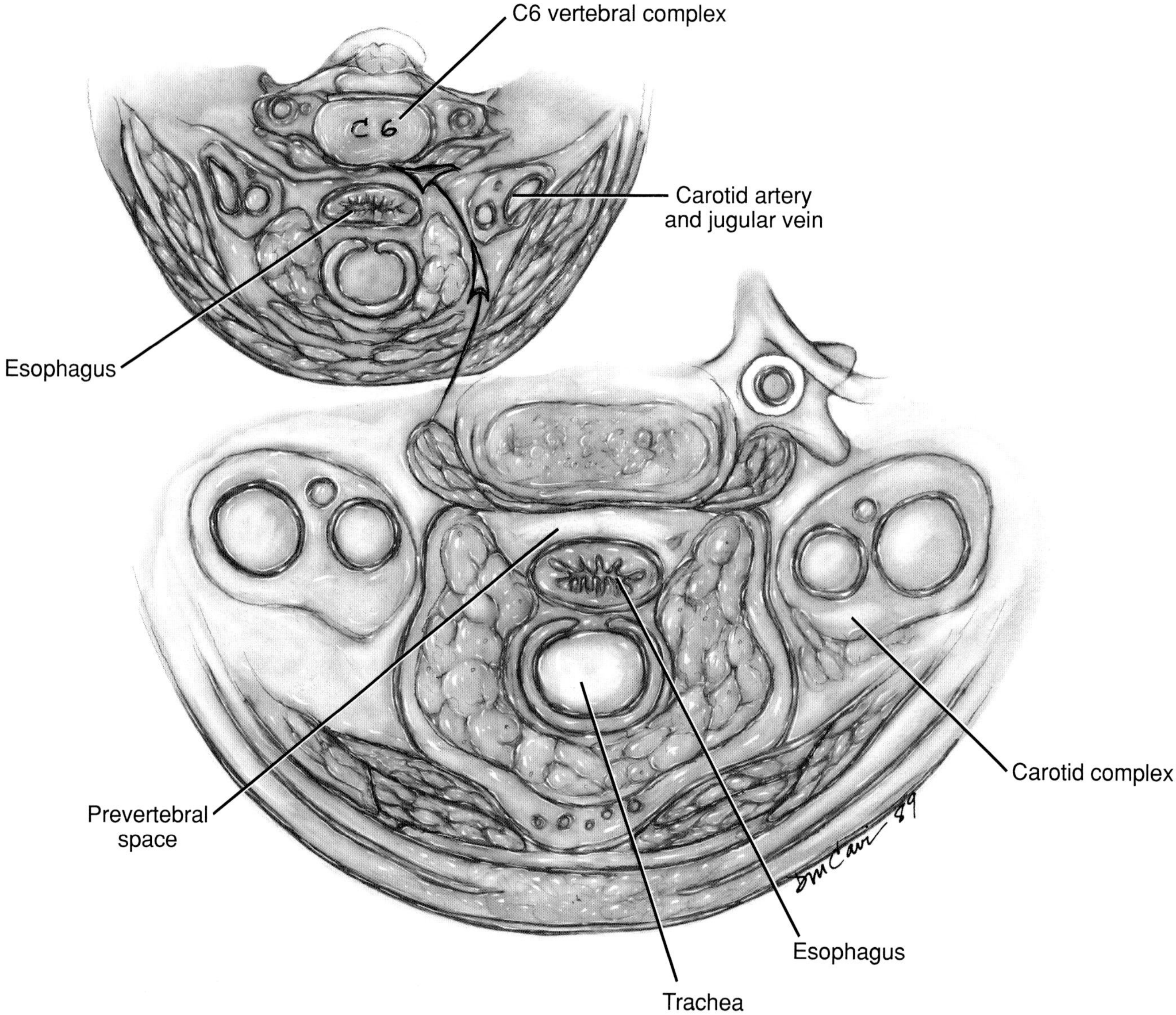

Figure 10.4. Operative approach medial to carotid sheath.

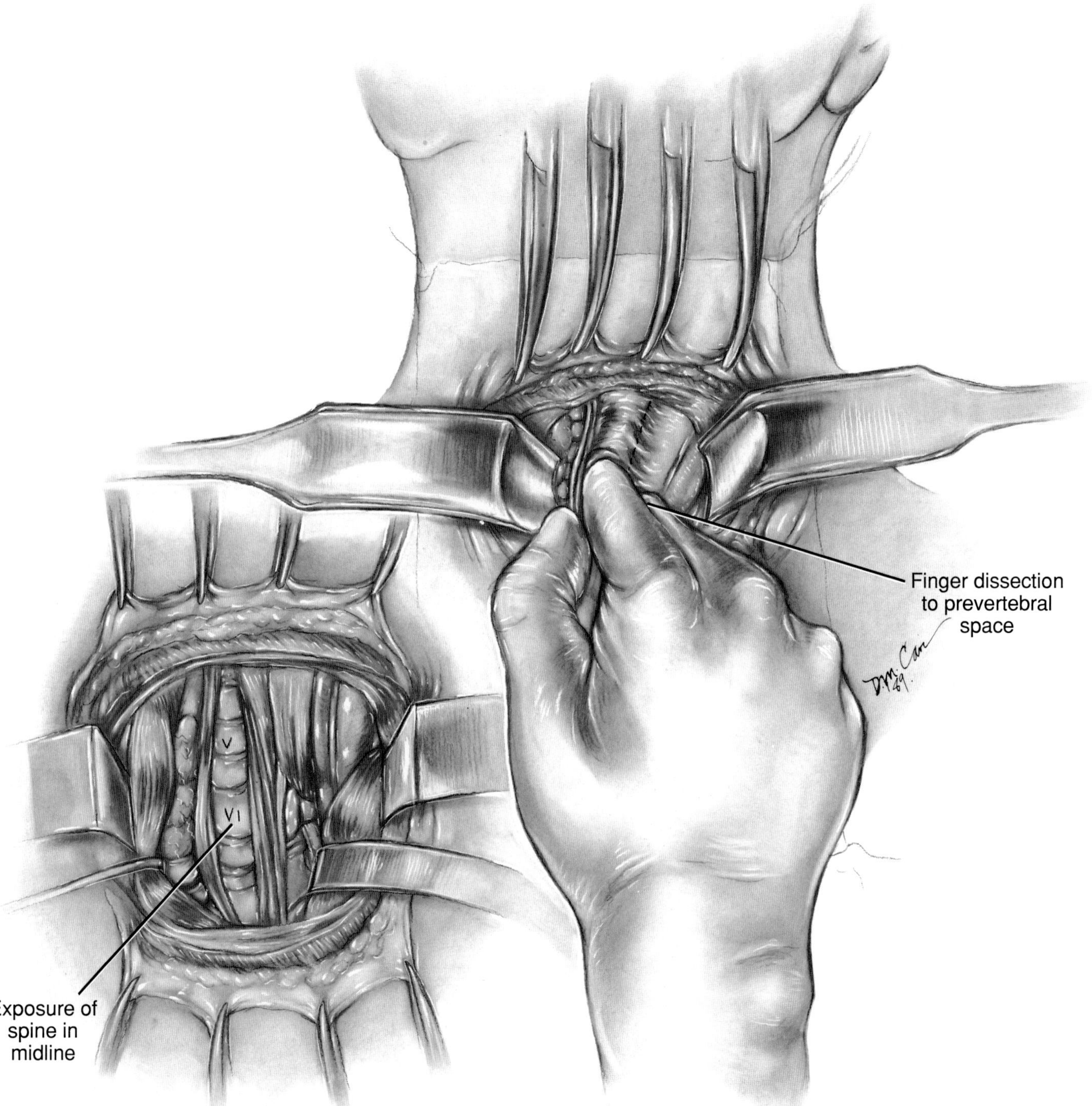
Finger dissection
to prevertebral
space
V
VI
Exposure of
spine in
midline

Figure 10.5.

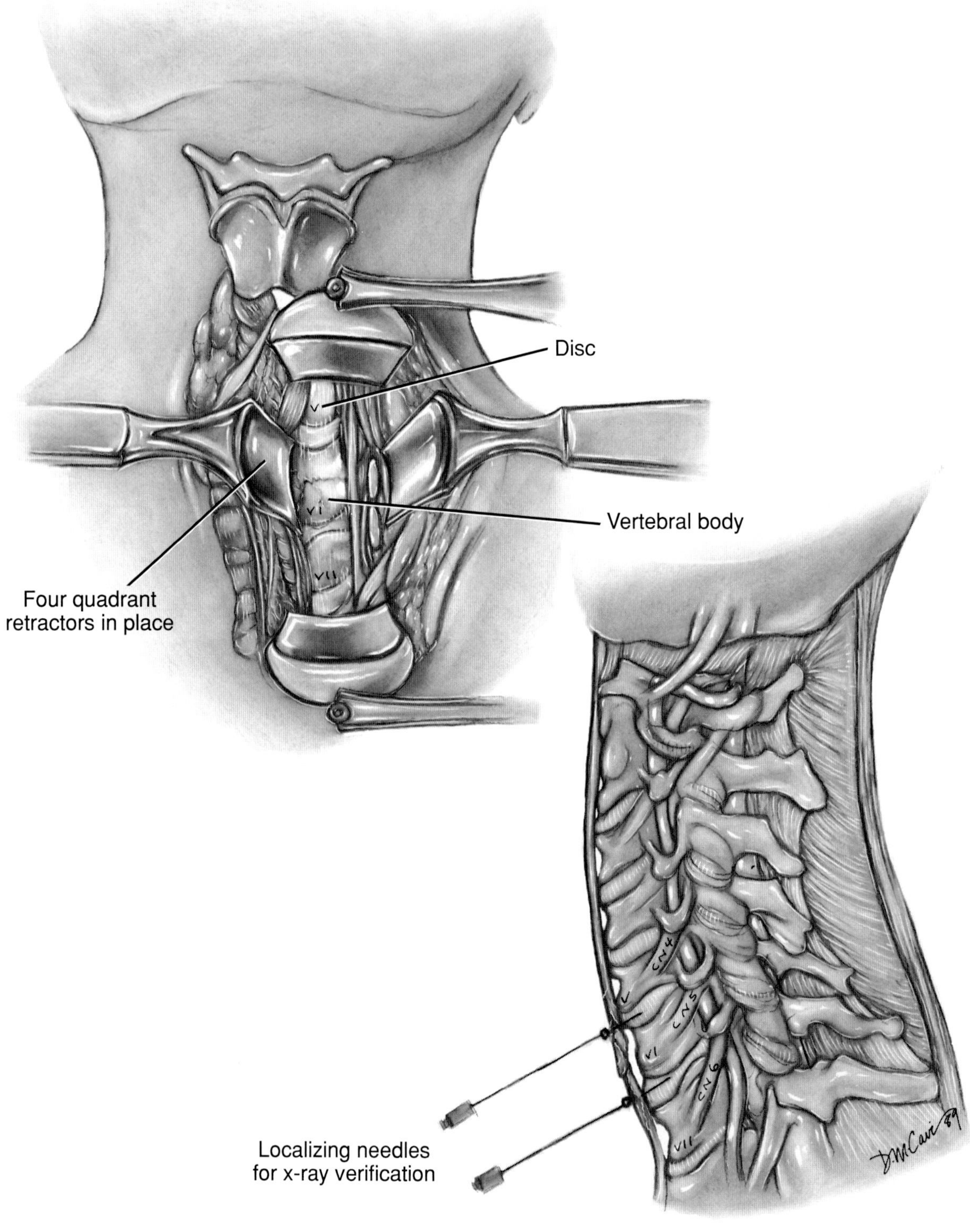
Disc
Vertebral body
Four quadrant
retractors in place
V
VI
VII
CN4
CN5
CN6
Localizing needles
for x-ray verification

Figure 10.6.

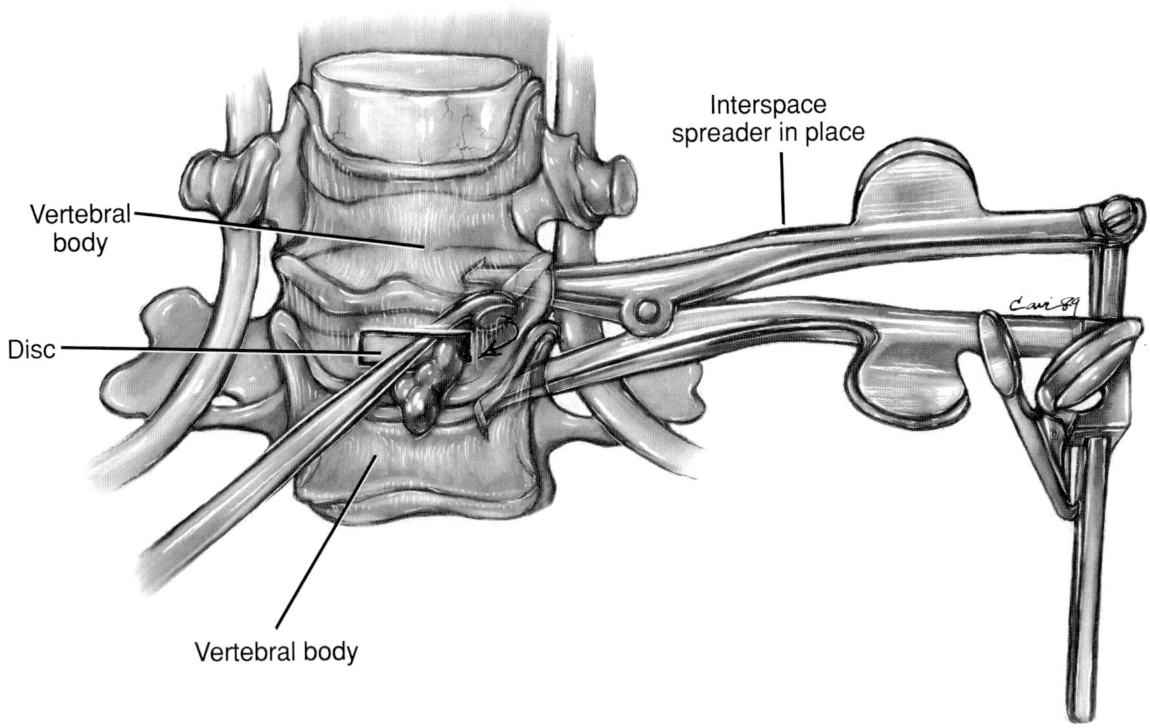

Figure 10.7. Removal of disc.

driven too far posteriorly (Fig. 10.8). If there is a free fragment disc that has herniated through the posterior longitudinal ligament, magnification makes it much easier to find that fragment. Careful inspection of the posterior portion of the incision will nearly always demonstrate a small hole with a tag of this tissue peeking through. The ligament is opened carefully with a #15 knife; gentle tugging will nearly always deliver the disc fragment. Since it is more common that the disc herniation is contained by the posterior longitudinal ligament, an opening into the canal is not always necessary. If discectomy without fusion is planned, then the operation is complete at this point. All that is required is to remove the retractors and close the skin; no other sutures are necessary.

If anterior fusion by the Robinson approach as well as disc removal is the goal of surgery, the next step is to measure the interspace. With a malleable probe, it is possible to measure the height, depth, and width of the space to be grafted. The height of a properly prepared interspace should be at least 5–6 mm. If it is not, then it is necessary to continue to curette or drill until the proper size space is obtained. Do not curette through cortical bone into the vertebral body. This has the potential of allowing collapse. The width is normally 11 or 12 mm, and the depth 12–15 mm. The plug to be fashioned should be of appropriate width and height but need not be the entire depth of the body. A plug 4 or 5 mm less in depth is quite acceptable.

Hip Incision

During the original preparation and draping, the opposite iliac crest has been appropriately prepared. The skin towel should expose the crest from the anterior superior iliac spine back about 6 cm. The bone graft will be taken just behind the spine, but a sufficient area should be exposed to allow some latitude in choosing the appropriate width for the graft. The graft should not be taken from the spine itself, for this will

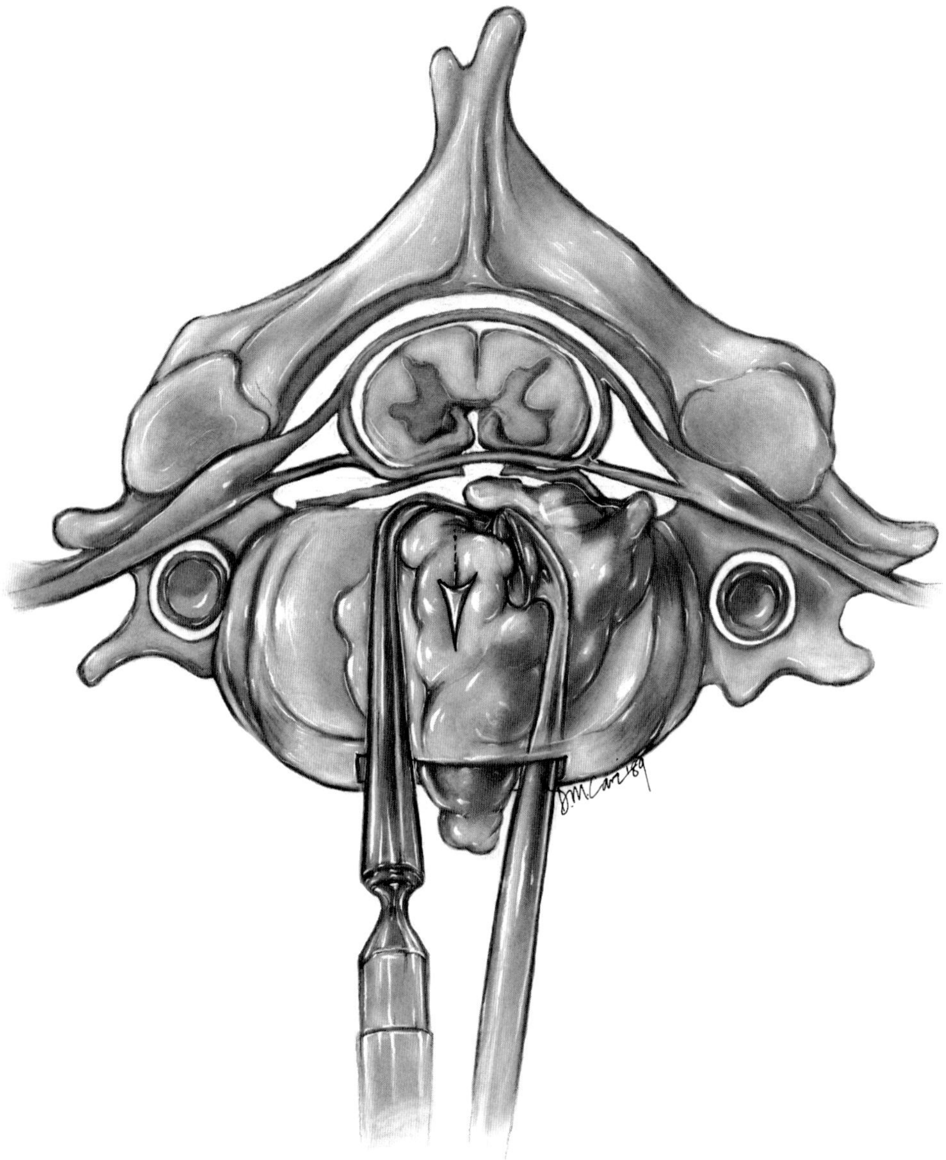

Figure 10.8. Removal of disc.

usually be too wide. A skin incision is made at the superior margin of the crest so that the closure is not immediately over the crest. The incision is deepened until the facial attachments of the muscles on the crest are exposed. Self-retaining retractors should be put in place to expose the crest. An incision is made along the midline of the crest. This will allow the muscles to be scraped away in a subperiosteal fashion. The midline incision is then undercut back to the inferior and superior margins of the crest over a distance of 2 or 3 cm. This may be done with a knife or with a Cobb elevator. A true subperiosteal dissection should be obtained. If this is done, there will be little bleeding. A subperiosteal dissection of the muscle down the sides of the ilium is then carried out, exposing a depth of about 2 cm. An oscillating saw is then used to cut the appropriate size plug (Fig. 10.9). It is better to remove as little bone as possible. Therefore, the block should be cut to near the appropriate size. The crest can be marked with about 1 mm of additional size for height, and then the appropriate plug cut through the full thickness of the crest with the oscillating saw. The cuts are carried down 12–15 mm so that an appropriate size block of bone averaging 6–8 mm in height and 12–15 mm in depth, the width of the crest, is obtained. Especially in large males, the crest near the anterior spine may be too wide for the interspace, and the width should be measured to choose the appropriate place for the block to be harvested. A small straight osteotome is used to cut across the block of bone at the base. The block is then sized with a rongeur, so that there is an absolute fit. All dimensions of the site to be grafted should be obtained again, and the graft fashioned to fit exactly. Very little hemostasis in the incision is required. Some bone wax will usually solve any troublesome bone bleeding. The hip wound is closed by reapproximating the muscular facial attachment in the midline of the crest. If there is much bleeding, a suction drain for 24 hours can be used. Otherwise, the subcutaneous tissue and skin are closed, usually with a subcuticular stitch, so that no stitch removal is required.

Attention is returned to the neck, and the graft is put loosely in place to be certain it is approximately the right size. Twenty pounds of weight are then applied to the traction, distracting the interspace. A properly sized graft can than easily be fitted. If there are problems, it is usually better to enlarge the graft site slightly rather than to weaken the graft by too much rongeuring or thinning. If there is a serious discrepancy in size, then either the site to be grafted must be significantly enlarged or the graft itself should be reduced. The graft should not be reduced below 6 mm in height. The bone is now tamped in place under direct vision. The impactors that have been designed for this are invaluable in allowing proper graft placement without risk of fracture of the graft. The graft should be countersunk underneath the lips of the vertebral body by 1–2 mm and should be firmly in place. Once it is in position, the weight should be removed from the traction, and the anesthesiologist asked to flex the neck to be certain the graft is solidly seated. The self-retaining retractors are then removed, and if hemostasis is adequate, which is usually the case, the closure is simple. It is wise to check the carotid artery as soon as the retractors are out and to inspect the esophagus to make sure no injury has occurred. Closure requires only a subcutaneous platysmal layer and a subcuticular stitch in the skin.

Postoperatively, the patient should be maintained in a metal brace for 6 weeks to 3 months. The period of time in the brace depends on what is seen concerning maturation of the fusion as judged by x-ray. The patient is not allowed to ambulate until the brace is available.

The Robinson fusion is extremely successful in relieving symptoms promptly. This is because no attempt is made to curette away posterior ridges and the spurs. As the fusion solidifies, the spurs will slowly disappear. However, relief of radicular symptoms is immediate and is probably related more to the distraction produced by the graft than to any removal of spurs.

Cloward Anterior Fusion

The Cloward anterior fusion technique is more radical in its approach than the Robinson fusion. However, the basic principles are the same; i.e., the exposure of the vertebral column is identical, though a somewhat more extensive exposure of the prevertebral space is required for the insertion of the Cloward instruments. Once the self-retaining retractors are in place and the interspace is exposed, the disc is removed in the same way as for a Robinson fusion. Disc removal does not have to be as complete because a much larger bony removal is contemplated and this will accomplish the final removal of remnants of the disc. When the disc is satisfactorily removed so that there is no possibility the drill will force a disc fragment posteriorly into the spinal cord, the depth of the interspace is measured with the gauge supplied with the Cloward instruments. Then the Cloward drill is set for the appropriate depth. The possible techniques are several: a midline fusion can be performed, or smaller drills can be used to carry out exploration and fusion, which is offset so it is more unilateral. The choice of these techniques will depend on the patient's symptoms.

Generally, a simple midline fusion is performed. With this operation the drill and drill guide are carefully centered on the vertebral body, with the center of the hole to be drilled in the middle of the interspace (Fig. 10.10). The drill guide has sharp spikes that will

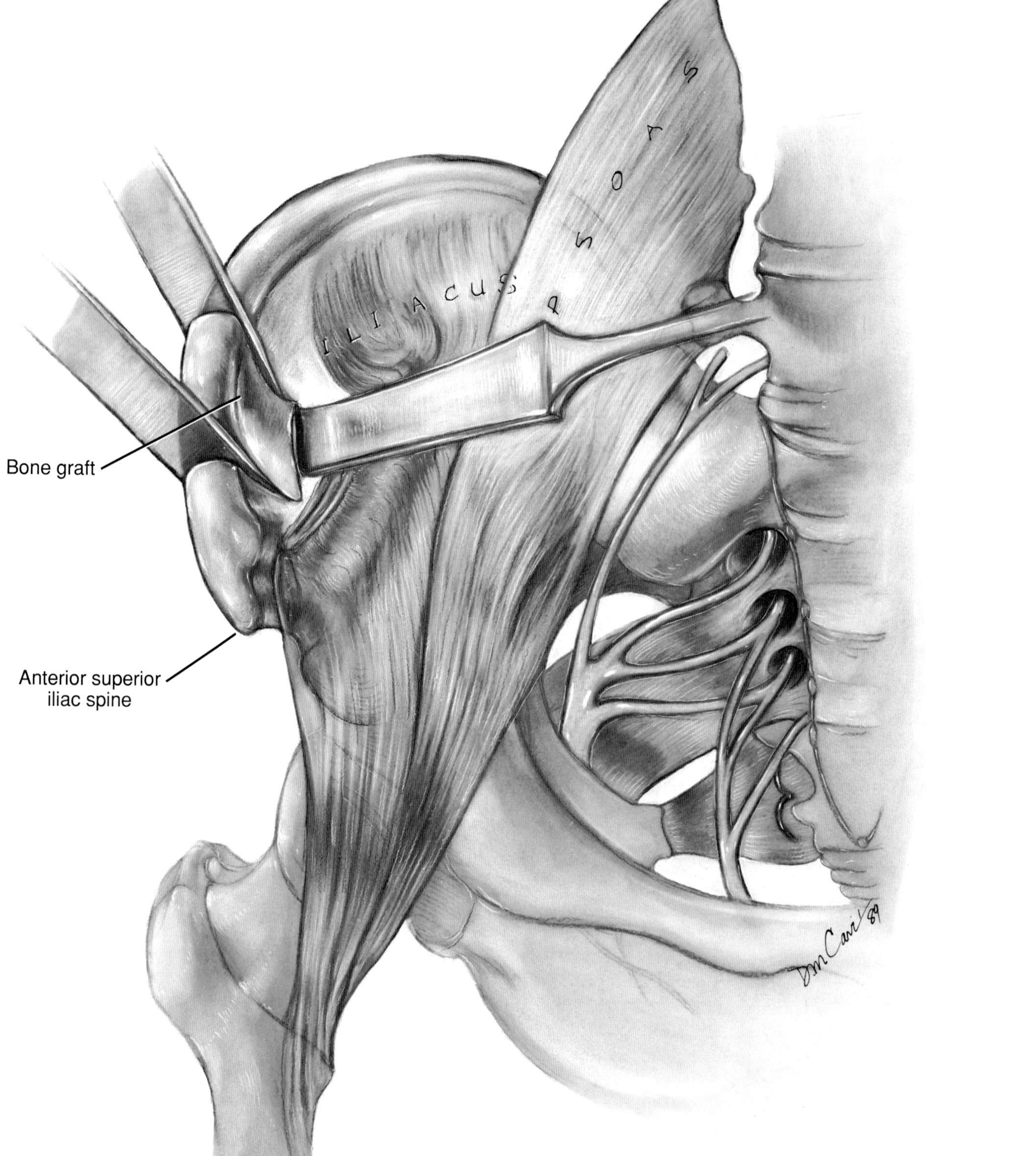

Figure 10.9.

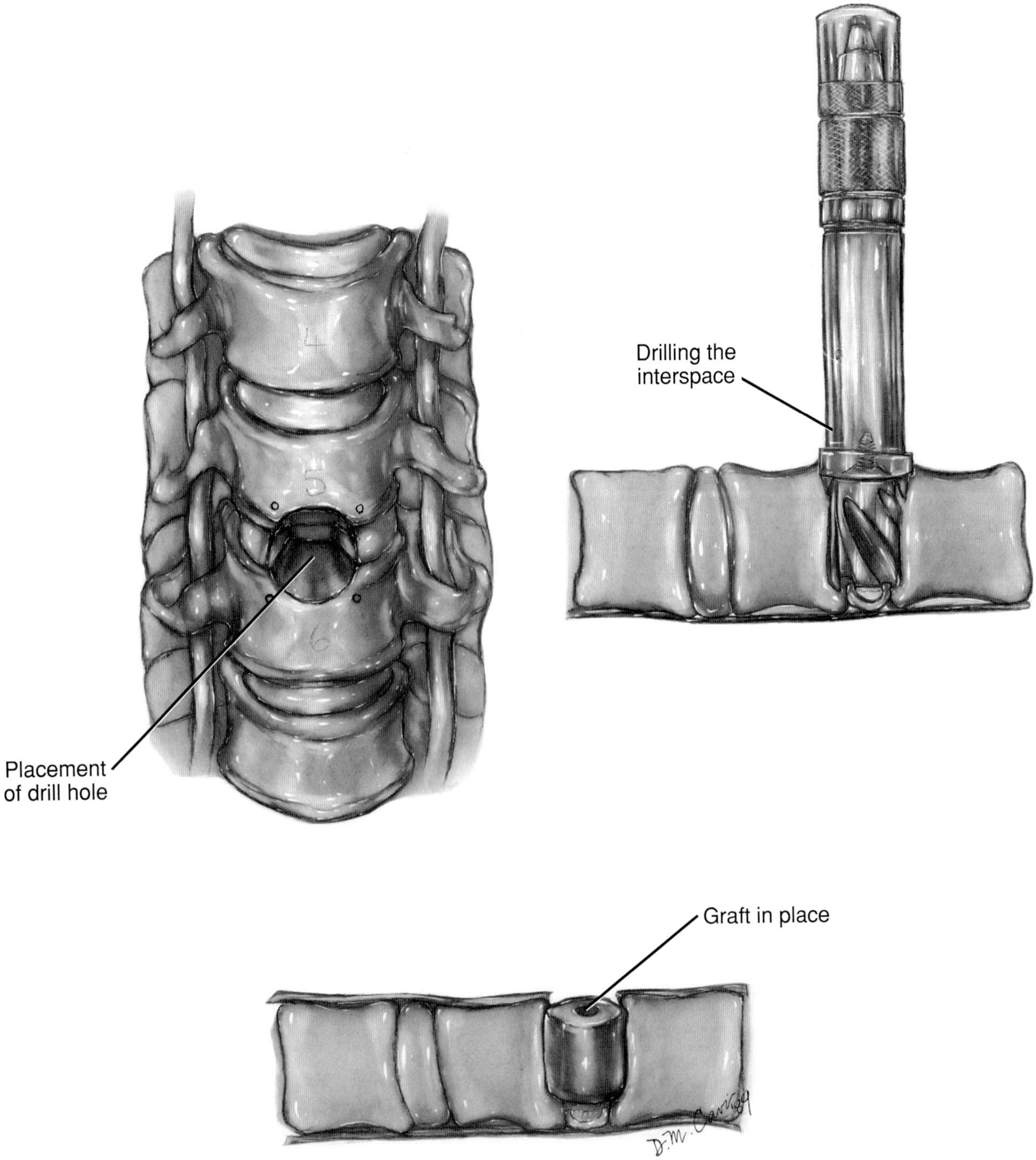
Drilling the interspace
Placement of drill hole
Graft in place

Figure 10.10.

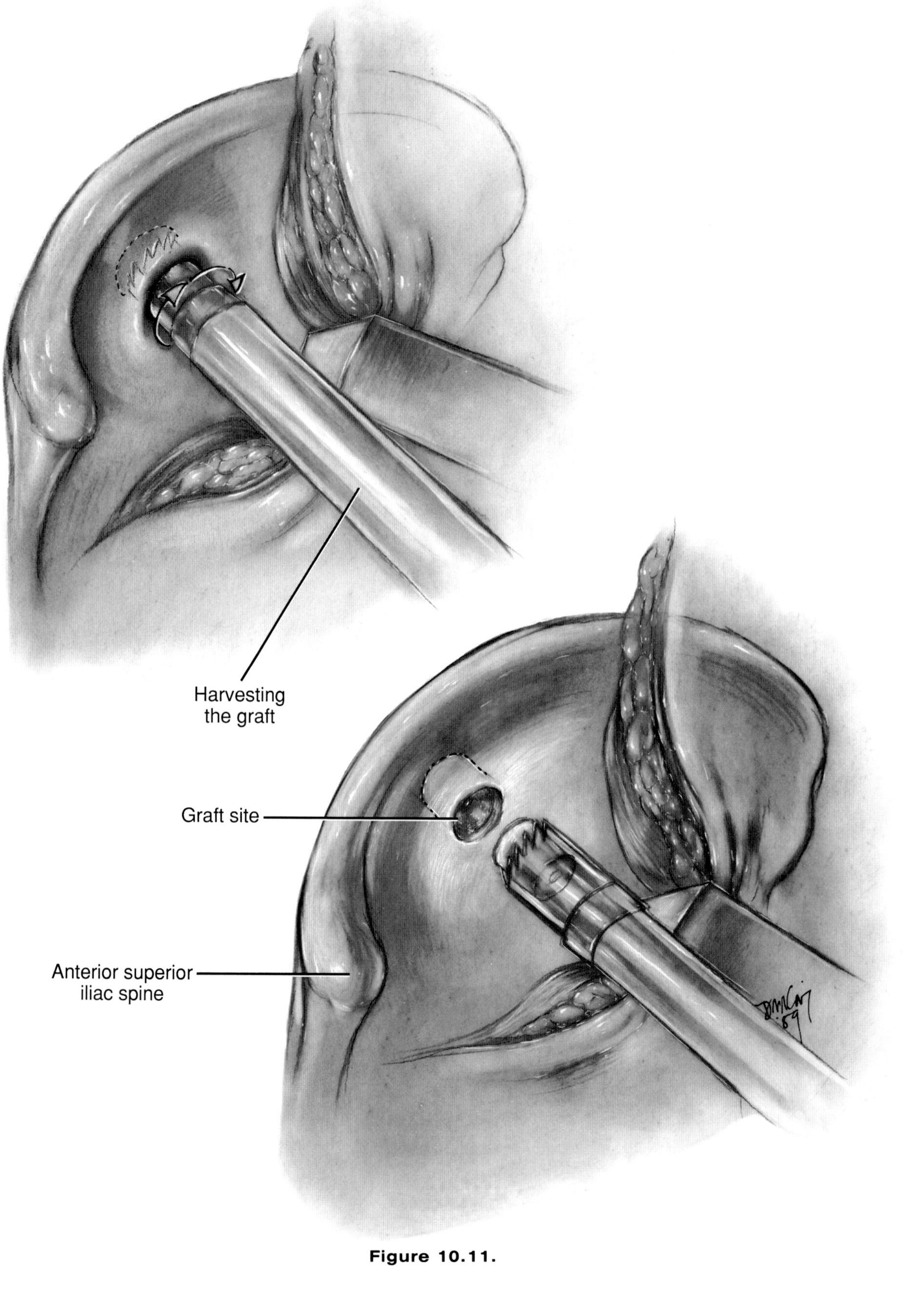
Harvesting
the graft
Graft site
Anterior superior
iliac spine

Figure 10.11.

hold it to the body above and below the interspace to be drilled. Once it is positioned exactly, it should be taped lightly to seat these spikes, securing the drill guide. The guide ensures that the hole will be drilled in the proper place and provides a stop so that the drill cannot extend beyond the measured distance. It is conservative to set this guide at least 1 mm short of the posterior longitudinal ligament and use a curette to remove the remaining portion. It is extremely important that the position of the guide be checked with regard to its midline location, so that it is in the exact center of the interspace to be drilled. The only exception to this is when two interspaces are going to be drilled out. Then it is necessary to offset them so that the common body that will be drilled has no more than one third of each of the holes to be drilled. Otherwise, the entire body will be destroyed by the drilling. Placing two thirds of each drill hole on a body and one third to receive a single hole on the common body will solve this problem. The drill is then inserted, and the interspace and adjacent bodies are drilled away. This will leave a circular hole the full depth of the vertebral body with perhaps 1 mm of the cortical bone remaining posteriorly. Residual bone is removed with a curette. The drill should never be used freehand, no matter what the temptation. In the event the drilling is less than was planned and a second drilling is required, it is necessary to make sure that the guide is returned to exactly the same location each time it is removed to check the depth of the hole. When the drilling is complete, the bone should have been removed nearly to the posterior ligament. The small angled curettes supplied with the set can then be utilized to remove the remainder of the posterior rim. This will effectively remove any bony ridges present. The spurs underneath the nerve root can also be removed in a radical fashion by lateral curetting or by use of a high-speed drill. When the spurs are actually removed by drilling or curetting, the operating microscope allows the surgeon to carry out this maneuver under direct vision at all times.

Obtaining the bone for grafting requires an exposure similar to that described for the Robinson fusion (Fig. 10.10). Because of a slightly different technique, a more extensive exposure is required.

The Cloward bone dowels are taken from the iliac crest 1 cm or so behind the anterior superior spine. When they are taken directly beneath the spine, they may be too thick to fit well. The incision should be made parallel to the crest and just above it. The crest is exposed, and the interdigitating fibers of muscular attachments are divided carefully so that a subperiosteal dissection of the muscles from both the inside and the outside of the crest is possible. The Cloward drill is then fitted into the incision at a convenient flat spot, and the dowels are harvested by drilling through the whole thickness of the ilium. A large abdominal retractor on the pelvic side protects the bowel from perforation by the sharp Cloward drill, should it plunge through the bone. The dowel should be checked for appropriate size and shape. The cut edges of the bone should not be waxed, for this will retard bone healing. It is better to pack the area with a hemostatic agent that will allow scar formation and bone regeneration to fill the defect. The muscular attachments should be closed over the crest. No other muscle sutures are necessary. A drain is left beneath the muscle so that a painful hematoma does not form. Subcutaneous tissue and skin closure requires no special consideration.

Once the grafts are harvested, they should be immediately checked again for size. The appropriate holes have been cut from the cervical area as described. The dowels are placed over the hole, and the holes are spread with the interspace spreader. The dowels are then lightly tapped in place and countersunk 1 or 2 mm, depending on their height and the height of the hole cut in the bone through the disc space (Fig. 10.11). The least inaccessible hole should be filled first. Once the dowels are in position, the anesthesiologist can gently manipulate the neck to make sure they are well seated. Then the wound can be closed without drainage. Only stitches in the platysma, subcutaneous tissue, and skin are required.

SECTION 4

Cervical Spondylosis and Fracture

11

Decompressive Operations on Cervical Spine

Cervical Decompressive Laminectomy

Cervical decompressive laminectomy may be accomplished with the patient in the sitting or the prone position. The sitting position has several advantages: the blood runs out of the incision, the lesion is not obscured, and less suctioning is required. Instruments are directed up and down, parallel rather than perpendicular to the cord, so the risk of cord injury may be somewhat less. On the other hand, there is always the danger of air embolus. In the prone position, blood accumulates in the base, and the instruments are at least partially directed toward the cord, but there is no risk of air embolization. The preanesthetic preparation of the patient is much simpler, and it is easier to extend the incision downward if the need arises.

After the patient is positioned, the skin incision is planned to extend at least one level above and below the expected bone removal. This will ensure adequate exposure of the cord at either end of the laminectomy to be certain that no constriction occurs at the limits of bone removal. The incision is carried to the ligamentum nuchae in the midline. Aside from crossing veins, this should virtually be avascular, since it is through ligament. When the spines in the midline are reached, self-retaining cerebellar retractors are utilized to hold the margins of the wound back and expose the spinous processes. Adequate hemostasis can be obtained by electrocoagulation; there will be some skin bleeding, which is usually minor and will stop. The use of compressive skin clips is another way to stop this skin bleeding. Skin towels are not required. The attachments of the cervical muscles to the spine are then cut away. It is easier to begin at the bottom, since the bleeding will be less troublesome. This is particularly true in the sitting position. The bifid nature of the spines makes it difficult to obtain the same bloodless subperiosteal dissection possible in the thoracic and lumbar areas. However, if the attachments are carefully cut with a knife on the bone and the dissection begins in the proper plane, there is little bleeding except from crossing veins. Open 4×4 gauze sponges should be packed in the surgical space created to obliterate it and absorb the minor bleeding that occurs. By this point it is usually possible to identify accurately the cervical levels involved. This is done by counting from C2 and using the bifid appearance of the spines as seen at surgery and compared with x-rays to localize the position accurately (see Fig. 11.3). If there is any question, a lateral cervical spine film should be taken. A subperiosteal dissection of the muscle mass from the laminae should now be carried out by using small square cervical osteotomes sized to the cervical lamina. The large lumbar osteotomes are dangerous, since they are sharp enough and strong enough to cut cervical bone. The dissection should be carried out to expose the facet joints to the lateral margin. The surgical area is packed with gauze. It is always wise to leave tails of gauze hanging out of the wound rather than putting them underneath the muscle. It is not likely that a sponge could be left in a cervical wound, but it has happened, and leaving a part of the sponge out is a good habit. An identical procedure is carried out on the opposite side, and self-retaining retractors are then put in place. Angled cerebellar retractors are ideal for this purpose. They should be placed at the extremities of the wound, and the muscle should be satisfactorily retracted to the edge of the zygapophyseal joint. Immaculate hemostasis should be obtained throughout the operative site. There should be no bleeding when the laminectomy begins. The next step is to identify the extent of the cervical laminectomy accurately. This is easily done with this exposure by identifying C1-C2 and then counting down. Even when they are not exposed, it is a simple matter to reach C1-C2 with a palpating finger. The appearance of the first bifid spine is also a useful landmark and can be judged from the plain anteroposterior film. The spines of the laminae to be removed are then excised with a heavy bone-cutting rongeur. It is important that the bites be clean. The cervical laminae should not be twisted or pulled in order to remove bone or ligament. For the usual amount of bleeding it is unnecessary to apply bone wax. Occasionally, a diploic space will be unusually vascular, and then bone wax should be used. The laminectomy is begun at the lower level and carried to the upper limit of the required bony removal.

A double-action rongeur such as the Leksell is ideal. The instrument should not be placed in the spinal canal. The proper use is with two hands, with one squeezing the handles and the second propped underneath the instrument, applying pressure outward so that any slip is out rather than in. The instrument is used at a 45° angle, and the cutting jaws of the instrument are never placed beneath the laminae. In this way, the jaws of the instrument never intrude on the spinal canal below the level of the bone, and there is no chance of momentary compression of the spinal cord. The removal of the laminae continues in this way until it is complete. Usually, it is easiest to remove laminae and ligament together. The interlaminar ligaments attach on the upper margin of one laminae and run to attach at about midpoint of the laminae above. These ligaments should not be ripped out with the rongeurs but should be cut cleanly. If they do not cut cleanly with the rongeur bite, they can be held on the stretch and divided with a #15 knife.

Any venous bleeding that occurs in either the sitting or the prone position must be immediately controlled by coagulation or packing. The laminectomy is now extended via 45° cervical punches, which are utilized to widen the laminectomy, first on one side and then on the other. The laminectomy should be carried to the margin of the zygapophyseal joint, exposing the origins of the root sleeves. This will ensure that an adequate cervical decompression has been accomplished. This is the most likely place for venous bleeding to occur. Large bleeding veins should be coagulated with a low bipolar current. Temporary packing with cottonoid or small cotton balls followed by permanent packing with properly sized small strips of Gelfoam or other hemostatic agents will control the bleeding. Hemostasis must be absolute before closure.

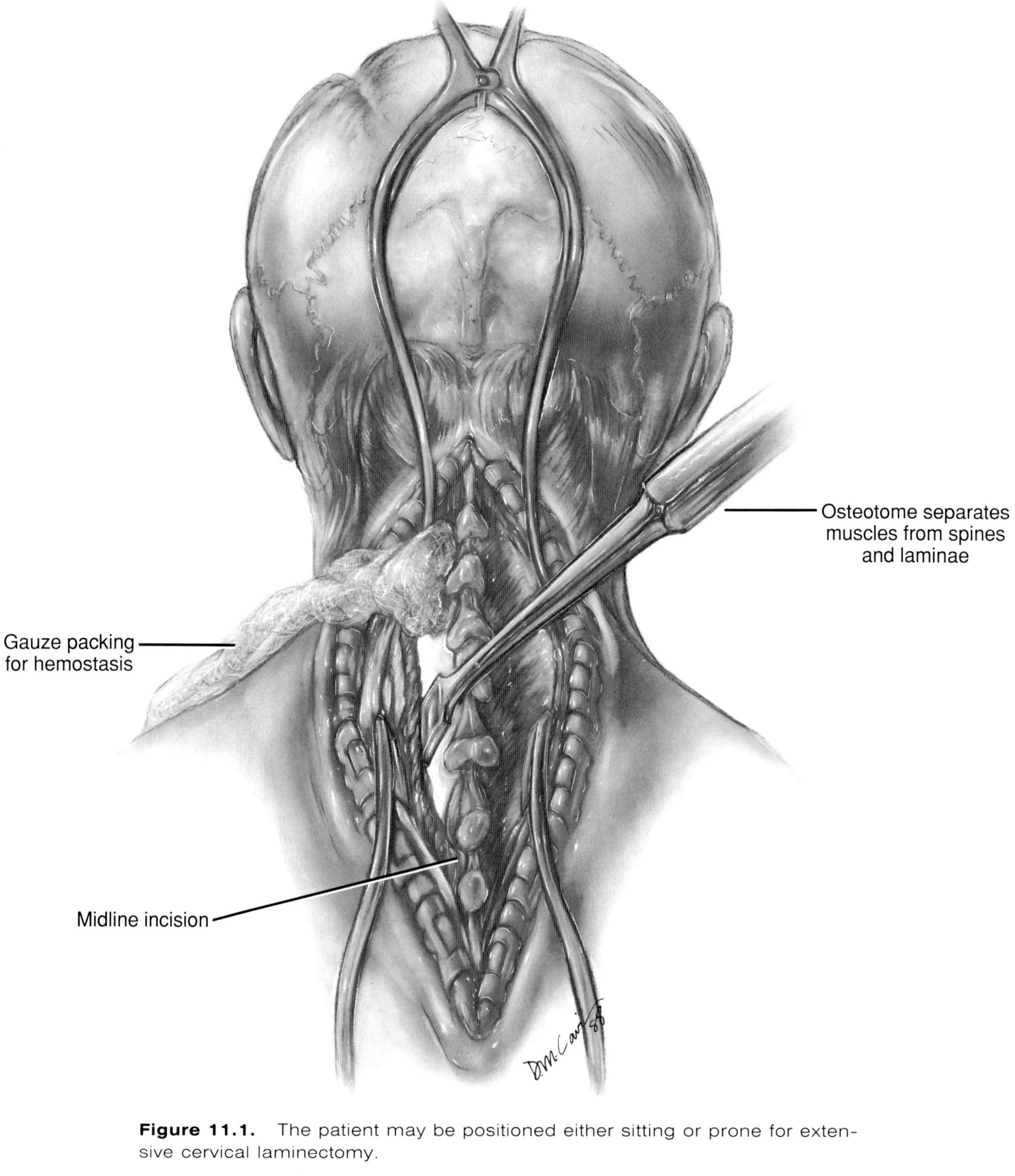

Figure 11.1. The patient may be positioned either sitting or prone for extensive cervical laminectomy.

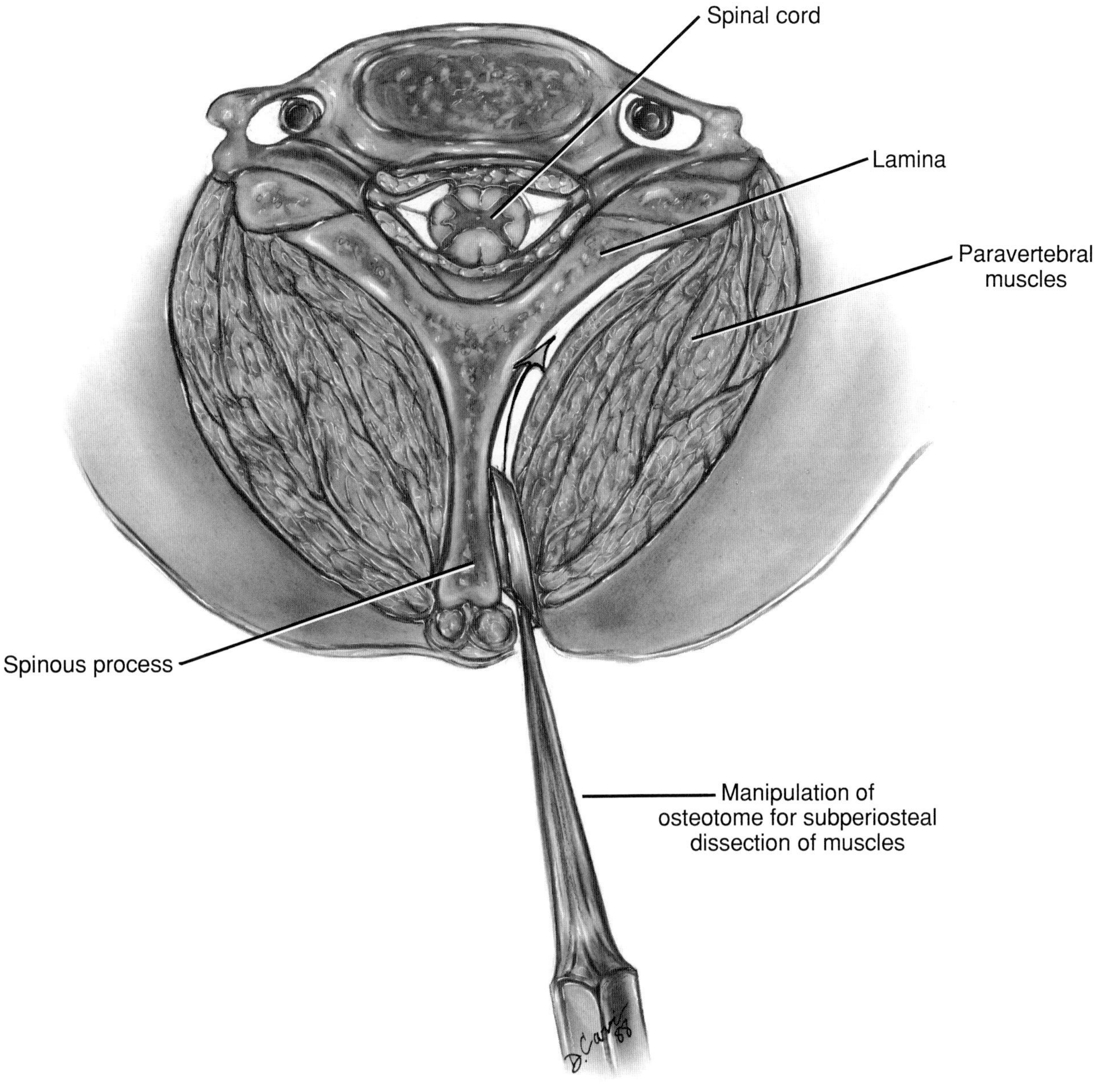
Spinal cord
Lamina
Paravertebral muscles
Spinous process
Manipulation of osteotome for subperiosteal dissection of muscles

Figure 11.2.

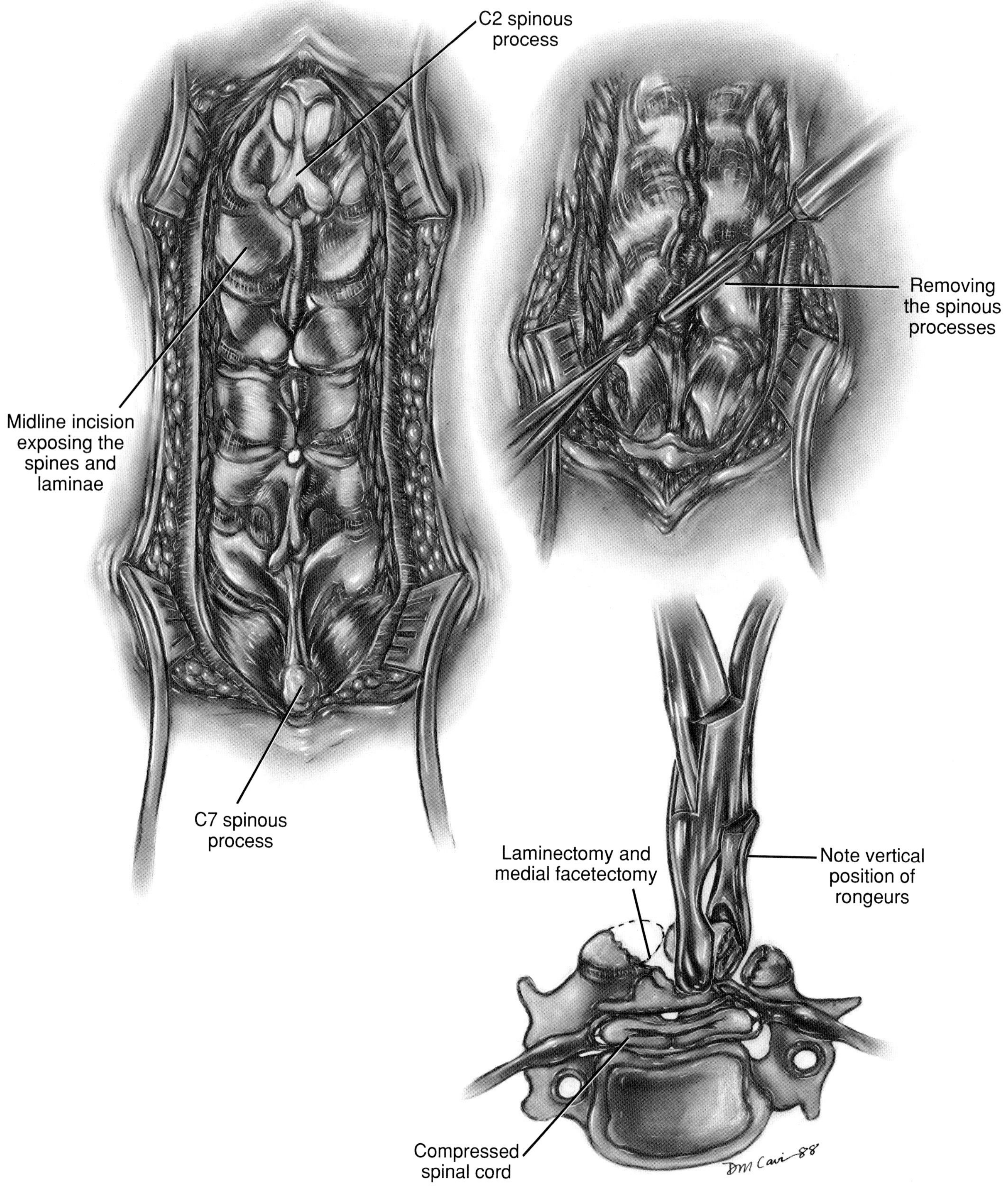
C2 spinous process
Removing the spinous processes
Midline incision exposing the spines and laminae
C7 spinous process
Laminectomy and medial facetectomy
Note vertical position of rongeurs
Compressed spinal cord
DM Cavi 88'

Figure 11.3.

Decompression for spondylotic myelopathy may be extended further. Some surgeons advocate only doing the bony decompression described. The dura may also be opened, leaving the arachnoid intact. This relieves any possibility of dural compression and also allows examination of the cord. It is important to leave the arachnoid intact. With the operating microscope the midline is identified and the dura is carefully opened with a #15 knife until the arachnoid is seen, then a small blunt grooved director is inserted and the dura is opened with a knife. This can usually be done without opening the arachnoid. The cord can be inspected, and the surgeon can then be certain that no further compression is present, and as long as the arachnoid is intact, the closure can proceed without any other special precautions. Some surgeons have recommended a more radical approach in which dura and arachnoid are opened and the dentate ligaments are sectioned. This adds little to the technicalities of the procedure but does increase the risk of cord injury, and there is a greater incidence of pseudomeningocele. If this maneuver is to be done, then the dural opening is still done as before, without entering the subarachnoid space. Then the arachnoid is opened from below upward in the midline with microscissors. Adhesions to the cord are coagulated and cut as required; then, with a small blunt dissector (the Rhoton #5 is a convenient size), the cord and roots can be easily reflected away, and the insertion of the dentate ligament beneath the dorsal root is divided with microscissors. It is not necessary to coagulate these structures. When sectioning is complete, a decision has to be made about closure of the dura. If the dura can be closed without compromising the cord, it is preferable to do so. Often, this is not the case, since the spinal cord will have migrated behind the actual posterior margin of the dura. In this case, a dural patch using fascia or a commercially available dural substitute is best. It is reasonable to leave the dura opened, a time-honored neurosurgical procedure, but reconstitution of normal anatomy with a commercially available dural substitute or facial graft is better. Hemostasis in the upper epidural space must be complete before closure of the muscle is done. Packing the gutters with strips of hemostatic agents such as Gelfoam will usually suffice. No sutures are placed in the muscle, but the cervical fascia is closed in the midline with heavy absorbable sutures. A subcutaneous tissue and skin closure is then routine. A subcuticular stitch will obviate the need for stitch removal and allow the patient to leave the hospital promptly.

Cervical Laminectomy for Spondylomyelotic Disease

The purpose of cervical laminectomy for spondylomyelotic disease is decompression of the spinal cord and decompression of nerve roots that may contribute to the symptomatology. The operations are performed with the patient under general anesthesia and in the sitting or the prone position. Patients with compromised spinal cords are susceptible to injury during intubation and positioning, so care must be taken to avoid manipulation of the neck. Physiological monitoring of cord function is a desirable adjunct to surgery. A skin incision is made in the midline to extend at least one segment beyond the expected decompression above and below. The skin incision is usually made from the occiput to the spine of C1. The incision should be taken to the spinous processes and the rim of the foramen magnum in the midline. The ligament and muscles should then be carefully cut away from the spinous processes with a #15 knife or a small electric knife. Self-retaining retractors put in place to stretch subcutaneous tissues and keep the ligaments and muscle on the stretch are helpful. The incision that separates muscle from bone should be on the bone insofar as possible so the subsequent removal will be truly subperiosteal. It is helpful to grasp the muscle to be cut with a ligament and stretch it laterally so that the fewest fibers possible are divided and the cleanest incision possible is made on the bone. It is easier to work from above down. As the incision proceeds, the newly created space should be packed with 4×4 gauze sponges to reduce the risk of air embolism in the sitting position and to control bleeding. The muscle incision should be made bilaterally over the entire area where laminectomy is contemplated, before the subperiosteal dissection is continued. One side is packed while the other is completed. Any significant bleeding points should be coagulated. The majority of the small bleeders on the muscle will stop during the packing. The subperiosteal dissection should then be completed with cervical osteotomes. I prefer the square osteotomes sized to fit the cervical laminae. Beginning at C2, the subperiosteal dissection is carried out, with the muscles scraped from bone to the lateral margins of the zygapophyseal joints. The arrangements of the cervical laminae make it unnecessary to carry out the angled dissections required in the lumbar region. The osteotomes are directed down the spinous process and directly out the lamina. The upper and lower margins of the laminae are freed of tissue by these maneuvers, which are perpendicular to the midline and parallel to the laminae. When one side is completed intact, the other side is also dissected free and packed. The packing should then be removed, and cerebellar-type self-retaining retractors utilized to expose the entire space. Hemostasis should be obtained at this point, and if there are any significant venous bleeders in patients in the sitting position, they should be immediately occluded with moist 4×4 gauze sponges while the hemostasis is obtained. Remember that air embolism can occur in the prone position if the patient's head is even slightly above the line of the heart. The laminae should now be identified. Since the spine of C2 is exposed, it is a simple matter to count for appropriate localization. Large bone-cutting rongeurs should be used to remove all the spines that are planned to be included in the laminectomy, leaving those that are not. This reduces the possibility that the laminectomy can be stopped short of the desired goals. The laminectomy then begins from the bottom of the incision upward. It is easiest to start in the midline at the lowest level and remove bone with a rongeur until dura or ligament is exposed. There are two possibilities for the bony removal. One is to take bone and ligament in single bites. A strong surgeon with sharp instruments can do this. If the ligaments are taken with the bone and torn away from their attachments laterally, excessive epidural bleeding is likely to occur, but clean bites with the bone occlude the epidural space and reduce bleeding to a minimum. Sometimes, the ligaments are quite adherent to bone and very difficult to dissect free. At other times, the bone comes off easily, exposing the ligament that will then be removed as a separate piece, as the ligaments attach from the upper margin of the laminae below, beneath the laminae above, and insert across at approximately the midpoint of the lamina. This ligament is usually not completely discontinuous but thinned at its point of major insertion. If the bone is removed without the ligament, the ligament should be excised with a knife as soon as bony removal is complete. The rongeur should not be placed within the cervical canal. It is used perpendicular to the laminae, and the lower jaw is inserted no further than the lower margin of the bone. One finger should be kept hooked under the instrument with steady pressure outward so that if there is a slip, the tendency is to slide out, not in. With the patient in the sitting position any epidural bleeding must be stopped promptly either by coagulation or packing. With the patient in the prone position it is less critical, for air embolism is not likely to occur, but the bleeding will obscure the operative field and must be controlled promptly for this reason. The majority of the laminar bone is removed in this way until the entire dura is exposed. Then, with small angled cervical punches, the laminectomy can be widened to the exits of the dural root sleeves. If foraminotomies are required because of radicular symptoms, they are carried out in the manner described for foraminotomy by using a high-speed drill, a small cervical punch, or a curette. The drill provides wide foraminotomy with the least possibility of injury of a nerve root. Doing foraminotomies after laminectomy is much easier because the exact location of the root is seen and the foraminotomy can be tailored to the beginnings of the root sheath. Multilevel foraminotomies do increase the risk of spinal instability but, if required for the relief of symptoms, should be performed. A second-stage anterior fusion will be needed in the small number of patients who will become unstable. Epidural venous bleeding is most likely to occur with the lateral extensions of the laminectomy. Bipolar coagulation or hemostatic packing will control such bleeding. Be careful not to coagulate around the roots. With the patient in the sitting position, such venous bleeding must be controlled immediately, and the bleeding point should be occluded with moist cotton while the packing or coagulation is readied. It is usually not necessary to open the dura in cord compression from spondylotic disease. If you do wish to explore the spinal cord, one way to do so without compromising the space available to the cord by closure of the dural incision is to open the dura without opening the arachnoid. With the aid of magnification the dura is opened in the midline, with the arachnoid left intact. The arachnoid is dissected free with a small blunt dissector over a few millimeters, and a grooved dural director is then put in place so the dura can be opened safely with a #15 knife, and the director will separate dura from arachnoid. The opening should be in the midline and then at the extremities of the bony incision, and incisions should be made perpendicular to the midline to allow

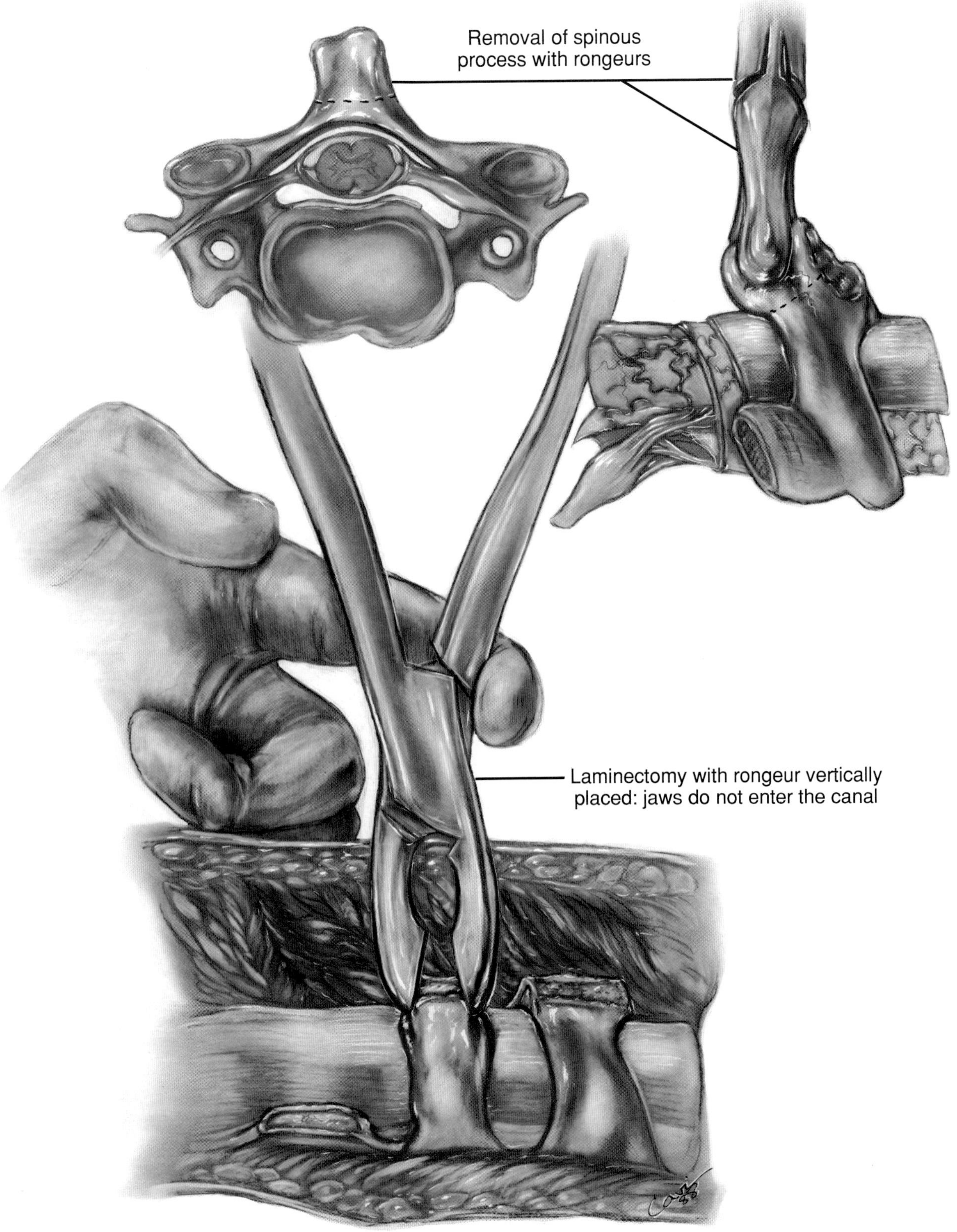
Removal of spinous process with rongeurs
Laminectomy with rongeur vertically placed: jaws do not enter the canal

Figure 11.4.

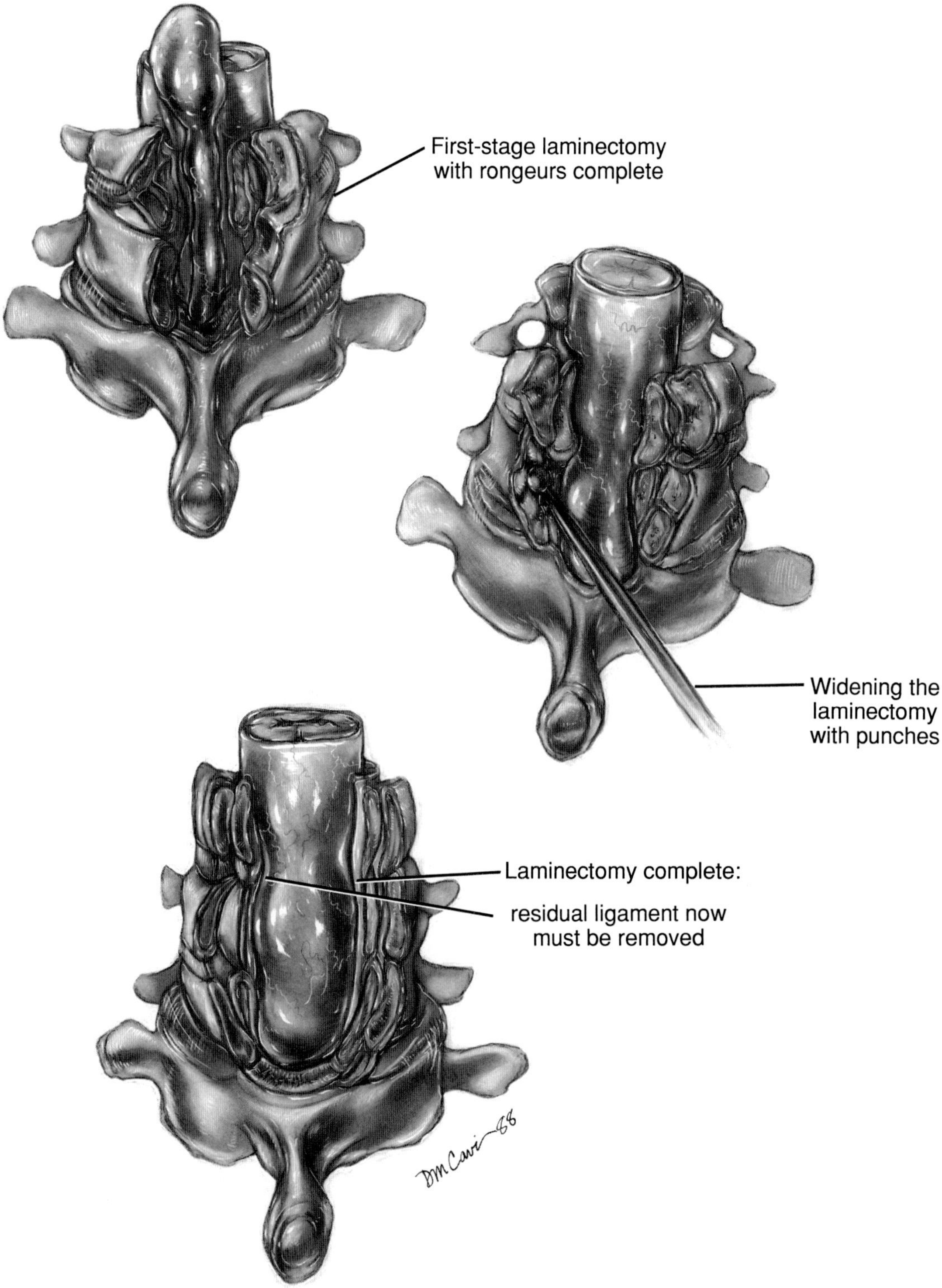
First-stage laminectomy with rongeurs complete
Widening the laminectomy with punches
Laminectomy complete:
residual ligament now must be removed
DM Cavi 88

Figure 11.5.

flaps of dura to be developed laterally. If the arachnoid is intact, there will be no need to close the dura. If there is a problem with lateral hemostasis, the dura can be sutured to the muscle immediately above the zygapophyseal joint to occlude this venous bleeding. If bleeding is not a problem, then nothing needs to be done about closure. This maneuver will allow the spinal cord to be inspected almost as well as with the arachnoid open. If the arachnoid is inadvertently opened during these maneuvers, the dura should be closed. If there is any possibility of compromise of the cord by the dural closure, a patch will be required.

The last step is verification that the cord is adequately decompressed and that there is no possibility of additional compression at the upper and lower margins of the laminectomy. Hemostasis is checked again, and the cervical musculature is closed in the midline by closing the ligamentum nuchae only. No stitches are required in the muscle. Closure of the skin and subcutaneous tissue is routine.

Robinson Fusion for Spondylotic Myelopathy

Robinson fusion for spondylotic myelopathy is done in the same general way as described for simple discectomy and fusion for unilateral radioculopathy (see Chapter 10). The procedure is the same until the disc is removed. Then, since decompression of the spinal cord is the principal goal, it is necessary to remove the posterior ridges carefully. To have adequate vision, it will be necessary to be certain the interspace is open, preferably widened to about 6 mm. This can usually be done while retaining margins of cortical bone, except with the most degenerated and collapsed interspaces. As soon as the interspace is properly exposed and the anterior disc is removed, an operating microscope is brought into the field and utilized for removal of the posterior ridges. These ridges are usually not extremely hard bone, and they can usually be removed with small curettes. Angled curettes of 1 and 2 mm are perfect for this purpose. The posterior longitudinal ligament is left intact, and the ridges are curetted under direct vision. They can also be removed with a high-speed drill using a small diamond burr (Fig. 11.6). The use of the drill in a cervical interspace is a job for an experienced spine surgeon who routinely uses this instrument, and great care must be taken to remove the ridges without injury to any other structures. The two great risks are extending the resection too far posteriorly, lacerating the dura, or extending it too far laterally, drilling into the vertebral artery. In most instances, the ridges can be removed without traversing the posterior longitudinal ligament. In these cases of spondylosis, the dura and this ligament are often tightly adherent, and it is easy to lacerate the dura if the ligament is removed. Should a dural laceration occur, it can be sealed by occluding it with a small amount of fat taken from the subcutaneous tissue of the neck. When the graft is seated on top of the fat, an adequate seal should occur. A cerebrospinal fluid leak through the neck wound is a catastrophe, and you must be certain the seal is good before closure can proceed. The Robinson anterior decompression is most commonly utilized for one- or two-level spinal cord compression. Multiple levels can be fused individually. Sometimes, total corpectomy is necessary if the compression extends over the entire body. The details of replacement of the body are in Chapter 12. If more than two levels of compression are present, a posterior decompression may be substituted as easier even when the principal problem is anterior. The ideal patient for the anterior operation has a single-level bar. When two or more levels are done, it is not necessary to take special precautions about the placement of the grafts because the Robinson fusion does not disrupt the integrity of the body. It is necessary to remember that the protective posterior lips of the vertebral body have been removed, so the surgeon must be especially careful in tamping the graft to the proper depth. Since there are several millimeters of leeway with this type of graft, driving it in too far is not a common problem. Should this occur, it is recognized immediately at the time of surgery and can be remedied simply by extracting the graft and replacing it. The risk of cord injury is small but real, and a postoperative film is taken to be certain placement is satisfactory, before the patient is awakened.

Posterior Cervicothoracic Osteotomy for Chin-on-Chest Deformity

For ankylosing spondylitis and occasionally for other seronegative spondyloarthropathies, it is necessary to place the patient's head in a more functional position. Many patients present with such pronounced cervical

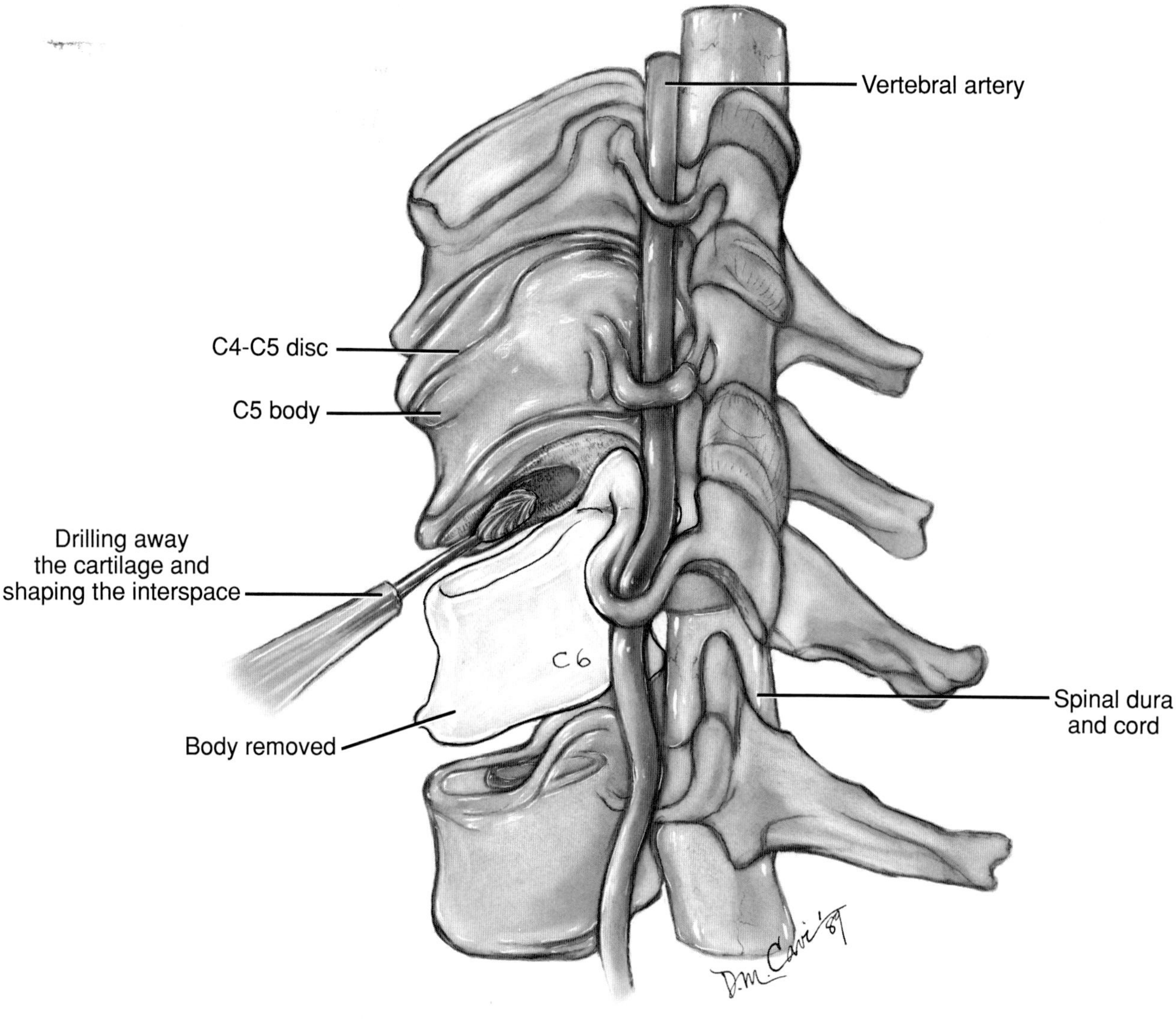

Figure 11.6.

kyphotic deformities that they are unable to ambulate while looking straight ahead. The patient should be in a standing position with the knees straight for examination. The major indication for performing a closing wedge osteotomy in the cervicothoracic area is failure to extend the neck up to the midline to view the horizon. If the major part of the deformity is in the thoracic or the lumbar spine, then the placement of the osteotomy should be at the L2-L3 level. The approach in this chapter pertains to the patient with the major part of the deformity in the cervicothoracic area.

The time-honored approach has been that of Urist, recently popularized by Simmons. It is an osteotomy performed with the patient under local anesthesia, as the initial published experience revealed a 10% risk of intraoperative death and a 30% incidence of intraoperative neurological deficit when the procedure was performed under general anesthesia. Most patients with ankylosing spondylitis at the stage in their disease when they require cervicothoracic osteotomy have had their ribs spontaneously fused to their thoracic spines, thereby eliminating active chest expansion. They are totally dependent on their diaphragm for

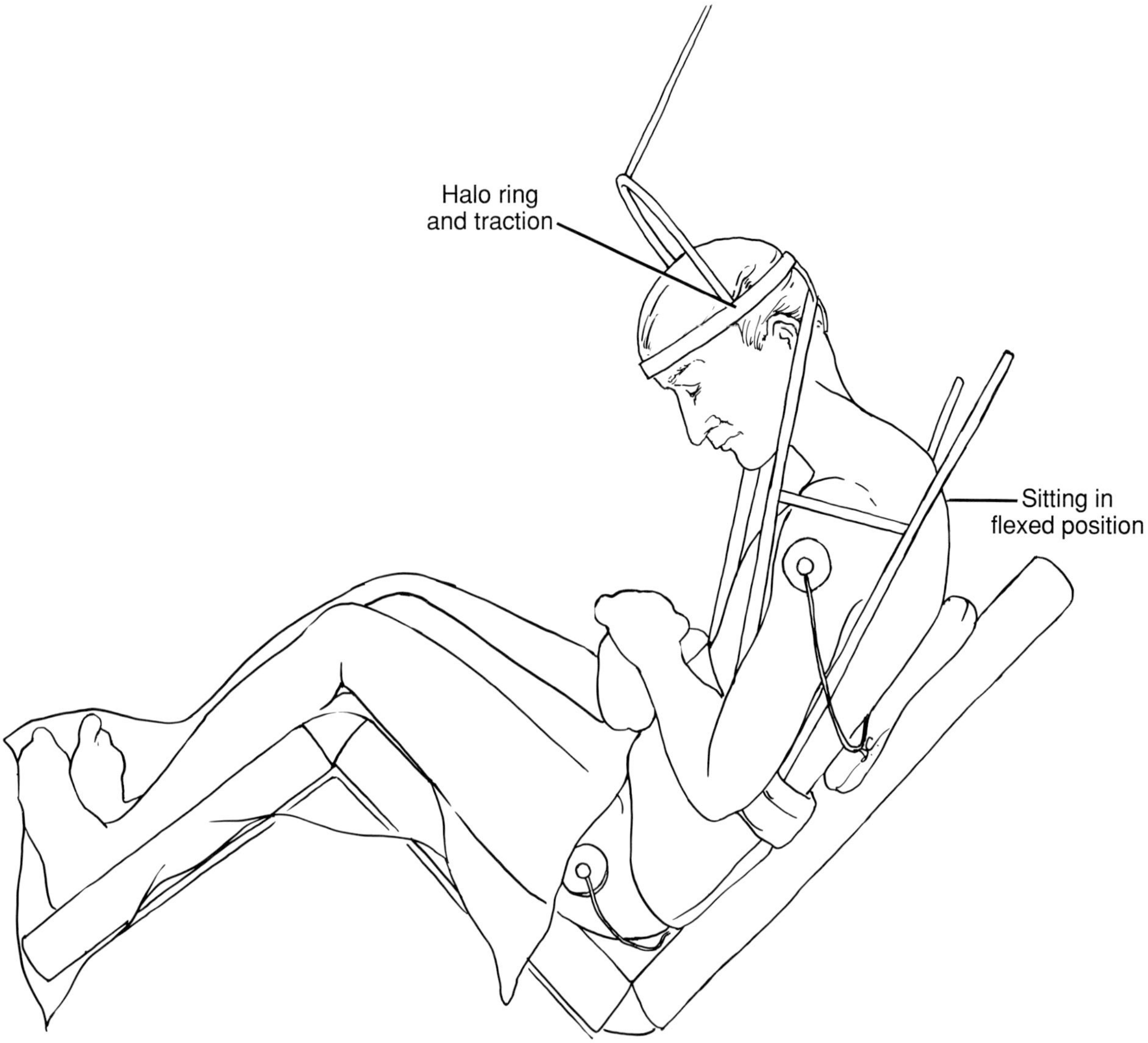

Figure 11.7. Position for correction of chin-on-chest deformity.

breathing and tend to be susceptible to such postoperative pulmonary complications as pneumonia.

Technique of Cervicothoracic Osteotomy

The C7-T1 area is chosen for the osteotomy, as the vertebral arteries usually enter the foramen transversarium at C6. An osteotomy superior to the C6 level would tend to apply traction on the vertebral arteries with secondary vertebrobasilar ischemia. The cervicothoracic area has proved to be the safest location for the osteotomy. Multiple osteotomies throughout the thoracic spine can be performed, although this is usually associated with higher neurological complications.

The patient is placed in a halo-pelvic device preoperatively. As the procedure is performed with 1% Xylocaine anesthesia, the halo is usually placed 1 day prior to the operative procedure to preserve as much local anesthetic as possible for use during the operative cervicothoracic correction. The patient is placed on an operating table in the sitting position with the cervicothoracic area exposed and with the patient in 10 pounds of traction. The patient's pelvic device is already hooked up, as after the cervicothoracic osteotomy, the degree of instability is significant. It is unwise to perform a destabilizing osteotomy and then be in the difficult position of trying to hook up the pelvic device. It is much safer to have the halo-pelvic device in place and then merely to have to make minor adjustments to stabilize the neck. The cervicothoracic area is prepped and draped with the patient in the sitting position. The paraspinal muscles are dissected off the posterior elements from C5 to T3. Care is taken to dissect the transverse processes of T1. These are the key anatomic landmarks in localizing the site of the osteotomy at C7-T1. Note that the interspinous ligaments and the ligamentum flavum are usually totally ossified. The bone is usually more brittle than normal, although it is not good for purchase of wires or instrumentation. Most investigators utilize simple wiring techniques inferior and superior to the osteotomy but rely on the halo-pelvic device for stability. A standard laminectomy is performed by utilizing Leksell rongeurs, exposing the cervical spinal cord from C7 to T1. The C8 nerve roots are then completely unroofed, and the C7 pedicles are completely undercut. The most common mistake made in the surgical procedure is to fail to decompress the C8 nerve roots. Specific attention should be made to intraoperative complaints of paresthesias along the ulnar border of both arms or even complaints of intrinsic weakness during closure of the osteotomy. A C8 neurological deficit is the most common complication of the procedure. For this reason, we perform a very meticulous decompression of the spinal cord and the C8 nerve roots prior to the correction. Occasionally, a patient's C8 nerve roots are irritated and extremely painful. To remedy this, cotton and Gelfoam soaked in Xylocaine are applied over the inflamed nerve foot.

Usually, there is minimal bleeding and excellent hemostasis, as the patient is in the sitting position. The patients usually have nasal prongs and oxygen administered during the operative procedure, but the patient must be awake enough to be able to provide continuous neurological feedback during the correction. The procedure conceptually involves a closing osteotomy involving the posterior elements. Simultaneously, the anterior elements are corrected with an opening osteotomy. The hinge of correction is at the level of the posterior longitudinal ligament at C7-T1. With gradual correction the patient can be given nitrous oxide, which is self-administered via a breathing mask. When the patient is sufficiently sedated, he or she will spontaneously drop the nitrous oxide mask, and the correction can be obtained. With an assistant holding the halo on both sides, the patient's occiput is directed in a posterior fashion, and anterior pressure is directed on the superior portion of the thoracic spine. The spine is gently hinged at the C7-T1 area with direct visualization of the exposed neural elements. Usually, there is some redundancy or wrinkling of the dura as the osteotomy progresses and the spinous processes at C6 and T2 become closer together. A wire is then passed from C6 to T2 and, when the desired amount of correction is completed, secured. A lateral radiograph is taken to document that avulsion of the anterior longitudinal ligament and an opening osteotomy have occurred at C7-T1. The key biomechanical complication to prevent is translation at the C7-T1 area, either anteriorly or posteriorly. With the appropriate amount of correction, bone graft is placed along the posterior elements from C7 to T2. It is extremely important to save all of the bone during the decompression laminectomy, as the patient's iliac crest cannot be utilized at this point in the operative procedure. Place Gelfoam over the exposed neural elements to prevent any bone graft from coming in contact with the spinal canal. Most investigators also find it helpful to have placed the closing stitches in the fascia prior to the osteotomy. This is because after the correction the wound is extremely deep and hard to work in with the patient under local anesthesia. Sometimes, the skin has to be closed in a horizontal fashion to close the wound. A dressing is applied and a small suction drain is utilized. During the closure, continuous monitoring is made of the patient's neurological status. If there is any difficulty, then the amount of correction is diminished. The average amount of correction is 50°. It is not unusual to be able to achieve up to 70° of correction at the cervicothoracic area if this is required to bring the neck in a vertical position.

After closure of the posterior cervicothoracic wound and application of a dressing, the patient's halo-pelvic device is then secured in the corrected position. It is useful actually to have the patient stand by the side of the operating table at this point to better adjust the brace. This also provides the surgeon with the ability to finely tune the amount of correction to ensure that the patient can indeed look straight ahead and have good visibility of the horizon while in the standing position with the knees straight.

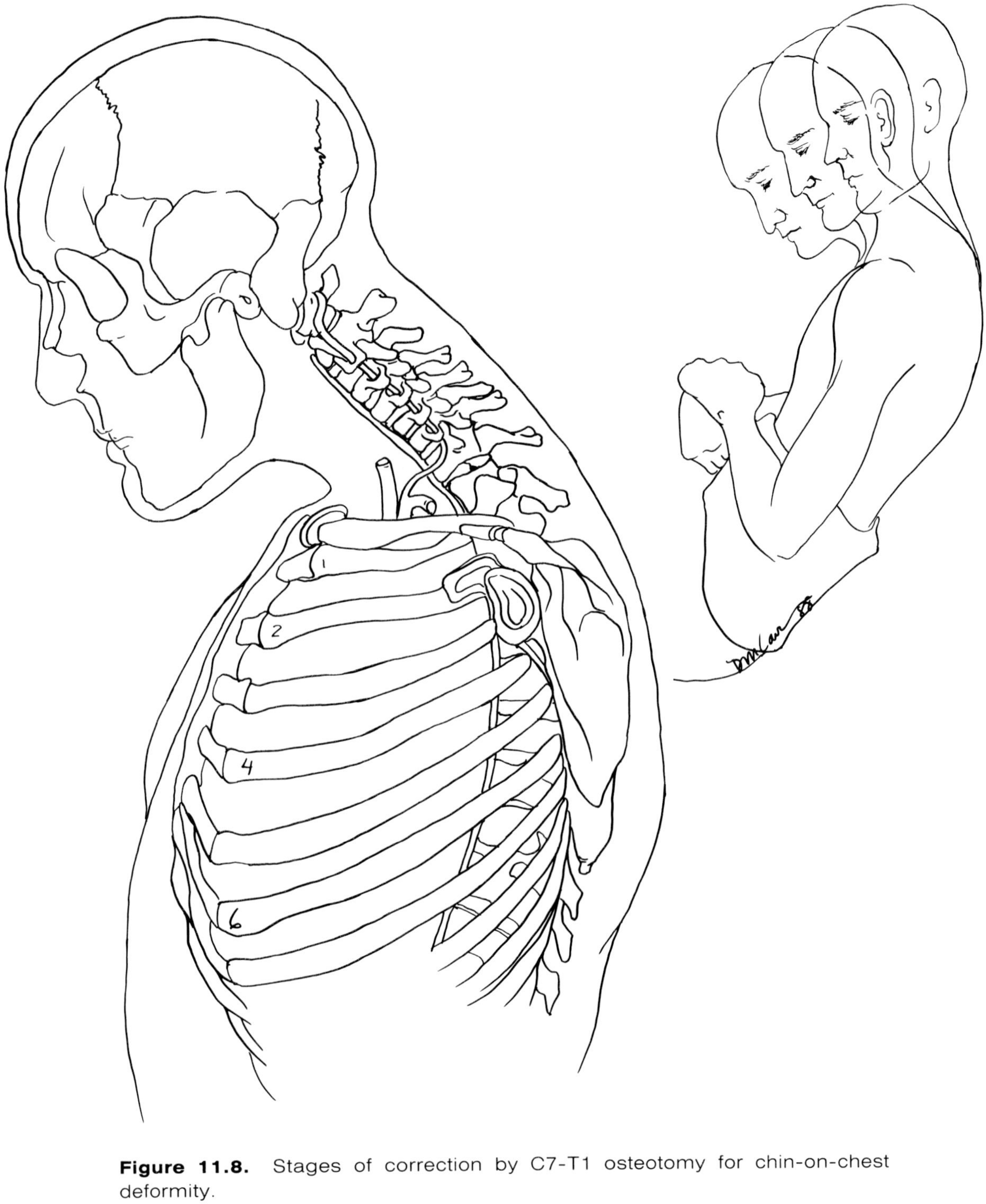

Figure 11.8. Stages of correction by C7-T1 osteotomy for chin-on-chest deformity.

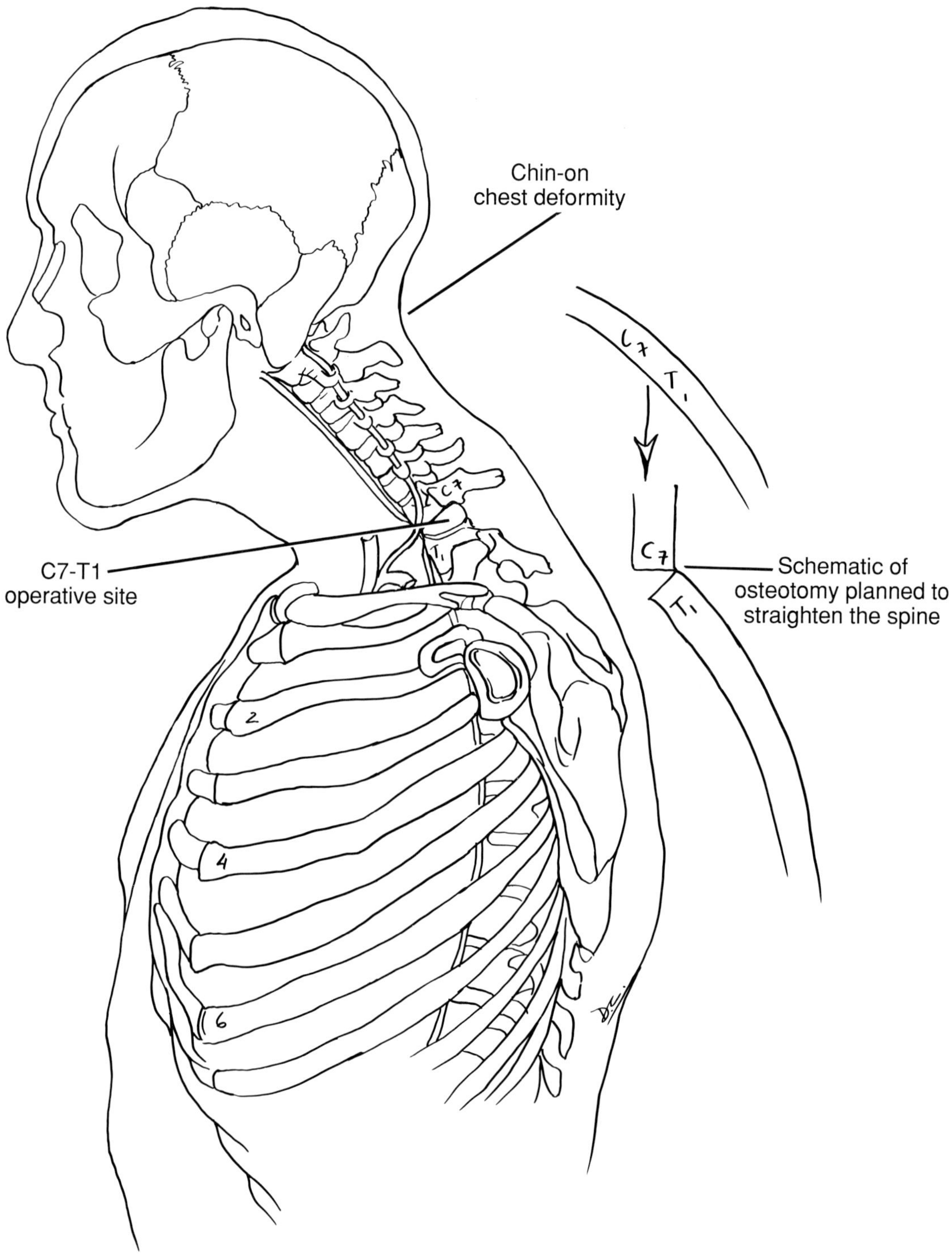
Chin-on
chest deformity
C7-T1
operative site
Schematic of
osteotomy planned to
straighten the spine

Figure 11.9.

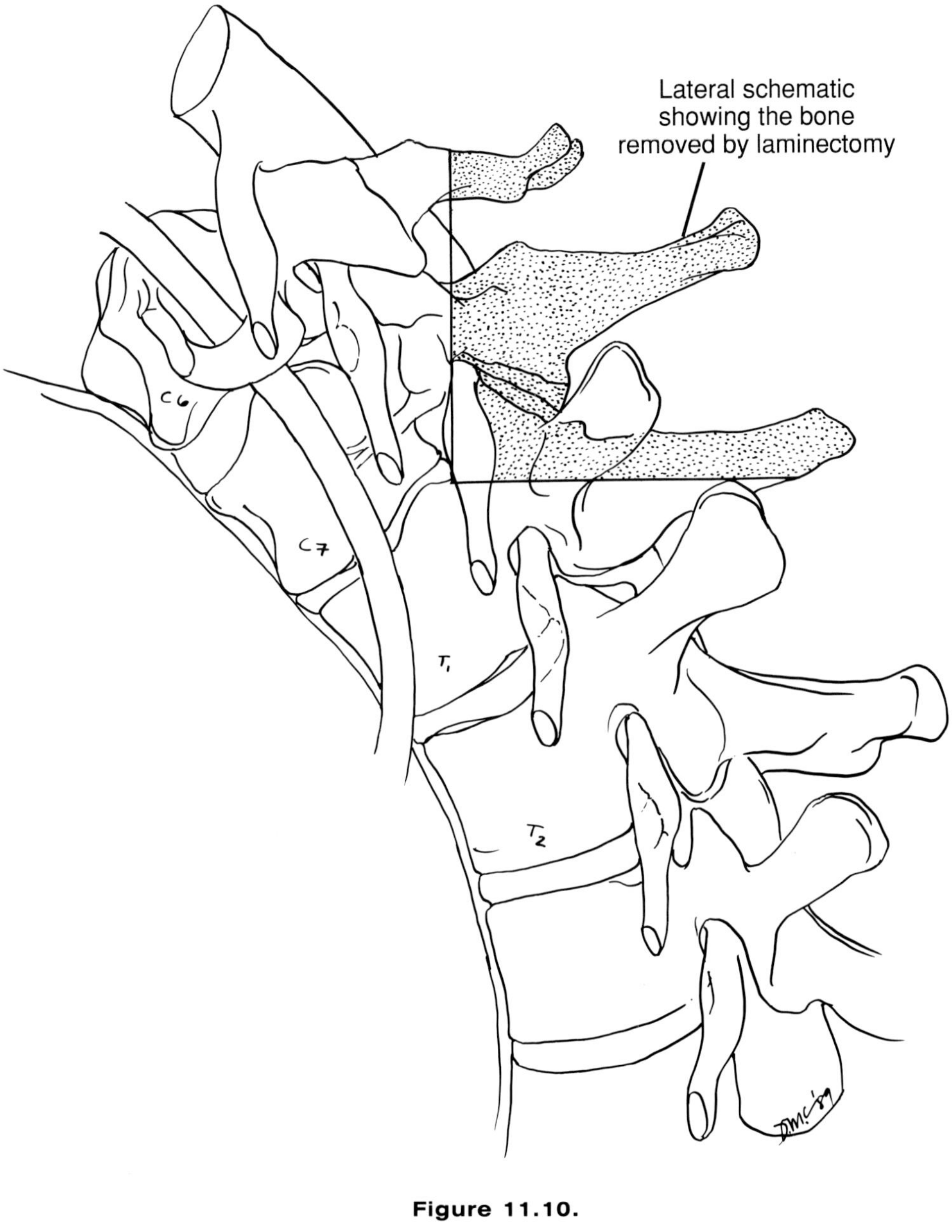
Lateral schematic
showing the bone
removed by laminectomy
C6
C7
T1
T2

Figure 11.10.

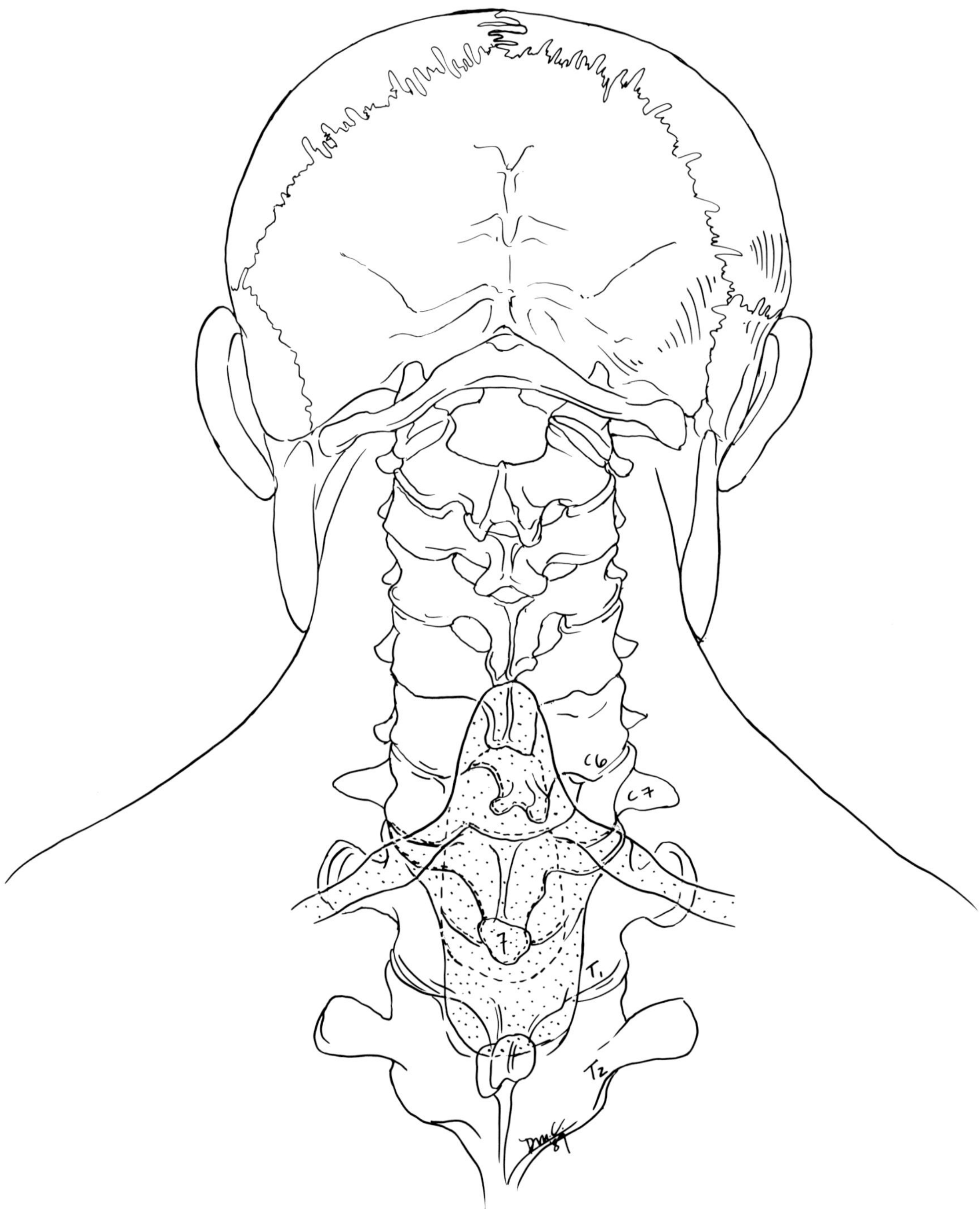

Figure 11.11. Schematic of posterior decompression showing relationship of laminectomy, foraminotomies, and neural elements.

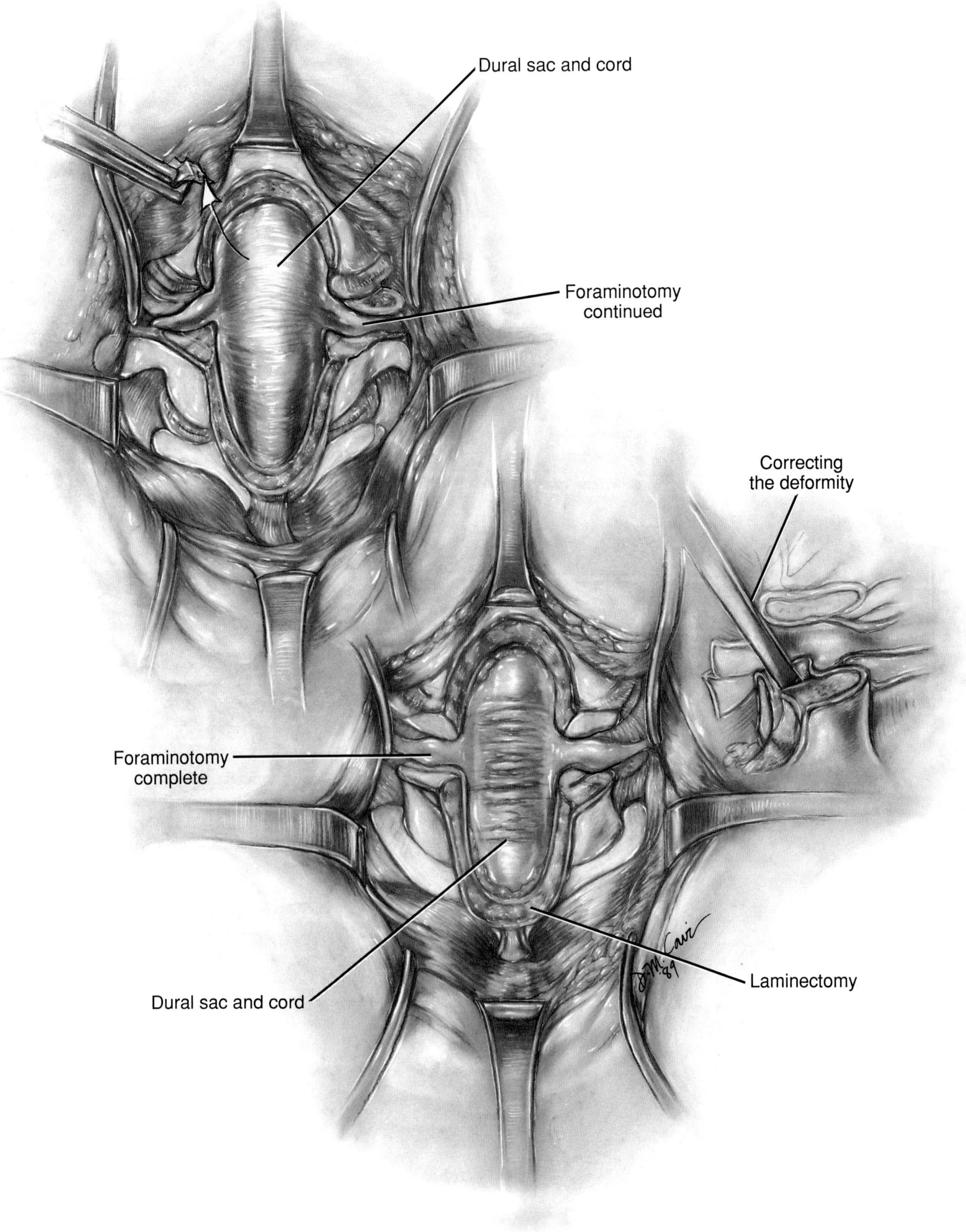
Dural sac and cord
Foraminotomy continued
Correcting the deformity
Foraminotomy complete
Dural sac and cord
Laminectomy

Figure 11.12.

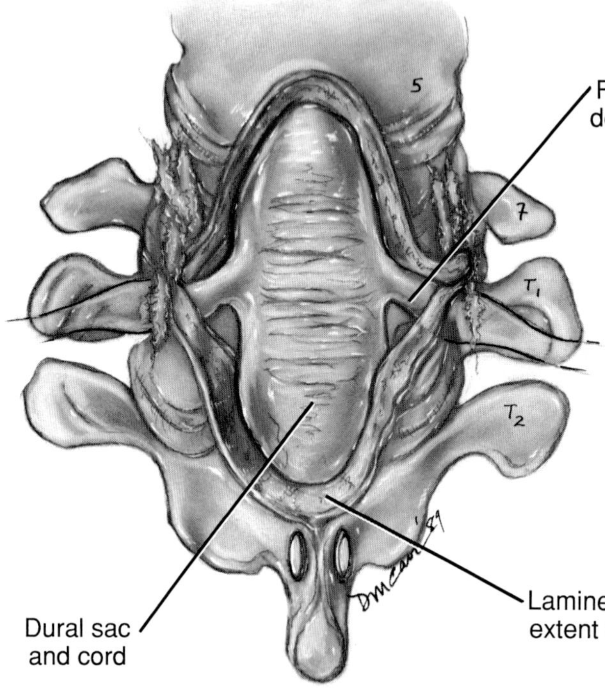

Figure 11.13.

The surgeon has to be careful not to overcorrect the deformity, as the patients with occipitocervical fusion and fusion of the thoracolumbosacral spine have no ability in the other parts of the spine to compensate for overcorrection of the deformity.

The incidence of nonunion is extremely small, provided the halo-pelvic immobilization is continued for a 3-month period. Perform lateral tomography and flexion-extension radiographs to ensure that a solid fusion has occurred. At 3 months postoperatively, if the patient has a nonunion, it is treated by performing an anterior cervical fusion with insertion of the iliac strut graft at the C7-T1 osteotomy site. This can be safely performed with the patient under general anesthesia at 3 months, as the patient now has an adequate amount of working distance from the chin to the chest to allow for safe intubation.

12

Anterior Cervical Corpectomy for Spinal Cord Compression

Patients who are candidates for anterior cervical corpectomy for spinal cord compression may have suffered trauma, have a bony tumor, or have developed severe deformities secondary to spondylotic change or an oddity such as calcification of the posterior longitudinal ligament. The decision to use the anterior approach for decompression of the cord is usually made when the demonstrated compression is principally anterior and when it is relatively localized to one or two bodies. More extensive resections can be done, but grafting is harder. Operations are done with the patient under general anesthesia in the prone position, with cervical traction utilized. Halter traction is satisfactory, but skeletal traction is more reliable. Care should be taken during intubation to maintain the neck in a neutral position, and physiological monitoring throughout the procedure is helpful (Fig. 12.1).

If a single body is to be removed, a transverse incision will suffice. If the bony excision is to be larger, then an incision along the anterior border of the sternocleidomastoid is desirable. Subcuticular closure results in little cosmetic difference between the two. The location of the incision can be judged by palpating the lateral tubercle of C6 in most patients. If there is any question about incision placement, an x-ray taken

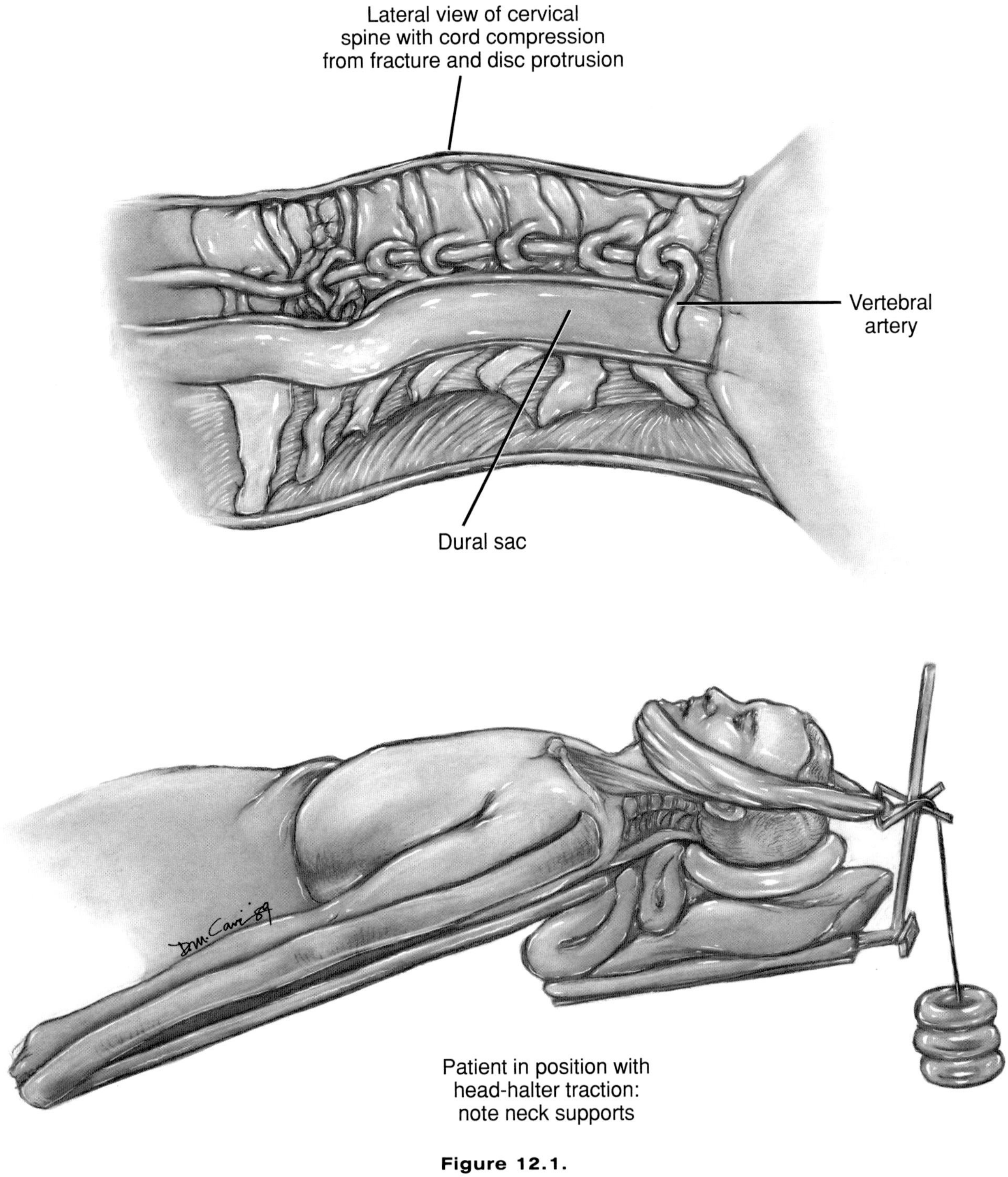

Lateral view of cervical spine with cord compression from fracture and disc protrusion
Vertebral artery
Dural sac
Patient in position with head-halter traction: note neck supports

Figure 12.1.

with an external opaque guide in place will identify the proper incision point. This is critical if a transverse incision is used, but it is of much less importance if a vertical incision is used. The transverse incision should extend from near the midline to 1 or 2 cm beyond the medial border of the sternomastoid. A convenient skin crease will help hide the incision. The vertical incision should be at and parallel to the anterior border of the sternocleidomastoid and extend for a centimeter above and below the expected length of the bony excision. Right-handed surgeons naturally approach from the right side. However, long experience with the Smith-Robinson fusion suggests that the complication of hoarseness occurs less commonly when a left-sided approach is used. After the skin is opened, the platysma should be divided, and the areolar plane anterior to the sternocleidomastoid entered. The dissection along the anterior border of the sternomastoid is virtually bloodless and can be done bluntly. It requires nothing more than inserting two forefingers and spreading to reach the prevertebral space. This is done with a carotid sheath and its contents moved laterally, with the midline laryngeal and pharyngeal structures remaining on the medial side. Occasionally, the dissection cannot be performed bluntly because of crossing veins that are branches of the external jugular. These should be identified, isolated, tied, and divided before the blunt dissection. The superior and inferior thyroid veins and arteries may be encountered in the depths of the incision. Perservation of these vessels is desirable, but those that impede the midline exposure should be isolated, tied, and cut. As long as the blunt dissection is gentle, there is little risk of injuring these large, tough vessels. The omohyoid muscle will cross obliquely for exposures at the C5-C6 and C6-C7 levels. It should be isolated and retracted out of the field, if possible. If it is not, it simply is divided and hemostasis is obtained in the cut muscle margin by electrocoagulation. Thyroid retractors are then utilized to retract the larynx and pharynx medially, exposing the anterior surface of the vertebral column. When the surgeon is in the proper plane, this should result in the immediate development of the prevertebral space that is filled only with loose areolar tissue. Kutner dissectors are a handy way to develop this space. Occasionally there will be large traversing veins, but more commonly there is nothing in the space that is vascular or neural. It is important to be positioned behind the esophagus, and care must constantly be taken to protect the esophagus from either sharp or blunt dissection. The operation can be done with hand-held retractors, but the procedure requires a great deal of precision drilling, and I think it is better to have self-retaining retractors that provide both exposure and protection for surrounding structures. The Cloward retractors designed for this purpose are ideal. The blunt blade of proper length is inserted on the medial side, and the sharp blade is utilized with the teeth in the anterior paravertebral muscles. One retractor is used for lateral exposure, and this is inserted first. The blunt medial blade should be exactly at the level of the planned bony incision. Then, another Cloward retractor is placed vertically to provide superior and inferior exposure. Both of these blades should be blunt. As soon as the retractors are in place, it is important to check the carotid pulse above the retractors to make certain the carotid is not being compromised, and then it is necessary to be certain that the retraction on the esophagus is broadly spread. An x-ray should be taken either now or before the retractors are put in place to be certain about the levels to be resected. When the extent of the bony removal is identified, the interspaces at the upper and lower margins should be easily accessible by the exposure. If they are not, it is necessary to continue the dissection up and down until both are widely exposed. The anterior longitudinal ligament is then incised along the margins of the disc that bound the projected graft and cut across laterally near the insertions of the paravertebral muscles (Fig. 12.2). When these muscles are reasonably lateral in their position, nothing needs to be done to them. When they are near the midline, they should be lifted from the anterior surface of the vertebral column laterally to the margin of the body. This can be done with an electric knife or with osteotomes. The muscles may need to be cut transversely at the level of the disc space. The discs should be removed piecemeal with disc rongeurs back to the posterior longitudinal ligament. The body or bodies should now be removed. Several techniques are available for the corpectomy (Fig. 12.3). The high-speed drill is probably the fastest way to remove the body and, in experienced hands, the safest. With magnification the drill can be used to wipe away bone and shape the channel for the subsequent graft. Laterally, vertebral bodies should be

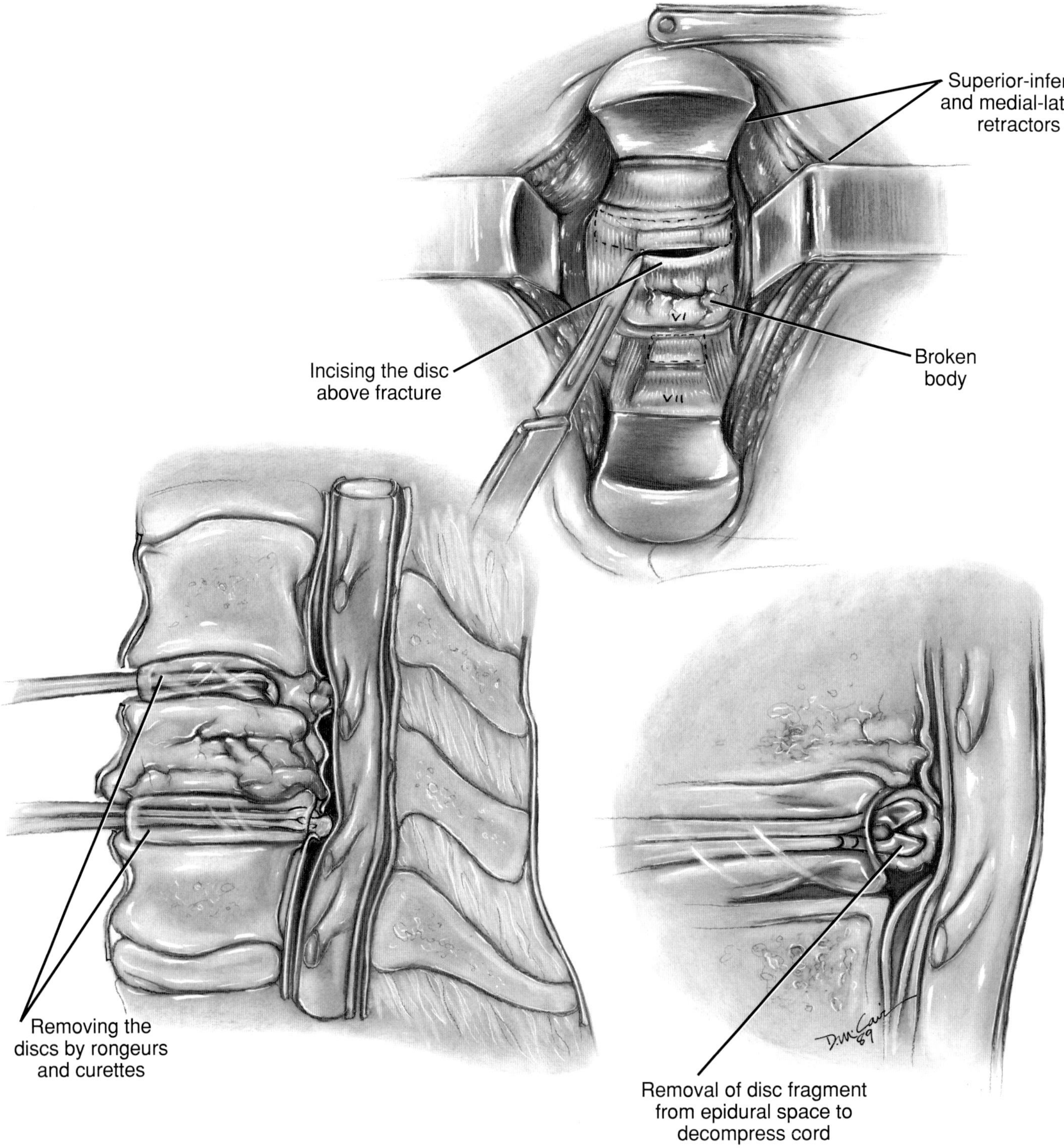
Superior-inferior
and medial-lateral
retractors
Incising the disc
above fracture
Broken
body
VI
VII
Removing the
discs by rongeurs
and curettes
Removal of disc fragment
from epidural space to
decompress cord

Figure 12.2.

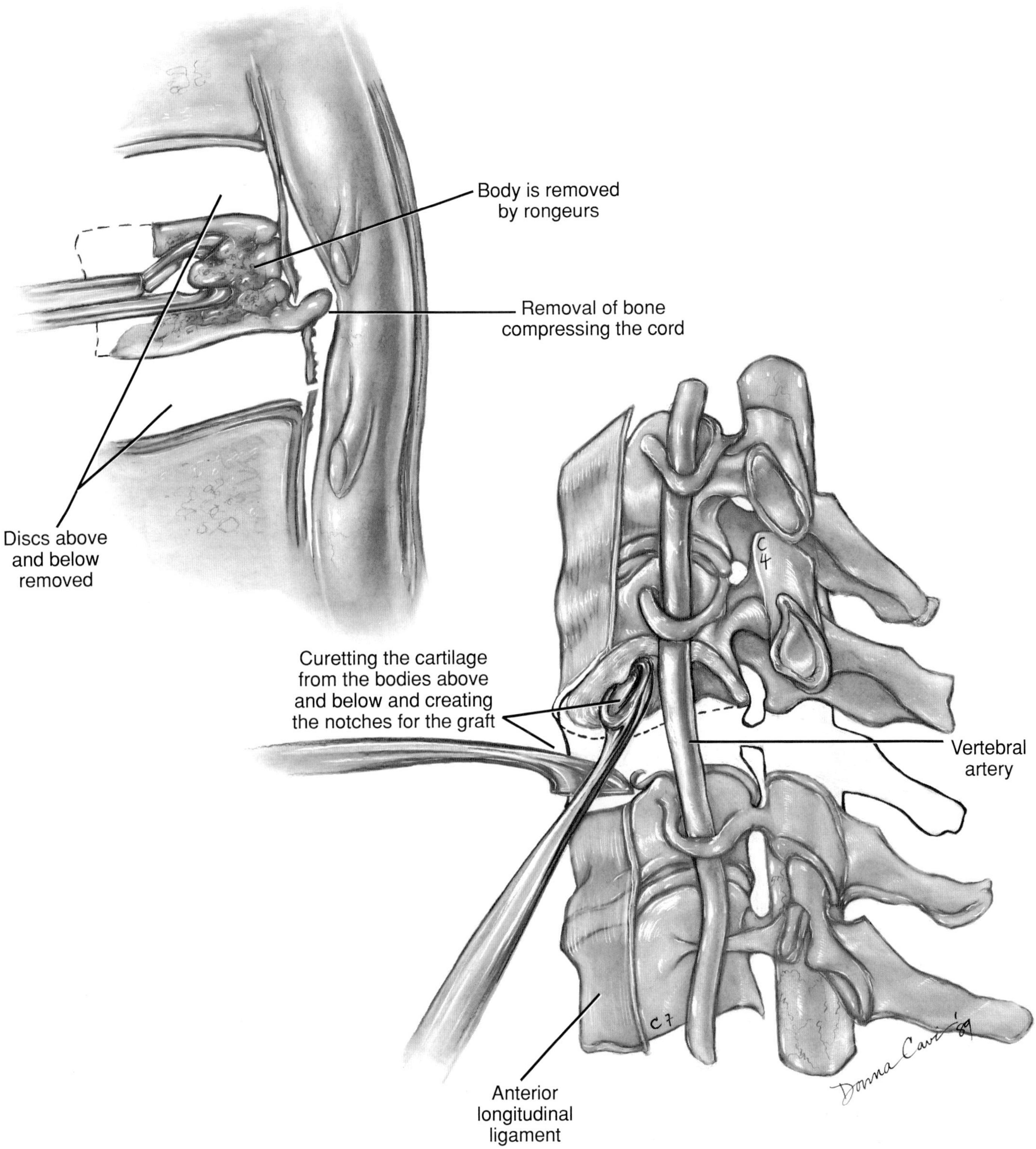
Body is removed
by rongeurs
Removal of bone
compressing the cord
Discs above
and below
removed
Curetting the cartilage
from the bodies above
and below and creating
the notches for the graft
Vertebral
artery
C4
C7
Anterior
longitudinal
ligament
Donna Cavi '89

Figure 12.3.

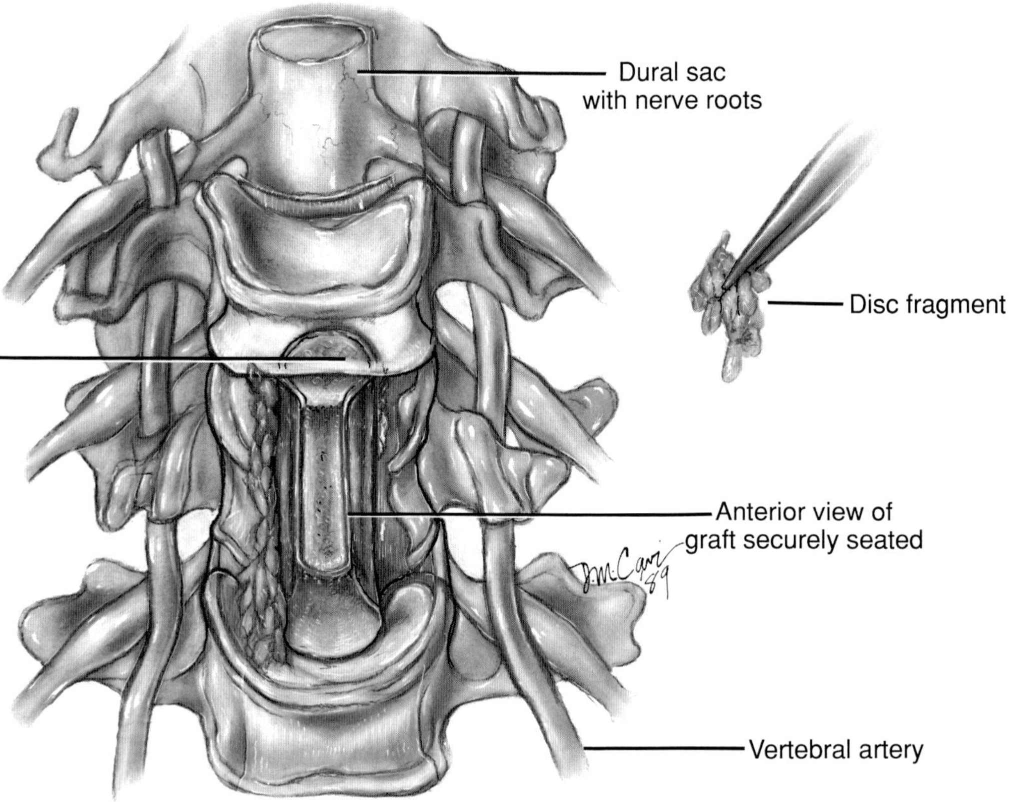

Figure 12.4.

left intact at approximately the lateral margins of the dural canal. The drill can be used to skeletonize the body posteriorly. The very thin rim left posteriorly can then be lifted up with rongeurs or curettes and removed. The dura is often quite adherent to a calcified posterior ligament; this posterior dissection must be done carefully, since it is easy to enter the dura. Any dural lacerations should be repaired if possible, and when they cannot be sutured, they should be occluded with a small amount of fat or muscle. The cut omohyoid is a good source of muscle that can be slipped into a small dural opening. The bodies can also be bitten away with rongeurs, but the limited exposure makes it difficult to put rongeurs that are large enough for the task into the incision. Angled cervical punches can be used to remove the posterior rim, rather than curettes. When serious spondylosis is the problem or with calcified posterior longitudinal ligaments, magnification adds safety to the procedure. When rongeurs have been employed, once the major bony removal is complete, the microscope should be brought into the field, and the removal of the posterior ridges with curette or drill should be undertaken under direct magnified vision. When the drill is employed, the microscope should be used throughout. If only the ridges are to be removed, it is not necessary to resect entire bodies. In this case, the bony removal is begun at the interspace and is extended only to the extent required for total removal of the ridges above and below. The end of the operation should see complete removal of all bone and ligament that are compressing the spinal canal from the front (Fig. 12.4). If there is an associated radicular compression, the bony removal can be extended to include the anterior spurs underneath the root. This should be done under direct vision, and magnification is helpful. The high-speed drill or a small angled curette is used.

Irrespective of the size of the bony removal, accurate fitting of the graft is essential. The lateral walls should be dressed until they are smooth and even. Curettes or the drill should be used to undercut the anterior surface of the bone and create an overhang 2–3 mm deep. This should be 1–2 mm from the anterior surface and include the whole width of the body down to a point 1–2 mm from the posterior surface. This channel provides strong cortical bone anteriorly and posteriorly to anchor the graft. Identical channels are made above and below. The length of the graft is then measured, the width of the channel is obtained, and the depth of the channel is measured carefully. The length should be such that the graft is 1–2 mm smaller than the undercut channel but is longer than the defect in the external surface of the bodies. This must be sized precisely so that the graft is not too long to be inserted but is long enough to be wedged firmly in the channel and not dislodged anteriorly (Fig. 12.5).

The graft should now be harvested from the opposite iliac crest. A skin incision is made directly over the crest that is 1 cm longer than the length of the graft that should be taken. The interdigitating fibers of the muscles of the crest are divided down to bone, and a careful subperiosteal dissection is carried out. A graft of this type should be taken well back from the anterior superior iliac spine where the width of the crest is relatively uniform. If the spine is included, then one part of the graft will often be wider than another, and the graft will be difficult to shape and fit properly. The appropriate area on the crest should be identified and measured. A graft should be cut that is 1 or 2 mm longer than the length needed. However, there is no reason to remove an excessively large piece of crest for this procedure. The graft length is carefully marked, and an oscillating saw used to cut the graft to the appropriate size. Remember to cut outside the measured marks to avoid reducing the graft size. The approximate depth should be marked with an osteotome, and then the graft removed by using sharp osteotomes to cut the inferior margin. This should be done with light blows of a hammer to avoid breaking this large graft. The bone thus freed should come loose in the wound and can be removed for shaping. Hemostasis can easily be obtained by use of thrombin-soaked Gelfoam, which will allow some regeneration of bone and is better than waxing the cut bone edges, which will reduce regeneration. The wound is closed with a suction drain. Closure requires only apposition of the fascia and muscular fibers along the crest. Subcutaneous and subcuticular skin closures will eliminate the need for suture removal. The channel should now be remeasured, and the graft carefully measured and marked for shaping. The shaping is best done by hand or with a high-speed drill. A small vice on the table is handy to help the shaping with the drill. Remember to hold the bone with a sponge or something with a rough surface while rongeuring the edges. It is very easy for the bone to slip from gloved fingers. Repeated checks may be necessary to be certain that the graft is being fitted properly. When it appears to be perfect in configuration, 20 pounds of traction should be placed on the neck to obtain some distraction, and the graft should then be slid into place by placing either the lower or the upper margin in the channel and then tamping the other end lightly until it slides into position (Fig. 12.5). When the graft is firmly seated, remove half the traction weight, and check to be certain that it is stable. The graft should remain in place as the anesthesiologist gently flexes, extends, and rotates the neck. With short grafts of no more than one body, the postoperative immobilization can be with a metal two- or four-poster brace. For larger grafts of more than one body, skeletal fixation may be necessary; immobilization in a halo until incorporation of the graft is demonstrated by x-ray is wise with large grafts. The type of postoperative stabilization must be decided by the surgeon, based on the demonstrated stability of the graft. Various fixation techniques with plates, screws, and other metal appliances have been advocated. Remember that all these metal appliances will be immediately behind the esophagus, and if any protruding edges are present, the wall of the esophagus may be eroded at some later date. None of the devices for fixation can be considered standard technique, but many are satisfactory in the hands of those who understand their principles and uses.

Once the graft is firmly seated and the surgeon is satisfied with its appearance and stability, the retractors are removed. The carotid pulse should then be checked to be certain the carotid is not injured and the wound is irrigated thoroughly. Closure requires only a layer in the platysma, a subcutaneous layer, and a subcuticular stitch. The patient must be immobilized postoperatively until the brace can be applied. During post-anesthetic recovery, sandbags at the side of the head should be adequate. The patient

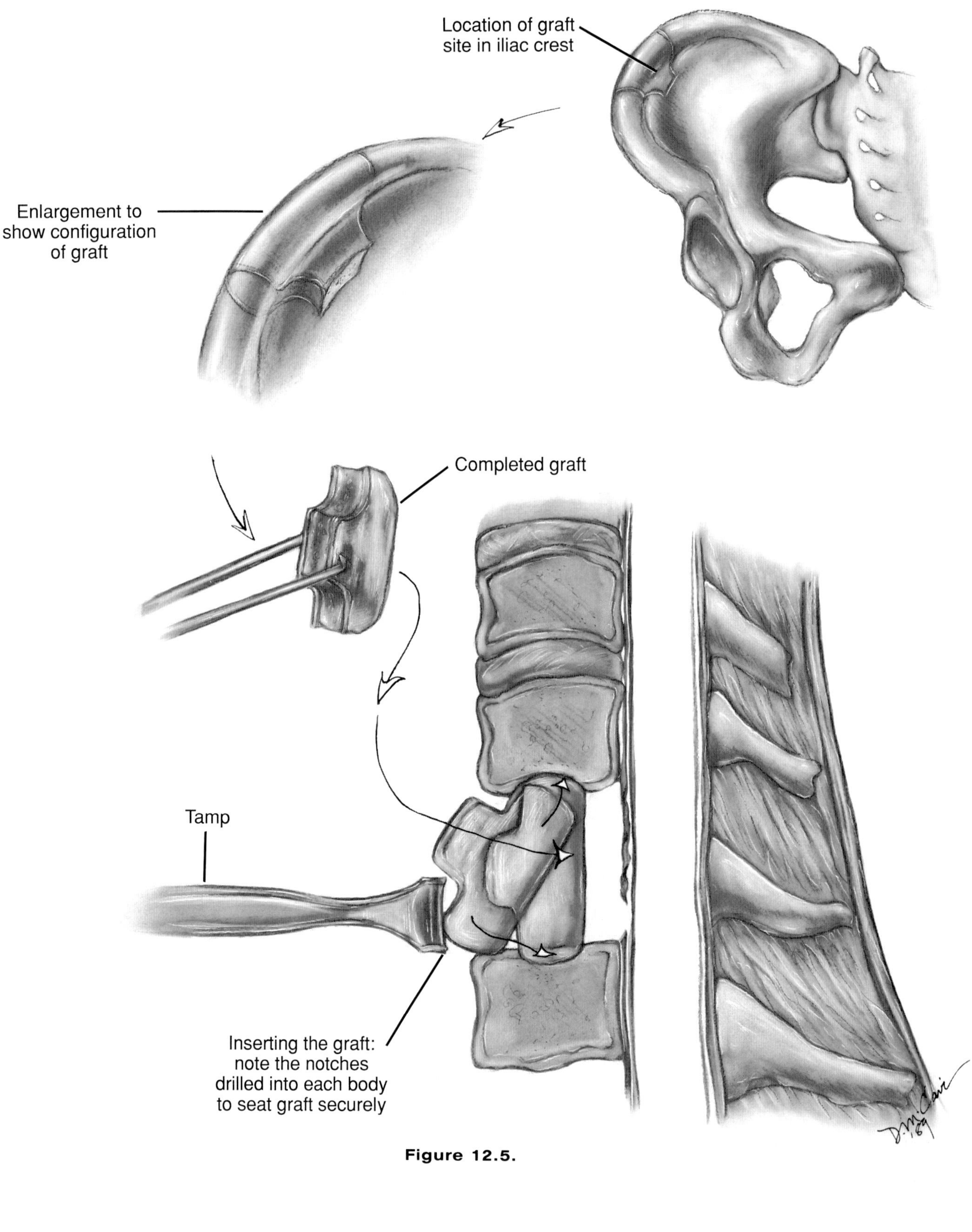
Location of graft
site in iliac crest
Enlargement to
show configuration
of graft
Completed graft
Tamp
Inserting the graft:
note the notches
drilled into each body
to seat graft securely

Figure 12.5.

should not be allowed to be elevated or out of bed until awake enough to apply a metal brace. If a halo is to be utilized, it should be applied immediately after surgery, with the same anesthetic used. Verification of the graft position at the termination of surgery is desirable, and it is wise to check graft position at least once before the patient leaves the hospital.

Metastatic Tumors of the Cervical Spine

Metastatic tumors involving the cervical spine present a special challenge with regard to stabilization. The surgical procedure required consists of an initial posterior spinal fusion with a second-stage anterior methyl methacrylate stabilization following corpectomy and tumor removal.

The procedure begins with placement on an operative wedge frame while the patient is awake. Thirteen pounds of skeletal traction are applied through Gardner-Wells tongs. The neurological status is checked before the patient is anesthetized. Spinal cord monitoring is used throughout the procedure. The patient is turned on the operative wedge frame into the prone position, and monitoring is again checked to ensure normal potentials. The posterior aspect of the cervical spine and the posterior iliac crests are prepared and draped. A 6-cm graft is taken from the right posterior iliac crest, utilizing the outer table and the bulk of the cancellous portion of the bone (see Chapter 16). Following exposure via a midline incision, the posterior elements from C1-T1 are completely dissected free of soft tissue (see Chapter 16). The posterior elements that have evidence of tumor involvement should be removed if it will not interfere with the fusion. The high-speed drill is used to make a hole through the junction of the spinous process and lamina at every level to be fused. A lateral x-ray is obtained to document the appropriate cervical levels. A Chandler towel clip or right-angle drill is used to make a smooth hole in the bases of the spinous processes. Two Drummond buttons are placed in the lowest two spinous processes, and a 20-gauge wire is passed through and around the other spinous processes. The posterior wires from the lowest level are then tightened to the wires of the next to highest level, and the posterior wires of highest

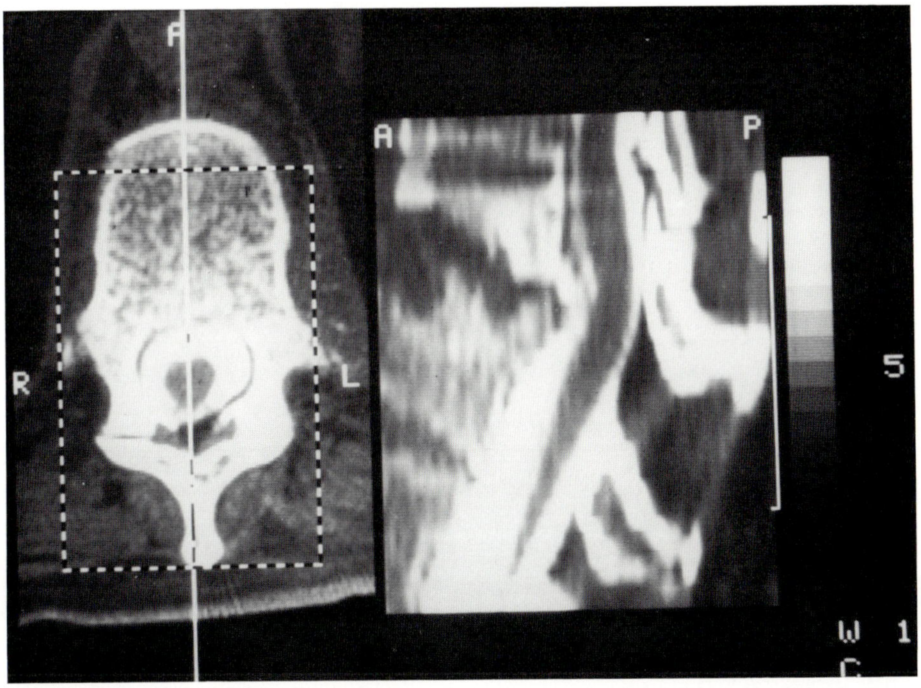

Figure 12.6. A pathological fracture on the thoracic spine from breast metastases is demonstrated. The need for anterior decompression is obvious. Appropriate treatment will be radical resection of the two involved vertebral bodies with block fusion.

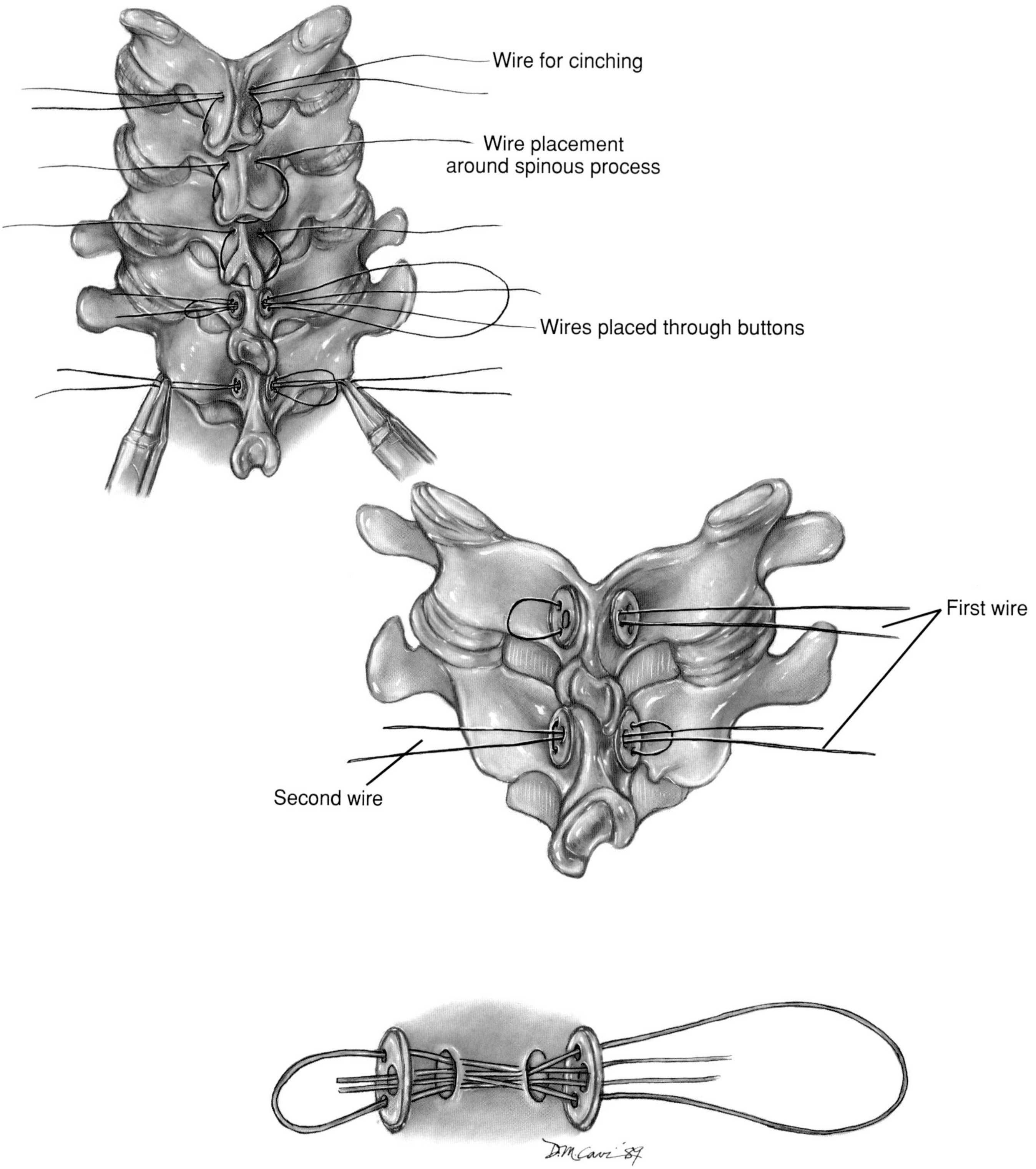

Detail of button-wire relationships

Figure 12.7.

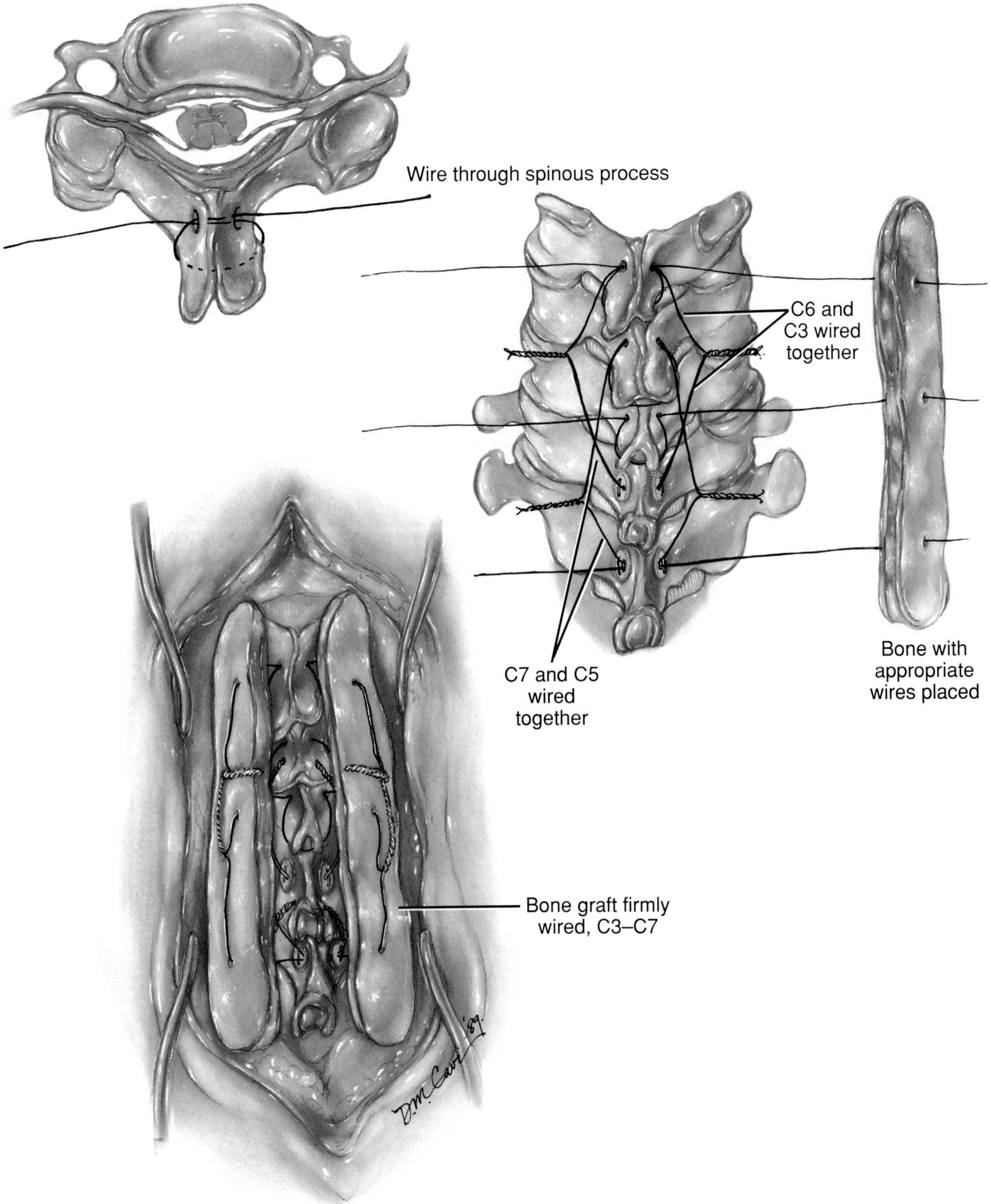
Wire through spinous process
C6 and
C3 wired
together
C7 and C5
wired
together
Bone with
appropriate
wires placed
Bone graft firmly
wired, C3–C7

Figure 12.8.

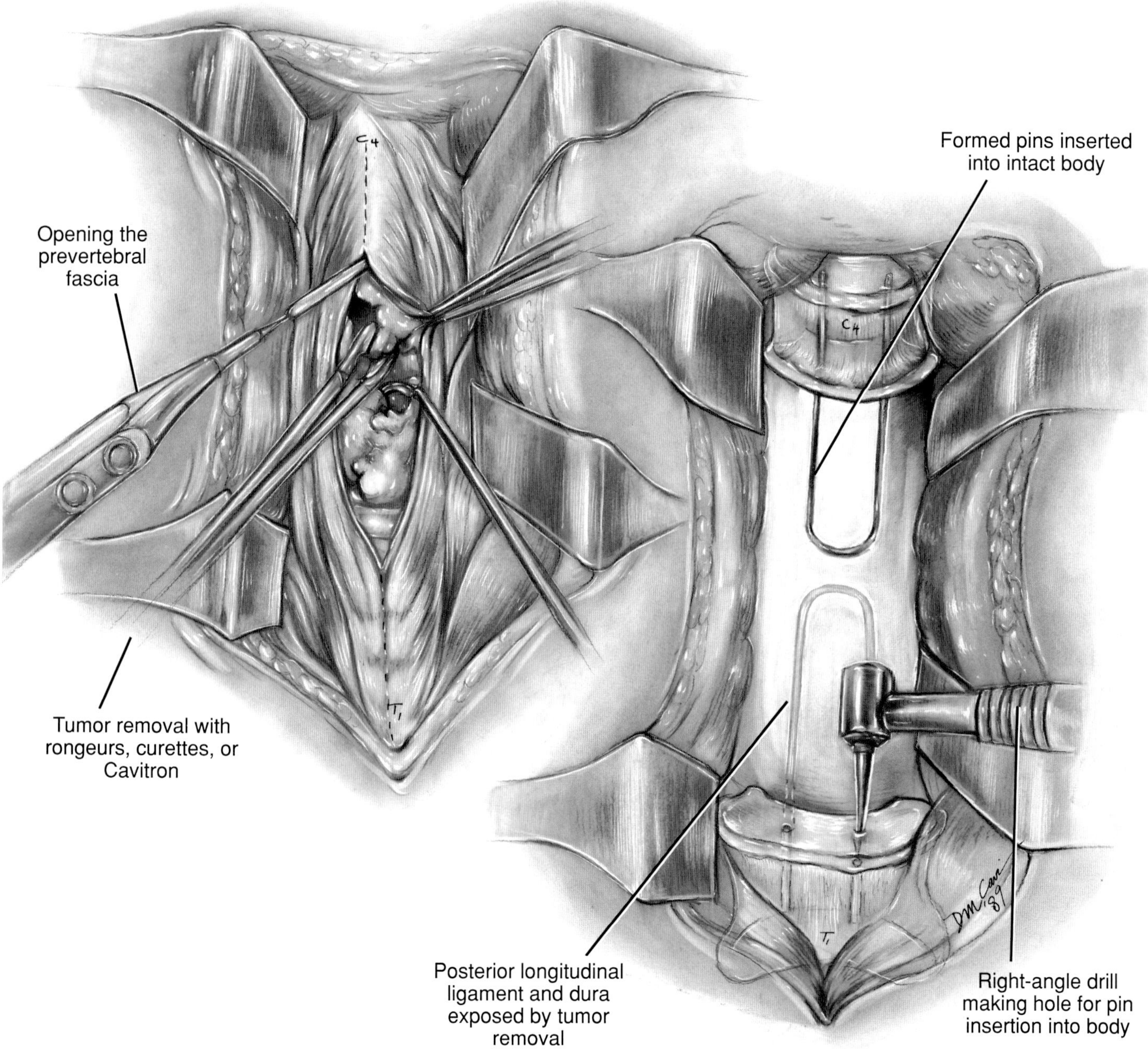
Opening the prevertebral fascia
Tumor removal with rongeurs, curettes, or Cavitron
Formed pins inserted into intact body
Posterior longitudinal ligament and dura exposed by tumor removal
Right-angle drill making hole for pin insertion into body
C4
T1

Figure 12.9.

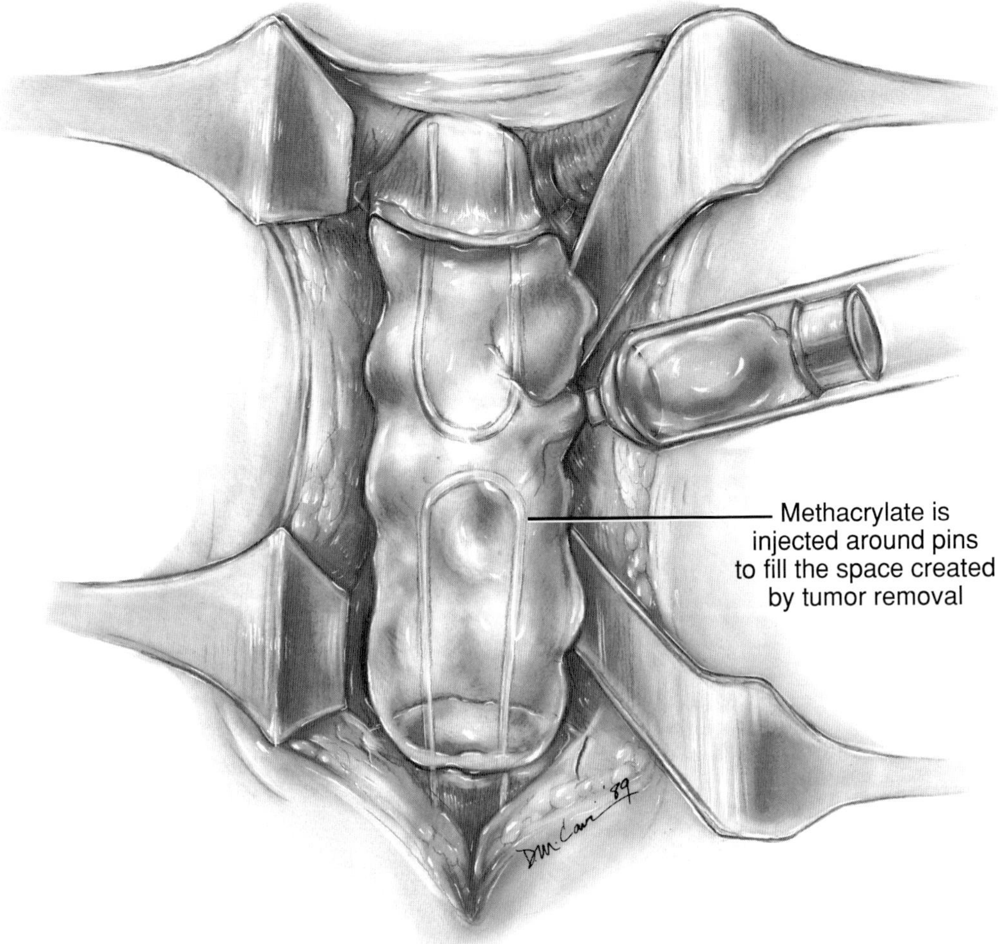

Figure 12.10.

level are tightened to the wires at the next to last segment. This provides a stable construction. The midline tethering construction provides immediate stability to the vertebral units included in the wiring. Next, corticocancellous bone grafts are tightened down into place with wires connecting the highest, lowest, and middle spinous processes. Three holes drilled into the bone graft ensure that the bone graft is secured properly. After the wires are maximally tightened, two transverse wires through the grafts at either end are used to increase the rotational stability.

Following closure of the posterior wounds, the patient is turned in the supine position. By using an oblique incision anterior to the border of the sternocleidomastoid, the neck is entered as described in Robinson's approach to the anterior cervical spine (Chapter 10). The length of the incision is dictated by the extent of the corpectomy. The anterior border of the sternocleidomastoid is isolated following incision of the platysma. The carotid artery is retracted laterally, and the trachea medially. The deep cervical fascia and pretracheal fascia are entered and exposed. With the electrocautery, a midline incision between the longus coli muscles is made, and the tumorous bone is exposed. With angled curettes, pituitary forceps, and ultrasonic dissector or laser, the necessary corpectomy is performed (Fig. 12.9). Bone and disc are removed, leaving a normal body above and below and dura behind. A right-angle dental burr is used to make two holes in the end plates of these bodies. An

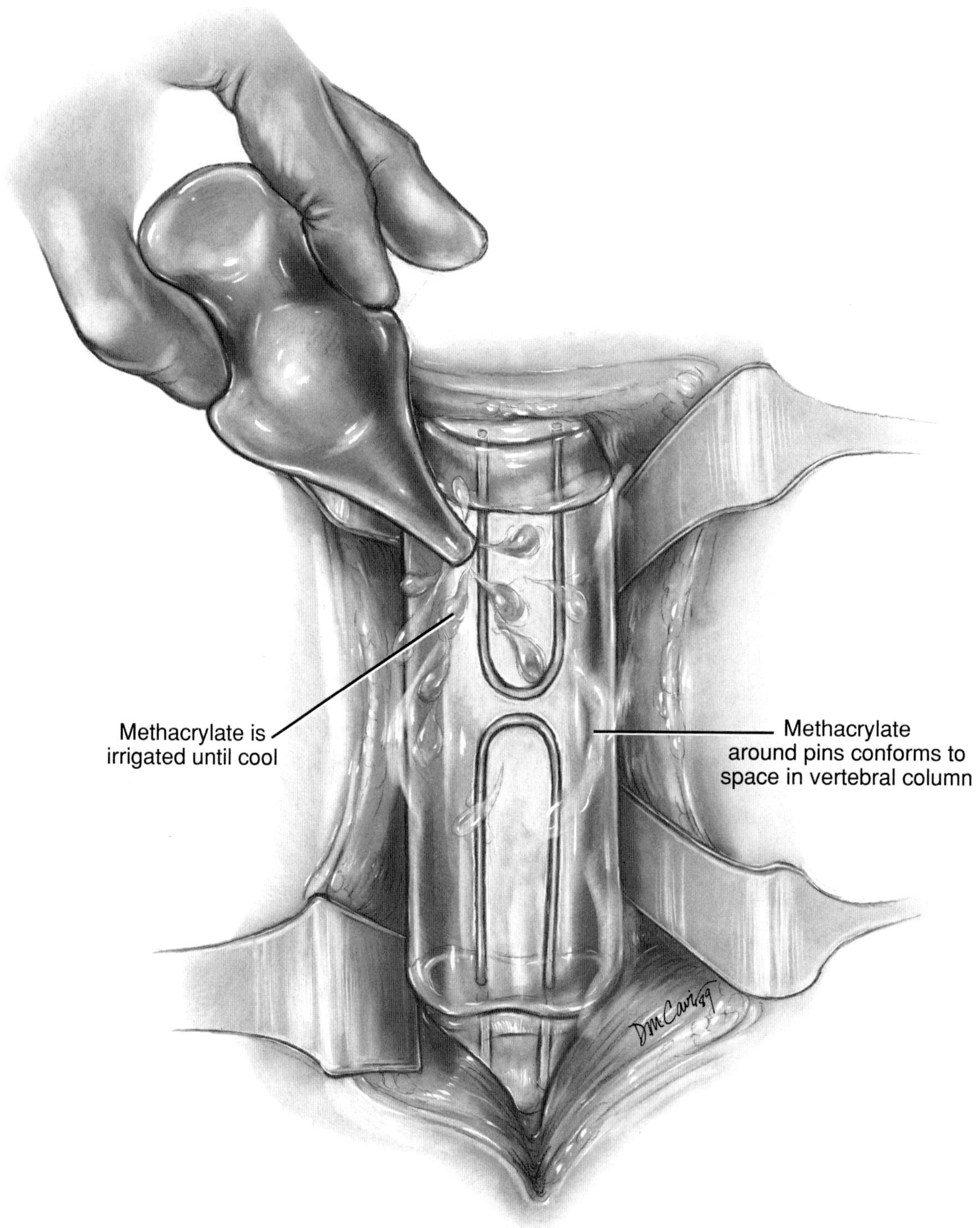
Methacrylate is
irrigated until cool
Methacrylate
around pins conforms to
space in vertebral column

Figure 12.11.

18-gauge wire fashioned in the shape of a "U" is inserted through the lower holes and secured by penetrating the upper body. The lower body is also entered with a second "U"-shaped wire. A Gelfoam pad is placed over the dura. Following this, the polymethyl methacrylate is prepared and placed in the defect from C4 to T1 (Fig. 12.10). The plastic is irrigated to disperse the heat from the exothermic reaction while it hardens (Fig. 12.11). When the process is complete, retractors are removed and both the carotid and the esophagus are checked. The platysma is closed with interrupted sutures, followed by skin closure.

Postoperatively, the patients are placed in a halo vest for 2 months. Stability is verified before the halo is discarded.

13

Transscalene Approach to Lateral Structures of Neck

The transscalene approach is used to expose the vertebral artery, transverse processes, pedicles, and cords of the brachial plexus from the third through the seventh cervical segments. The major indication is for neoplastic destruction of the lower two cervical vertebrae with involvement or compression of the vertebral arteries. This approach, as opposed to the traditional Robinson anterolateral approach, facilitates proximal and distal control of the vertebral artery. It is performed through an anterior transverse incision placed in a skin fold in the neck from the midline to several centimeters posterior to the posterior border of the sternomastoid muscle. The incision is deepened to the platysma, which is grasped between forceps at the lateral aspect of the incision and divided in line with the skin incision while being bluntly elevated from underlying structures. The sternomastoid muscle is then isolated by clearly demonstrating its anterior and posterior borders. The deep surface of the muscle is freed from the carotid sheath and other underlying structures so that a finger can be pressed under the belly of the sternomastoid. Using this finger to protect the underlying structures, sharply transect the sternomastoid muscle and retract the divided segments

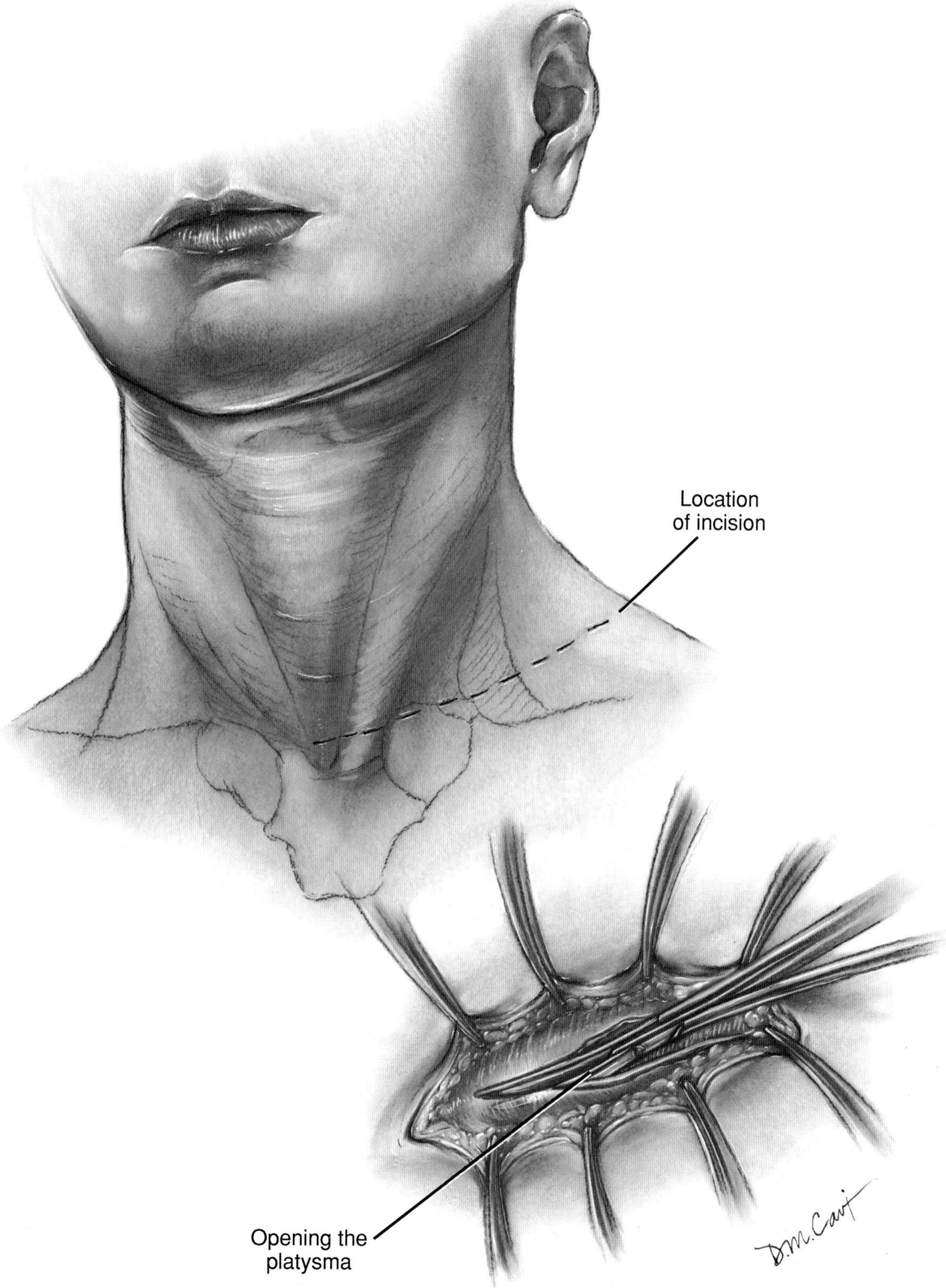

Figure 13.1.

superiorly and inferiorly. In a similar fashion, divide and transect the omohyoid muscle lying deep to the sternomastoid. An alternative incision can be parallel to the sternomastoid, which is retracted laterally rather than cut.

The structures now exposed are: the anterior scalene muscle, the phrenic nerve that lies on the surface of the anterior scalene muscle, and the cord of the brachial plexus that emerge from under the lateral wall of the anterior scalene muscle. Carefully mobilize the phrenic nerve throughout the limits of the incision, and gently retract it anteriorly with tapes. Attention is then directed toward identifying and mobilizing the medial and lateral borders of the anterior scalene muscle without damaging the cords of the brachial plexus. The cords of the brachial plexus usually emerge from beneath the lateral border of the anterior scalene muscle and travel between the anterior and middle scalene muscles. However, the cords can emerge through the body of the anterior scalene muscle; therefore, it is important to identify clearly all of the cords of the brachial plexus before proceeding further. Once the brachial plexus cords are identified and protected, sharply divide the anterior scalene muscle several centimeters inferior to the site of the exposure desired. Then, being careful not to damage the vertebral artery as it extends between the bony foramen and the transverse processes of the second through the sixth cervical vertebrae, dissect and severe the origin of the anterior scalene muscle from the anterior tubercle of the transverse processes. The superior portion of the muscle is then excised.

If the pedicles are to be exposed, identify and place tapes around the vertebral artery both proximal and distal to the area of desired exposure for arterial control. The adventitia of the vertebral artery is intimately adherent to the periosteum of the foramen transversarium. With sharp dissection, the colli muscle is reflected medially, and the remaining fibers of the scalene muscle are reflected distally and laterally. This exposes the transverse processes, pedicles, neural foramen, and nerve roots.

Removal of bone over the vertebral artery and foraminotomy are both difficult maneuvers. The usual reasons for vertebral decompression are arteriovenous fistula or vertebral ischemia caused by a large compressive spur. The techniques are the same for both exposures.

It is unusual to operate on an arteriovenous fistula. Intravascular techniques usually suffice. When direct surgery is required, it is important to identify the site of the fistula. The exposure must be sufficient to allow control above and below. First isolate the vertebral artery between the subclavian and the C6 transverse process, and place a vessel loop around it. Expose the vessel in the foramen transversarium above the fistula, and remove bone until the vessel can be circumscribed. The bone is often densely adherent to the vessel, with the periosteum literally fused to vessel wall. This is a difficult dissection. When it is complete, pass another loop at this level. Then remove bone between the two loops until the artery is mobilized from its bed in the bony canal. If bleeding is a problem, the vessel can be occluded. Remember the presence or absence of a competent opposite vertebral artery must be verified by angiography before this operation is begun. The venous plexus is stripped until the fistula is found. The ideal solution is direct repair of the arteriotomy with a fine arterial suture, 5-70. Sometimes, only isolation and packing or trapping are possible. When hemostasis is adequate, the wound is closed with a drain.

At C1-2-3 the lateral approach is employed. Otherwise, the principles are the same and no other modifications in technique are required.

When foraminal decompression is the goal, the operation is slightly different. Proximal and distal control are less critical. Arterial bleeding can always be stopped by direct compression in the bony canal. Bone removal must be complete at least one level above and below the spur to be removed. Removal of two levels provides better mobilization. An adequate decompression includes the anterior and lateral bony walls of the foramen transversarium. The vessel is mobilized from its bed and controlled with one- or two-vessel loops. Remember the cervical roots are exiting immediately posterior to the vessel. They must be identified at each level. The bony spurs are then identified on either side of the disc space. The spurs are drilled away with protection of the root and the dural sac. Fine rongeurs can be used, but the drill is safer. Bone is removed until the vessel is no longer compromised, and both cord and root are decompressed. There are much easier ways to achieve foraminal decompression, so most surgeons do not use the lateral approach for spur removal alone. The

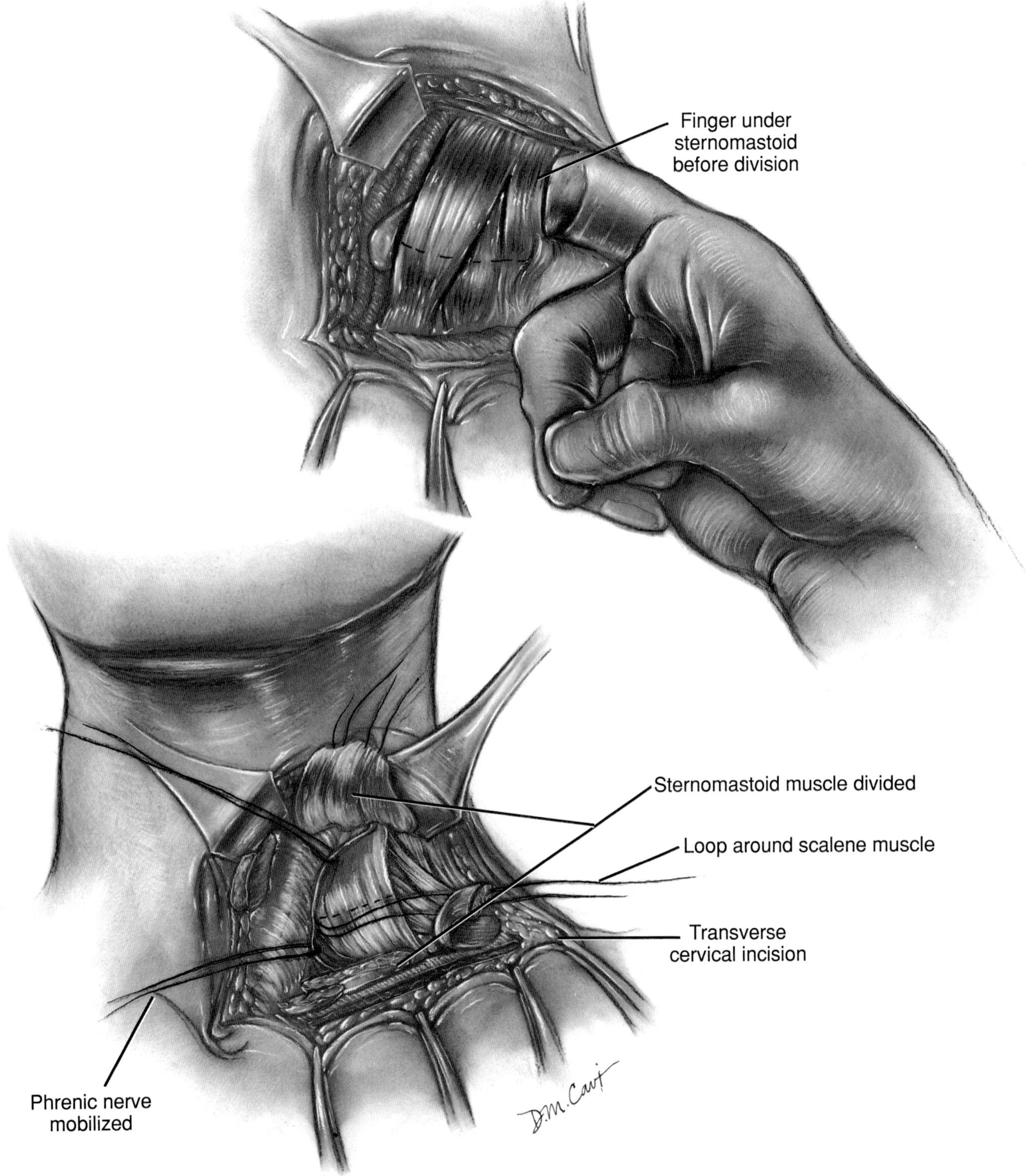
Finger under sternomastoid before division
Sternomastoid muscle divided
Loop around scalene muscle
Transverse cervical incision
Phrenic nerve mobilized
D.M. Cart

Figure 13.2.

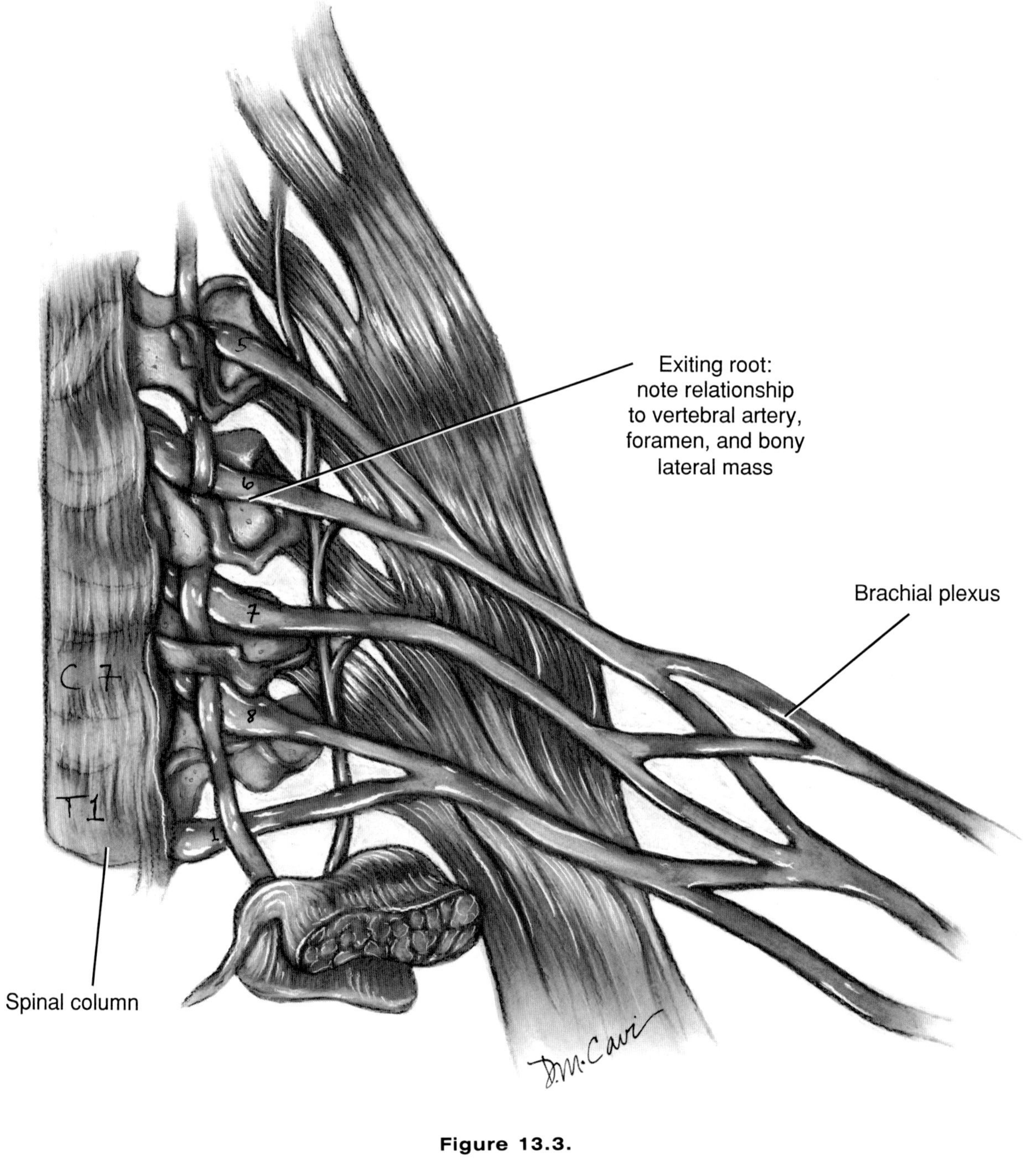
Exiting root:
note relationship
to vertebral artery,
foramen, and bony
lateral mass
Brachial plexus
Spinal column
C 7
T1
5
6
7
8
1

Figure 13.3.

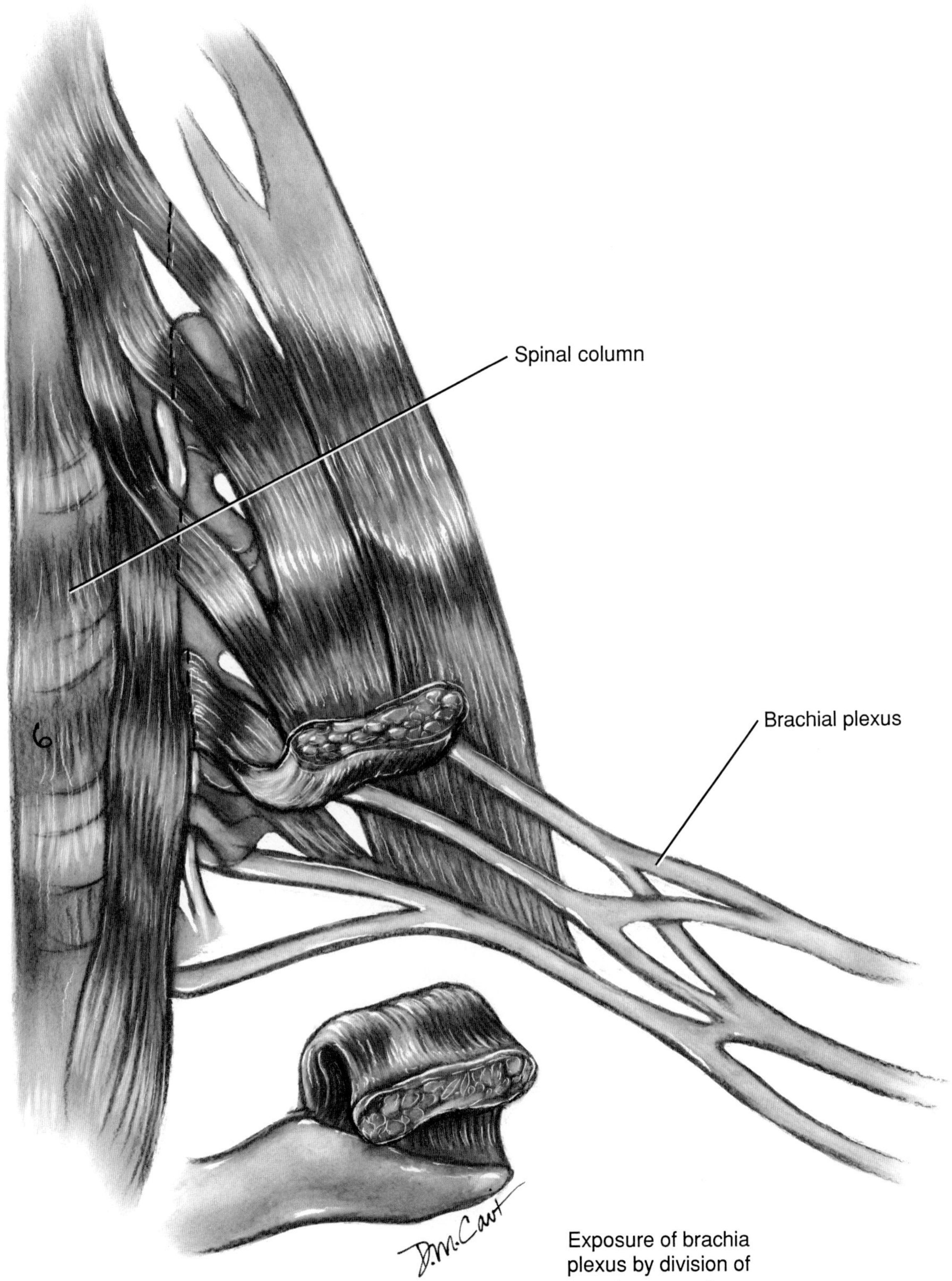

Exposure of brachia plexus by division of scalene muscles

Figure 13.4.

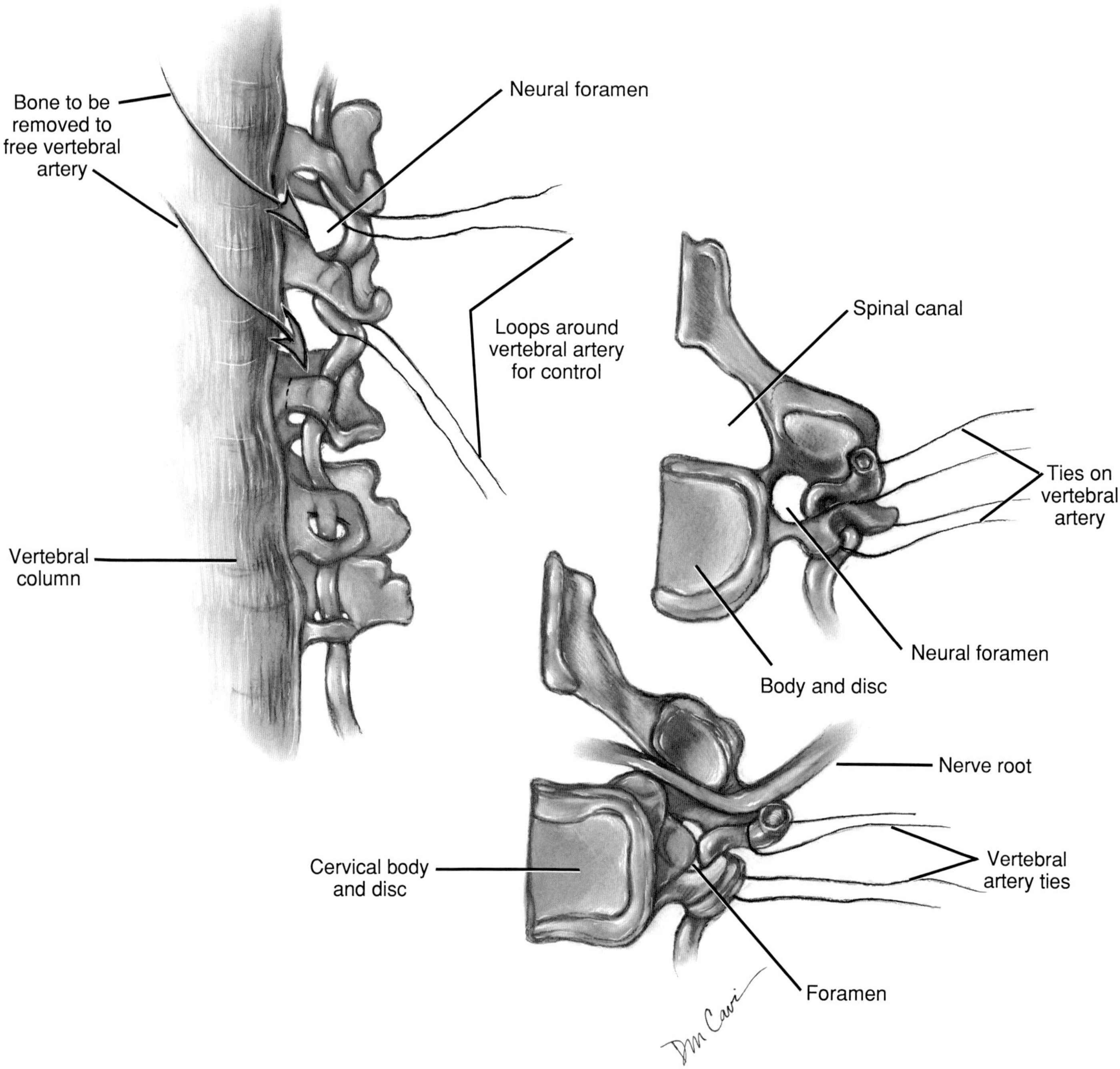

Figure 13.5.

artery is replaced in its bed. Closure over a drain is routine.

During closure a drain is left to the depth of the resected portion of the anterior scalene muscle. The omohyoid, sternomastoid, and platysma muscles are reapproximated, and the skin is closed with fine interrupted sutures. Postoperative management is similar to that for the Robinson anterolateral approach.

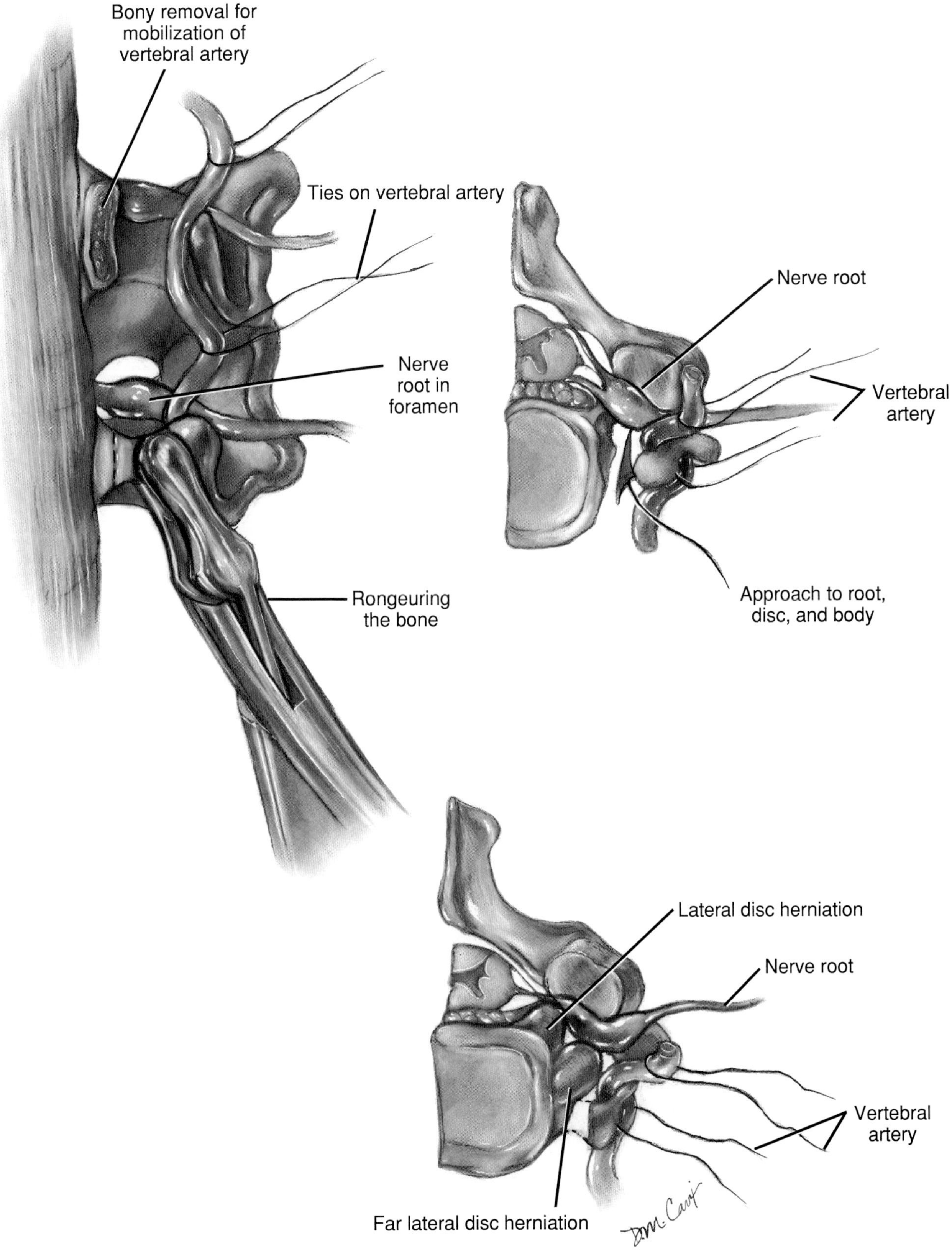
Bony removal for mobilization of vertebral artery
Ties on vertebral artery
Nerve root in foramen
Rongeuring the bone
Nerve root
Vertebral artery
Approach to root, disc, and body
Lateral disc herniation
Nerve root
Vertebral artery
Far lateral disc herniation

Figure 13.6.

14

Anterior Operations on Upper Cervical Spine

Anterior Retropharyngeal Approach

Indications for Procedure

Occasionally, it is necessary to perform anterior decompressive surgery superior to the C3 vertebrae. This approach is useful for tumors needing biopsy at C2, for anterior decompression of the spinal canal, and for anterior stabilization with the use of bone grafts. The anterior retropharyngeal approach to the upper cervical spine achieves exposure sufficient for extirpation and stabilization of lesions involving the atlas and axis. The exposure is accomplished entirely extramucosally. It is a cranial extension of the anterior cervical approach described by Robinson and Smith in 1955 and can be used for spinal canal decompression as well as strut graft stabilization for posttraumatic deformities and cervical tumors. This extensile approach was originally developed by Southwick and Robinson and published by Riley in 1973, who included dislocation of the ipsilateral temporomandibular joint to increase exposure, a step necessary for only two patients in our series. Sufficient exposure can be achieved without dislocation of the temporomandibular joint except in those patients with such profound instability that extension of the spine and rotation of the skull to the opposite side are contraindicated. Adequate exposure can be achieved through a smaller skin incision than that described originally.

Surgical Technique

The patient is transferred supine to an operative wedge turning frame, and careful neurological examination is performed. Somatosensory evoked cortically recorded spinal cord monitoring potentials are utilized from this point forward throughout the operative procedure. Gardner-Wells tongs with 10 pounds of skeletal traction are utilized rather than a head halter, which would extend too far interiorly around the mandible. The neck is extended maximally with the patient still awake, but it is extended only to the degree that does not cause neurological symptoms or spinal cord monitoring potential changes. This position is designated as maximal neck extention, and it is not exceeded at any time throughout the operative procedure. Fiberoptic nasotracheal intubation is performed with the patient under local anesthesia. After the airway is secured, the patient undergoes general anesthesia. The mouth is keep free of all tubes—no oral airways or esophageal stethoscopes are permitted in the mouth, as any depression of the mandible inferiorly increases the difficulty of the exposure.

A modified Schoebringer incision is utilized. The vertical limb is extended inferiorly along the sternomastoid border as needed, depending on the amount of cervical spine exposure required. A transverse incision is made beneath, parallel to the mandible through the platysma muscle, and the superior medial, inframedial, and lateral flaps are elevated in the subplatysmal plane. The incision is made on the patient's right side if the surgeon is right-handed. In contrast to the Robinson-Smith exposure to the midcervical levels, which is usually performed on the patient's left side, the extrapharyngeal exposure to the atlas and axis is sufficiently superior to the right recurrent laryngeal nerves that there is no increased morbidity with the right-sided exposure. The exposure is a superior extension of the standard Smith-Robinson exposure to the midcervical spine; therefore, only the specific modifications allowing visualization of the atlas and axis are described. The surgeon should be thoroughly familiar with the facial planes traversed by the Smith-Robinson anterior approach: (1) the superficial fascia of the platysma, (2) the deep investing fascia of the platysma, (3) the superficial layer of deep cervical fascia, (4) the alar or pretracheal fascia, and (5) the prevertebral fascia.

The marginal mandibular branch of cranial nerve VII is found by ligating and retracting the retromandibular veins superiorly. The common facial vein is continuous with the retromandibular vein, and the branches of the marginal mandibular nerve usually cross the vein superficially and superiorly. By ligating the retromandibular vein as it joins the internal jugular vein and keeping the dissection deep and inferior to the vein as the exposure is extended superiorly to the mandible, the superficial branches of the facial nerve (VII) are thus protected.

The anterior border of the sternocleidomastoid is mobilized by longitudinally transecting the superficial layer of deep cervical fascia. This allows location of the carotid sheath by palpation of the carotid arterial pulse. The submandibular gland is resected with care taken to suture the duct in order to prevent fistula formation. The jugulodigastric lymph nodes from the submandibular and carotid triangles can be resected and sent for frozen section histological analysis at this point if neoplasm is suspected. The posterior belly of the digastric muscle and the stylohyoid are identified (Fig. 14.1). Retraction superiorly at the base of the origin of the stylohyoid muscle can cause injury to the facial nerve (VII) as it exits the skull. The digastric tendon is divided and tagged for later repair. Division of the digastric and stylohyoid muscles allows mobilization of the hyoid bone and the hypopharynx medially. This maneuver helps keep the exposure out of the nasopharynx, hypopharynx, and esophagus, which are considered contaminated spaces. If the hypopharynx is inadvertently entered, a nasogastric tube should be passed immediately by the anesthetist while the surgeon visualizes the hole in the hypopharynx. The hypopharynx is closed in two layers with absorbable sutures. Parenteral antibiotics are added to the routine prophylactic antibiotic regimen with a spectrum against anaerobes. In this situation, the nasogastric tube is left in place for 7–10 days postoperatively to help prevent esophageal or hypopharyngeal leakage or fistula formation, which can lead to mediastinitis. Complete mobilization of the hypoglossal nerve from the skull base to the anterior border of the hyoglossus muscle is done. The nerve is retracted superiorly throughout the remainder of the procedure.

The dissection then proceeds to the retropharyn-

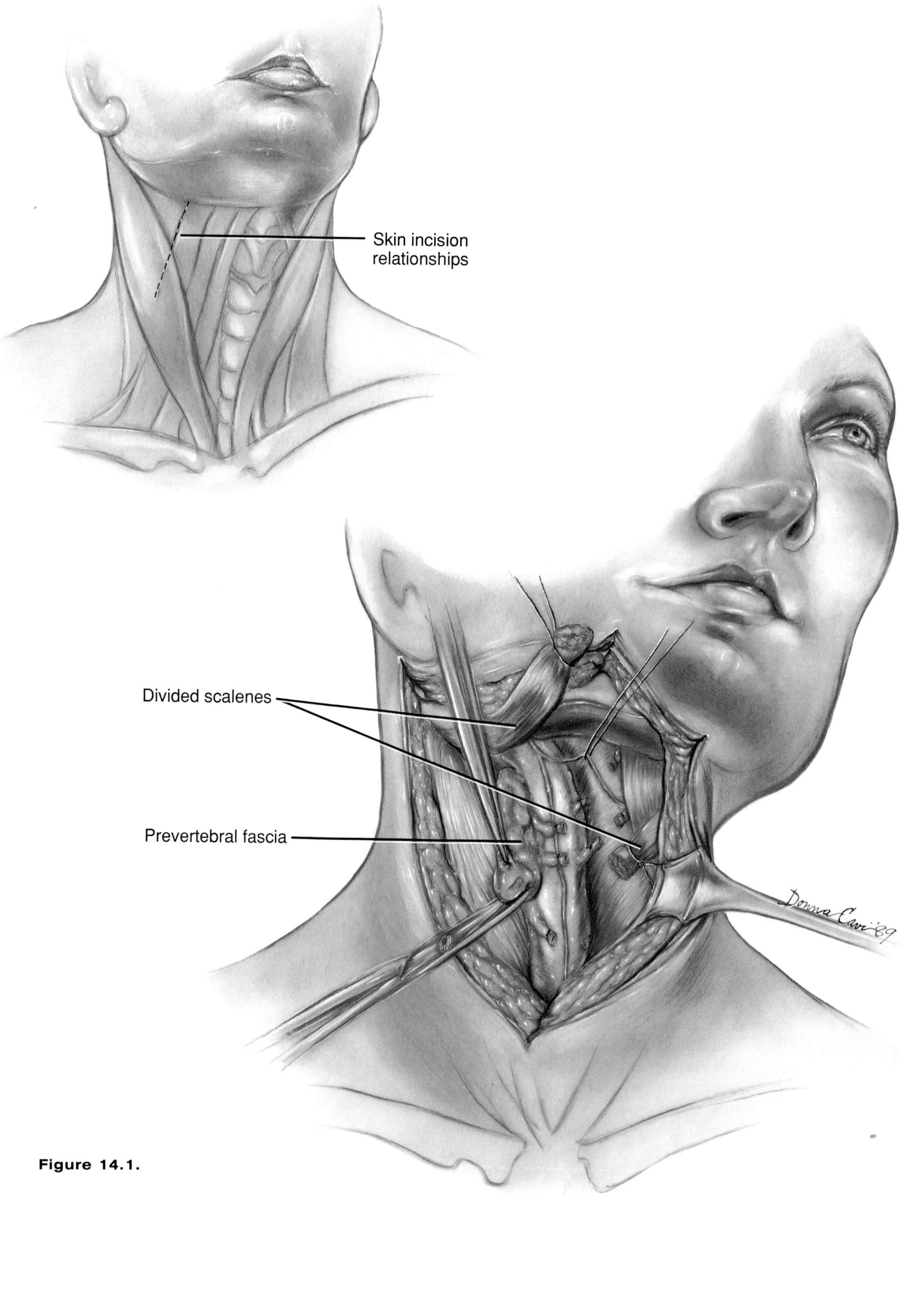

Skin incision
relationships
Divided scalenes
Prevertebral fascia

Figure 14.1.

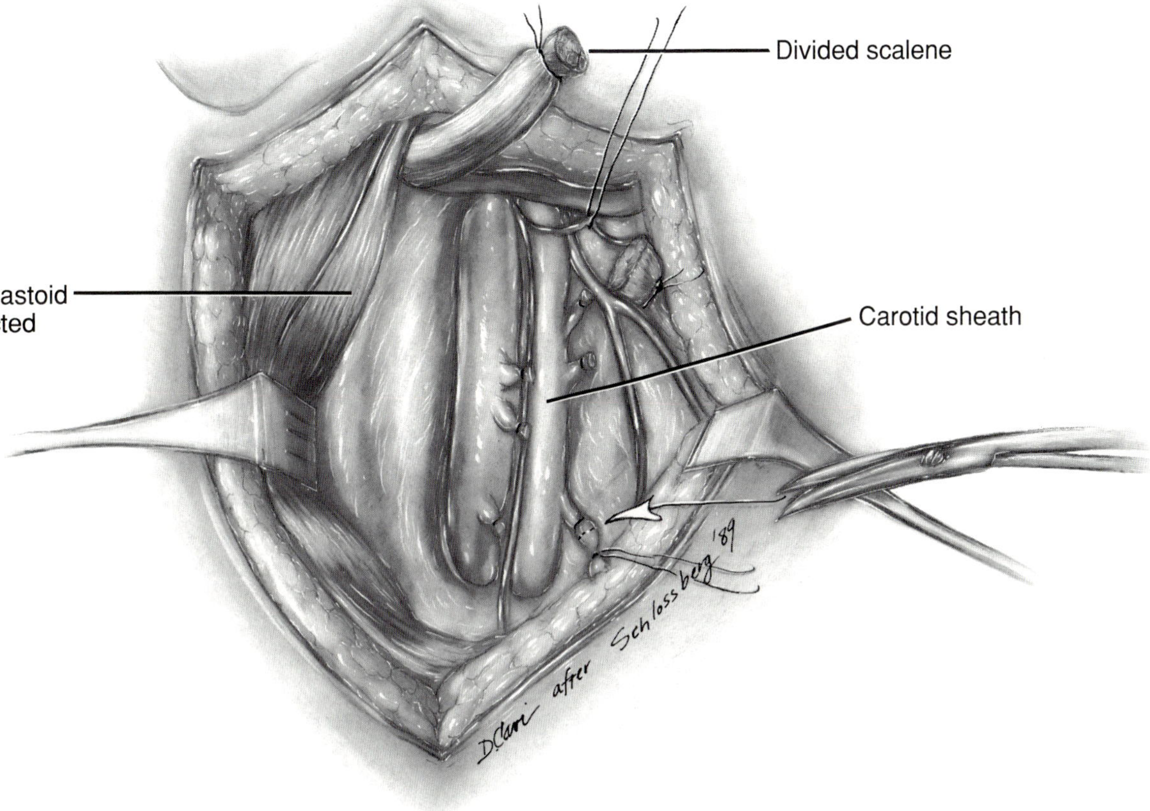

Figure 14.2. Approach to prevertebral space.

geal space, between the carotid sheath contents laterally and the larynx and pharynx anteromedially (Fig. 14.2). Superiorly, exposure is facilitated by ligating the tethering branches of the carotid artery and internal jugular vein. Beginning inferiorly and progressing superiorly, ligating the following branches of these vessels will help mobilization of the carotid sheath laterally: (1) superior thyroid artery and vein, (2) lingual artery and vein, (3) ascending pharyngeal artery and vein, and (4) facial artery and vein. The superior laryngeal nerve is immobilized from its origin near the nodose ganglion to its entrance into the larynx. We have been able to preserve the superior laryngeal nerve; the deficit of transection of the superior laryngeal nerve is a loss of high-pitched phonation. The prevertebral fascia is transected longitudinally, exposing the longus colli muscles that course longitudinally. It is very important at this point to gain orientation of the midline by noting the attachment of the left and right longus colli muscles as they converge toward the anterior tubercle of the atlas. The degree of head rotation toward the side should be gauged by palpation of the anterior point of the jaw. If possible, head rotation is eliminated, as the fusion usually involves the anterior C1 arch. It is important to maintain surgical orientation regarding the midline of the cervical spine as the longus colli muscles are detached from the anterior surface of the atlas and axis. This orientation is maintained throughout the anterior spinal cord decompression in order to extend the decompression laterally enough to decompress the spinal cord, yet not so far laterally as to enter the vertebral arteries. The atlanto-occipital membrane is not violated, but the anterior longitudinal ligament is sacrificed. The approach is principally utilized for tumors but is occasionally utilized for removal of a fractured odontoid when fusion is planned. The transoral route is used more commonly for straightforward problems of the odontoid. This approach is advantageous for tumors. The anterior decompression is usually initiated by performing a C2-C3 discectomy, unless the tumor has destroyed the disc space also. Visualization of the C2-C3 uncovertebral joint helps confirm the orientation of the midline, and the discectomy provides depth perception by visualization of the posterior longitudinal ligament with very minimal blood loss. The tumor is removed by the most appropriate measures. The Cavitron is very helpful, a laser may be useful, and en bloc resection of some of these tumors may be possible. A high-speed drill is utilized for the corpectomy of residual C2. The blood loss during the anterior C2 corpectomy can be minimized by generous use of thrombin-soaked Gelfoam sponges, bone wax, and bipolar cauterization of feeding vessels (localized preoperatively by carotid and vertebral arteriography). In cases without cranial settling (basilar invagination of the odontoid), the odontoid can be retained to lock in the superior aspect of the strut graft. A fibular or tricortical iliac strut graft is fashioned in the shape of a clothespin. The two prongs of the "clothespin strut graft" are placed superiorly to straddle the anterior arch of C1. The inferior edge of the graft is tamped into the superior aspect of the C3 vertebral body, which is undercut to help obtain stability.

Closure is begun by the reapproximation of the digastric tendon. Section drains are then placed in the retropharyngeal space and in the subcutaneous space. They are brought out through stab incisions beneath the cervical flap. The platysma and skin are sutured in the standard fashion. If the spinal instability has been created by the pathological process or the anterior decompression, then a posterior cervical stabilization and wiring are indicated. The patient is kept in skeletal traction until the posterior stabilization can be performed.

The patient is awakened while in the supine position, and neurological examination and spinal cord monitoring potentials are documented. The patient is transferred to an intensive care unit bed with the head elevated 30° to reduce the retropharyngeal edema. The patient is kept intubated for 48 hours postoperatively. At this time, flexible nasopharyngoscopy is performed.

These patients require a halo vest or halo cast for 3 months postoperatively, until there is radiographic evidence of fusion of the anterior strut graft.

Transoral Approach

The usual reasons for approaching the C1-C2 area through the mouth are: os odontoideum; odontoid fracture; basilar impression, either congenital or from rheumatoid arthritis; and tumors of the lower clivus. Before this route is chosen, the stability should be assessed and a decision made about whether posterior stabilization will be required. The risks of infection when fusion by the transoral approach is utilized are too great to warrant this technique on a regular basis. When the transoral approach is required, it is more likely that posterior stabilization will be necessary either before or after the transoral procedure. It is commonly chosen when the principal compressive mass is anterior and when adequate decompression cannot be obtained by posterior surgery with or without stabilization.

The operation is carried out with the patient under general anesthesia in a supine position and with the patient's head either flat or extended approximately 15°. Oral intubation is important. A special tongue retractor that keeps the tongue out of the way and incorporates the endotracheal tube is mandatory for this procedure. Remember to release pressure on the tongue every 45 minutes (measured by the clock) throughout the operation. One member of the team should be assigned this measurement, to remind everyone that the tongue retractor should be released.

Following adequate intubation, the tongue retractor is put in place, and the posterior pharynx is exposed. C2 can often be palpated through the mouth, but it is not necessary to do so. The soft palate should be divided, and if the lesion is high, it may also be necessary to bite away some of the hard palate. A midline incision is made from the approximated area of C2 up to about the midpoint of the clivus. The exposure is such that an incision from the upper and lower extremities will just about expose C2-C1 and the lower clivus. Great care must be taken to preserve the pharyngeal mucosa without injury. All of the dissection should be carried out in the retropharyngeal space. The muscles and ligaments attached to the skull base and upper cervical vertebra can be extremely adherent. They are also very vascular, and an electric knife is a good way to carry out this

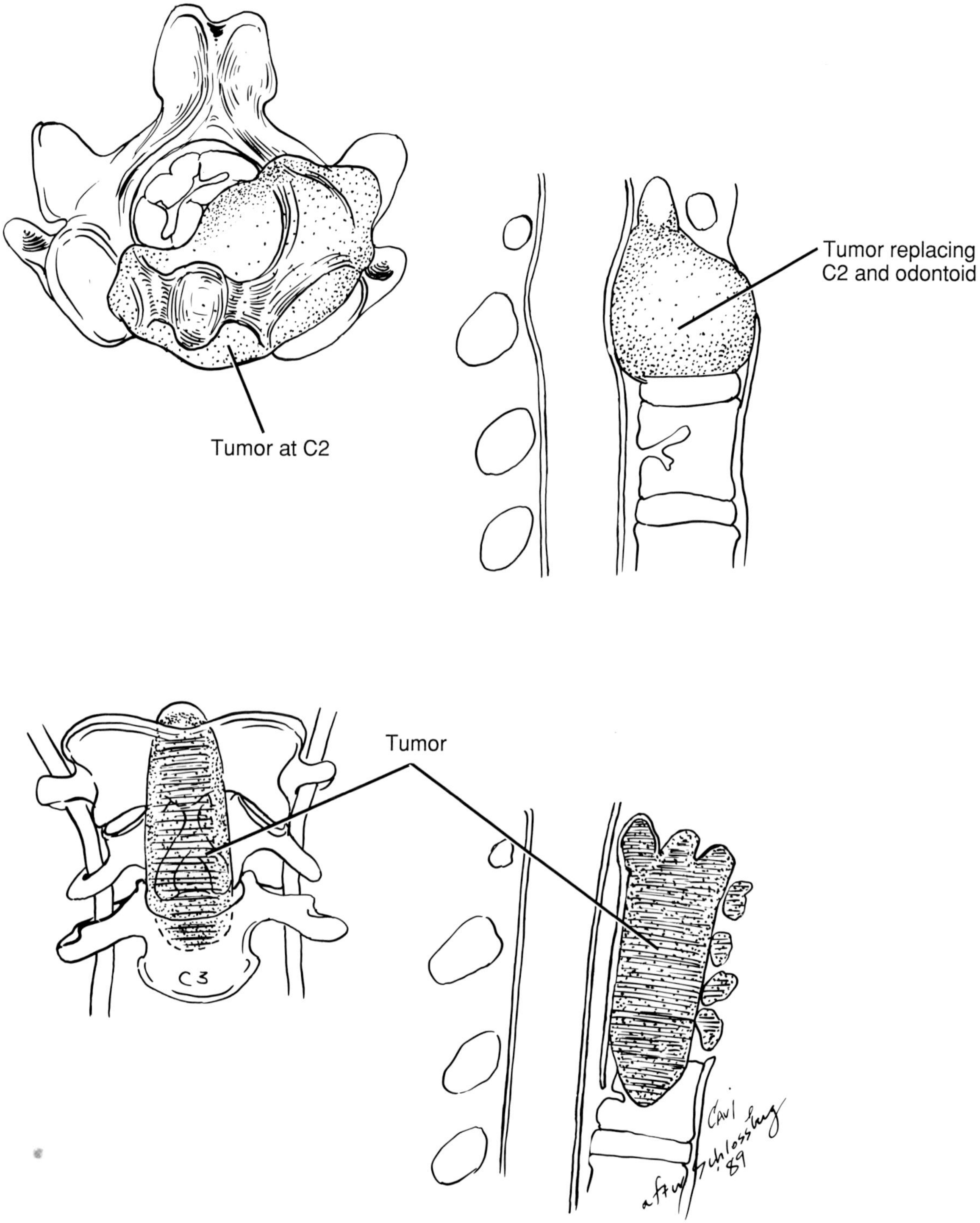

Figure 14.3.

dissection; care must be taken, however, not to injure the pharyngeal mucosa with it. As the muscles are dissected laterally, the spines and laminae of C1-C2 become apparent. The arch of C1 should be exposed as far laterally as possible. This will also allow the lower third of the clivus to be exposed, and then the body of C2 can be added to the exposure. What is then done depends on the pathological anatomy (Fig. 14.3). The high-speed drill is used to remove whatever bone contributes to the compression or is fractured. This may include the arch of C1, the odontoid portion of the body of C2, and/or the lower clivus. Often, there is a good deal of soft tissue associated with the abnormalities. This is particularly true with rheumatoid arthritis and may also be true with the Chiari malformation. This pannus should be removed until decompression of the cervical medullary junction is certain. The ultrasonic dissector is an excellent way to remove this firm tissue. It is extremely important not to enter the subarachnoid space. Cerebrospinal fluid leak will compromise the pharyngeal suture line and greatly increase the risk of infection. If the subarachnoid space is entered, a watertight closure should be obtained; a lumbar drain should be placed before the patient awakens and kept in place until the suture line is thoroughly healed.

Once all of the bone is removed and decompression is adequate, the wound can be closed. The retropharyngeal tissue should be closed in the midline with heavy absorbable sutures. The pharyngeal tissue can be closed as a single layer with absorbable sutures.

When the dura has been opened widely, either by the surgeon or by the destructive process, and the clivus extensively removed, it may be necessary to perform more elaborate reconstruction. There are several techniques available for muscle flap interposition and watertight reconstruction of the retropharynx. These are difficult, specialized procedures and should not be undertaken by anyone who is not skilled in their application. Many are still in evolution.

15

Cervical Spine Stabilization with Trapezial Osteosynthetic Plate Technique

The introduction of the anterior approach to the cervical spine by Robinson and Smith in the 1950s made the anterior elements of the cervical spine accessible. Anterior decompression of the cervical spinal cord has been made possible, and stabilization procedures for trauma and tumors have been performed with a variety of materials. Anterior cervical plating has not found widespread acceptance, although it allows for rigid fixation and stabilization in reconstructive cases where a corpectomy has been performed for metastatic primary tumor. A rigid construction can be made with methyl methacrylate and reinforced with a posterior fusion in primary decompression or a salvage situation.

A number of systems of equipment and surgical techniques have evolved over the past 20 years. At the present time, the surgeon can choose between an H-shaped plate from Synthes or the trapezial osteosynthetic plate that has been popularized by Caspar. Indications in Europe have included degenerative cervical spondylosis, fracture, and tumors. At the present time, we believe that the plate system has the most beneficial use in reconstructive cases where more conservative measures of stabilization have failed.

Because of the risk of cervical spinal cord injury

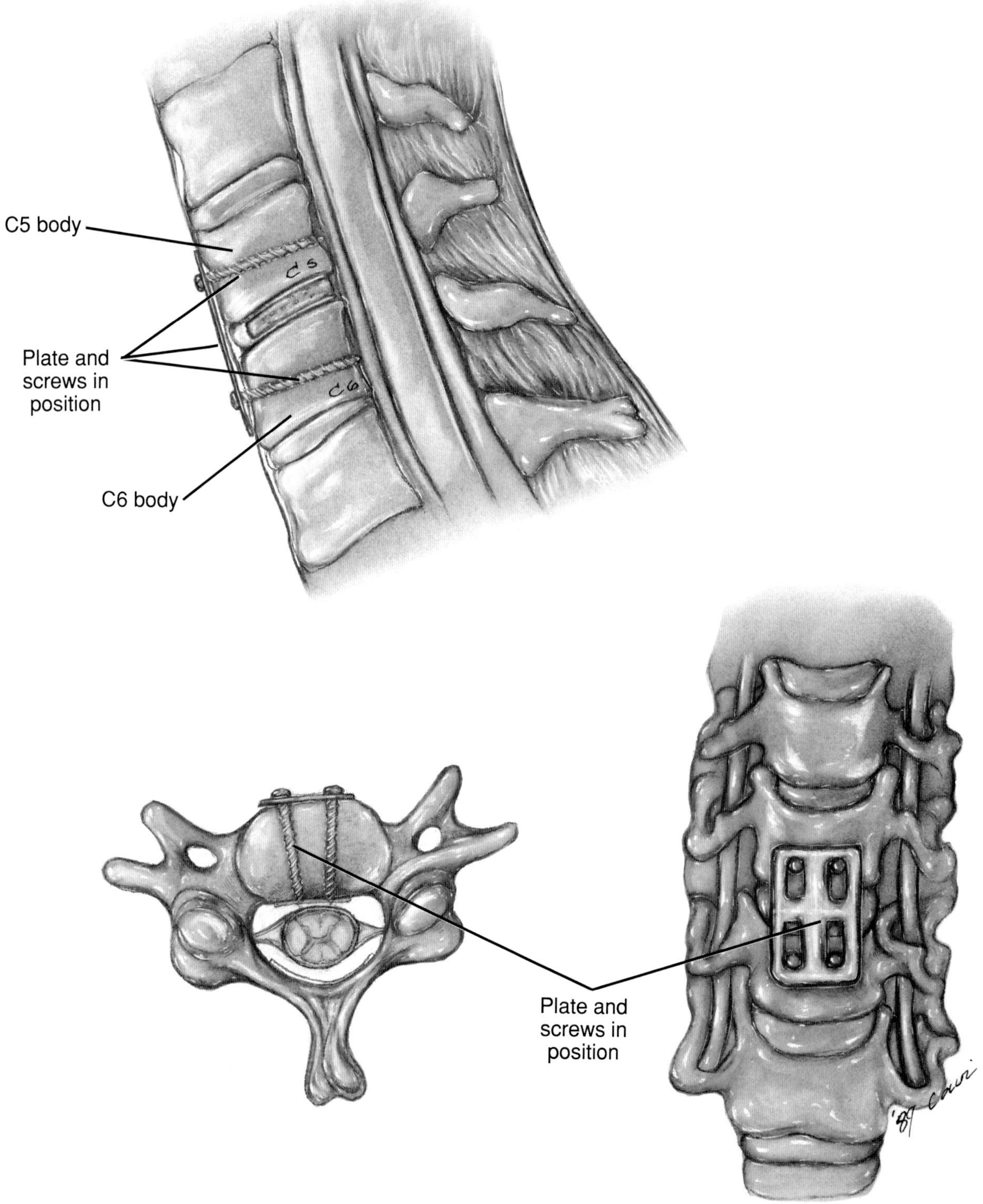
C5 body
Plate and screws in position
C6 body
Plate and screws in position

Figure 15.1.

from screw placement and the risk of esophageal rupture from improper plate placement, the surgeon must become familiar with the procedure before using it in the operating room. It is important to utilize x-ray control for placement of the screws. An exacting surgical technique is necessary to minimize risk and maximize benefits.

A classic anterior approach can be utilized and has been described previously in Chapter 10. If the patient has an unstable cervical spine, the procedure can be performed in cervical traction on an operative wedge frame. It is necessary to position the intraoperative x-ray monitor prior to scrubbing and draping the surgical field. The surgeon should be able to obtain sagittal and lateral direction x-rays throughout the procedure.

A transverse incision can be used on the left or the right side of the neck. Surgical exposure of the affected level should be done as described. After the level of the corpectomy has been defined on x-ray, a discectomy is performed of intervertebral discs a level above and a level below that of the pathology. A corpectomy can then be performed as described in the previous chapters. Loupe magnification can be utilized during the corpectomy to prevent injury to the dura, should the posterior longitudinal ligament be removed or violated.

After a complete corpectomy has been performed, a piece of Gelfoam may be necessary to protect the dura from any methyl methacrylate that may be placed as a spacer. The plate size must be determined under x-ray control. Position must be performed with x-ray to prevent malpositioning of the plate.

The plate must be appropriately contoured to the levels above and below the area of the corpectomy (Fig. 15.1). After the plate is positioned under x-ray control, it can be held by the assistant, and the appropriate angle drill guide can be placed in the apertures to allow for placement of the drill. The surgeon must use an adjustable drill under x-ray control. A 2.0-mm drill is used for the 3.5-mm screws. A single-hole drill guide can be used under radiographic control. The drill should not be placed into the spinal canal, disc space, or end plate in order to prevent injury or pullout of the screw. After the initial screw hole is drilled, a blunt 15.0-cm × 1.8-mm K-wire can be placed in the slot under x-ray control and used to stabilize the plate further. The second drill hole should be drilled at the same level as the first, and another blunt K-wire placed. After the plate is positioned, the inferior screws can be drilled in a similar manner with drill guide and x-ray control.

The blunt K-wires and plate should be removed, and the screw length determined with the depth gauge. At the present time, the thread length of an 18.0-mm screw is 16 mm long with a 2.0-mm head. The length of the screw head must be taken into account to prevent the screws from being too short, which would increase the risk of pullout. If a measurement of 18.0 mm is obtained with the depth gauge, a 20.0-mm screw is necessary to prevent pullout. As a margin of safety, 1.0 mm can be subtracted, which would equal a 19.0-mm screw in this example.

The anterior cortex of the vertebral bodies can be tapped prior to mixing the methyl methacrylate and placement of the plate. The surgeon may use a small fine wire mesh and Gelfoam to protect the spinal cord and to prevent extrusion of the methyl methacrylate posterior to the longitudinal ligament. Before the methyl methacrylate is placed, the appropriate screws and plate should be selected and available to place as the methyl methacrylate cures. A shorter locking screw can be selected to stabilize the methyl methacrylate construction and can be placed as the methyl methacrylate cures.

After the spacer is placed in the corpectomy defect, the plate is placed under x-ray control, and the screws are positioned and tightened in a smooth manner. The posterior longitudinal ligament and the epidural space provide the margin of error.

At the end of the placement of the plate and screws, a hard-copy radiograph should be obtained after position is checked on the intraoperative fluoroscope (Fig. 15.1).

A closure in layers can be performed with a drain placed to prevent postoperative hematoma formation. A closed suction drain can be utilized for 27–48 hours.

Concomitant posterior stabilization with iliac crest bone graft, utilizing the triple-wire technique, is recommended to allow for maximal stabilization but can be minimized because of the immediate stabilization of the anterior plate. Factors such as the quality of the bone and the patient's overall medical condition must be considered, and a two-poster brace may be appropriate without the posterior fusion.

Indications for this procedure are limited. The procedure should be reserved for complex reconstructive cases where more conservative forms of immobilization and reconstruction have failed and neurological deficit is present or impending.

16 Posterior Cervical Fusion below C2

Southwick Wiring and Fusion

Indications for Surgical Procedure

This Southwick wiring technique was developed in the late 1950s by Southwick working with Robert Robinson. The procedure is indicated in patients who have had prior laminectomies in the cervical spine and who have continued instability. In addition to postlaminectomy kyphosis and iatrogenic conditions, the Southwick wiring technique has been applied to patients with the disruption of posterior elements from fractures and tumors.

Surgical Techniques

With the patient in the prone position in skeletal traction, it is important not to have the patient's neck too far extended. A slight amount of flexion will allow less overlap of the facet joints and facilitate the passage of the facet wires. The posterior elements are stripped across the levels of the desired fusion by a midline approach. The facet joints are meticulously dissected, and the facet joint capsules are removed with rongeurs. It is important to avoid the venous plexus lateral to the facet joints; freely use the bipolar cautery in this area. Place a Freer elevator within the facet joint while the tunnels are being made for the wires. A $\frac{1}{16}$-inch burr or drill is then directed in an inferior and lateral direction through the inferior articular process toward the Freer elevator within the joint. The inferior ⅛-inch of the facet joint is utilized to provide the purchase for the wire. After placement of the burr hole through the involved levels of the fusion, a cervical wire is passed from one facet joint to its inferior counterpart. Use of a narrow hemostat is essential to grasp the 22-gauge wire within the facet joint and draw it through. For one-level instability at C5-C6, for example, two lateral wires from C5 to C6 will provide excellent immediate stability. For more than one-level instability, segmental wires are passed. For example, a desired fusion at C4, C5, C6, and C7 usually requires one wire on each side, with each through the facet joints at C4, C5, C6, and C7. Posterior iliac crest bone struts are then harvested. The bone graft usually encompasses the full cancellous thickness of the ilium including the outer cortical table. Four holes are then made with a 1/16-inch burr through each posterior iliac strut graft. Each segmental wire on each side is then passed through the iliac strut bone graft. The wires are then tightened down, and this provides loops around a full-thickness posterior iliac bone graft, which then secures it to each involved vertebra from C4 to C7. The excess amount of wire is then secured to an inferior intact spinous process, or the wires can be twisted together. We do not advocate simply cutting the excess wire after segmental attachment to the graft, as this provides no stability from one vertebra to the next.

The key distinguishing feature of the Southwick wiring is that it provides an oblique construction from the lateral facet joints to an inferior intact spinous process, so that the lines of stabilizing force are oblique rather than in a straight sagittal direction, as with the standard Rogers wiring. There is no biomechanical advantage to the use of sublaminar wires. There is a significant risk of iatrogenic neurological deficit with the passage of wires into the spinal canal. A definite advantage of the Rogers and the Southwick wiring techniques is that they obviate the risk of passing wires into the canal. Depending on the amount of preoperative instability, patients are placed postoperatively either in a Halo vest for 2 months or in a two-poster orthosis for 2 months.

Triple-Wire Fusion

The triple-wire cervical fusion technique was developed to serve patients with intact posterior elements who have not undergone extensive laminectomy, often for trauma or degenerative instability. The Southwick facet fusion is better for patients who have had multiple-level decompressive laminectomies.

Surgical Technique

The patient is placed in the prone position in skeletal traction with the neck as close to neutral as possible. A slight amount of flexion is acceptable, but extension must be avoided. Physiological monitoring of spinal cord function is a useful adjunct. The muscles and fascia are stripped from the spinous process and laminae according to standard techniques. The zygapophyseal joints are dissected and the joint capsules removed with drills or rongeurs. This fusion does not require the wide lateral dissection of the Southwick technique, nor does destruction of the facet have to be as complete. Incorporation of the facet in the fusion will be advantageous, however. A right-angled drill, heavy towel clip, or channeling device is then used to make a hole through the junction of the lamina and the base of the spinous process of each level to be fused (Fig. 16.4). Be certain to have all ligament and muscle removed from the spinous processes circumferentially so nothing will impede bony growth. It is important to stay well above the dura but still be in the center of the base of the spinous process so that a good purchase is obtained. The high-speed drill is then used to decorticate bone from spinous process and laminae. Wires are successively passed through and around these holes. A midline tethering wire of 20-gauge stainless steel is utilized (Fig. 16.4). The extent of the fusion should be judged by the space or spaces to be immobilized. Redundant bone above and below may interfere with adjacent motor segments and may be a cause of postoperative pain.

Wire placement is critical. A 20-gauge wire is passed through the upper hole, looped around the spinous process, and returned through the same hole. The wire is then directed to the lower hole, passed through it, looped below the spinous process, and returned through the hole to the same side as the upper end of the wire to be tied (Fig. 16.5).

Two 22-gauge wires are then passed through the same holes, through the bone grafts bilaterally, and then tied. This creates rotational stability as two large iliac strut grafts are compressed against the posterior cervical lamina. Cancellous bone is then packed in

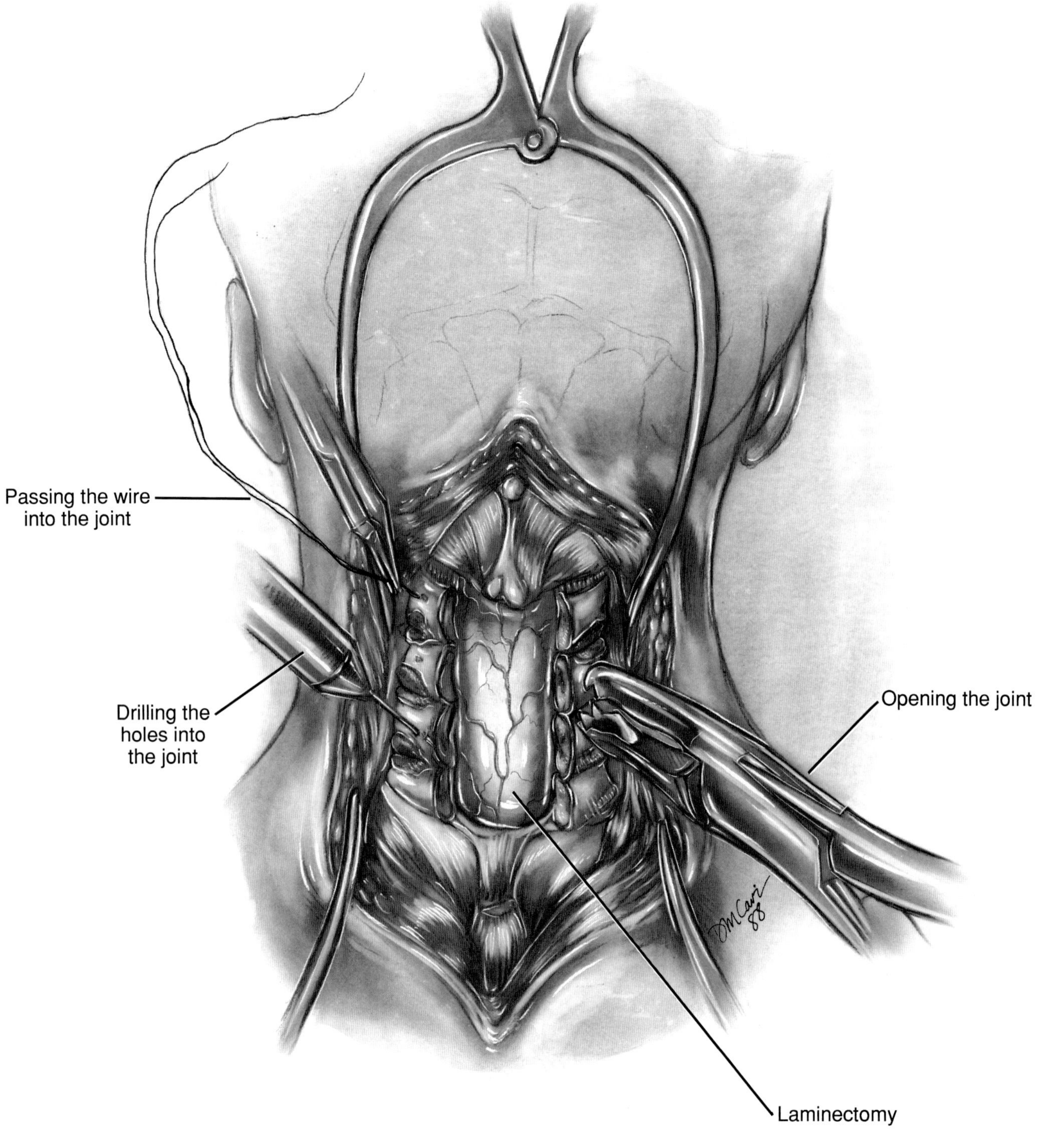
Passing the wire into the joint
Drilling the holes into the joint
Opening the joint
Laminectomy

Figure 16.1.

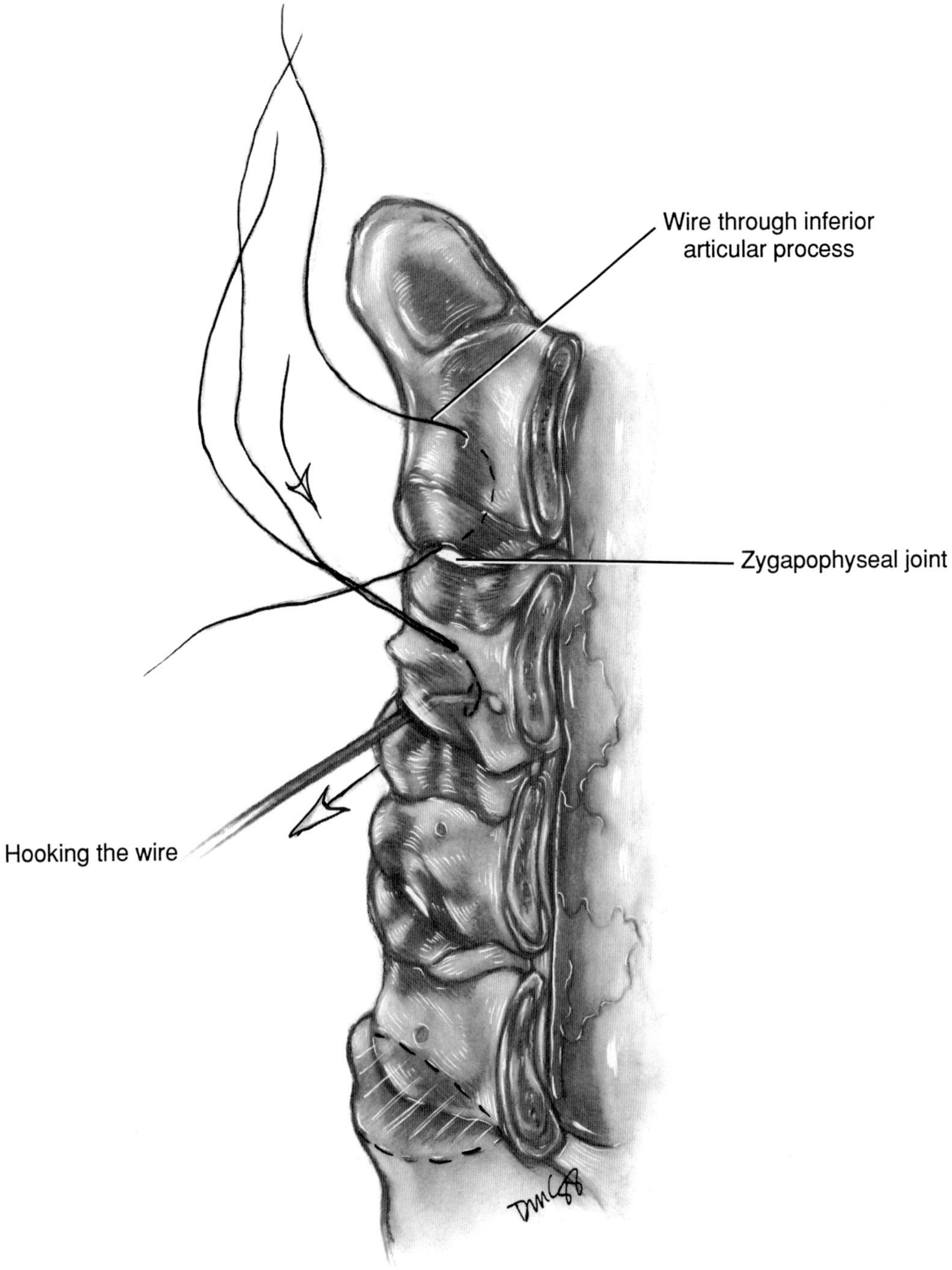

Figure 16.2.

and around the fusion and the facets. The construction is stable, but in order to improve the chance of fusion, the patient is usually immobilized in a two-poster metal brace for 6–8 weeks after the operation. Final stability is checked at 3 months postoperatively by flexion and extension lateral cervical spine roentgenograms.

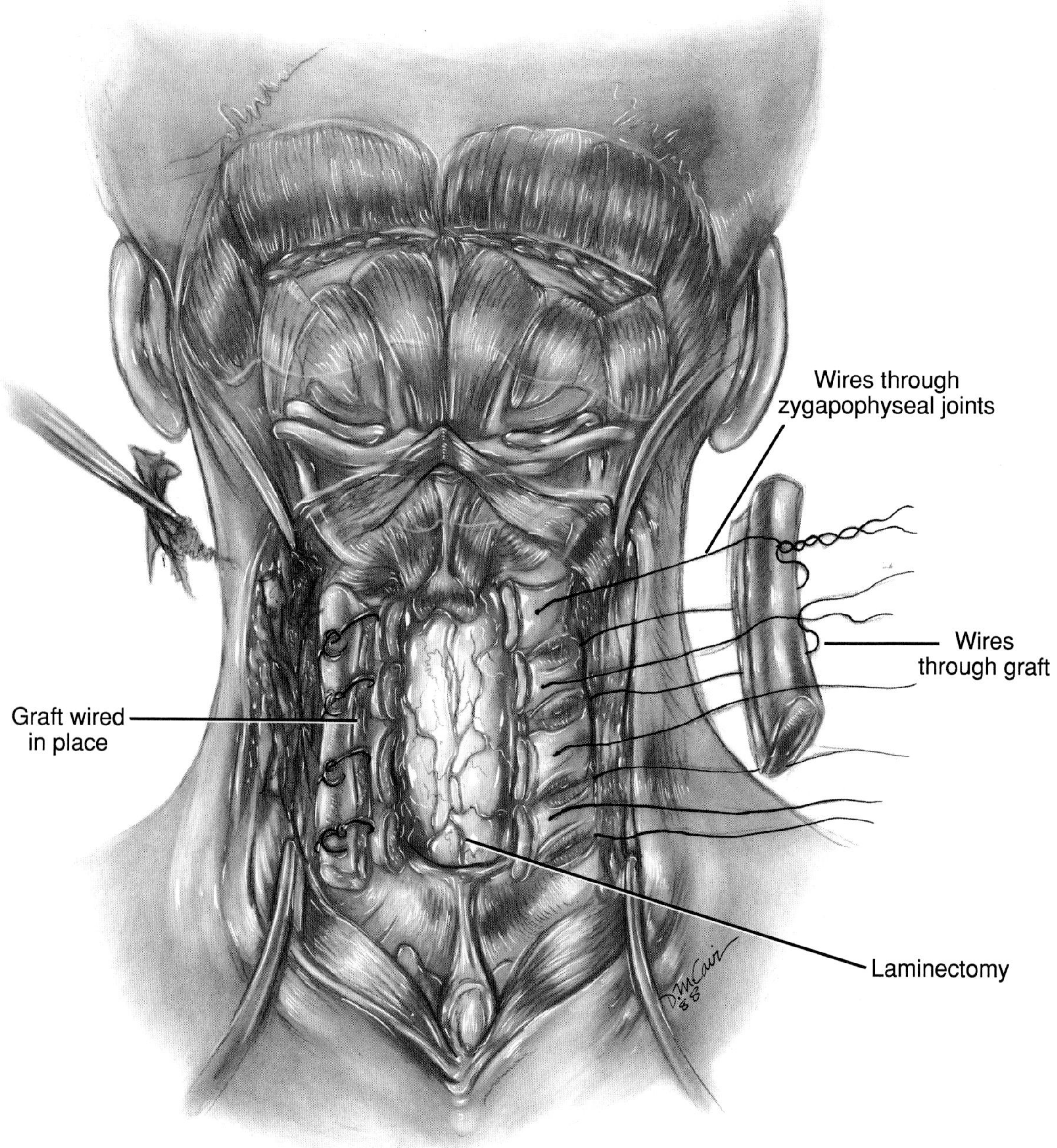
Wires through
zygapophyseal joints
Wires
through graft
Graft wired
in place
Laminectomy

Figure 16.3.

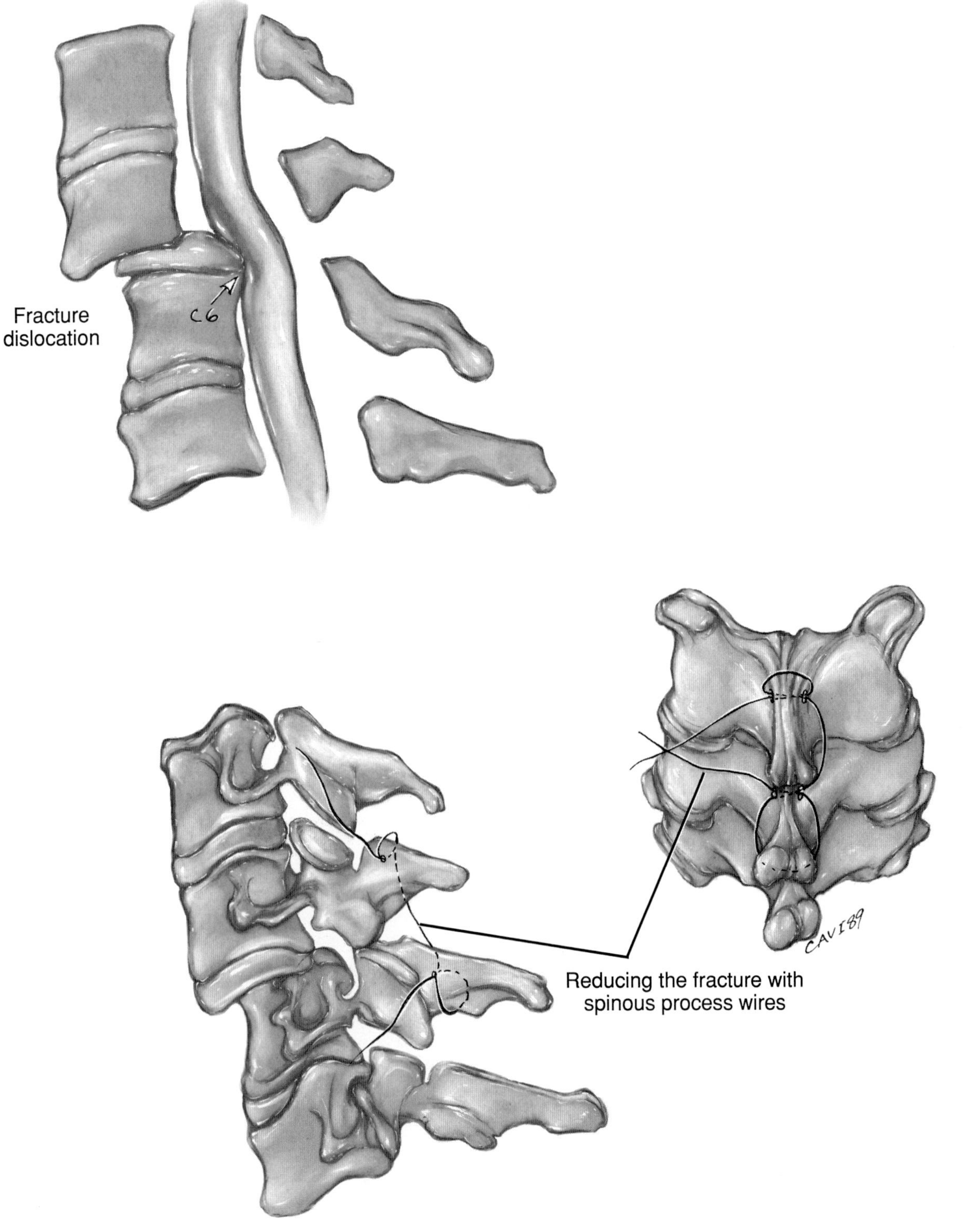
Fracture
dislocation
C6
Reducing the fracture with
spinous process wires

Figure 16.4.

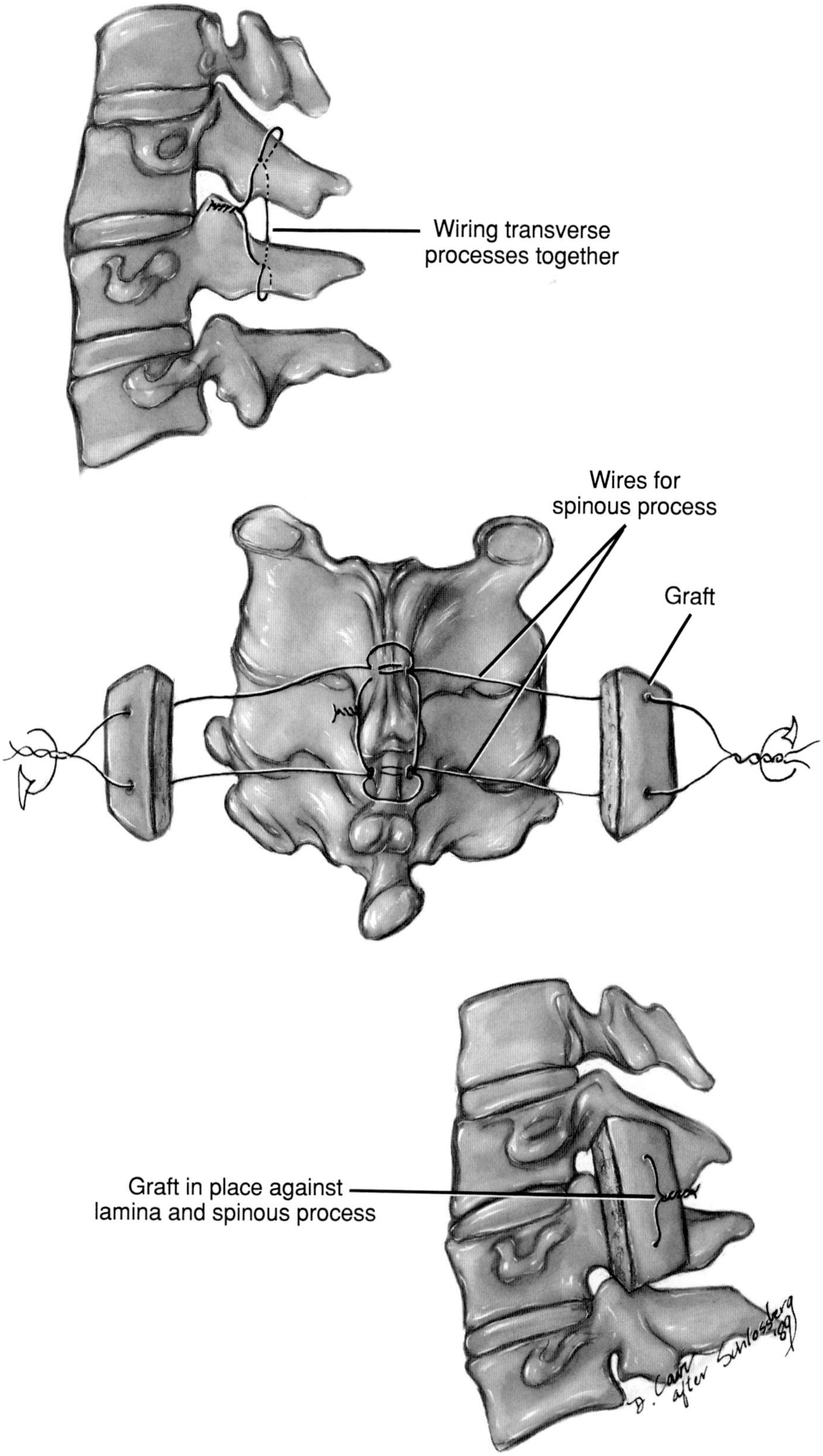
Wiring transverse
processes together
Wires for
spinous process
Graft
Graft in place against
lamina and spinous process

Figure 16.5.

17

C1-C2 Decompression and Fusion: Posterior Approach

Occipital cervical instability is a common complication of odontoid fracture, os odontoideum, rheumatoid arthritis, and the Chiari malformation (Fig. 17.1). More uncommonly, it complicates achondroplasia and other forms of basilar impression. Instability may be demonstrated by movement during flexion/extension x-rays at either the occipital-C1 junction or between C1 and C2. Surprising degrees of motion and slippage are possible without the development of neurological deficits. When neurological abnormalities occur, there may be varying combinations of lower cranial nerve dysfunction and spinal cord compression. Hoarseness, difficulty swallowing, diminished voice volume, and sleep apnea all occur. Motor deficits are more prominent than sensory deficits, and quadriparesis in varying degrees may be present. The neurological deficit may be accentuated or precipitated by head movement.

The goal of surgery is stabilization. It is critical to be certain what is moving so the decision about whether occipital incorporation into the fusion is required can be made before the operation begins. It is also impor-

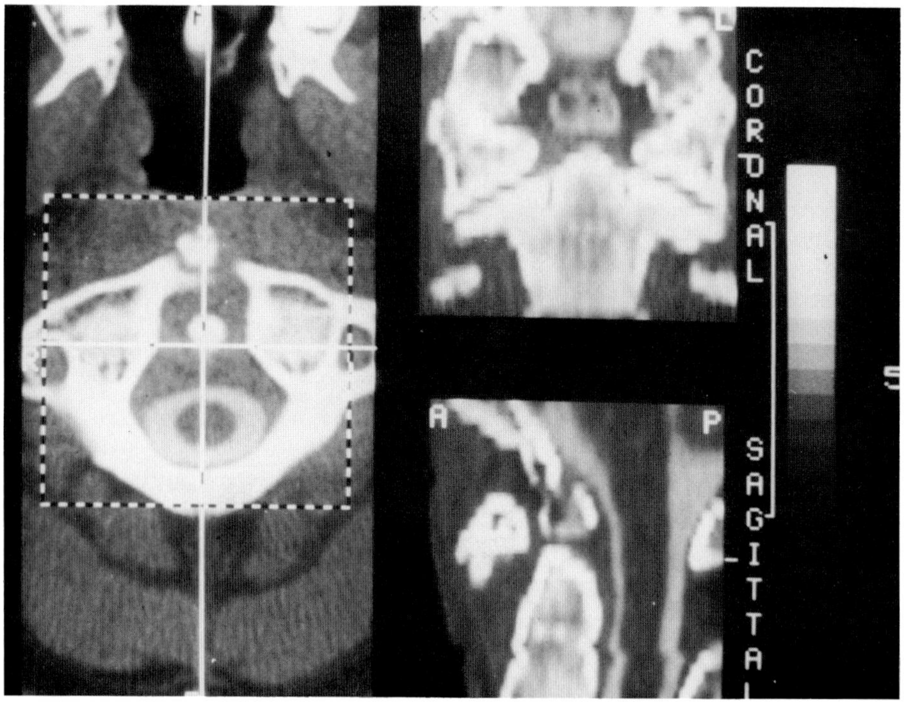

Figure 17.1. Typical picture of os odontoideum is seen. Posterior cervical fusion at C1-C2 will be adequate.

tant to determine whether any posterior decompression will be required, because this may modify the technique of fusion.

The operation is done with the patient in the prone position in skeletal fixation or skeletal traction (Fig. 17.2). The techniques of anesthesia and positioning are important. If the patient is strikingly unstable, a fiberoptic intubation is desirable. Spinal cord monitoring throughout the intubation is helpful. Turning the patient to the prone position is critical and probably the most dangerous part of the procedure. We use the operative wedge frame so that the patient's neck position does not have to be disturbed after intubation. The patient is intubated on the frame, awake and with the spinal cord being monitored. Skeletal traction is applied, and the patient is turned in the wedge frame to maintain a stable neutral position of the neck. The position should be neutral to external inspection, and this should be verified by x-ray before the surgery begins. Adjustments to the traction may be necessary to provide perfect alignment. In patients who are less unstable, it is reasonable to use routine skeletal pin fixation techniques following standard induction of anesthesia.

Following the neutral positioning, the area of the neck and both posterior iliac regions are prepared and draped for surgery. A midline skin incision is made from well up on the occiput down to the spinous process of C3. The muscles are divided in the midline until the spinous process of C2 is identified and the occipital bone is found (Fig. 17.3). The deep retractors are progressively advanced to maintain the exposure of the operative field. A subperiosteal dissection of muscles from spines and laminae is then carried out, beginning at C2, then including the occiput, and finally incorporating C3 into the exposure. The electric knife is a convenient way to carry this out and greatly reduces blood loss. As long as the dissection is carried out only on the laminae and spinous processes over bone, no injury to spinal cord or nerves can occur. Gentle use of osteotomes is also acceptable. The electric knife is employed to cut the muscles from the bifid spine of C2 and then to dissect the muscles from the spinous process and lamina bilaterally (Fig. 17.4).

There are large venous plexuses at C1 and C2 that are far lateral. It is wise to carry the dissection out to the limits of the zygapophyseal joints but not beyond and not between, to avoid these veins. When C2 is exposed, a deep retractor is put in place to maintain that exposure, and the muscles are cut away from the occiput in the same way. This exposes C1, leaving some of the muscles intact over C1. They are then dissected from C1, with care taken not to extend the dissection too far laterally in the region of the vertebral artery. Angled cerebellar retractors will serve well, though many other types have been described and are available. The retractors will now expose the occiput, the arch of C1, the spine and laminae of C2, and a variable part of C3. Sometimes, decompression by partial removal of the arch of C1 is required. This can be done with rongeurs, leaving stumps of C1 for the eventual fusion. If no bony removal is required, the procedure is continued with careful removal of all of the soft tissues from C1, C2, and the occiput. This must be done meticulously, and the cortical bone then scarified with the high-speed drill.

All is in readiness for the wires. The first step is to make a hole through the base of the spinous process of C2 (Fig. 17.4). This can be done with a tenaculum or with a right-angle drill. One wire will be passed through C2. The second set of wires must be placed around the arch of C1. A doubled wire is passed blunt end first from inferior to superior around the arch of C1 (Fig. 17.5). The process is duplicated on the opposite side. The free ends of the wire are passed through the loop, and the two wires are cinched tightly to C1. A second wire is doubly passed through the base of the spinous process of C2; i.e., one end is passed from left to right, the other is passed from right to left, and the loop is passed around and inferior to the spinous process of C2. This is cinched tightly.

Now a graft must be harvested from the iliac crest. This technique is identical with those described in detail for other grafts. The cortical grafts do not have to be as large as those used in the lumbar region. To harvest the graft, a curvilinear incision is made lateral to the posterior superior iliac spine and the sacroiliac joint from the rim of the ilium down into the sacral region. Remember that the cluneal nerves are easy to injure with a transverse incision. The incision is carried through muscle to bone, and the muscle scraped away, exposing the posterior surface of the ilium. A high-speed drill, oscillating saw, or osteotomes may be used to harvest appropriate grafts. You should

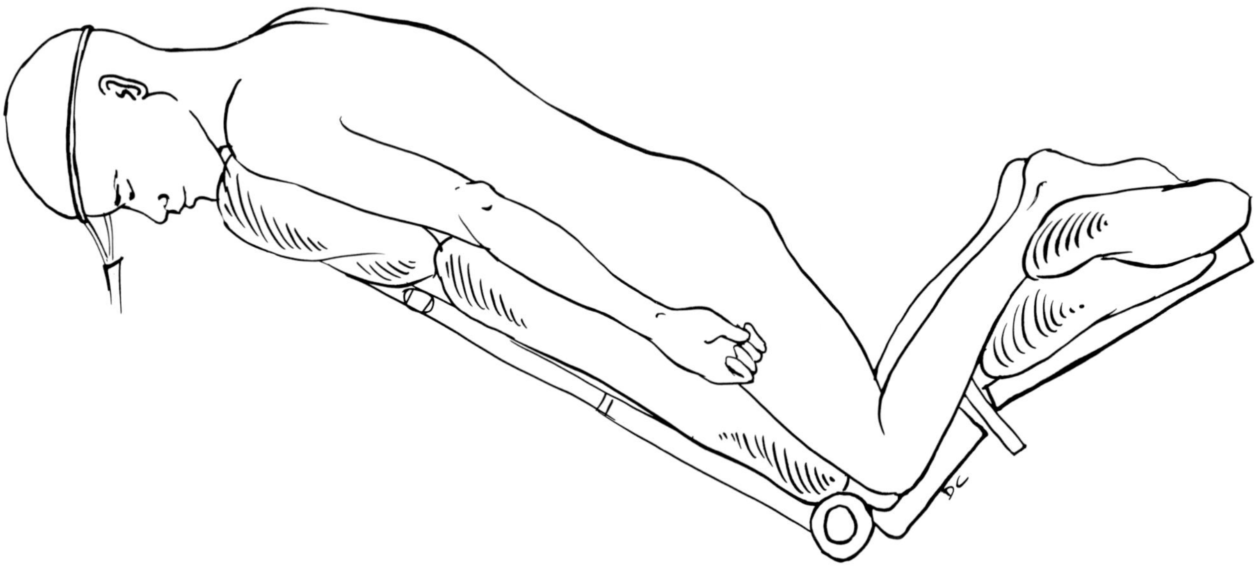

Figure 17.2.

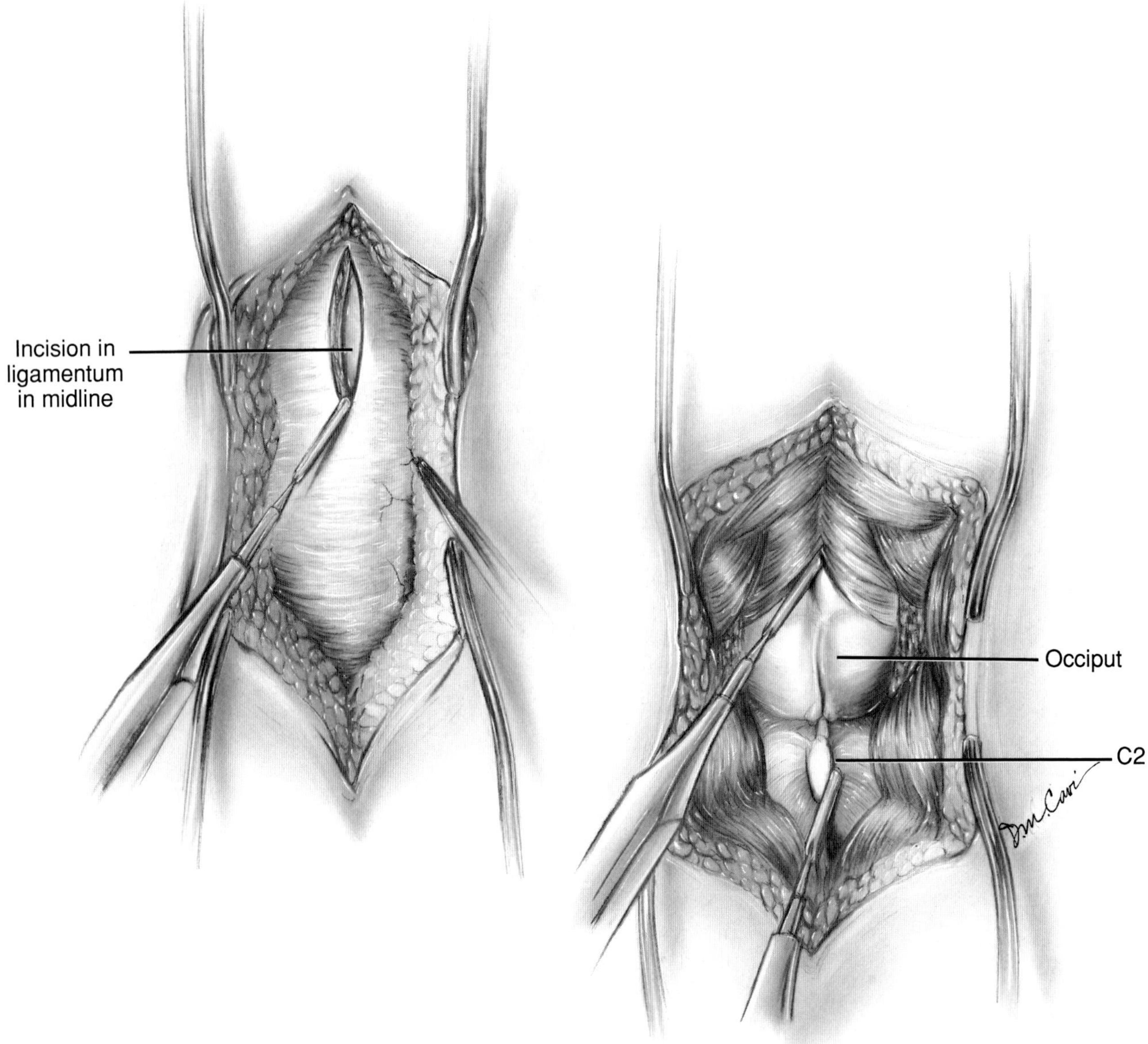

Figure 17.3.

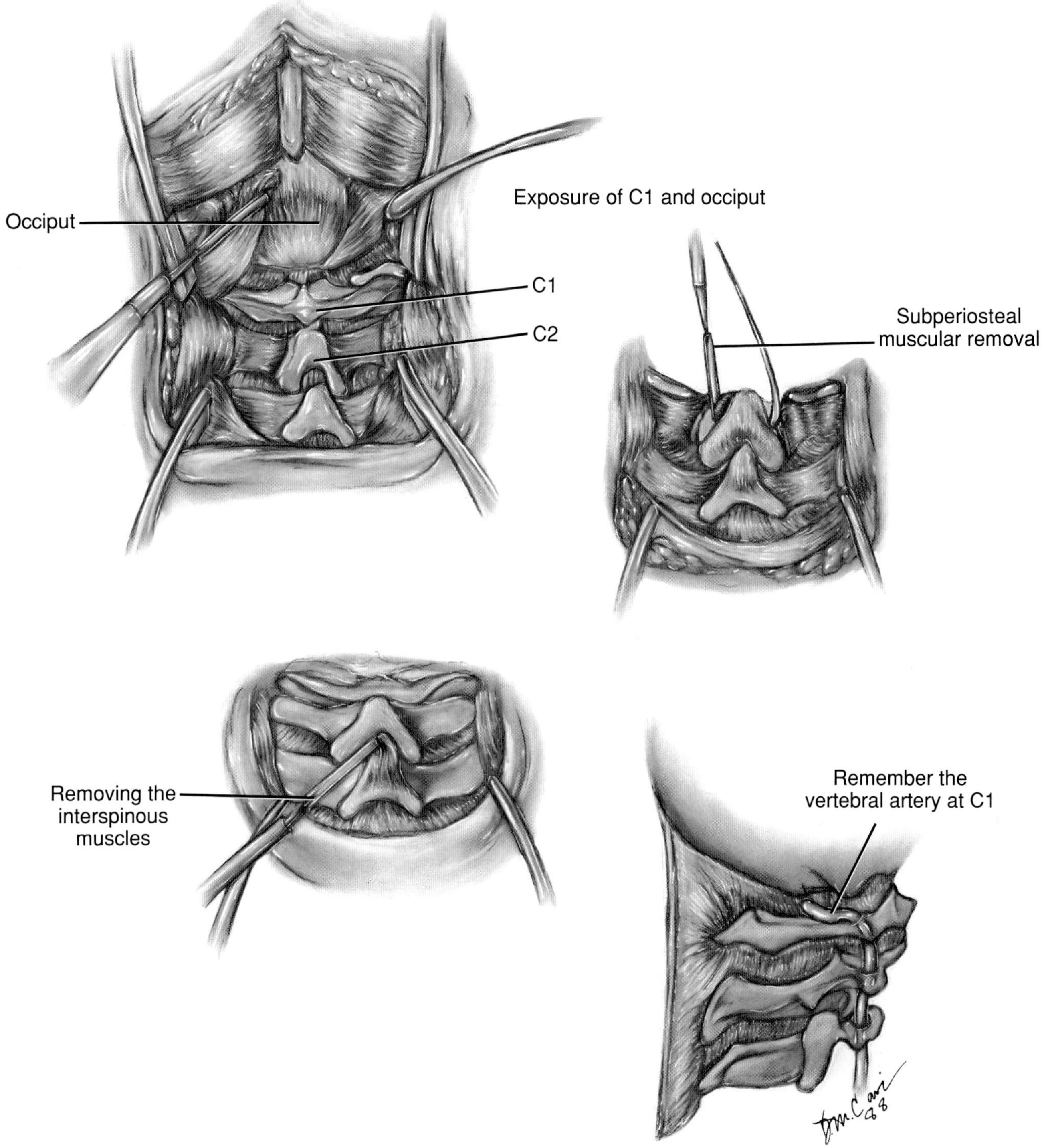
Occiput
C1
C2
Exposure of C1 and occiput
Subperiosteal muscular removal
Removing the interspinous muscles
Remember the vertebral artery at C1

Figure 17.4.

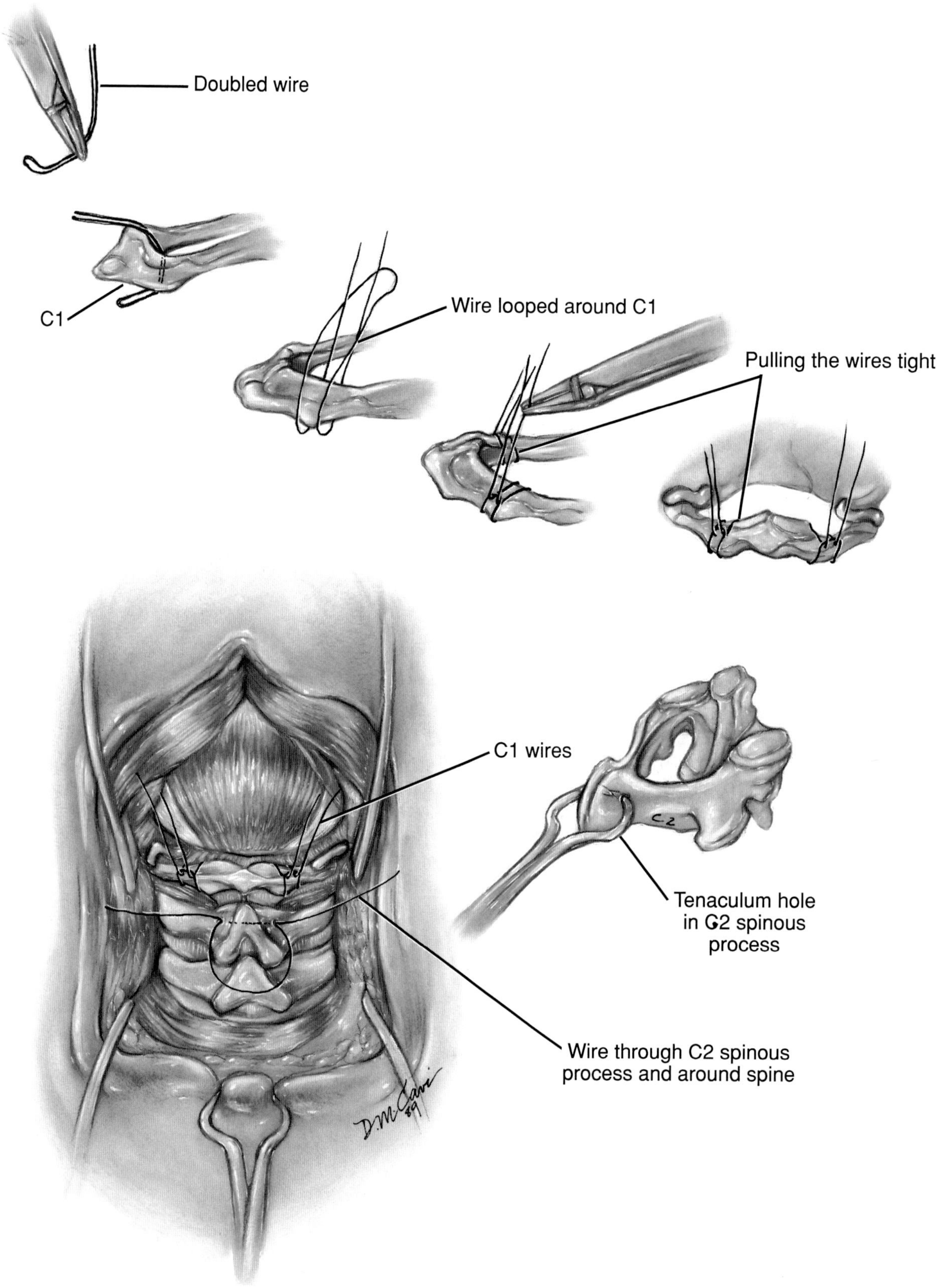
Doubled wire
C1
Wire looped around C1
Pulling the wires tight
C1 wires
C2
Tenaculum hole
in C2 spinous
process
Wire through C2 spinous
process and around spine
D.M. Cain
89

Figure 17.5.

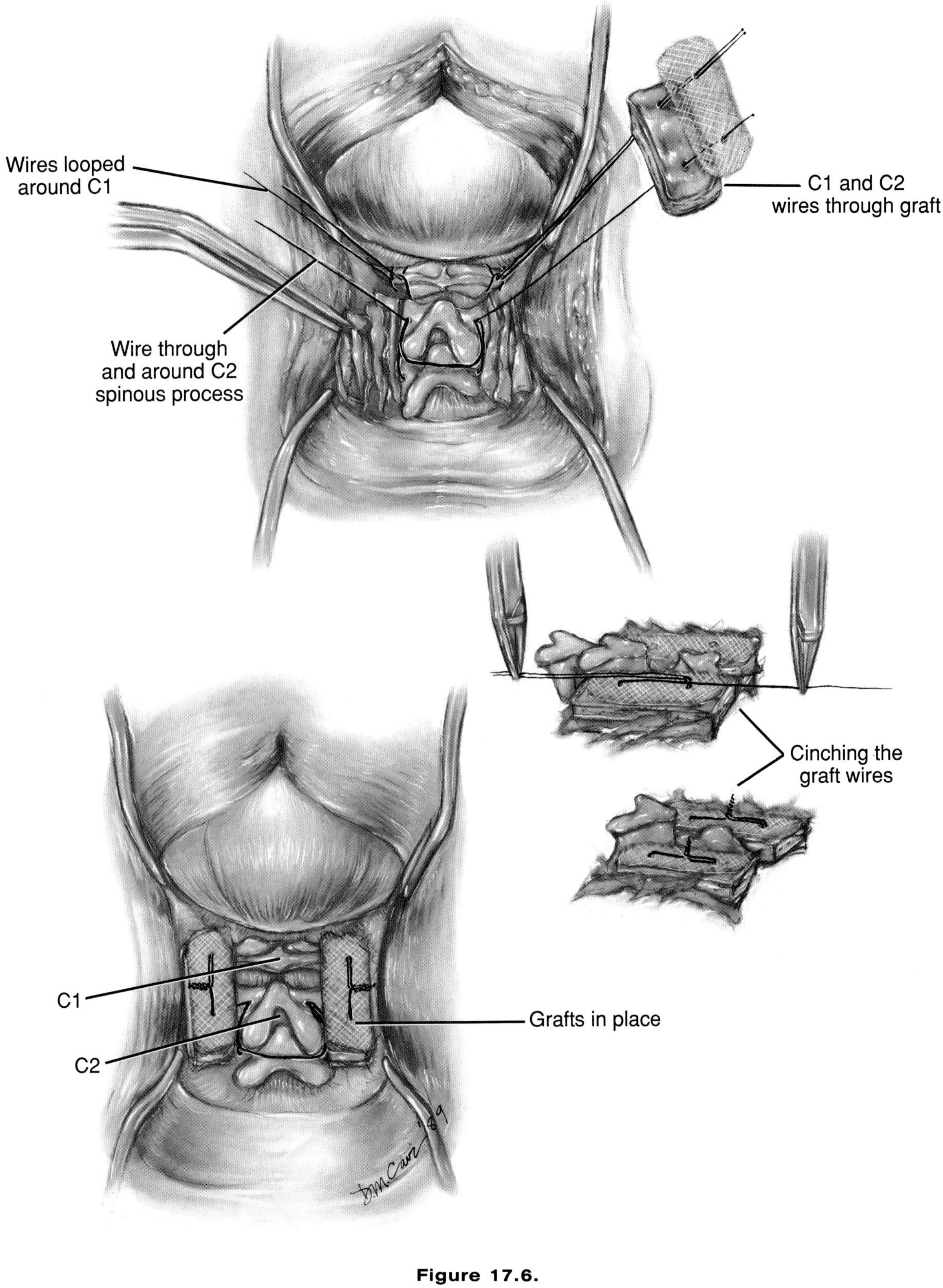
Wires looped
around C1
C1 and C2
wires through graft
Wire through
and around C2
spinous process
Cinching the
graft wires
C1
C2
Grafts in place

Figure 17.6.

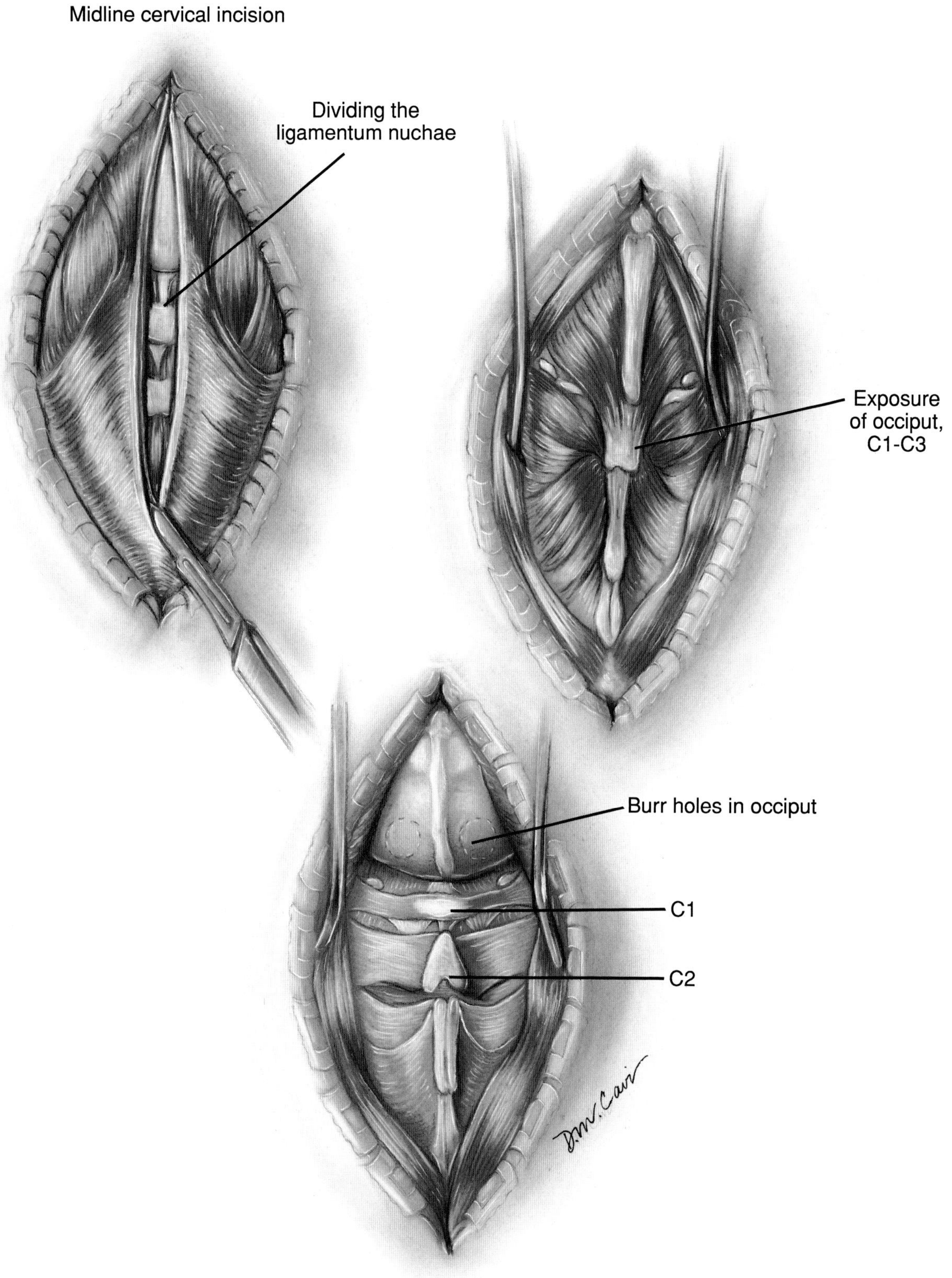
Midline cervical incision
Dividing the ligamentum nuchae
Exposure of occiput, C1-C3
Burr holes in occiput
C1
C2

Figure 17.7.

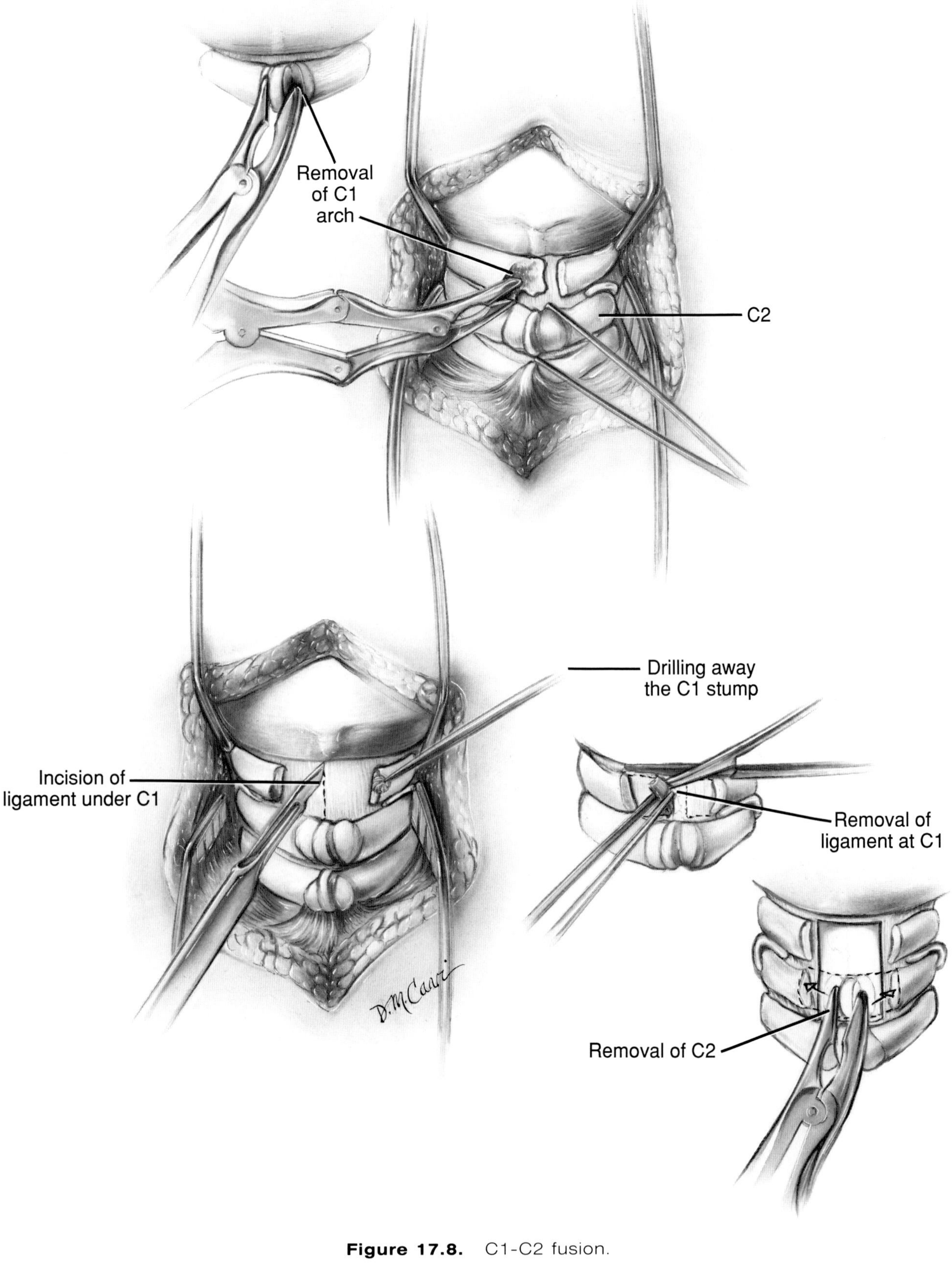

Figure 17.8. C1-C2 fusion.

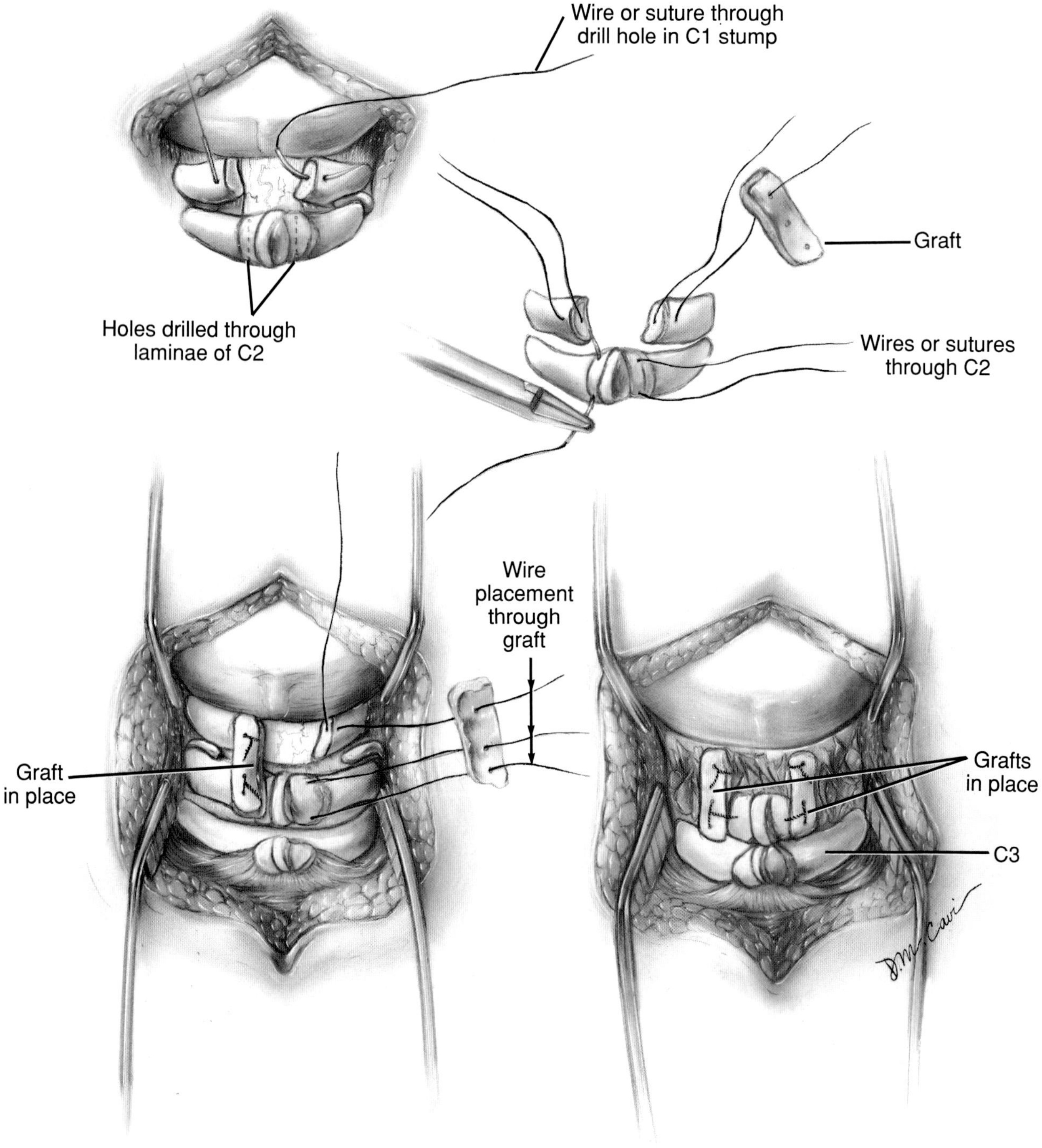

Wire or suture through drill hole in C1 stump
Graft
Holes drilled through laminae of C2
Wires or sutures through C2
Wire placement through graft
Graft in place
Grafts in place
C3

Figure 17.9.

measure the distance required to cover C1-C2 completely. If the occiput is to be incorporated, the graft must be somewhat longer. A full-thickness cortical graft 4–5 mm thick is harvested, and some cancellous bone also is removed. Identical grafts will be necessary for each side. With appropriate measurement they can be cut almost exactly but then should be sized to fit perfectly. Two holes are drilled through the graft, at least several millimeters from the end, at a place through which the wires from C1 and C2 can easily pass. The C1 wires are passed through the upper holes bilaterally, the C2 wires are passed through the lower, and the grafts are slid tightly into place. The wires are then twisted to hold the graft. Cancellous bone is packed around the construction, and the wound can then be closed in layers without further special attention (Fig. 17.6).

When the occiput is to be incorporated, the technique must be somewhat different. In preparation, the rim of the foramen magnum is isolated, and blunt dissectors are utilized to free dura from the rim and from the occipital bone (Fig. 17.7). An Adson periosteal elevator makes an ideal tool. A high-speed drill is then utilized to make a hole through the bone but not into dura. It is critical to avoid a cerebrospinal fluid leak. If a leak does occur, the area can be packed with fat, and the wound closed especially carefully. The extra time invested to avoid a leak is worth the investment, however. When the hole is drilled, a doubled wire is passed blunt end first through the hole and then out the rim of the foramen magnum. The two loose ends of the wire are looped through it, as was done for the C1 wire. The process is repeated on the opposite side, and these two wires are cinched tightly to the foramen magnum. The technique of graft placement is varied, in that a longer graft is required and three holes are drilled—one for the occipital wire, one for the C1 wire, and one for the C2 wire. The three wires are then tied together over the graft after it has been slipped into position. This incorporates the rim of the foramen magnum and occiput and makes the hole construction solid and safe.

Another technique is to drill only part way through the occipital bone. This is commonly possible in large adults when the drill hole is angled so that it comes out in the foramen magnum about halfway through the bone. This greatly reduces the risk of cerebrospinal fluid leak. Sometimes, it is necessary to bite away a small amount of the foramen magnum in order to pass the wires. Remember that the rim of the foramen magnum must be scarified with the drill to improve the fusion process. Cancellous bone is packed all around the occiput, and the wound then closed over the construction.

Another variation occurs when the arch of C1 must be removed in order to afford decompression. The technique varies simply by drilling a hole through the cut end of C1. Be sure to leave enough that a solid construction can be obtained. The hole is drilled either full thickness or partial thickness through C1, depending on the dimensions of that structure. The wires are then passed, and the grafts put in place in exactly the same way as previously described (Figs. 17.8 and 17.9).

These grafts are solid, and most patients can ambulate in a firm brace, such as the typical two- or four-poster metal braces. When the patient is particularly unstable or if significant compression anteriorly is present, it is probably better to place them in a halo device postoperatively. This is usually applied in the operating room before the patient awakens, but it can be applied several days later. The former is more comfortable for the patient, but applying the brace a few days later means that the immediate postoperative period is safer in terms of extubation, aspiration, and general airway care.

SECTION 5

Thoracic Disc

18

Operations on Thoracic Disc

Transthoracic Approach

In the region between T5 and T10, the transthoracic removal of the thoracic disc is the simplest approach to be undertaken. The patient is positioned on the side as for a thoracotomy, with the right side up. A standard thoracotomy incision is made (Fig. 18.1). Remember that the ribs below the disc herniation will lead to the appropriate place; i.e., the T8 rib will lead to the T7-T8 disc. During a thoracotomy, it is common to remove one of the ribs, but this is not always necessary. Once the chest is open and the lung retracted, the ribs are counted and followed to identify both rib and neural foramen appropriately. The rib is followed to the neural foramen, and the paravertebral tissue is incised longitudinally, exposing the disc (Fig. 18.2). In most patients, the discs and bodies are easily seen. In obese individuals, a moderate amount of dissection may be necessary to identify the appropriate area. Follow the rib to the neural foramen and identify the disc. When all of the soft tissue is removed from the paravertebral area, the entire neural foramen with both ribs and both pedicles should be visualized. The disc should be exposed on both sides, and there should be no extraneous material on the bone to impede drilling (Fig. 18.3).

The easiest way to remove the bone to gain access to the interspace is with the high-speed drill. To gain access to the interspace, it is necessary to remove usually all of the pedicle above and sometimes some of the pedicle below. The head of the rib must also be removed. This will provide access to the entire neural foramen. When bony removal is complete, the

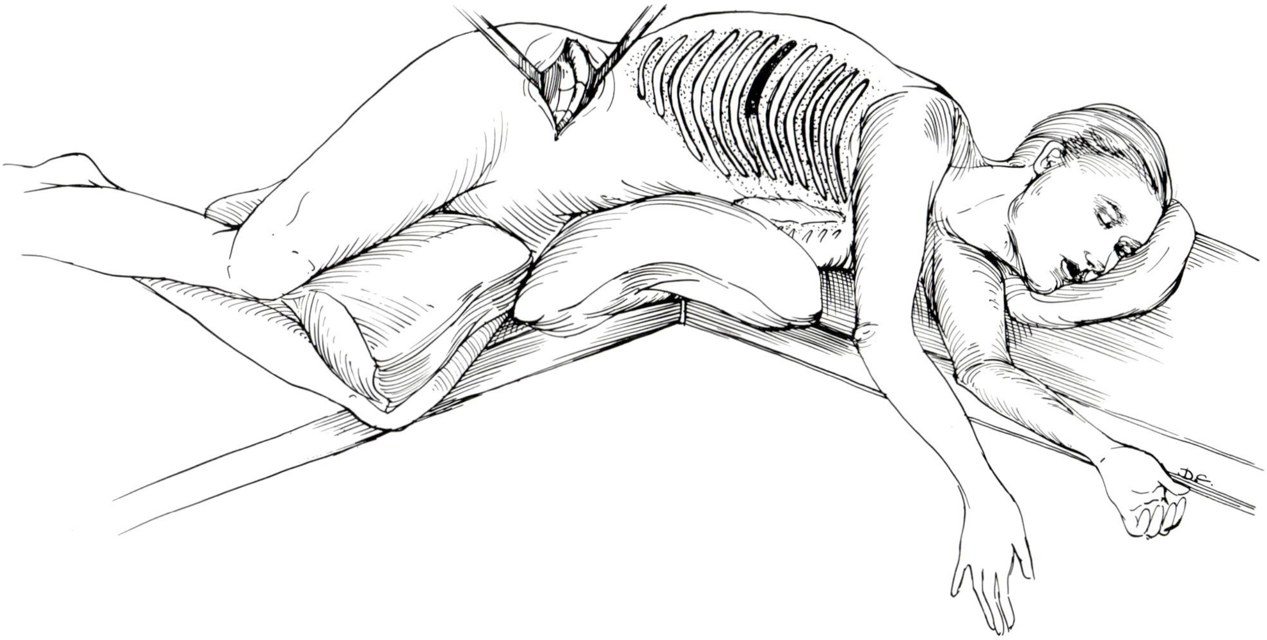

Figure 18.1.

interspace should be entered through a sizable incision as close to the posterior longitudinal ligament as possible. All degenerated disc material is removed. Frequently, the principal problem is compression by posterior bars, thickened annulus, and posterior longitudinal ligament. All this tissue needs to be removed. This is done by first removing all the soft tissue from the posterior quarter or third of the interspace. Then, the bony ridges are removed from side to side with the high-speed drill. The thickened ligaments and annulus may need to be cut away. Do not start laterally on the side of the exposure. It is better to proceed as far across the interspace as possible and drill away the ridges from the opposite to the ipsilateral side. If you begin on the side of the exposure, the decompressed dural sac will obscure vision and have to be retracted. By beginning as far to the opposite side as possible, you can avoid this problem and completely remove the bony and soft tissues under direct vision. As the decompression gradually progresses to the ipsilateral side, the dural sac will collapse into the decompressed area, thus ensuring that satisfactory removal has occurred. Before bony removal is complete on the ipsilateral side, it is important to continue to the opposite side until it is certain that all transverse compression has been removed. Then, the final drilling on the ipsilateral side allows the entire dural sac to collapse into the decompressed area (Fig. 18.4). Most surgeons favor a limited interbody fusion. Posterior materials have all been removed, and this should be continued until all degenerated disc material is absent from the interspace. The cartilage is breached, the remnant of the end plates is removed, and cancellous bone is exposed. Then pieces of the rib that has been removed are packed into the open area, with care taken not to constrict the spinal canal. If a rib has not been removed, the head of one of the exposed ribs can be taken to be utilized for the same purpose (Fig. 18.5).

It is extremely important not to cause a cerebrospinal fluid leak. A fistula into the chest is a major complication. If a cerebrospinal fluid leak does occur, try to close it with sutures, and if this is impossible, careful packing with fat or muscle will usually suffice.

The thoracotomy is closed in the usual fashion and requires no special care. Postoperatively, the patient should be kept in a brace for 3 months until the fusion heals.

Costotransverse Approach

The goals for the transthoracic and costotransverse approaches to removal of the disc are the same. The

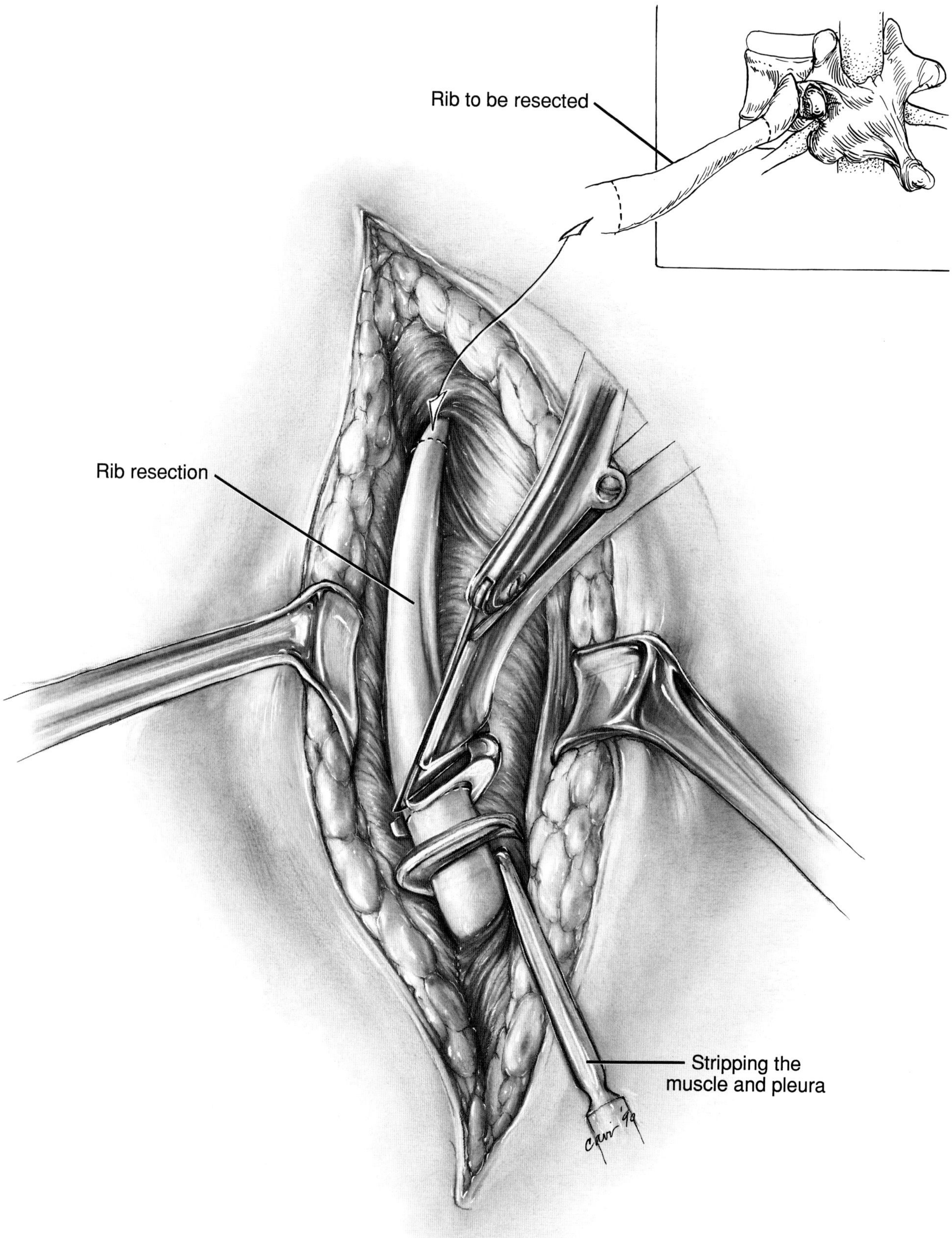
Rib to be resected
Rib resection
Stripping the
muscle and pleura

Figure 18.2.

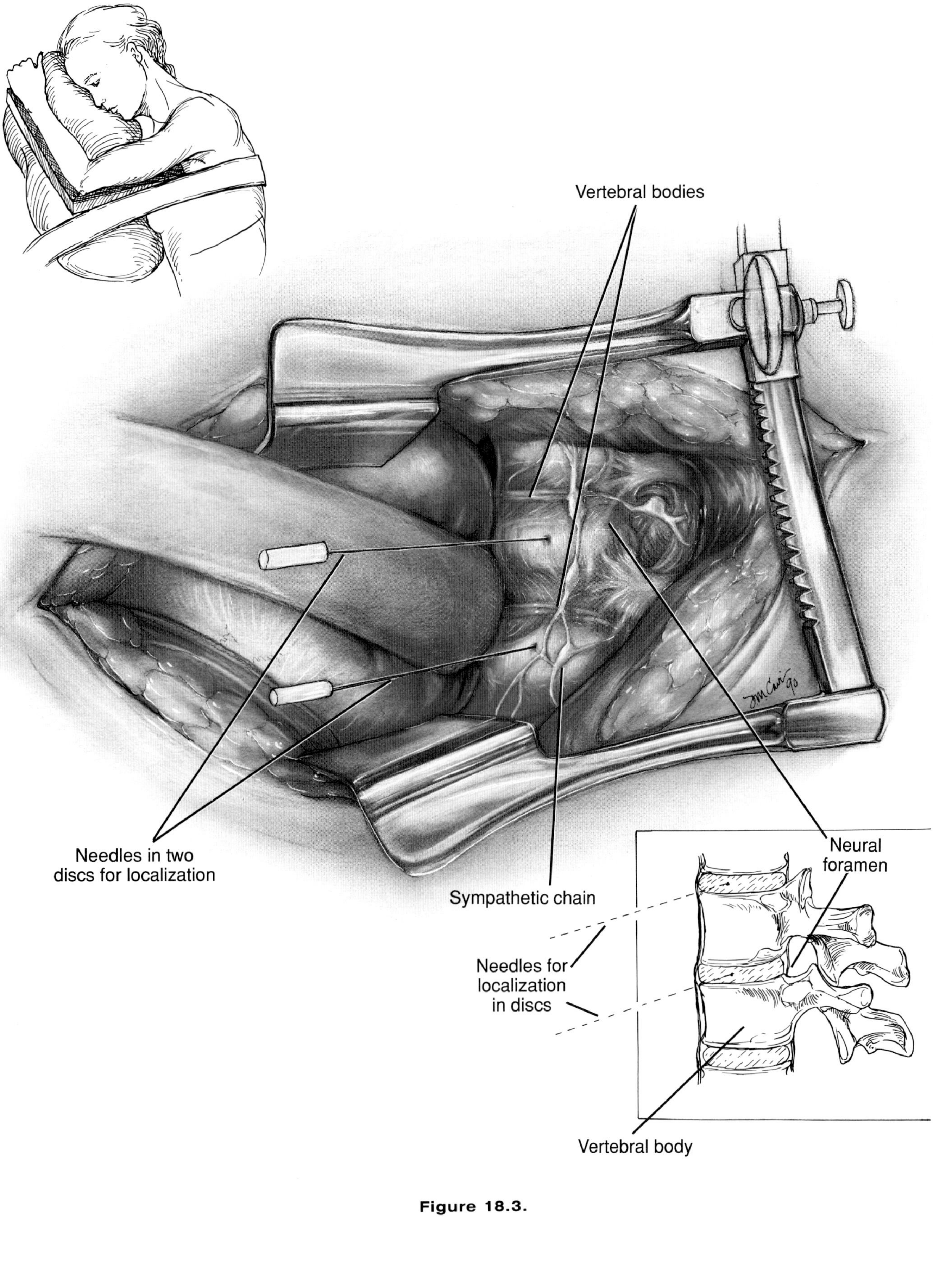
Vertebral bodies
Needles in two
discs for localization
Sympathetic chain
Neural
foramen
Needles for
localization
in discs
Vertebral body

Figure 18.3.

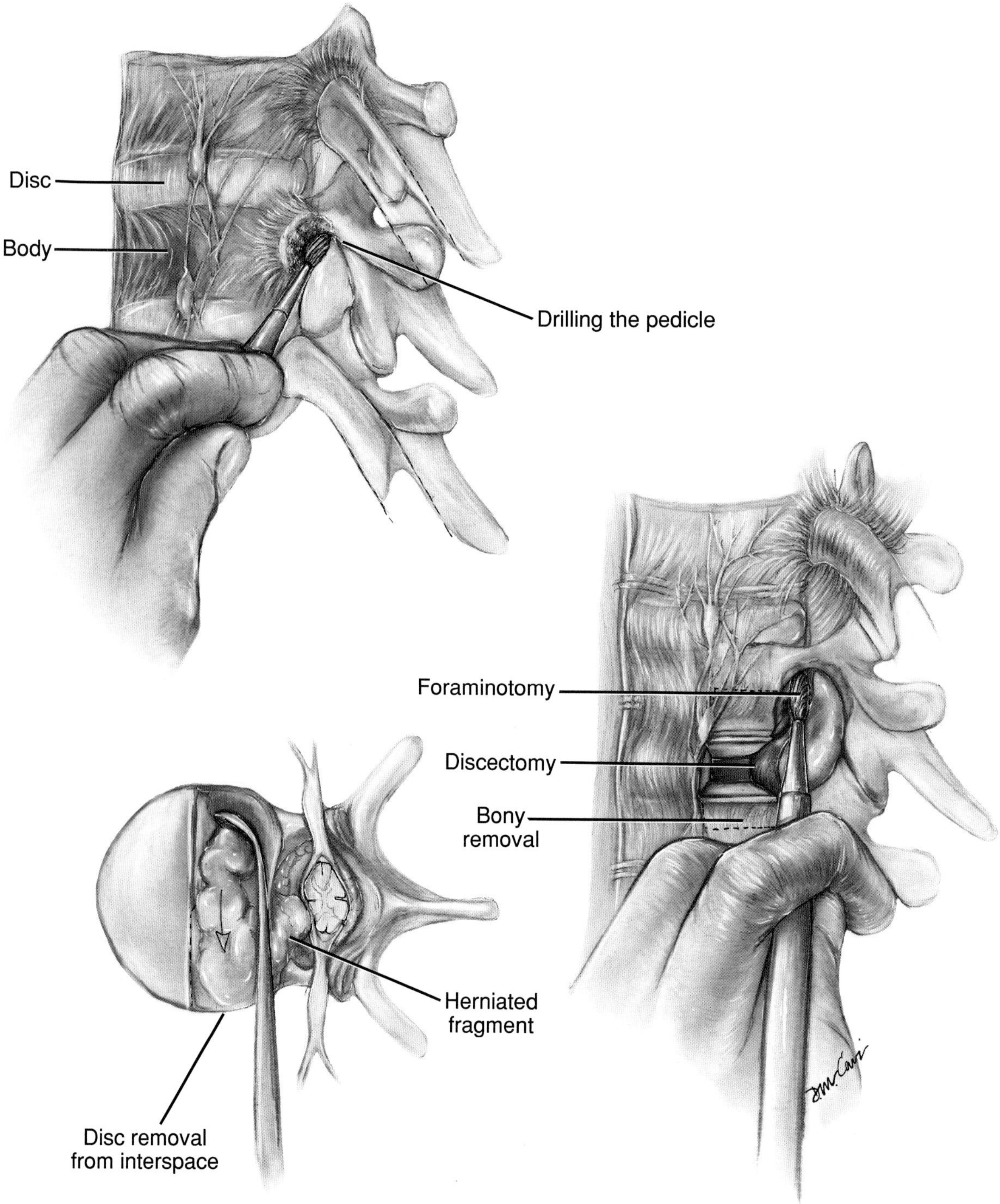

Disc
Body
Drilling the pedicle
Foraminotomy
Discectomy
Bony removal
Herniated fragment
Disc removal from interspace

Figure 18.4.

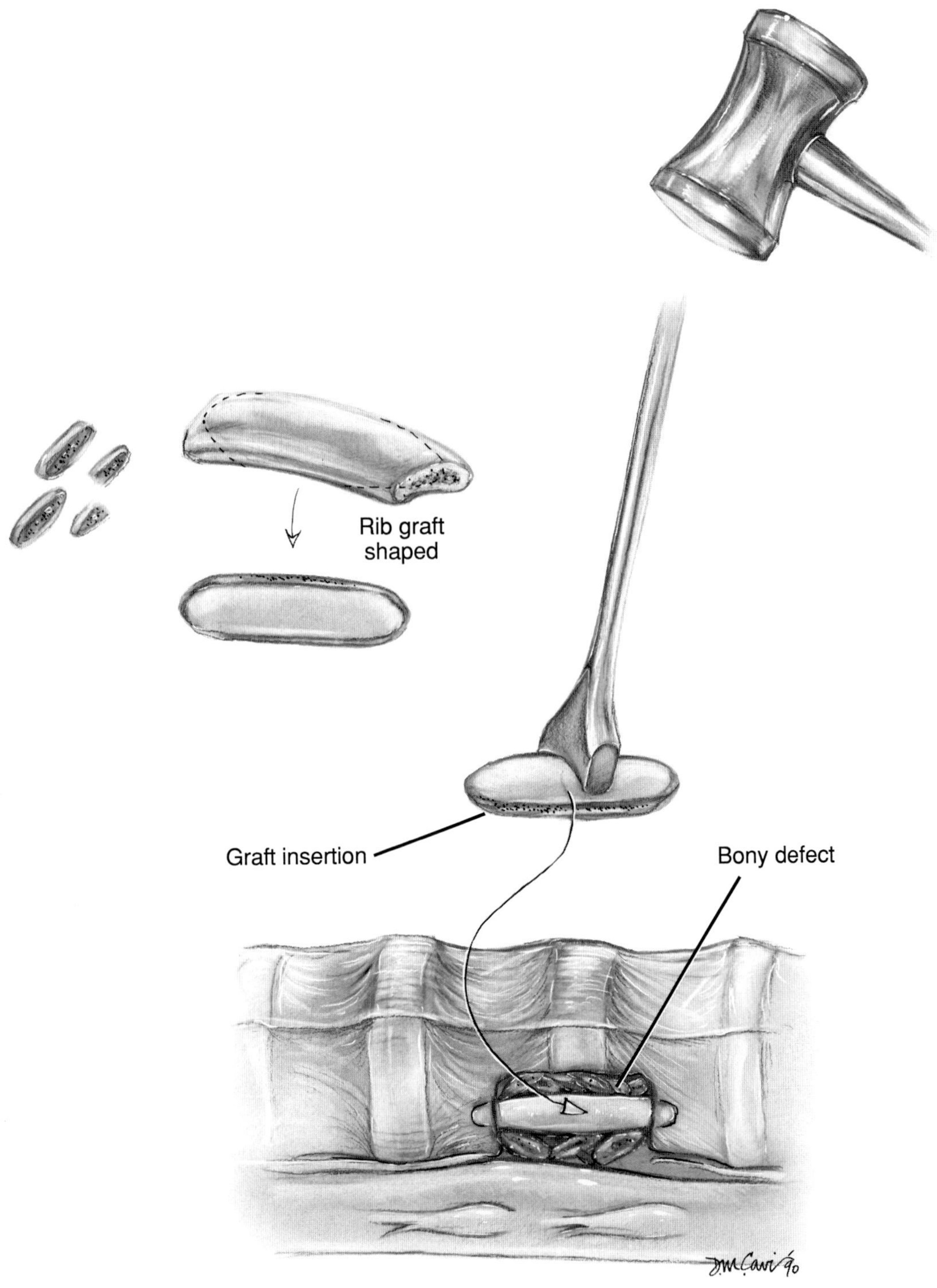

Figure 18.5.

costotransverse approach, however, is superior in the T10 through the T12 area and equally useful in the entire midthoracic region to the transthoracic approach.

The operation is carried out with the patient under general anesthesia and positioned semiprone, with one side of the chest elevated on a roll so that the side on which the incision is to be made is up about 15°. The incision is curvilinear. It should begin approximately at the midline and end at the midline. The apex of the curve should be centered on the rib to be resected. That depends on the location. Remember that the rib below the interspace leads to the involved area most reliably. The T8 rib will lead to the T7-T8 interspace. The apex of the curve should be about 10 cm from the midline. The incision is made down through muscle to the rib throughout its length. However, the paravertebral muscles should not be cut. It will be possible to work beneath them by elevating a thick flap. The dissection is carried from the most lateral portions of the incision on the surface of the rib toward the midline as far as possible. The ribs are followed to their articulation with the spinal column. This large flap is then retracted out of the way, and the whole rib is exposed. The next step is to isolate the rib in an extraplural fashion (Fig. 18.6). Standard instruments are used, and the rib is isolated as far medially as possible. A rib cutter is used to divide the rib near the lateralmost portion of the incision, and then the rib is stripped to its articulation. It may be possible to disarticulate the rib from its head in one piece, or it may be necessary to cut it and then remove the head separately. The pleura and other soft tissues are then mobilized from the vertebral column. The pleura is depressed in the bed of the resected rib, exposing the neural foramina above and below the disc space and the upper quarter of the vertebral body.

The pedicle obscuring access to the disc is then drilled away. It is usually necessary to take all the pedicle associated with the resected rib in order to expose the disc space satisfactorily. The lateral aspect of the annulus is then incised, and all degenerated disc material possible is removed. This gives free access to the disc space. In the event it is difficult to identify the neural foramen, following the neurovascular bundle of the resected rib toward the spinal canal will generally provide a ready identification. The high-speed drill is then utilized to drill away the posterior vertebral rim on either side. It is important to begin the drilling as far to the opposite side as possible. Otherwise, the dural sac will collapse into the drilling site, and retraction on the dura and potentially on the spinal cord will be required. As soon as the central portion of the canal is completely decompressed, be sure to proceed beyond the dural sac to the opposite side before removing the final portion of the disc and the ridges on the ipsilateral side to prevent this from happening. When the disc is entirely soft, it may not be necessary to drill at all. Simply removing the disc should be satisfactory. Most so-called thoracic discs, however, are thick bony ridges with thickened ligaments, and extensive removal with drill and sharp dissection is required for adequate cord decompression. All of this should be under direct vision, and there should be no question of complete cord decompression. Soft tissue and cartilage are then removed from the area of the vertebral body that has been drilled away until cancellous bone is identified. The remnants of the rib head are then packed into the defect, with care taken not to compress the spinal cord.

Closure of the wound is critical. This is a large, potentially painful incision, and anatomical closure is required. The pleura should be intact. If it has been opened, the anesthesiologist should inflate the lung, and the pleural tear is repaired while the lung is inflated. Put the stitches in place, inflate the lung, and tie the stitches. The chest tube is rarely required unless a major tear has occurred. The most critical aspect of the closure is anatomical reapproximation of the latissimus. This is critical to adequate function and a pain-free incision. Once the muscle layer is closed in anatomical fashion, the remainder of the closure requires no special care.

These operations are not commonly done. The surgeon may not be thoroughly familiar with the attachments of the muscles with the chest wall. Unless this is a standard operation for the surgical team, it is wise to study the anatomy of the region, before undertaking the operation, to be certain of the relationship of the rib, pedicles, neural foramina and disc, and the anatomical structures of the chest wall.

Transpedicular Approach

Removal of the thoracic disc via the transpedicular approach is performed with the patient under general anesthesia and prone, with the patient's head fixed in a skeletal fixation system. The table should be angled

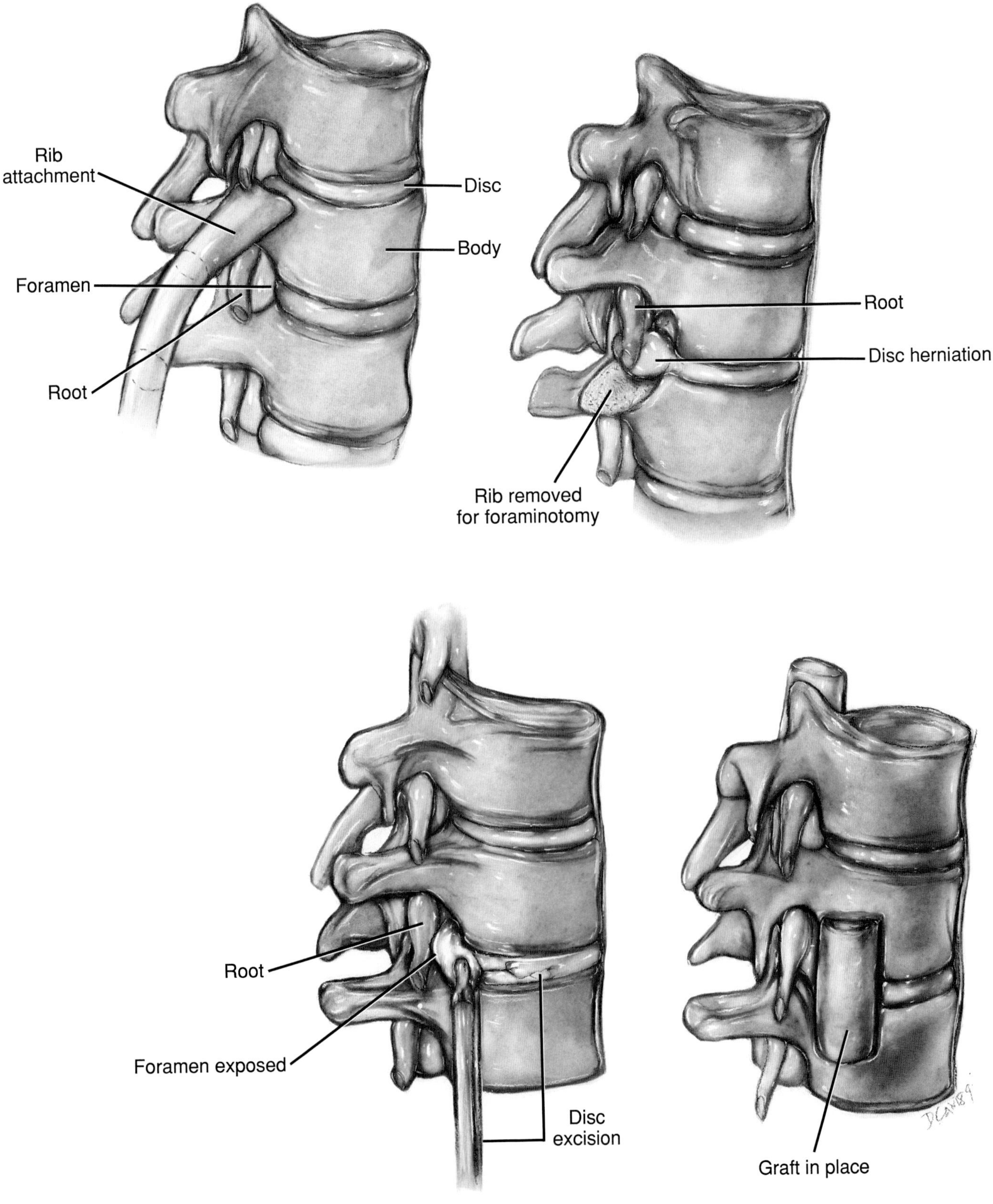
Rib
attachment
Disc
Body
Foramen
Root
Root
Disc herniation
Rib removed
for foraminotomy
Root
Foramen exposed
Disc
excision
Graft in place

Figure 18.6.

up 15°. A paramedian incision is made on the side to be excised. It may be necessary to work from both sides, and in that case, a midline incision is satisfactory. The exposure is performed as for any thoracic laminectomy. However, the incision must be longer, at least two segments beyond the expected area of resection, because of the lateral extension needed. The paravertebral muscles should be lifted off the posterior bony structures until the proximal ribs are exposed, the zygapophyseal joints are seen, and there is free access to the pedicle. It is not necessary to perform a laminectomy. If there is any question about localization, a film should be taken. The high-speed drill is then used to drill away the zygapophyseal joint, and the entire pedicle is removed to the level of the posterior aspect of the vertebral body. This will allow the mass beneath the spinal cord to be approached laterally without spinal cord retraction. Drilling should be continued until the interspace is evident and can be entered with disc rongeurs. As much material as possible should be removed from the interspace. When the problem is a truly herniated disc, this removal will provide adequate decompression of the cord. If there is a significant bony ridge, it will need to be drilled away. The bone and the thickened ligament can be removed slowly by a combination of drill and curettage over to the midline. With an asymmetrical process, a unilateral approach is all that is necessary. With a bilateral process, it may be necessary to repeat the procedure on the opposite side. The key is working from the most lateral aspect of the exposure so that no compression of the cord is allowed and no retraction of the cord is necessary. When the procedure is to be bilateral, it is much easier to perform a laminectomy and then drill away the bone, exposing the nerve roots.

Immaculate hemostasis is required, and hemostatics such as Gelfoam or Avitene will usually suffice. If the bone is bleeding, it can be waxed, but it is better to leave it so that bony fusion can occur. Stability should not be a problem because of the ribs, but posterior fusion can be added if indicated.

The wound is closed in the usual fashion without other special concerns.

SECTION 6

Congenital Anomalies

19

Chiari Malformation

Surgical treatment of a Chiari malformation is usually necessitated by a combination of symptoms that relate to cervicomedullary compression and/or syringomyelia. Typical symptoms include lower cranial nerve dysfunction, severe neck pain and headache, dysmetria and incoordination, spastic quadriparesis, spastic paraparesis with flaccidity of upper extremities, dissociated sensory loss involving the cervical dermatomes, and atrophy of shoulder girdle and upper extremity musculature, particularly the intrinsic muscles of the hands.

The diagnosis is now made with certainty by computed tomography (CT) scanning utilizing intrathecal contrast or by magnetic resonance imaging (MRI). The distorted cervicomedullary junction, tonsillar herniation, and compression can be appreciated with either study. The MRI is superior in demonstrating the syringomyelia.

The goal of surgery is decompression of the cervicomedullary junction and drainage of the syrinx, if present.

Surgical Procedure

The operation is carried out with the patient under general anesthesia and in either a sitting or a prone position. The sitting position provides easier access to the cervicomedullary junction for the surgeon and has the advantage of directing the instruments away from the cervical cord area. The major disadvantage is the risk of air embolism. The prone position avoids this risk but allows blood to pool in the depths of the incision, and the instruments are directed vertically

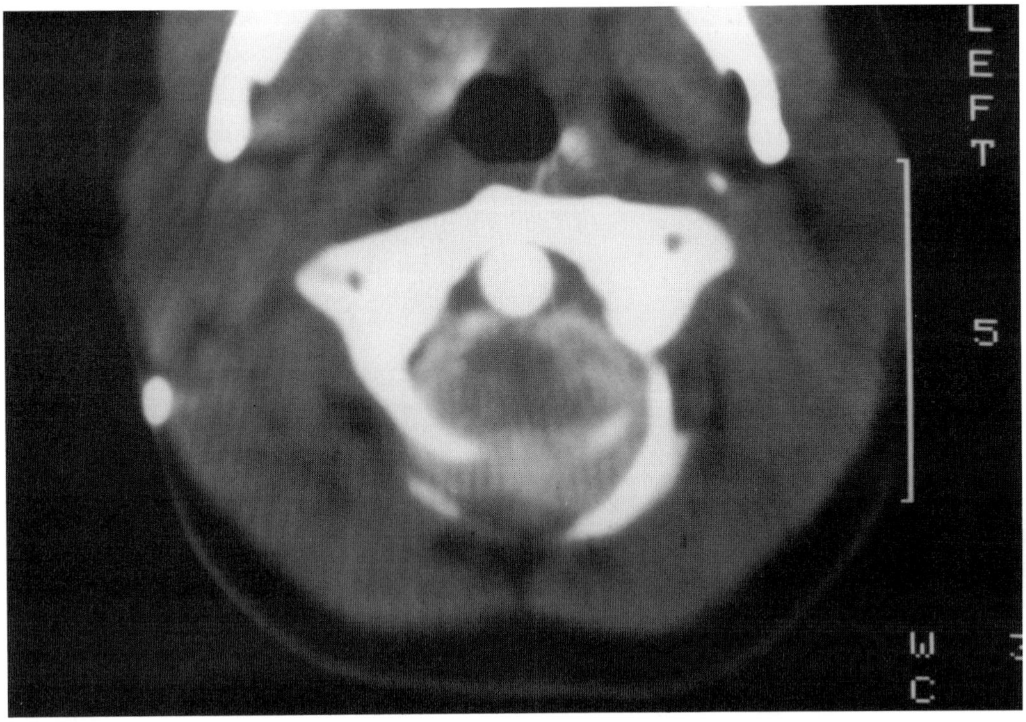

Figure 19.1. CT myelogram of Chiari malformation demonstrating tonsillar herniation into upper cervical canal with cervical cord compression.

toward the compressed neural tissue during removal of the arch of C1 and the rim of the foramen magnum.

The patient may be monitored during the procedure by utilizing evoked potential techniques. This is particularly important in achondroplastic children in whom the cord compression may be extreme.

Many prefer to carry out the procedure with adults in the sitting position and with children in the prone position. If the adult is hydrocephalic, which is rare, then the prone position is used.

The incision is made from the inion to approximately the spine of C3 in the midline. Skin hemostasis is obtained by the use of compression clips. When the approach is truly midline, there is very little bleeding until the spinous processes are reached. The muscle masses should be left intact, and crossing veins identified and coagulated before they are cut. The incision is carried to the occipital bone in the midline, down to the rim of the foramen magnum, onto the arch of C1 and to the spine of C2. Self-retaining cerebellar retractors are put in place, exposing the bone. A subperiosteal dissection of the muscles from the occipital bone is then carried out, exposing the entire rim of the foramen magnum from side to side. It is important to remember at this juncture that a dural graft will be necessary so that periosteum or cervical fascia is preserved. The periosteum should be reflected with the muscle so that its subsequent dissection as a watertight sheet is possible. The upper retractor is replaced, exposing the occipital bone. The arch of C1 has been exposed by the midline incision. The tissue adherent to the arch is grasped with fine forceps, and with a #15 knife, a subperiosteal dissection of these tissues from the arch of C1 is carried out. Once this is started, a small periosteal elevator can be employed for a blunt dissection, although it is just as easy to use the knife for sharp dissection. The lateral extent of the incision is signaled by the sudden appearance of loose areolar tissue and the vertebral venous plexus. Because an aberrant vertebral artery is a possibility, it is always wise to palpate occasionally during the dissection to be certain the vertebral artery is in its normal location. These newly created spaces are packed with gauze, and attention is turned to C2. The insertion of the cervical musculature is cut from the spinous process of C2. This should be done beginning as close

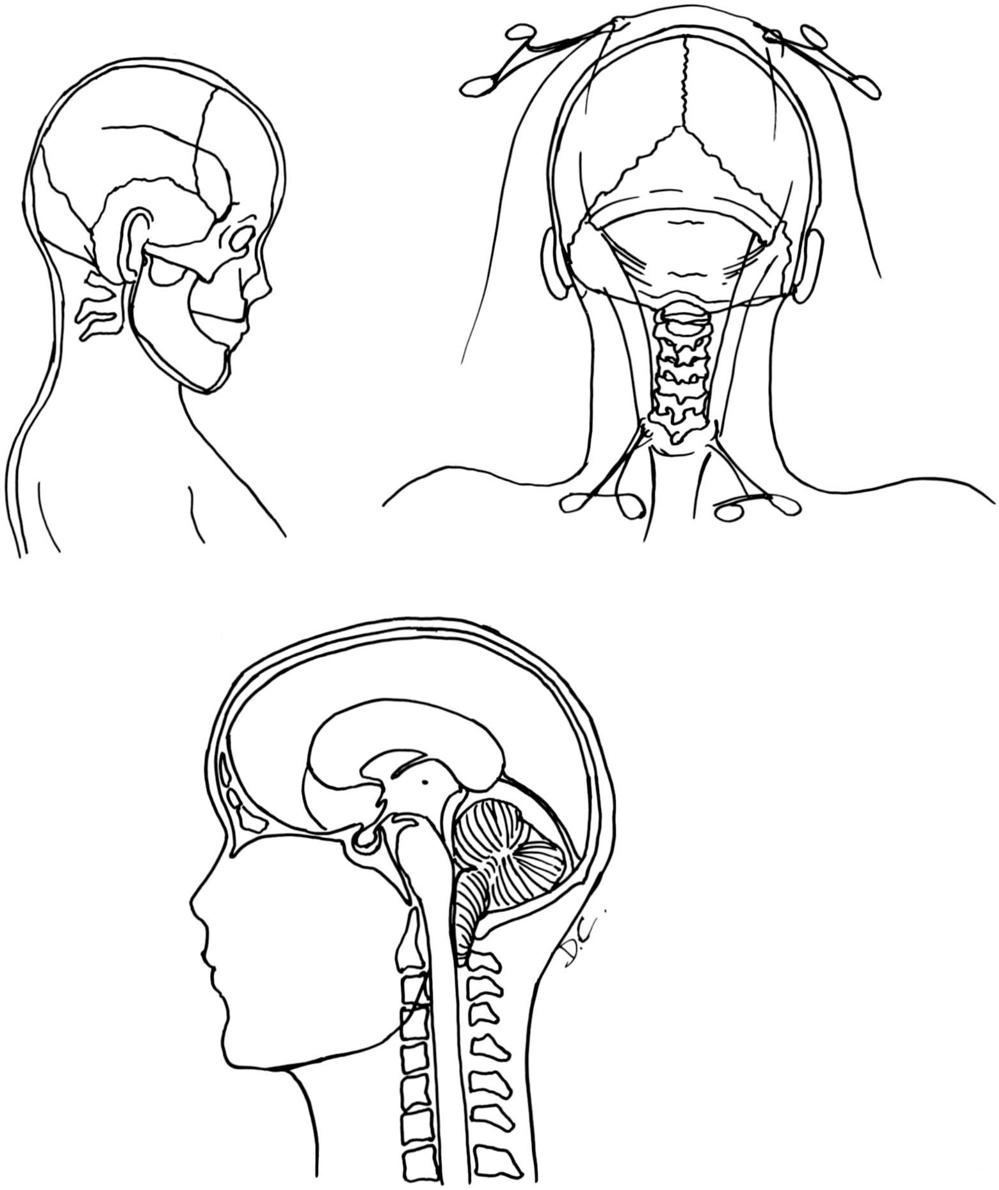

Figure 19.2. Sitting position for surgery on patient with Chiari malformation.

to the midline as possible; the fibers are divided in their tendinous attachment so that a subperiosteal dissection is possible. Small osteotomes are then utilized to scrape the muscle mass away. It is never possible to do this in a truly subperiosteal fashion, as can be done in lower spinal areas. Venous bleeding may occur but will usually stop with rapid packing. The lateral dissection should expose the zygapophyseal joints. The cerebellar retractors are then replaced, so that one exposes the occipital bone and the other lies in the juncture between C1 and C2, retracting the cervical musculature. In the event it is necessary to expose either the tonsils or the syrinx below the C2 level, the subperiosteal dissection of cervical musculature is extended down to the required level. With the imaging studies now available, the extent of

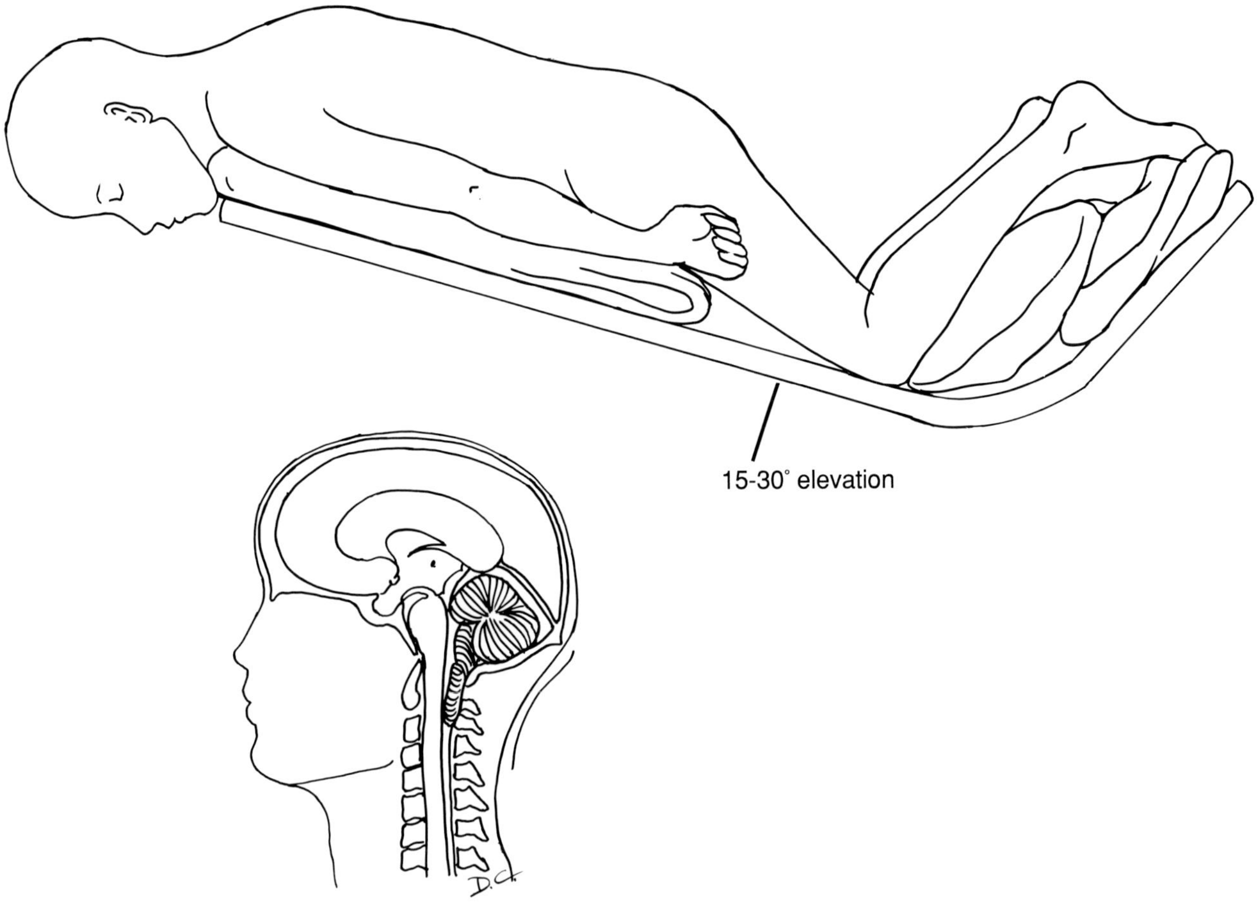

Figure 19.3. Prone position for surgery on patient with Chiari malformation.

the abnormality can be accurately assessed for surgery, and the required exposure gauged with certainty.

The bony removal begins in the posterior fossa. Burr holes are made on either side of the midline in the squamous portion of the bone, and rongeurs are utilized to connect the burr holes and remove the remainder of the posterior fossa bone, including the rim of the foramen magnum. It is extremely important that the rongeurs not be placed beneath the bone, except over the cerebellar hemispheres. There is little room, and significant neural compression can occur if the surgeon attempts to put the jaws of any of the biting instruments between bone and dura at the foramen magnum. The rongeurs are held vertically to the bone and reach the dura, but they do not extend under the rim. A high-speed drill can be used to remove bone. This requires a practiced hand. Unless it obscures the rim, the arch of C1 is left intact so that the upper cervical cord is protected while the heavier instruments or the drill are being used. Once the rim of the foramen magnum has been removed, the arch of C1 is rongeured away. It is important to free surrounding tissue from the bone so that the rongeur does not tear the fibrous connections of surrounding tissues to the arch. This can easily be done with the Adson periosteal elevator. The rongeurs are placed in a vertical fashion as was done with the rim of the foramen magnum, and the instruments are never inserted between bone and dura. The removal of C2 is less critical, and standard laminectomy techniques can be utilized. The extent of the bony removal is judged by the actual anatomical abnormality. The edges of the bone are waxed, and immaculate hemostasis is

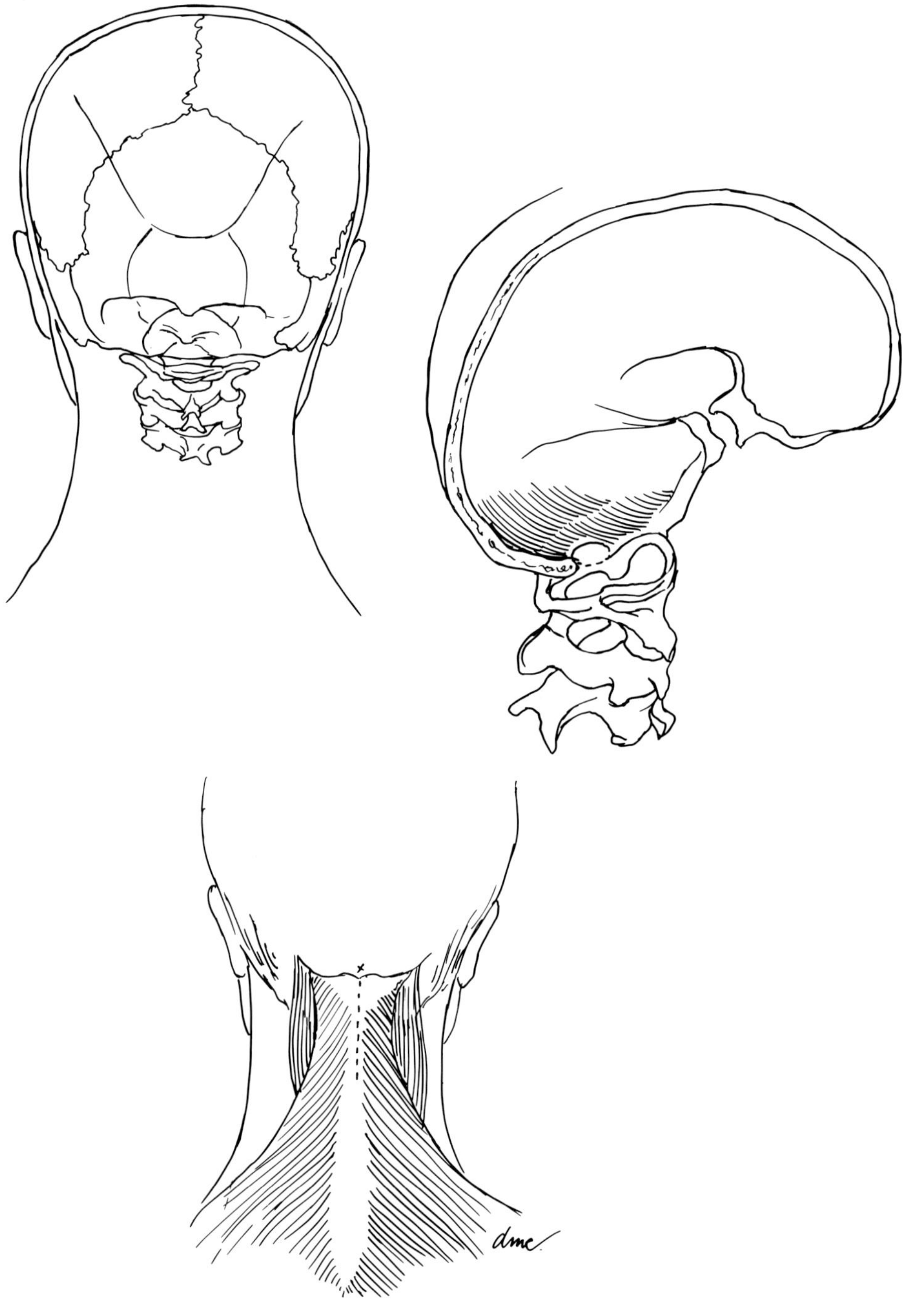

Figure 19.4. Midline incision.

obtained. The dura is then opened in the midline beginning at C2 and proceeding upward. Usually, it is possible to open the dura without opening the arachnoid. The operating microscope is brought into the field at this juncture in order to facilitate the removal without violation of the arachnoid. It is mandatory to open the dura. Usually, there is a tight constrictive fibrous band between the rim of the for-

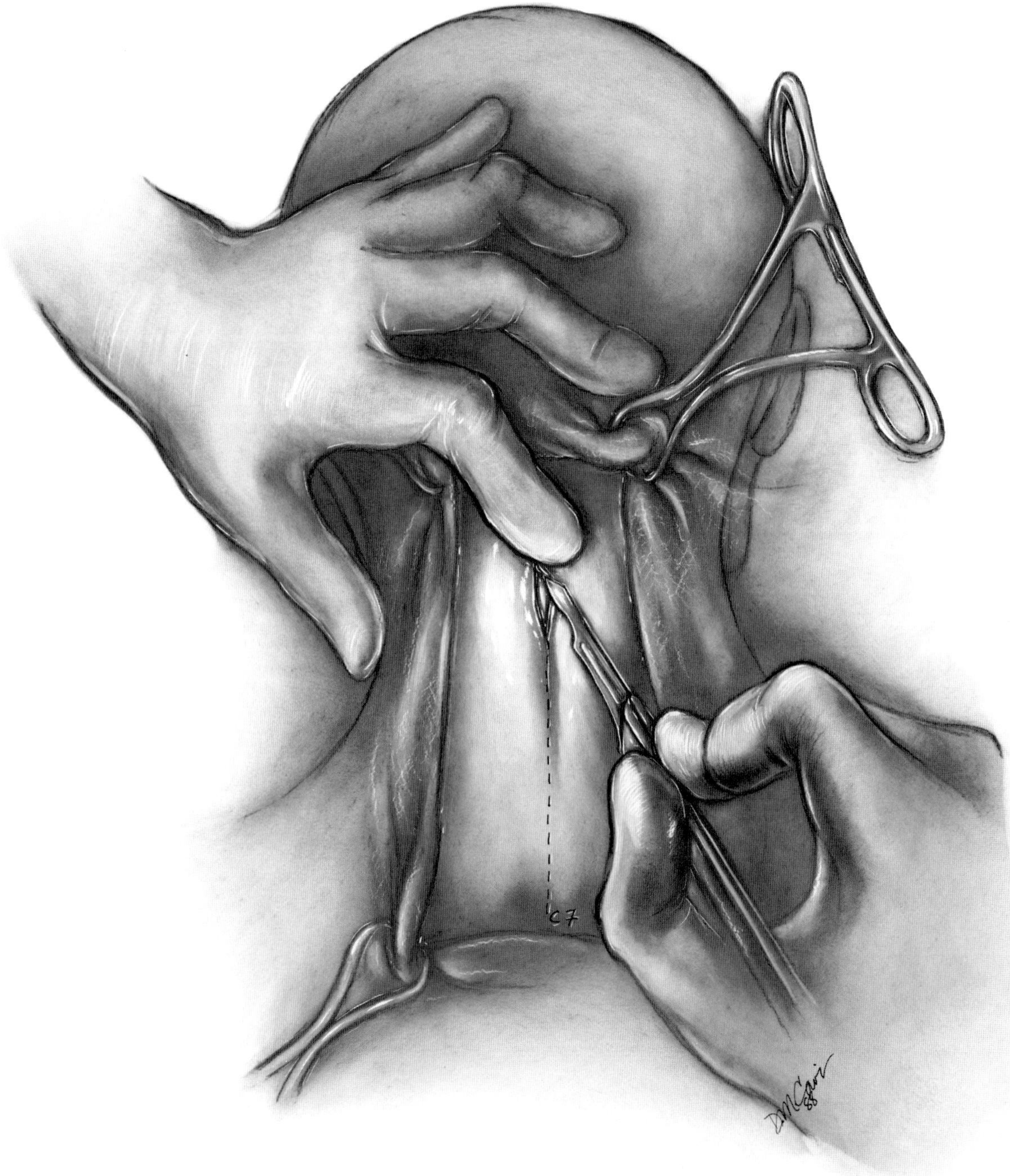

Figure 19.5. Midline cervical incision, with spinous processes exposed.

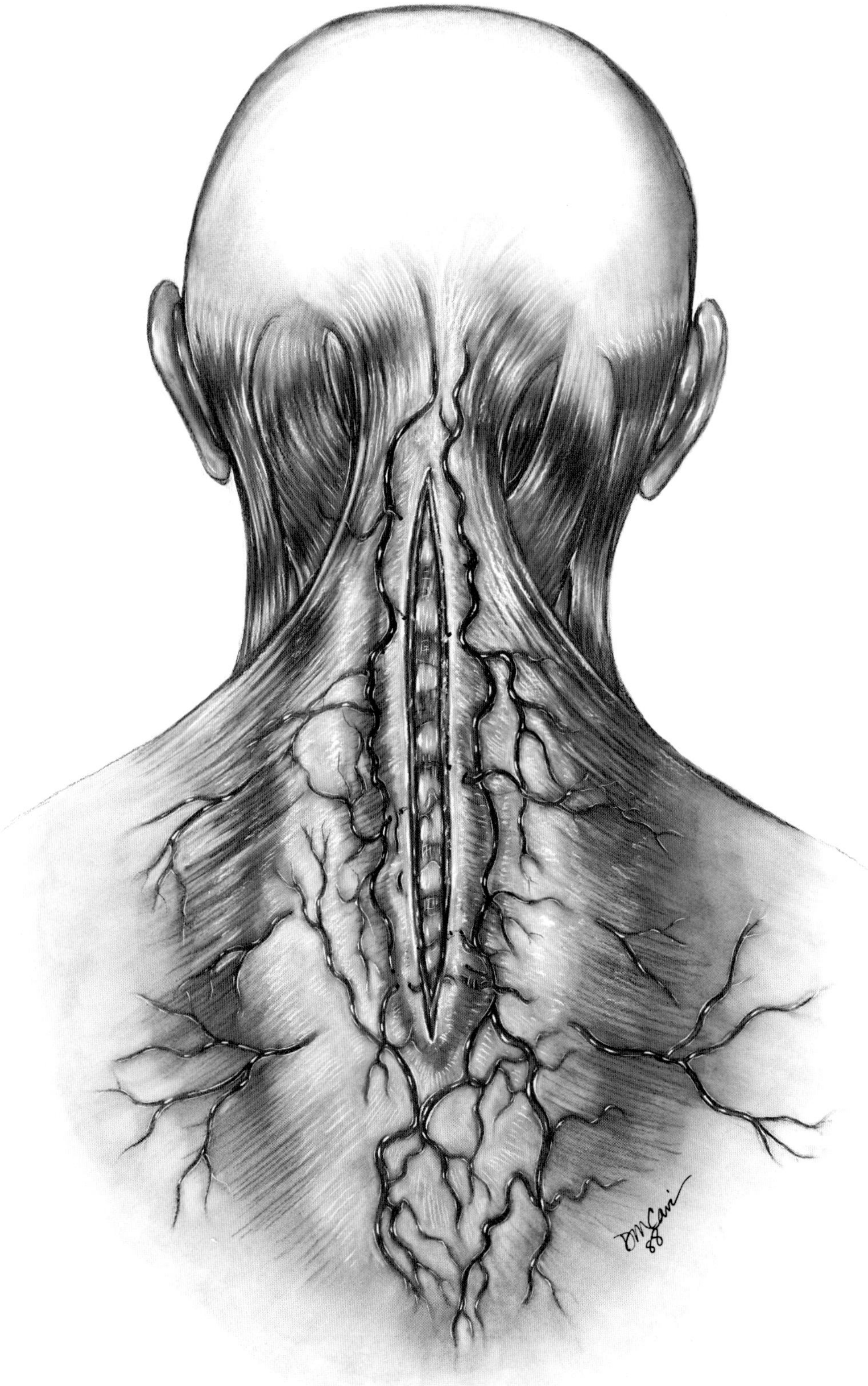

Figure 19.6. Midline cervical incision with occipital extension.

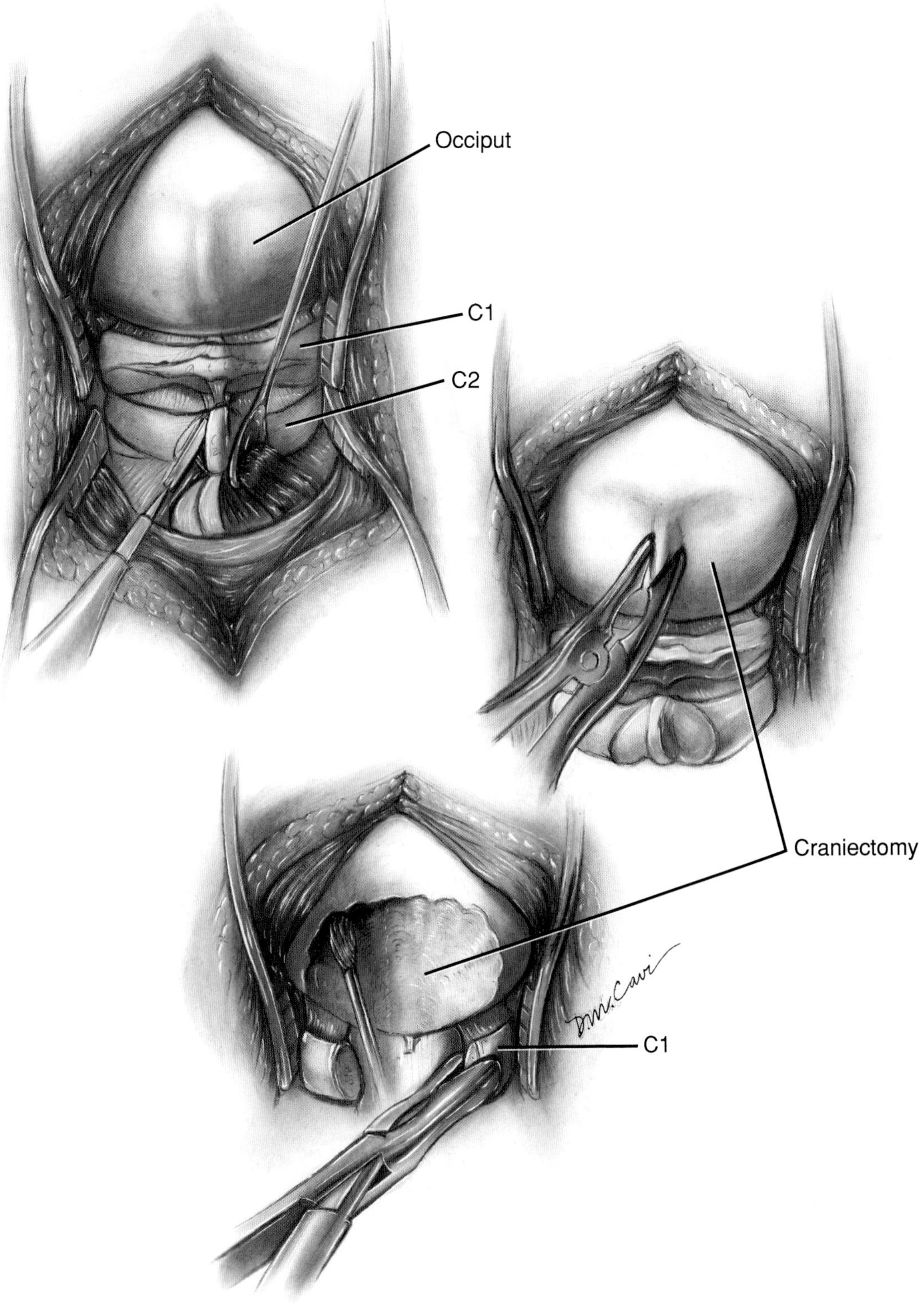

Figure 19.7.

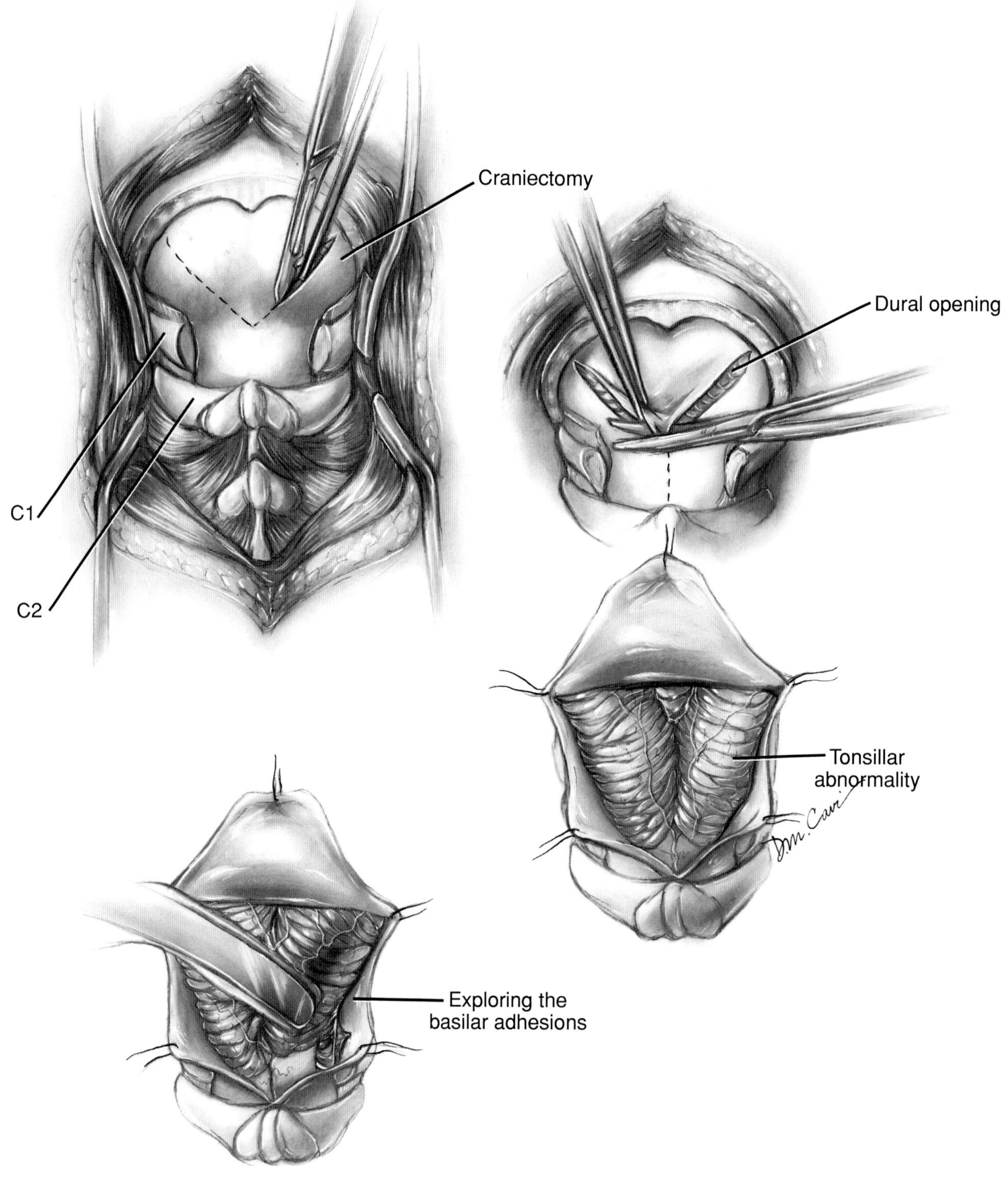
Craniectomy
C1
C2
Dural opening
Tonsillar abnormality
Exploring the basilar adhesions

Figure 19.8.

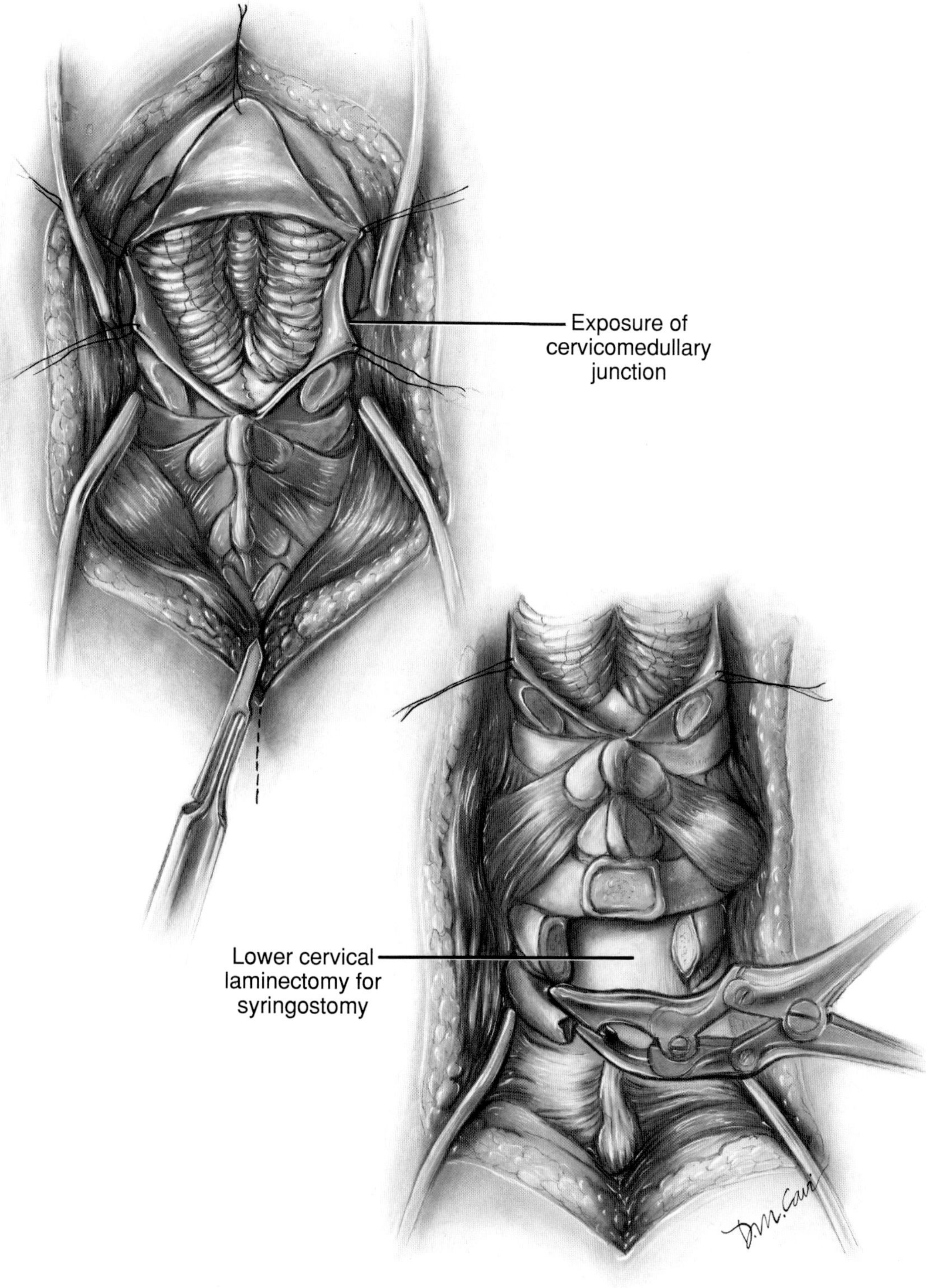
Exposure of
cervicomedullary
junction
Lower cervical
laminectomy for
syringostomy

Figure 19.9.

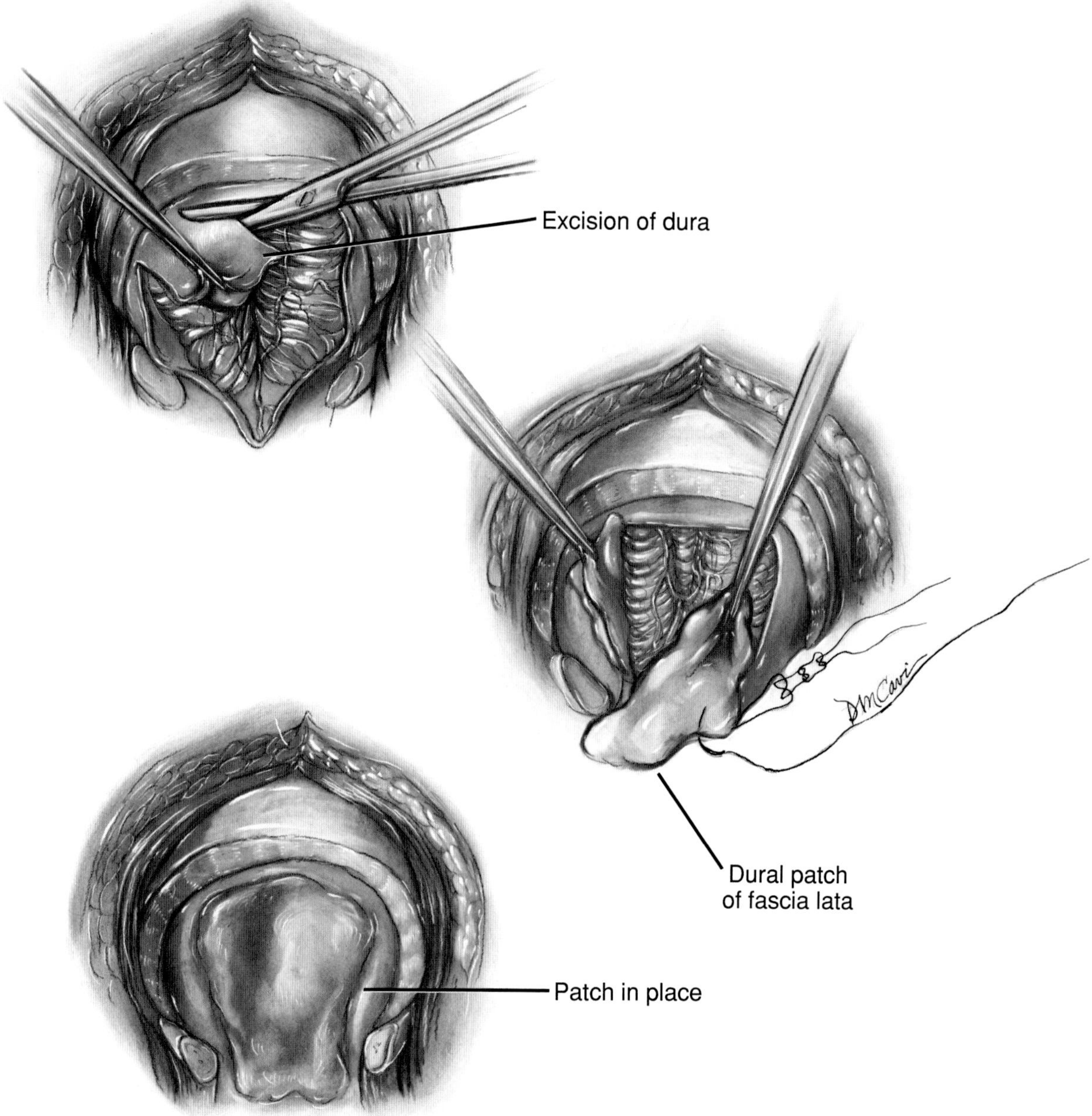

Figure 19.10.

amen magnum and C1, and unless this band of thickened dura is divided, decompression is incomplete. The dura is sutured back to the cervical musculature, creating a large diamond or rectangle and giving complete decompression. If no syrinx is present, this decompression is adequate, and nothing further needs to be done. There is no evidence that lysis of adhesions between tonsils and brain stem or opening the fourth ventricle will be of value unless obstruction of compression is present. When a syrinx is present, it is important to open the arachnoid and explore the obex. This may be difficult because there frequently are adhesions between tonsils, vermis, and brain stem. It may be necessary to remove a small amount of

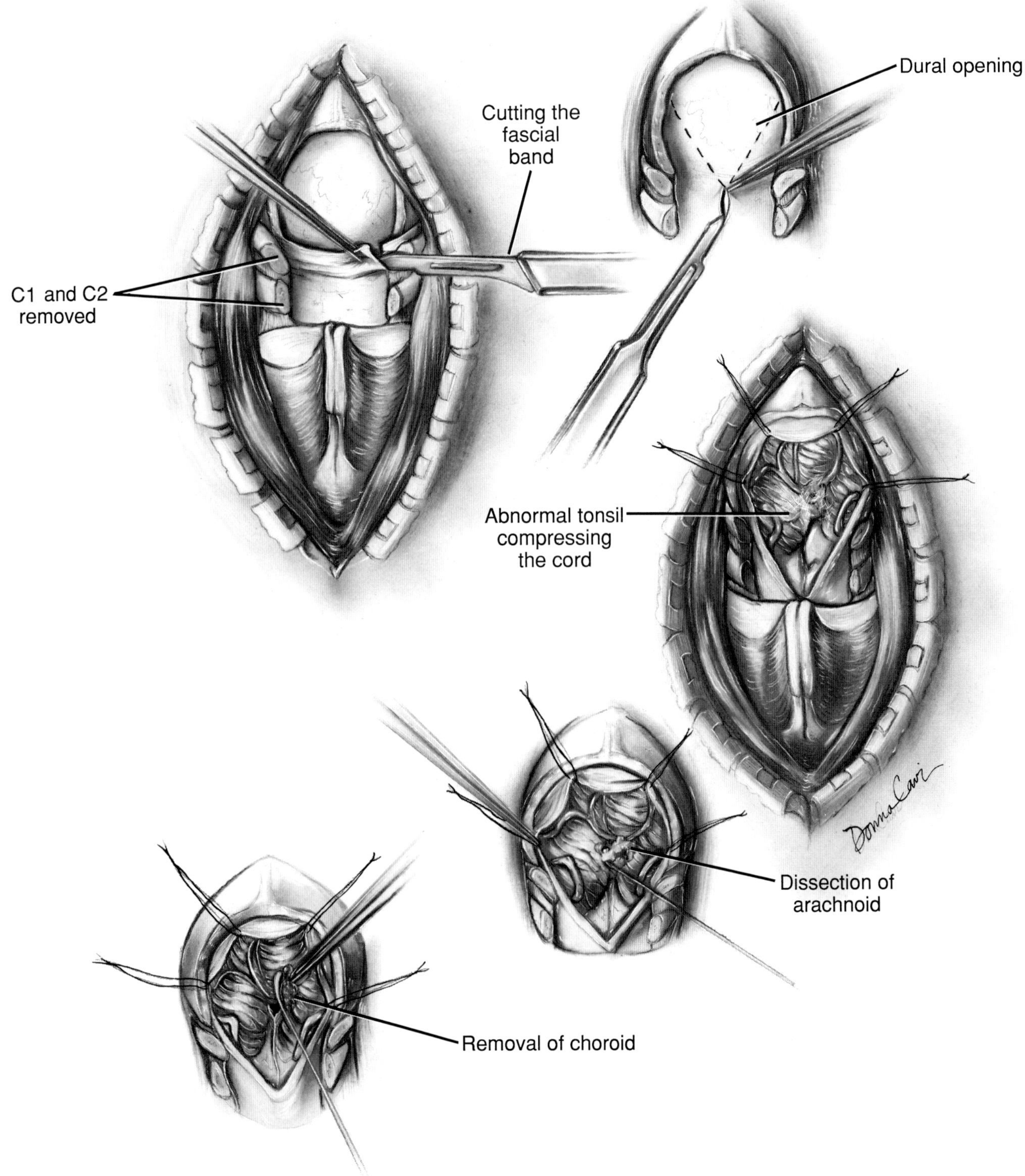
Dural opening
Cutting the fascial band
C1 and C2 removed
Abnormal tonsil compressing the cord
Dissection of arachnoid
Removal of choroid

Figure 19.11.

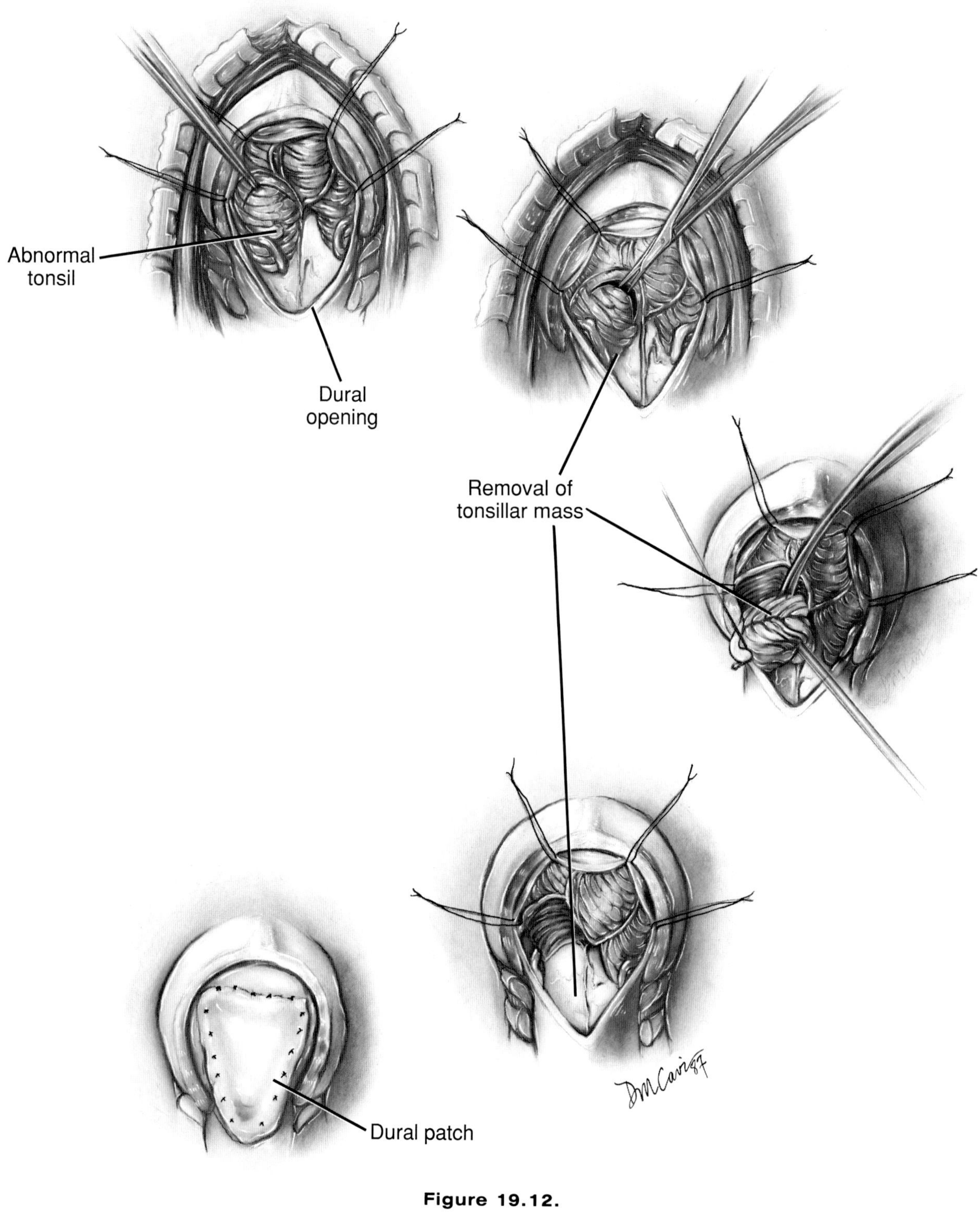

Abnormal tonsil
Dural opening
Removal of tonsillar mass
Dural patch
DMCair 87

Figure 19.12.

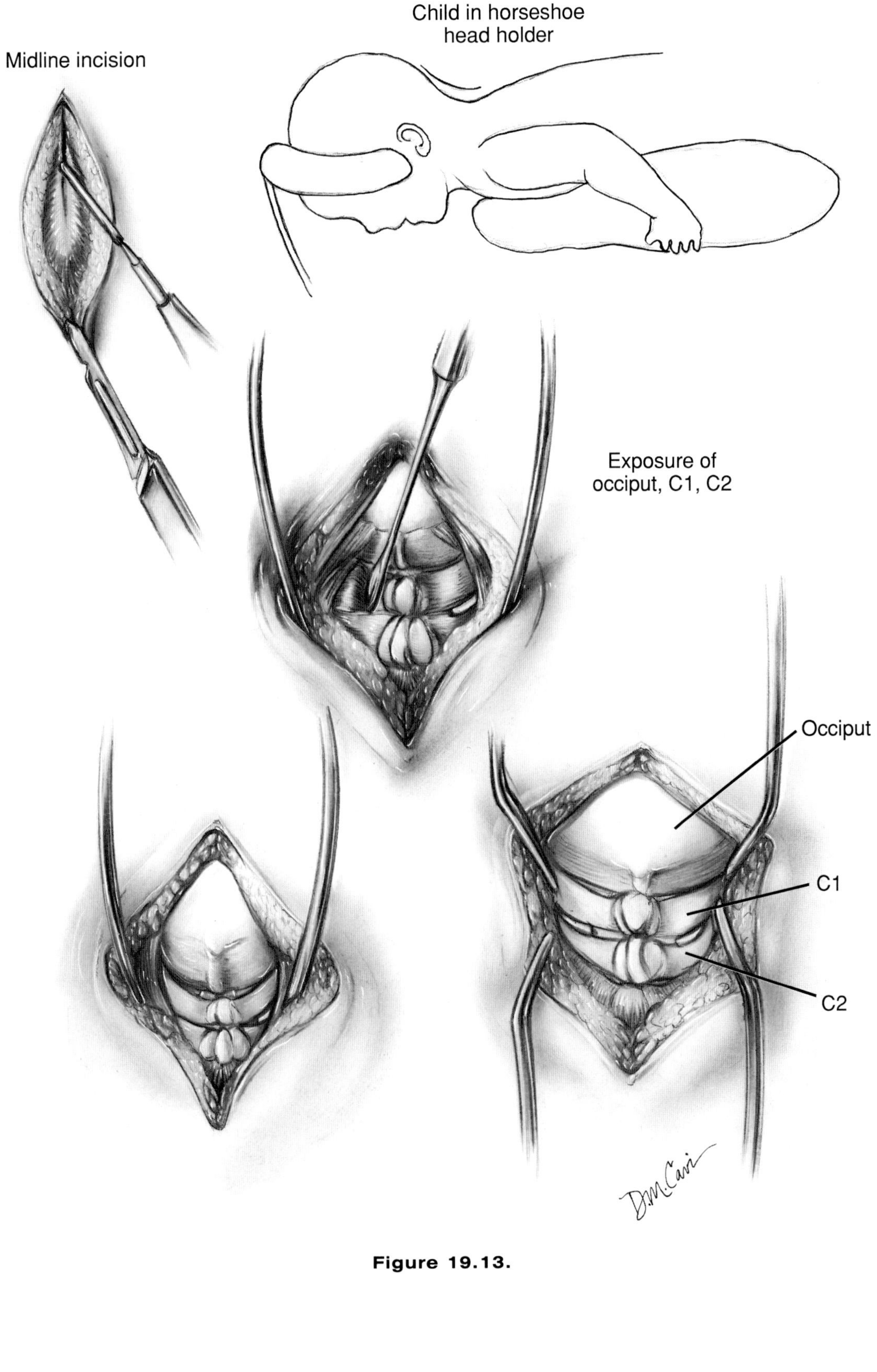

Child in horseshoe head holder
Midline incision
Exposure of occiput, C1, C2
Occiput
C1
C2
D.M.Cain

Figure 19.13.

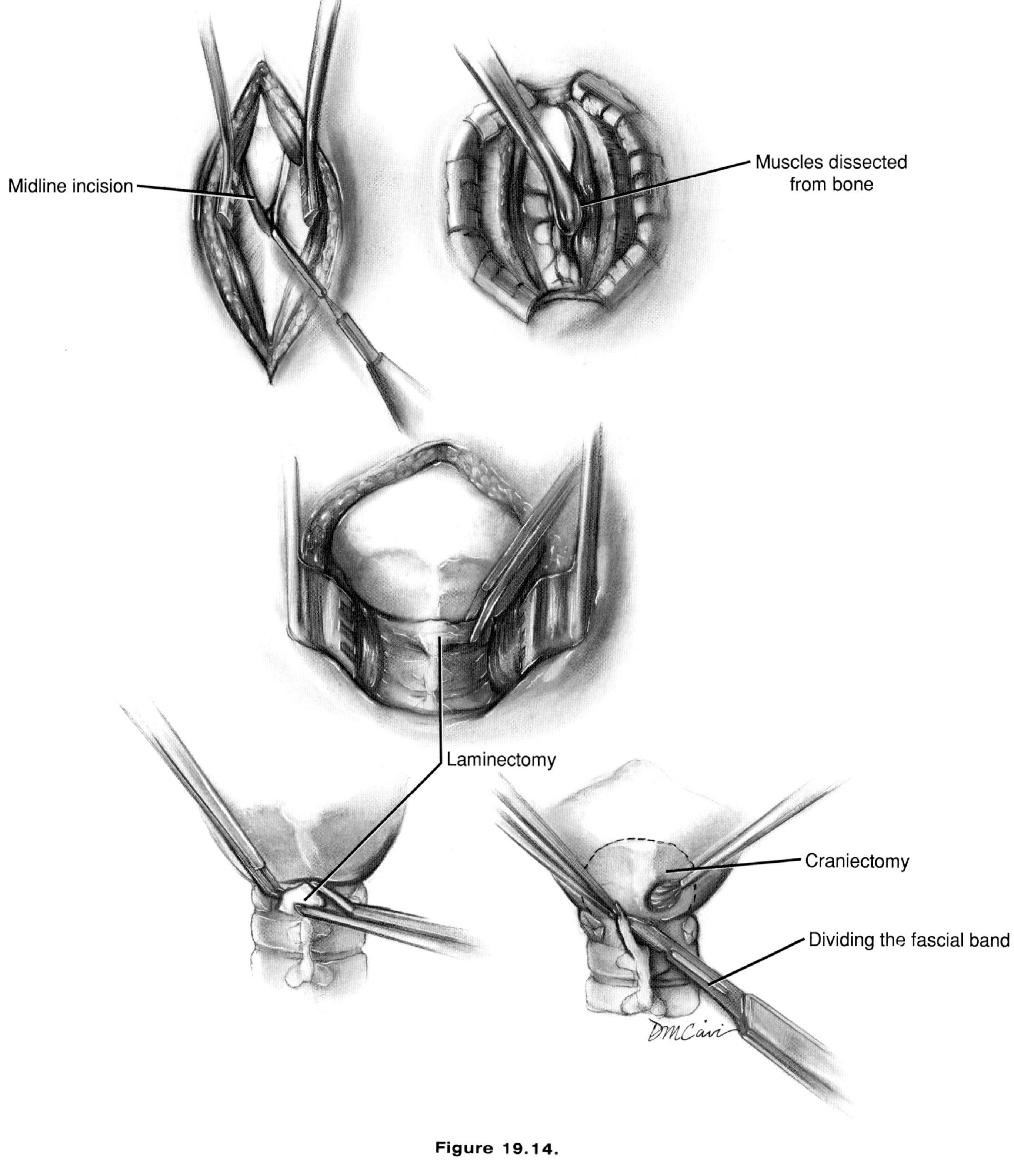

Midline incision
Muscles dissected from bone
Laminectomy
Craniectomy
Dividing the fascial band

Figure 19.14.

vermis or tonsil in order to find the fourth ventricle or to decompress the cervicomedullary junction. Occasionally, an open connection between the syrinx and the fourth ventricle will be found at the obex. When such a connection is present, it should be plugged with a small pledget of muscle. Such connections are rare, but when they are found, this is such effective therapy that it is always worthwhile to look for the opening. More commonly, there is no apparent connection, and in this situation there is no reason to attempt to manipulate an already-distorted brain stem and obex.

If a noncommunicating syrinx is present, there are two satisfactory forms of therapy. One is to extend the incision and carry out a laminectomy at the lowest extent of the syrinx. The other is to treat the syrinx by subarachnoid shunting at the level already exposed. The latter has the risk that a cord catastrophe

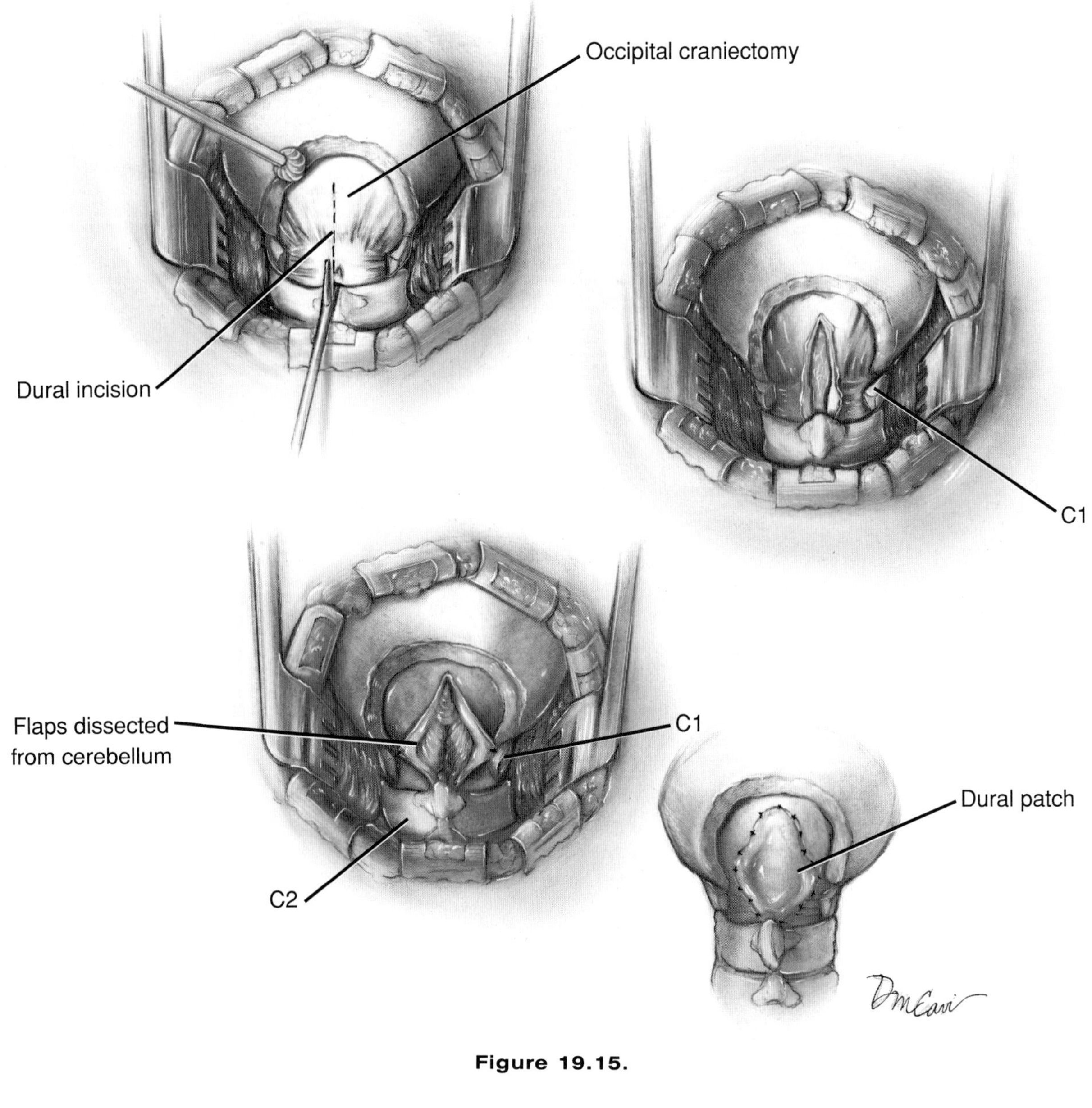

Figure 19.15.

is above the C3-C4 level, but it has the advantage of requiring no further exposure. In the usual situation, there will be a thinned area of the cord laterally near the dentate ligaments, which can be opened safely at the C1 or C2 level. A very small lateral incision is made through this thinned area with use of the microscope. Ventricular shunt catheters are then inserted into the syrinx. This can also be done through the posterior midline or any sufficiently thinned area. One is placed down as far into the cyst as it will freely pass and into the subarachnoid space in the cisterna magna. It is important that the catheter be in the subarachnoid space, not subdural. A second one is usually passed up in the syrinx and directed downward into the subarachnoid space. Both are sutured to a dentate ligament of the dura laterally. The same technique is used if the syrinx is exposed at its lower extent.

Closure is important. If the arachnoid has been left intact and no exploration or syringostomy has been done, then it is not necessary to do more than place a pledget of Gelfoam over the defect and close the muscle in layers. If the arachnoid has been opened, a watertight dural closure is needed. A patch must be used. Pericranium or cervical fascia are quite adequate, and a dural substitute of the surgeon's choice will be satisfactory. The muscle layers do not require extensive closure. Usually, it is satisfactory to bring the ligamentum nuchae together in the midline with a single layer of heavy stitches. The subcutaneous tissue is closed separately. It is necessary to obtain a tight closure of the muscles so that no cerebrospinal fluid leak can develop. The skin closure is at the discretion of the surgeon. These patients require no special postoperative care.

20

Syringomyelia

The goal of surgery in syringomyelia is to provide permanent decompression of the cyst with equilibration of the pressure within the cyst and the normal cerebrospinal fluid pressure. Three kinds of cyst will be encountered. Various cystic lesions accompany intramedullary glioma. Cysts will sometimes occur as late complications after trauma, and there is an idiopathic variety that may or may not be associated with Chiari malformation. The treatment of the cord tumor associated with the syrinx is described separately in Chapter 28. Traumatic syrinx and the cyst not associated with a posterior fossa abnormality are treated in the same way, while the cervical cyst associated with the Chiari malformation requires a more extensive surgical correction. The first diagnostic goals are to determine the presence or absence of tumor, the presence or absence of a posterior fossa malformation, and the extent of the syrinx. In the past, it was often necessary to carry out an extensive removal of bone to expose the entire length of the syrinx for exploration. With current imaging techniques, the presence of tumor is detected without this extensive surgery, and it may be possible to perform a limited laminectomy and drainage procedure. In such a case the laminectomy is carried out in the most dependent portion of the syrinx, if possible. In some portions of the cord, this will be more dangerous, and then the exploration and drainage should be performed at the widest area of cord dilatation. Several factors govern this decision-making process. In general, the surgeon should expose the cord below the C4 level to protect respiration. It is better not to enter the cervical enlargement or the lumbosacral enlargement, if possible. The upper thoracic cord is more dangerous to manipulate than lower down, and it is much more difficult to enter a syrinx where the cord is relatively normal in size than to enter a syrinx where the cord is greatly dilated.

Syringomyelia without Chiari Malformation

The operation for syringomyelia without Chiari malformation is carried out with the patient under general anesthesia in the prone position. A laminectomy is planned that will expose the cord over several segments where it is to be opened. It is preferable to have at least three segments available for exploration, since the thinnest area of the cord is difficult to localize by imaging and the cord surface may have blood vessels that make it difficult to incise if the surgeon's choice is limited. If an exploration for tumor is planned, then the laminectomy should extend at least one level above and below the extremities of the cyst. The laminectomy should be wide without entering the zygapophyseal joints. The weak paraspinous muscles that accompany this problem make subluxation likely if the stability of the spine is disrupted. The dura is opened in the midline with the aid of the microscope, and the arachnoid is preserved intact. If the syrinx is likely to be difficult to find, transdural sonography can be very useful. The dura should be sewn back to the paravertebral muscles for later watertight closure. The cord is then inspected throughout its exposed area with the arachnoid intact. The midline is explored to determine if the best access to the cyst is between the posterior columns and to look at the area of attachment of the dentate ligaments on each side. Often, the thinnest area of the cord occurs here between the dentate ligament and the corticospinal tract. Frequently, this is the best place to make the draining incision. An appropriately avascular thin area of the cord should be identified. Where the cord is extremely thin laterally is an advantageous place to put drainage tubes. If the cord is not thin laterally but is uniformly dilated, a myelotomy is best carried down the midline posteriorly.

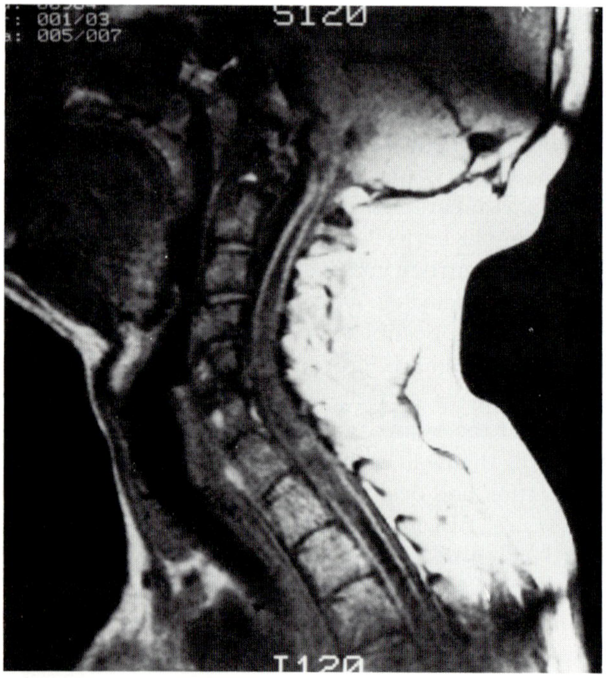

Figure 20.1. Magnetic resonance image demonstrating typical syrinx of cervical cord.

The cord is retracted medially, and an appropriately thinned area posterior to the dentate ligament is identified. This should be incised with microscissors or a sharp knife over a distance of at least 4 or 5 mm. The cord will immediately deflate and clear fluid should be obtained. If the fluid is not clear, a tumor is likely, and the operation must be changed to account for that possibility. When the fluid is clear, only drainage is necessary. Two drainage tubes should be inserted, if possible. Silastic ventricular catheters are satisfactory. They are sutured to the dentate ligament laterally with a small nonabsorbable suture, or they may be sutured to the dura on either side of the proposed midline closure if inserted between the posterior columns. The drainage end should be subarachnoidal, not subdural. Because of this the arachnoid need not be opened widely over the length of the syrinx. The tubes should be firmly attached to the dura so that they do not dislodge into the cyst at a later time and so occlude the opening. Shunts to pleura and peritoneum also are feasible.

The alternative to small myelotomy and tube drainage is a wide myelotomy over a long distance. These myelotomies are commonly carried out in the midline, and a segment of at least several centimeters is opened. Increasing the length of the myelotomy carries with it an increased risk of injury to the posterior columns but does reduce the chance that the drainage site will close. Some investigators have recommended marsupialization by suturing the cut pial margins of the posterior columns back to dura lat-

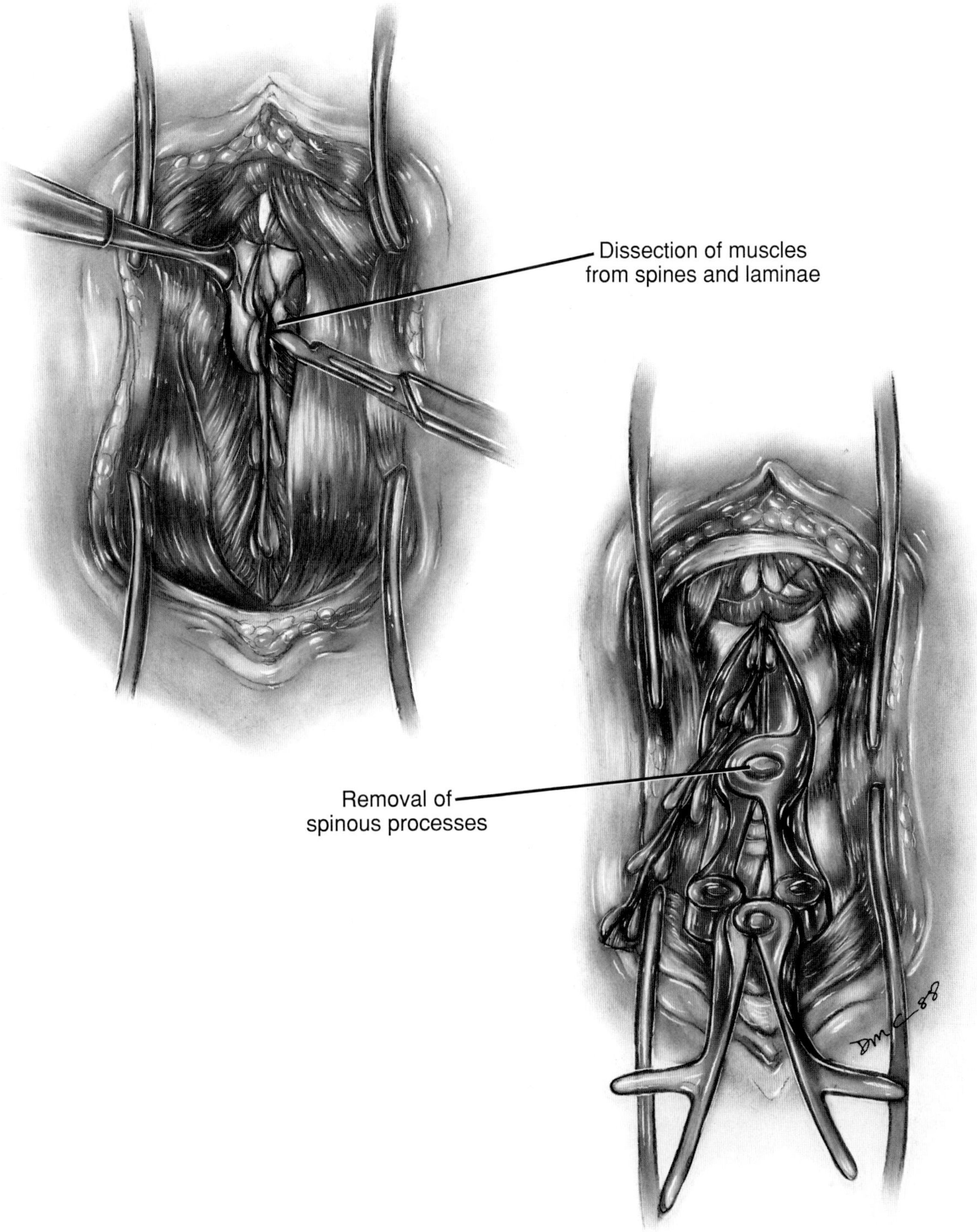
Dissection of muscles from spines and laminae
Removal of spinous processes

Figure 20.2.

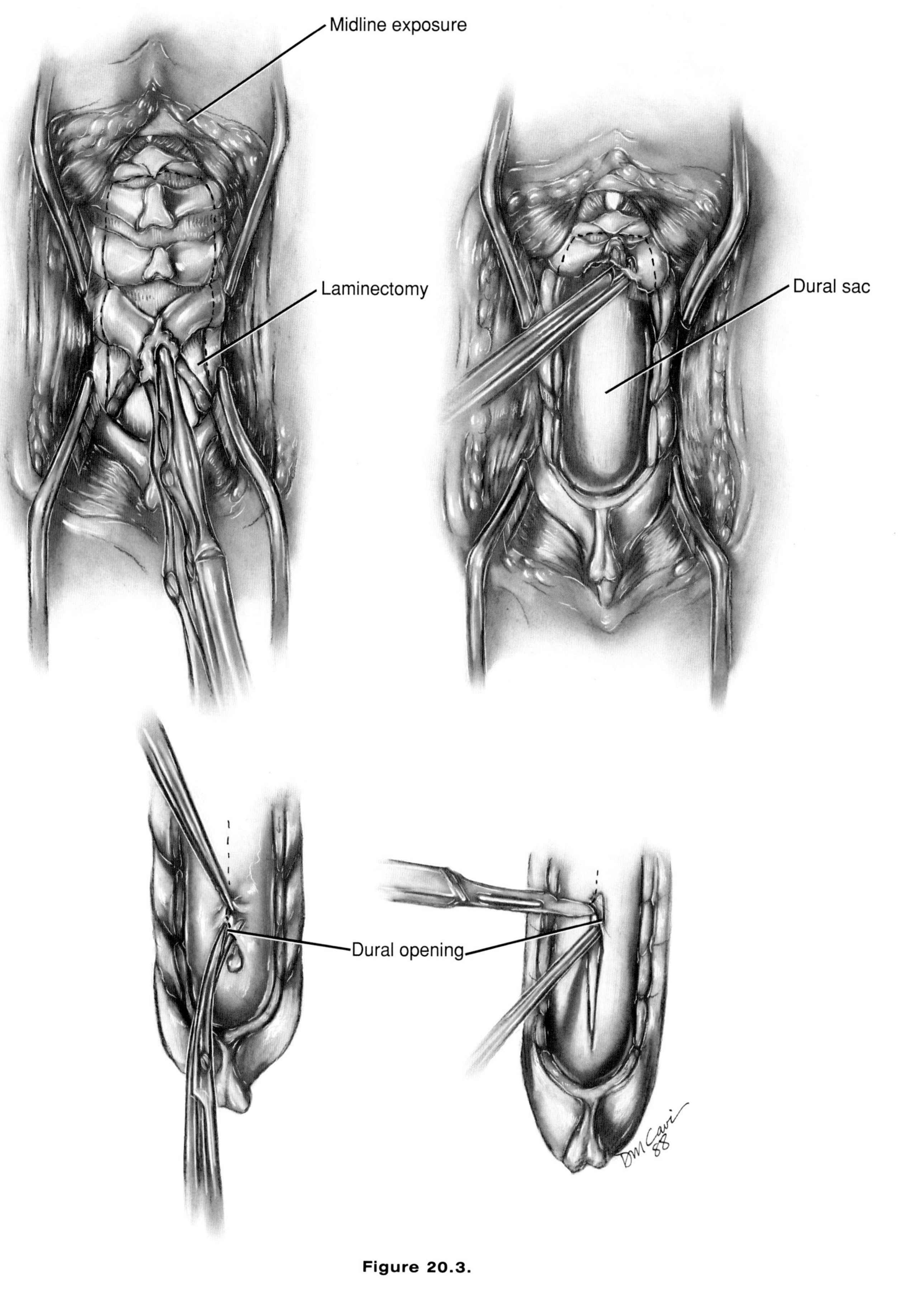

Figure 20.3.

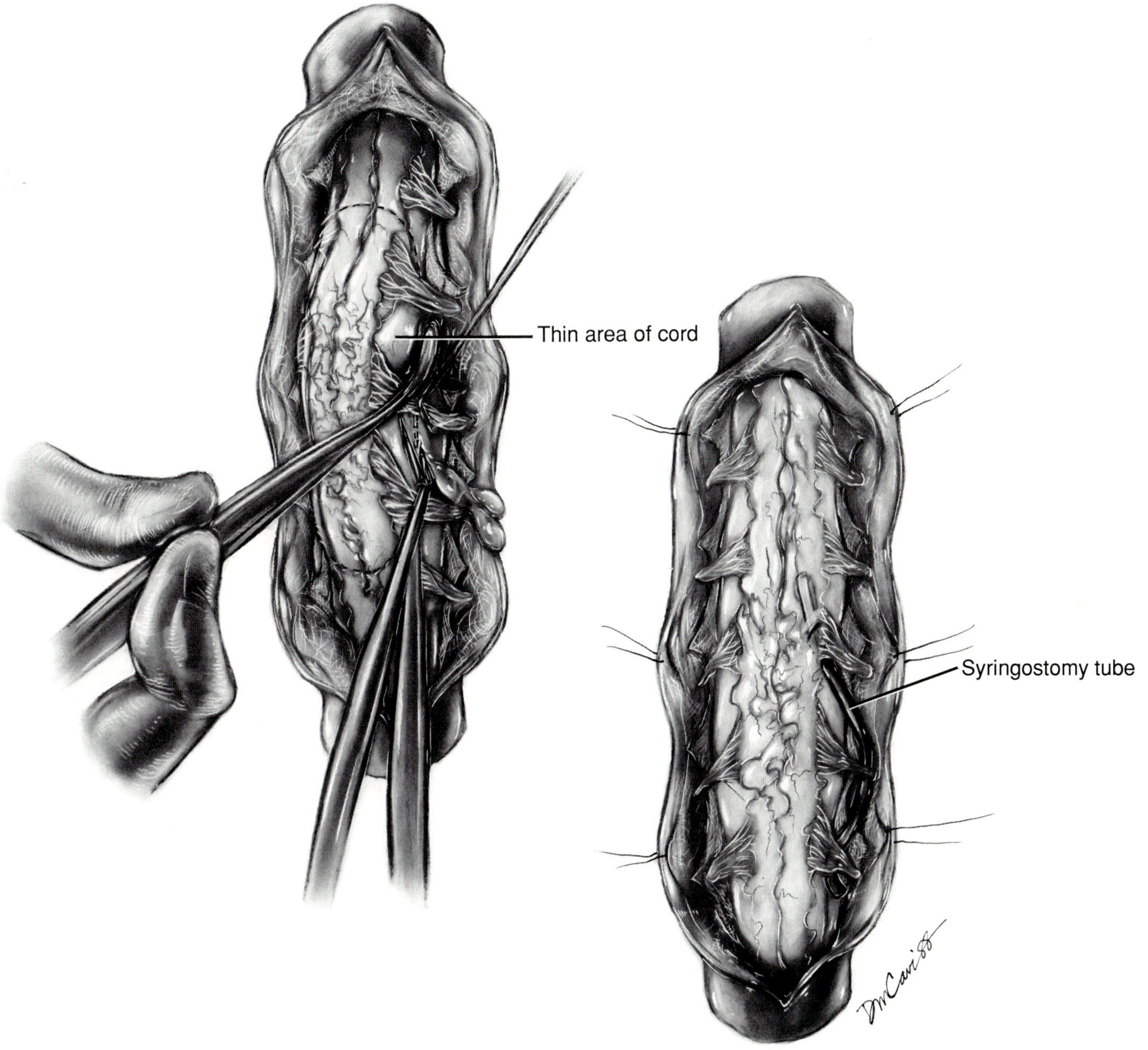

Figure 20.4.

erally, thus opening the cyst widely. There are no comparative studies of any of these techniques, and long-term follow-ups of tube drainage appear to be as satisfactory as any other technique devised.

Once the drainage tubes are in the subarachnoid space and secured, the dura is closed in a watertight fashion. No other special care is required for closure.

Syrinx Associated with Chiari Malformation

When a syrinx is associated with Chiari malformation, the procedure is modified to include exploration of the C1-C2 junction. The operation is identical with that described for the Chiari malformation. It is rea-

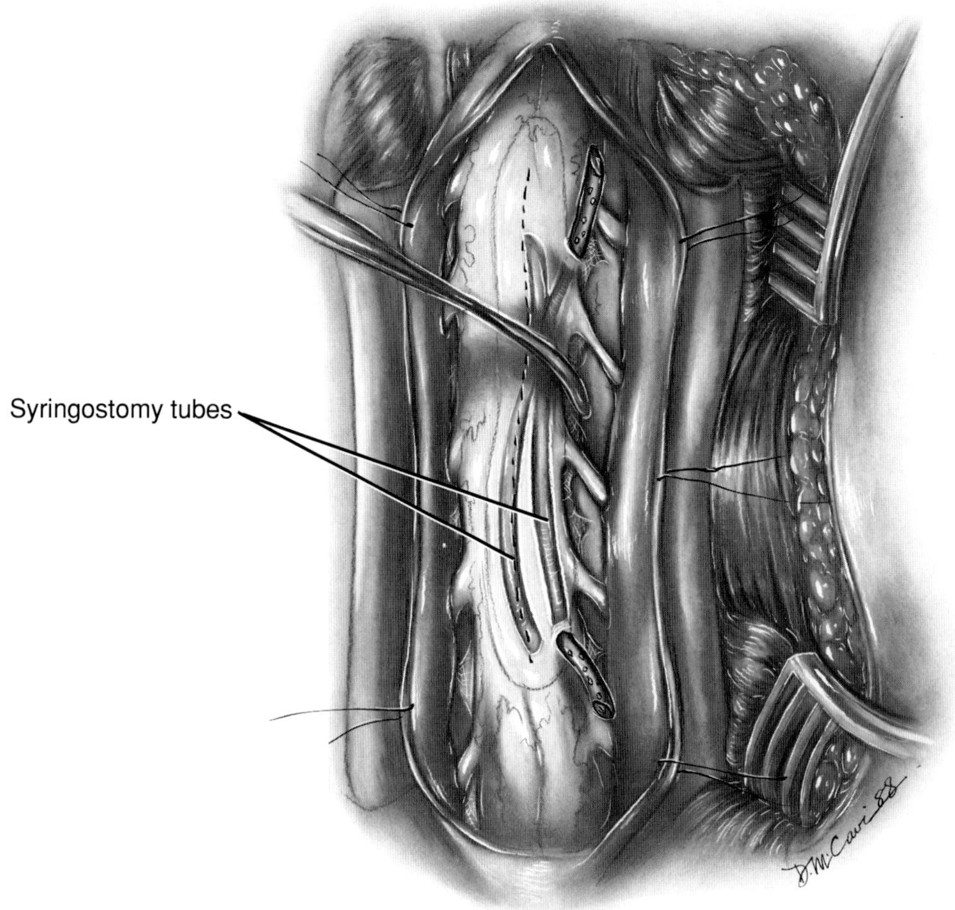

Figure 20.5.

sonable simply to drain the syrinx as just described, but release of cervicomedullary compression and the correction of hydromyelia, if present, offer an opportunity to correct pathology rather than treat the consequences only.

The operation may be done with the patient in the sitting position or prone under general anesthesia. The exposure for the posterior fossa and cervical cord is as described for treatment of the Chiari malformation and the isolated cervical syrinx. The goal of the posterior fossa exploration is twofold, i.e., decompression and exploration of a potential connection between the fourth ventricle and the hydromyelia. After the dura is opened, the posterior fourth ventricle must be explored. The first step is to elevate the tonsils so that the fourth ventricle can be seen. The roof of the obex is commonly a solid sheet of thickened, ballooned arachnoid. There may be adhesions between the tonsils and brain stem. These should be divided; opening the arachnoid roof provides access to the obex; subpial or en bloc removal of an abnormal, elongated tonsil may be required to provide access to the fourth ventricle. The abnormal tonsillar material may be very gliotic, and suction removal may be difficult. En bloc removal by sequential coagulation and division of the fibrotic brain may be required. When the fourth ventricle is exposed, the obex should be explored for an opening between the central canal and the fourth ventricle. If the opening is significant, it should be easily visible. A small, soft catheter, such as a ven-

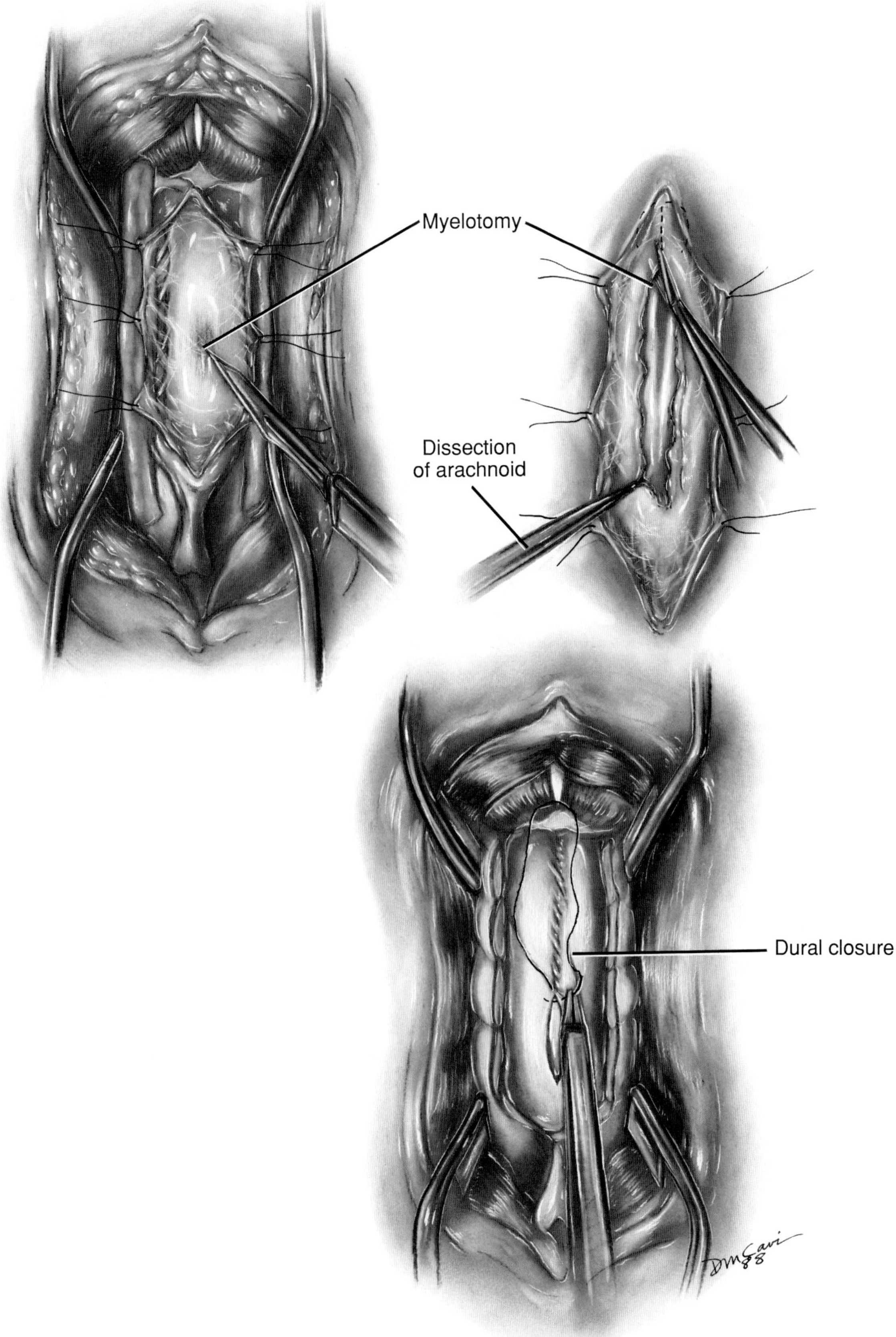

Figure 20.6.

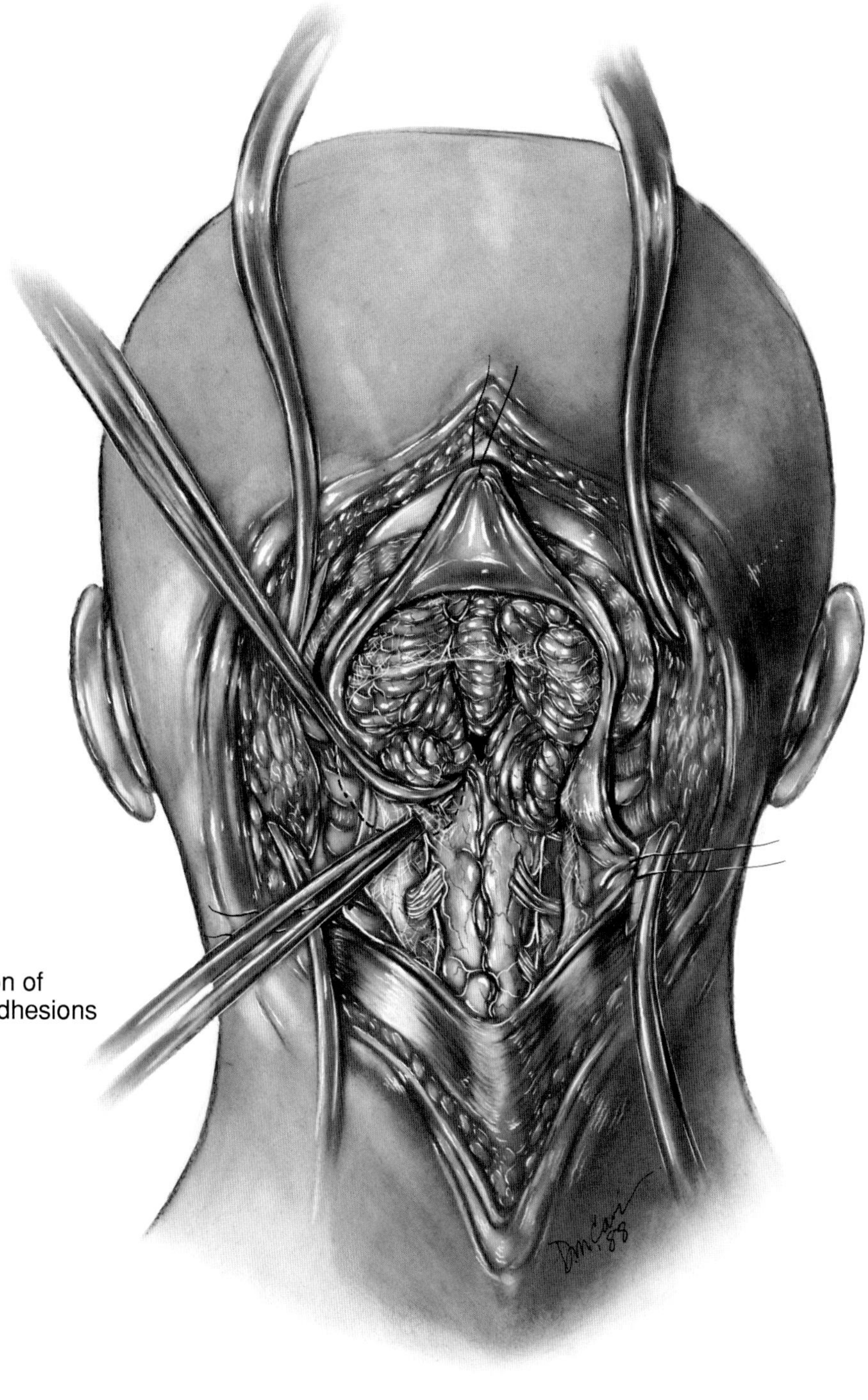

Figure 20.7.

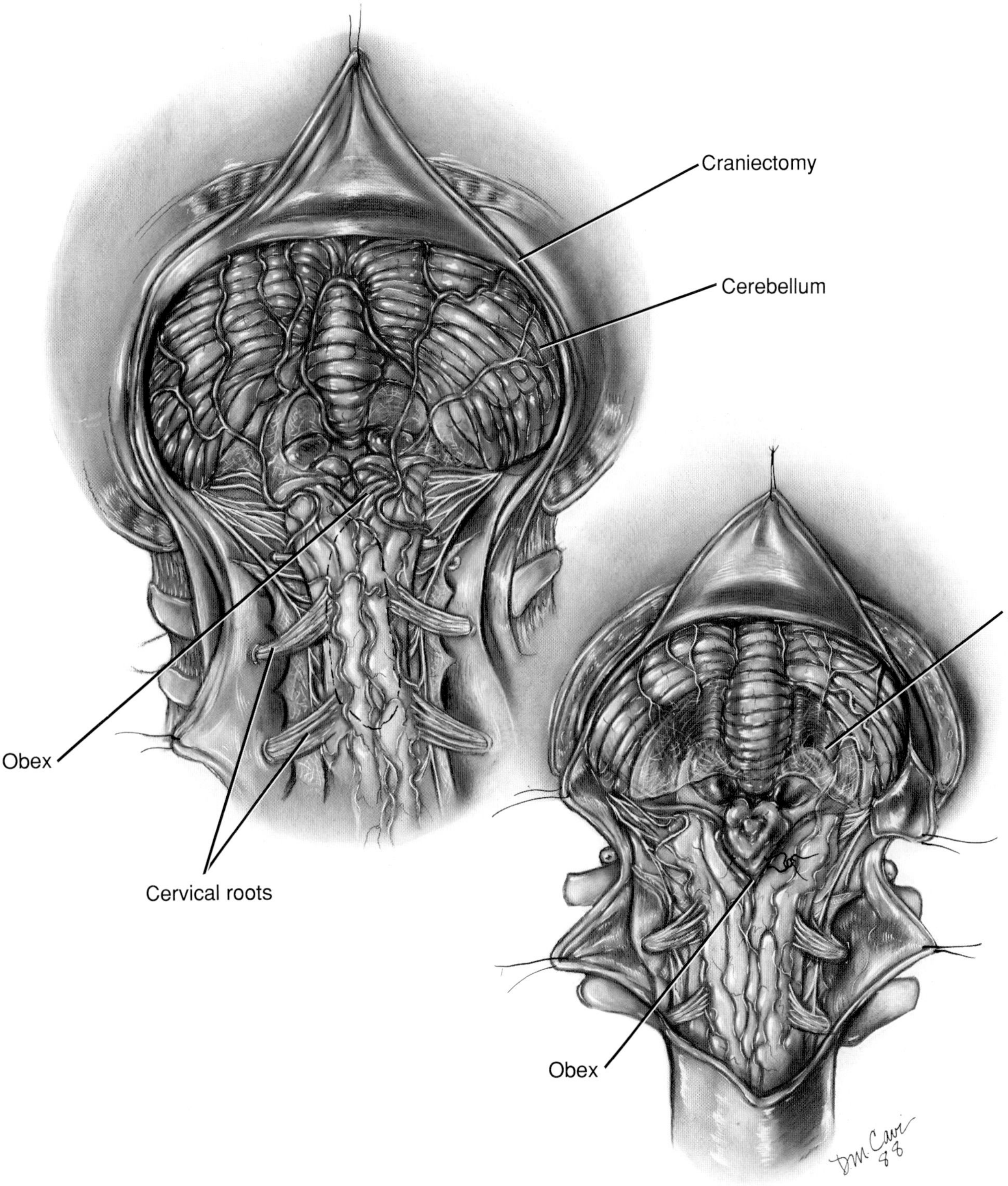
Craniectomy
Cerebellum
Adhesions
of tonsils
Obex
Cervical roots
Obex

Figure 20.8.

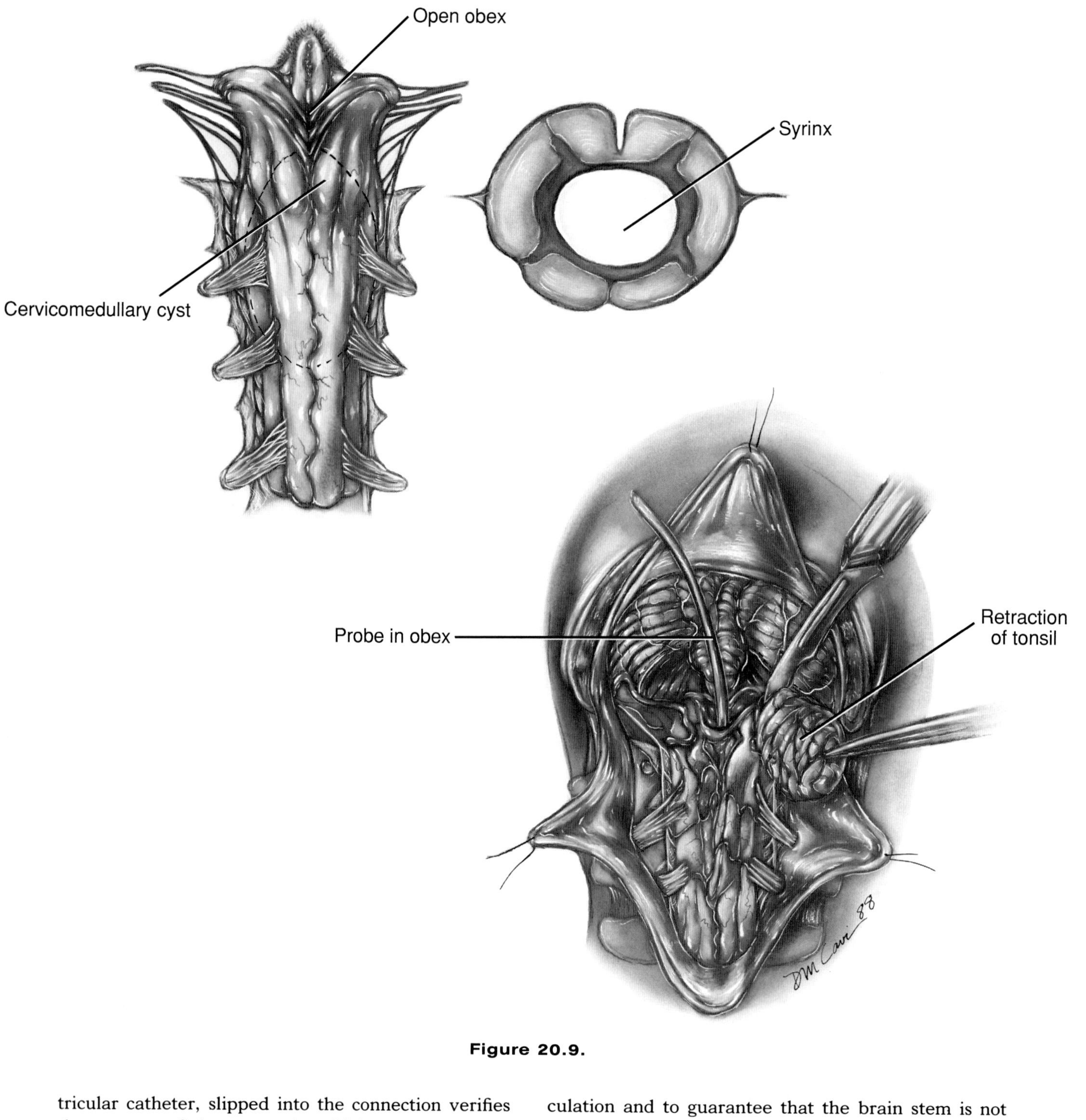

Figure 20.9.

tricular catheter, slipped into the connection verifies the patency of the connection. This catheter should not be forced. The opening can be closed by a small pledget of muscle or fat and occluded. The dura should be closed with a patch to allow adequate circulation and to guarantee that the brain stem is not compressed.

If no connection is found, the syrinx is attacked directly as described and shunted to the subarachnoid space. There are no special demands with this closure.

21

Diastematomyelia

Diastematomyelia is an anomaly that may occur in association with lipoma and the tethered cord syndrome or may present as an isolated abnormality. These anomalies usually occur in thoracic or thoracolumbar locations, but those associated with lipoma can also be purely lumbar. The basic abnormal structure is a spicule or band that divides the cord and may be bony or fibrous. Prior to computed tomography (CT) scanning or magnetic resonance imaging (MRI), the diagnosis of the nonossified anomalies was sometimes very difficult. Now the new scanning techniques demonstrate anatomy in great detail. Dilute intrathecal contrast will enhance the exactness of CT scanning, three-dimensional reconstruction is useful, and MRI is also an excellent way to delineate the nature and extent of the abnormality.

The operation is carried out with the patient under general anesthesia in the prone position. The midline laminectomy incision should be made so that the anomaly will be exposed one or two segments above and below. If there is an associated lipomatous mass, then the techniques utilized for the more conventional lipomas are employed until the spinal cord is exposed. When no lipoma is present, a laminectomy is carried out at least one segment above and below the malformation. Remember that other bony anomalies are often associated with these lesions and the laminectomy techniques must be predicated on the presence or absence of spinous and laminar anomalies. A laminectomy should then be done, exposing the dura above and below the abnormality that affects the spinal cord. Several kinds of anomalies may be encountered. There may be a fibrous or bony structure that connects the body anteriorly with the laminae posteriorly. This lesion may be extradural, and there

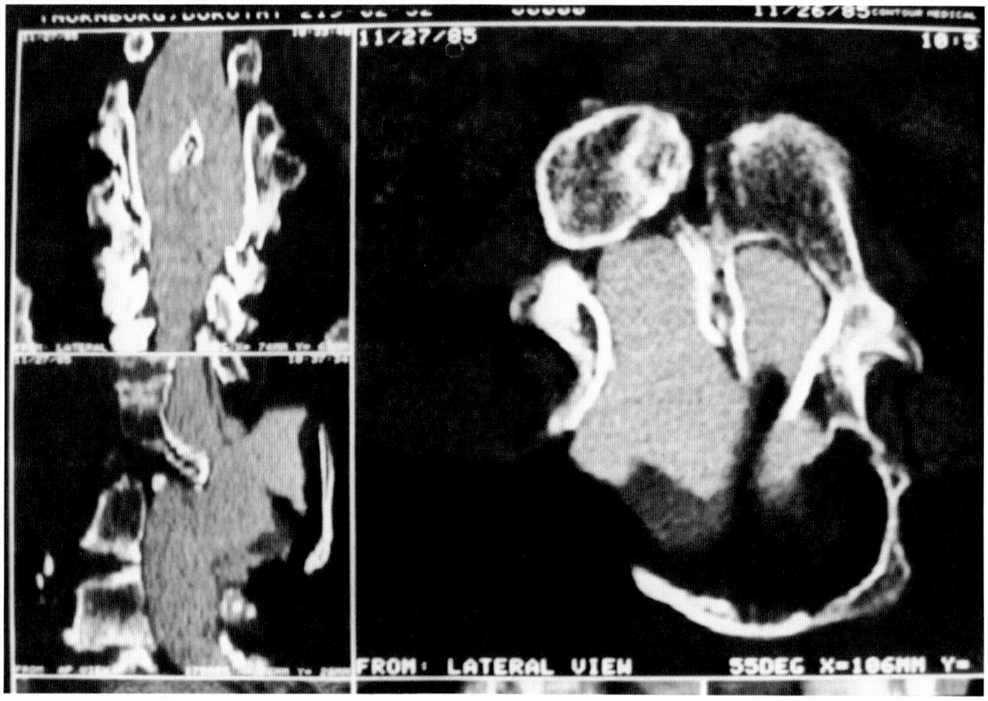

Figure 21.1. Typical features of diastematomyelia.

may be two intact dural tubes around the spicule. This is a rare situation, and when it is present, there usually is reduplication of the cord in each tube. The reduplication may be around the anomaly only, or it may extend for a long distance, perhaps even for the remainder of the dural sac. Sometimes, the spicule simply splits the cord, but occasionally, the encroachment may be asymmetric. Magnification and physiological monitoring make the surgery easier and safer. When the offending mass is completely extradural, the first step is to dissect it free from the dural tube by using a combination of sharp and blunt microdis-

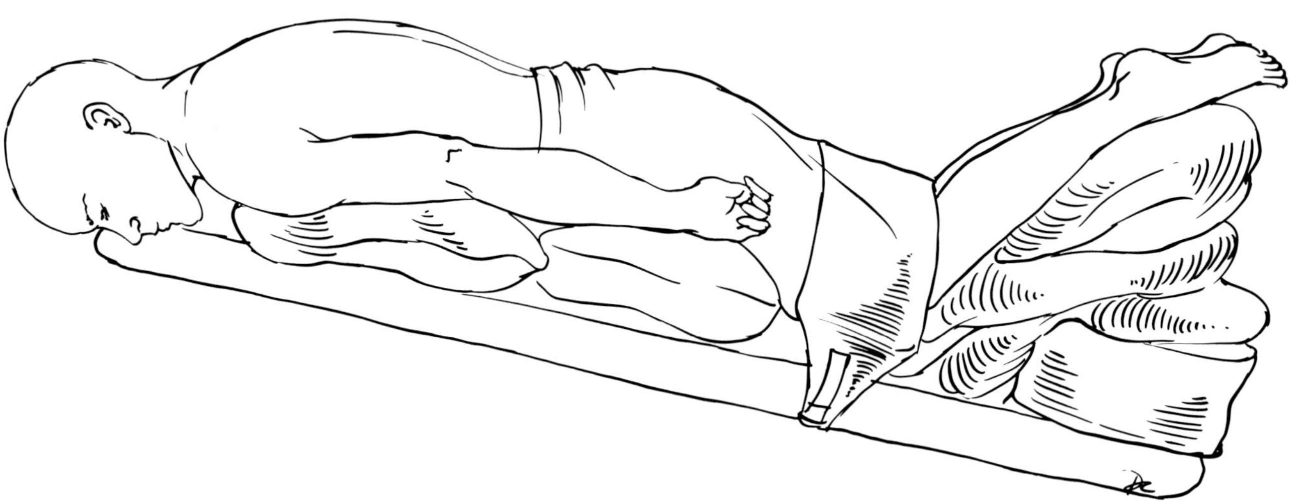

Figure 21.2. Patient prone with head elevated 15°.

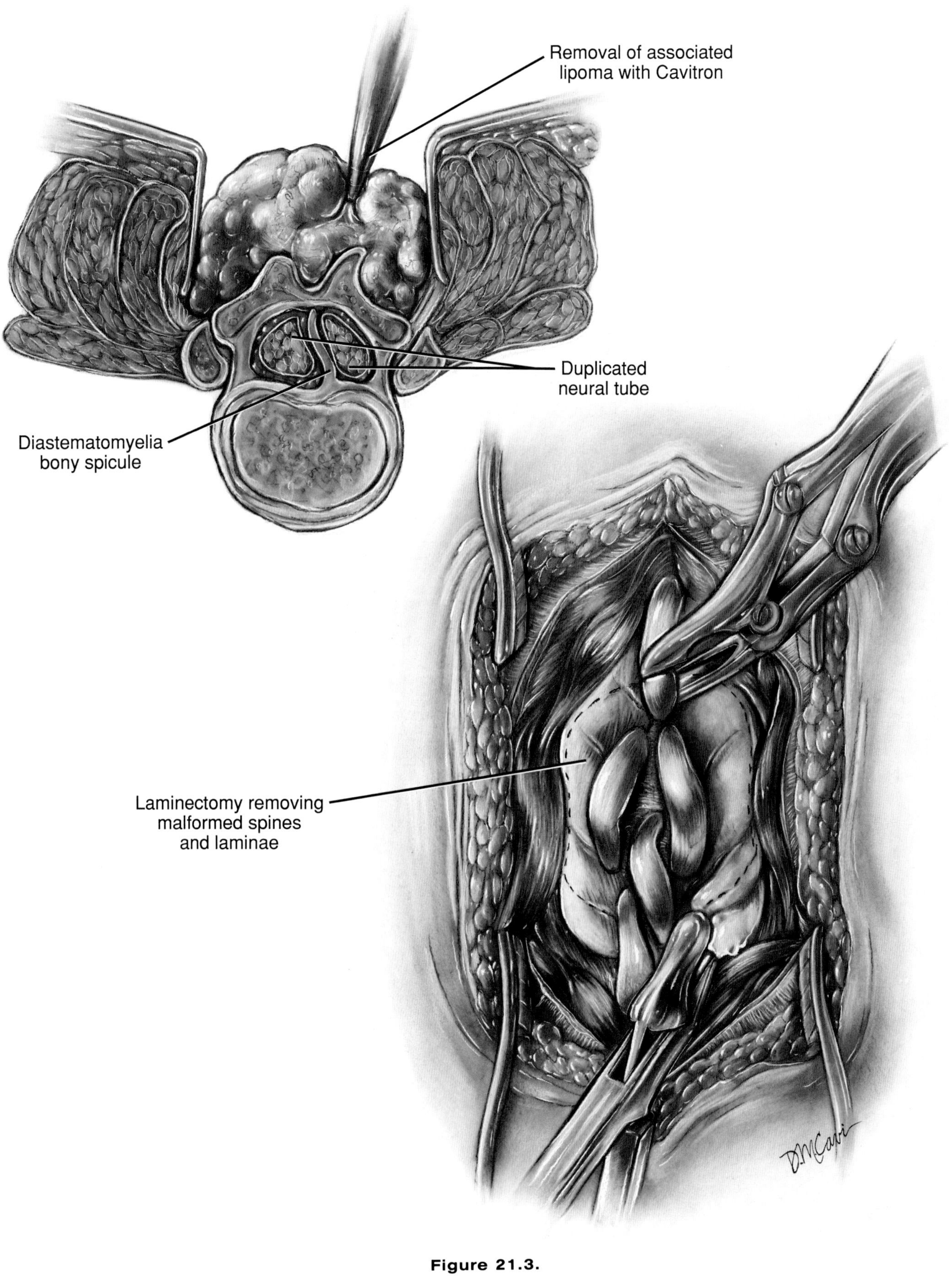

Removal of associated lipoma with Cavitron
Duplicated neural tube
Diastematomyelia bony spicule
Laminectomy removing malformed spines and laminae

Figure 21.3.

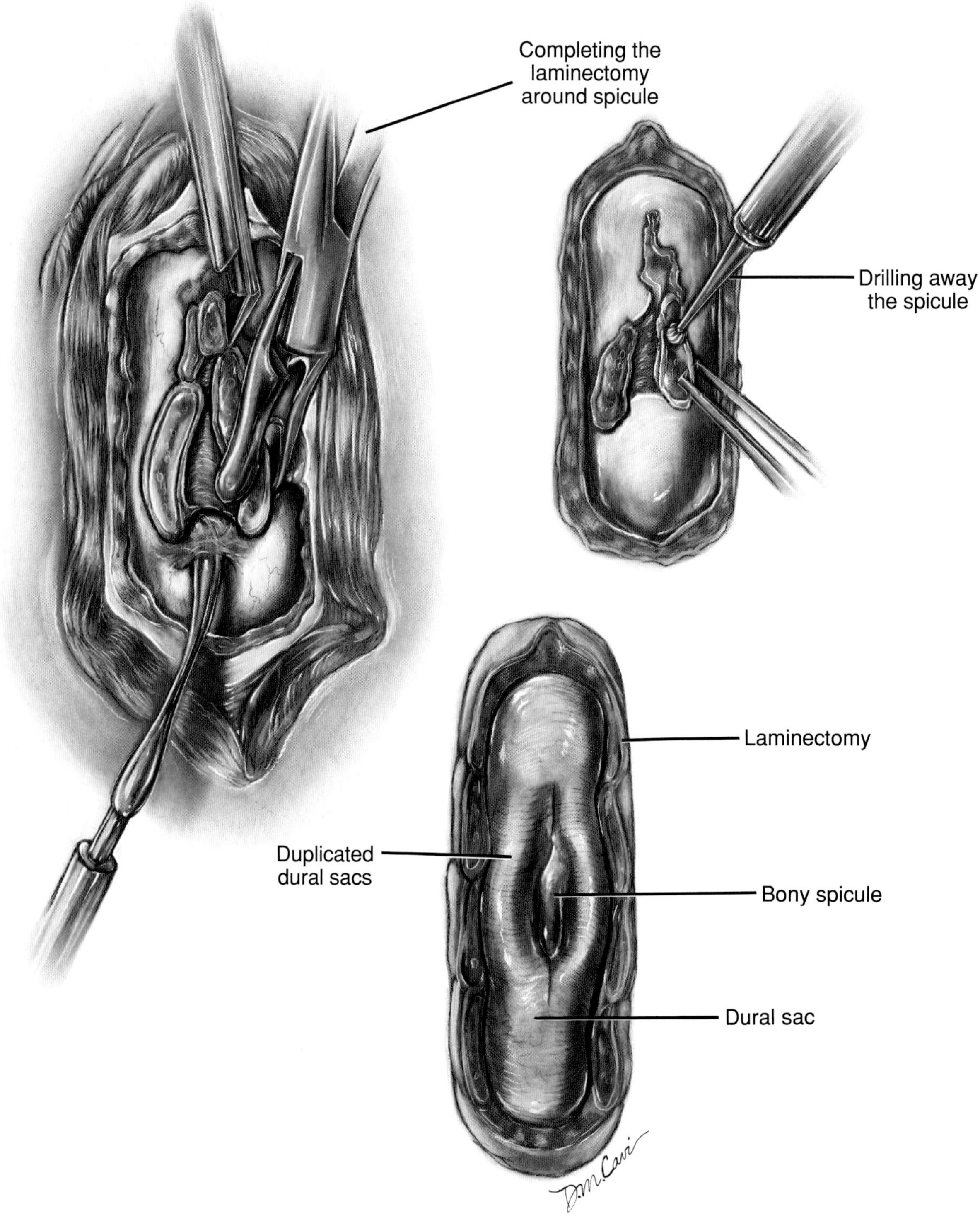
Completing the
laminectomy
around spicule
Drilling away
the spicule
Laminectomy
Duplicated
dural sacs
Bony spicule
Dural sac

Figure 21.4.

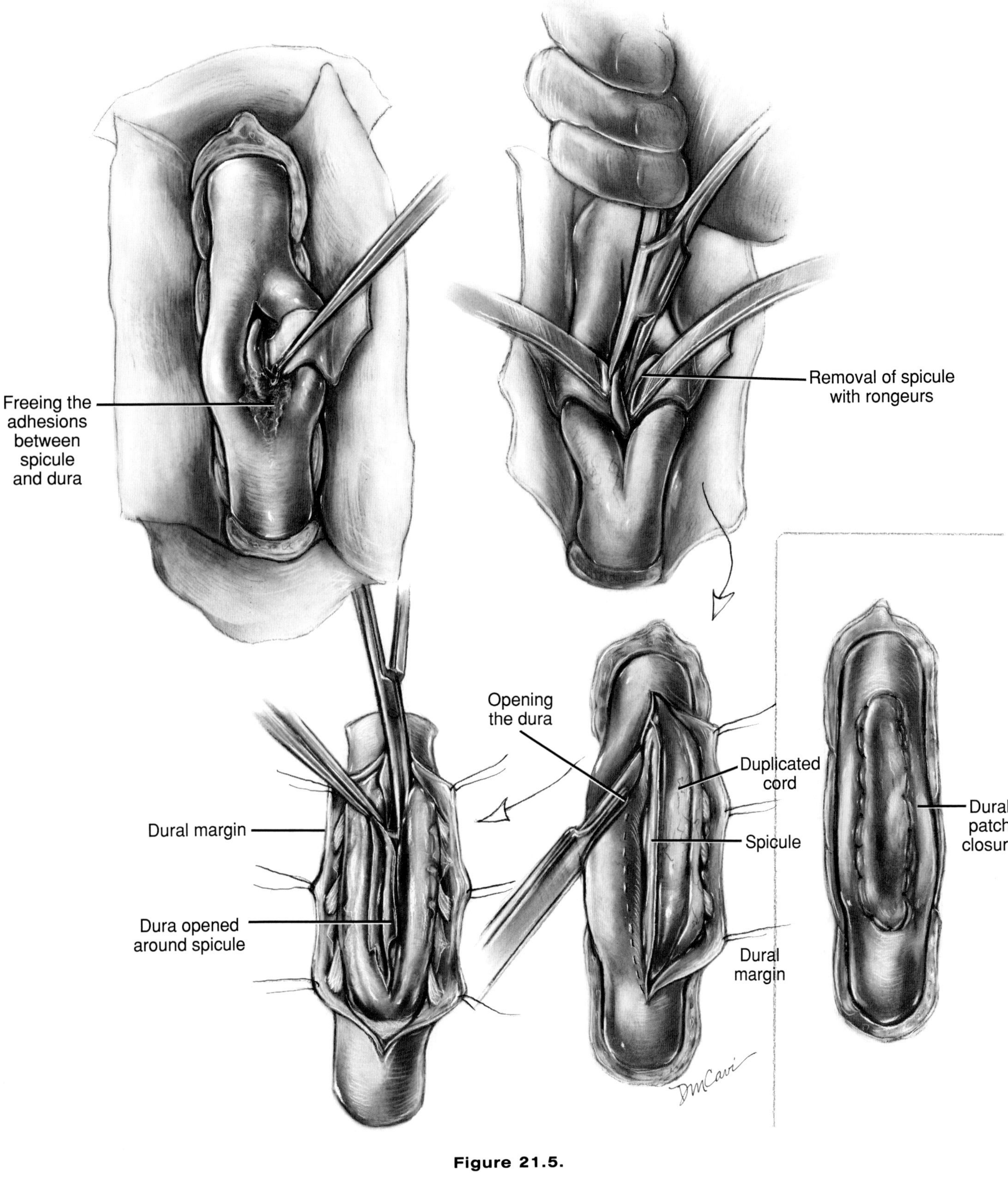
Freeing the adhesions between spicule and dura
Removal of spicule with rongeurs
Opening the dura
Duplicated cord
Dural margin
Spicule
Dural patch closure
Dura opened around spicule
Dural margin

Figure 21.5.

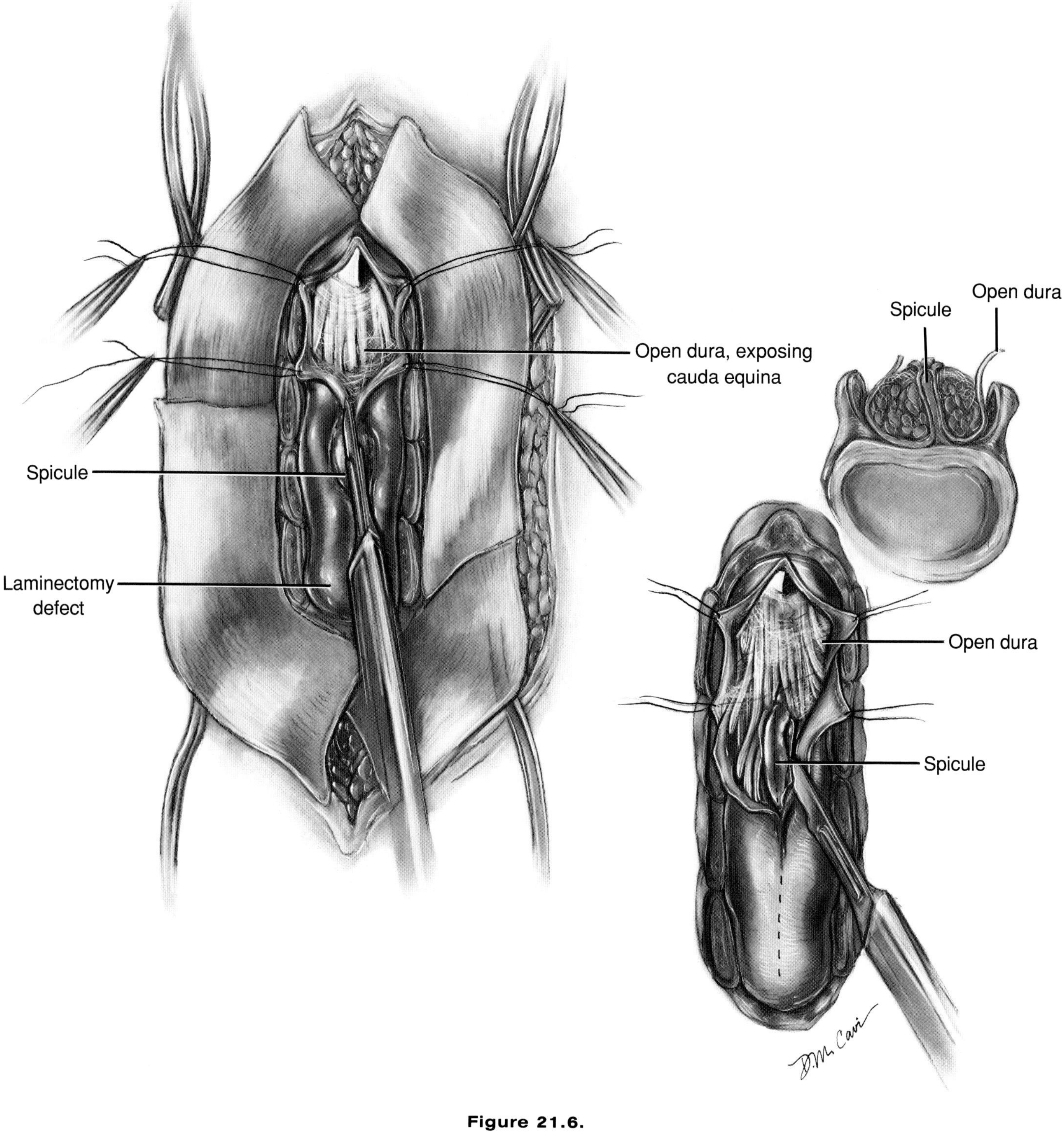

Open dura, exposing cauda equina
Spicule
Laminectomy defect
Spicule
Open dura
Open dura
Spicule

Figure 21.6.

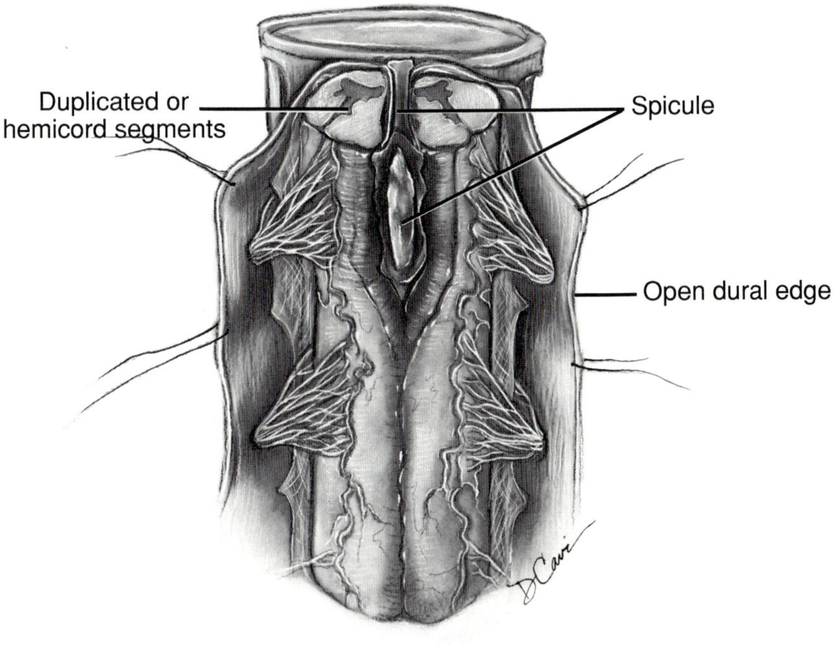

Figure 21.7.

section. The larger Rosen knives are excellent instruments for this. Sometimes, the bony spicule can be broken at the base by gentle manipulation with a rongeur. It is not safe to pass an instrument of any size into this very narrow space, but there usually is room to manipulate fine rongeurs to remove the bony spicule down to the vertebral body. The attachments of the dura to the body should be dissected free with a sharp dissector. If there is total duplication of the dural sac, it may be that removal of the extradural mass will provide adequate decompression and nothing further needs to be done. In most instances, duplication of the dural sac extends only a short distance. Then, it is important actually to open the dura and make certain that the tethering effect of the dural band is also gone. Under magnification the dura is opened above the defect down to it and below from the point where the dural duplication ceases. The dural incision is then carried out as medially as possible in each of the duplicated tubes, isolating the central stalk of dura that has surrounded the bony or fibrous spicule. This should be dissected free from the medial portions of the duplicated or divided cord. The redundant dura should be excised, and if there is room, the dura should be closed in the midline anteriorly. Frequently, there is enough dura that a small flap can be created on each side and the two flaps sutured easily in the midline, reconstituting the anterior dura. If the space is too small to do this, the anterior dura may be left open and simply excised down to the bone so no tethering of the cord can occur. Then the dura is closed posteriorly. If this can be done easily without compression of the cord, a primary midline closure is reasonable. If this cannot be done, a graft of fascia or artificial dural substitute should be utilized to achieve a watertight posterior closure. The closure requires no special care.

Intradural Tethering

The more common circumstance is that following laminectomy the surgeon is confronted with a single dural tube, and the tethering mass dividing the cord is completely intradural. When this is the situation, the dura should be opened under magnification. The dural opening should begin in the midline well below the intradural mass and be carried up until the mass is encountered. It should then be opened on either side as medially as possible and extended up over normal cord so that the transfixing structure with a small cap of dura is isolated. The small cap of dura provides a

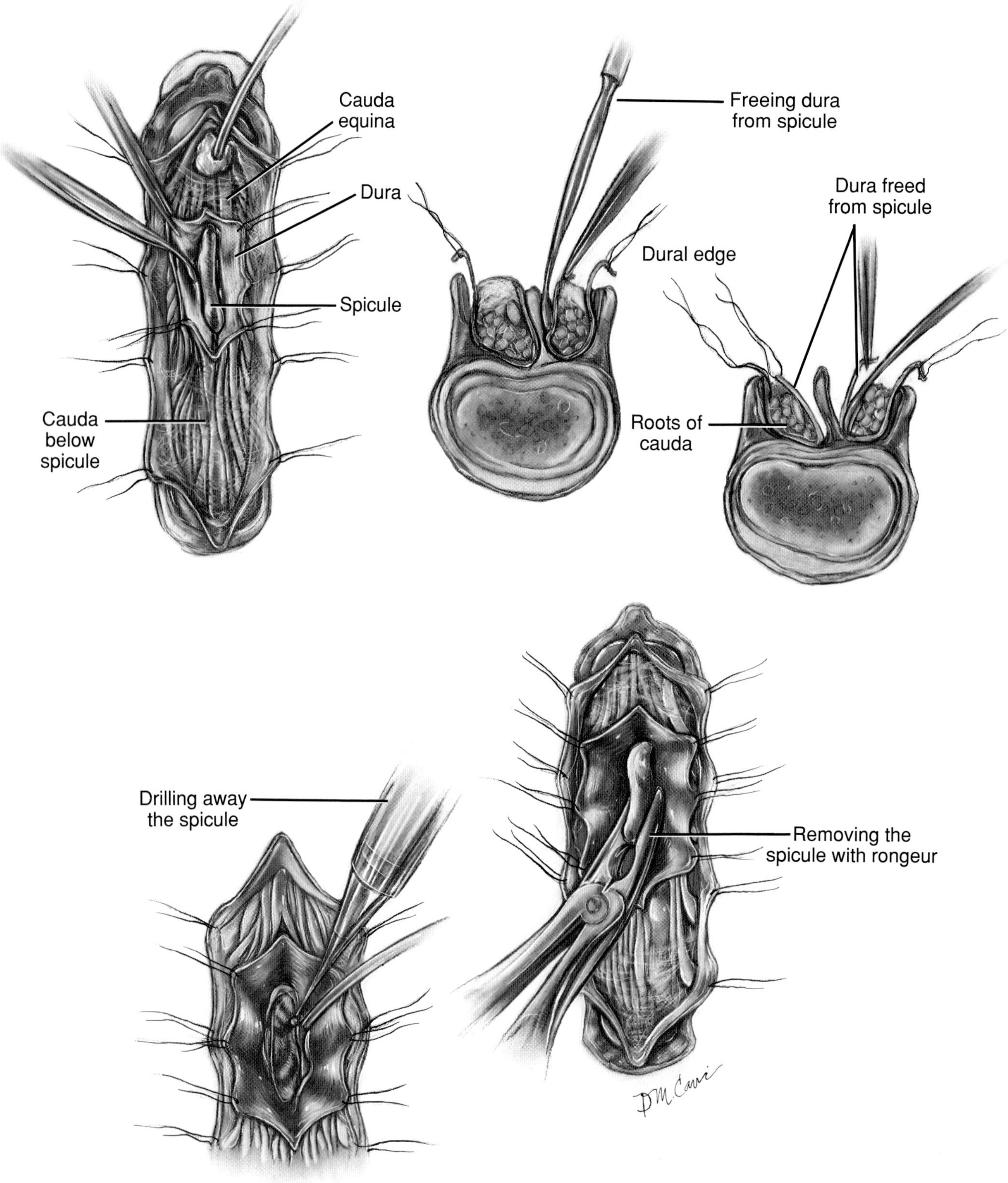
Cauda equina
Dura
Spicule
Cauda below spicule
Freeing dura from spicule
Dura freed from spicule
Dural edge
Roots of cauda
Drilling away the spicule
Removing the spicule with rongeur

Figure 21.8.

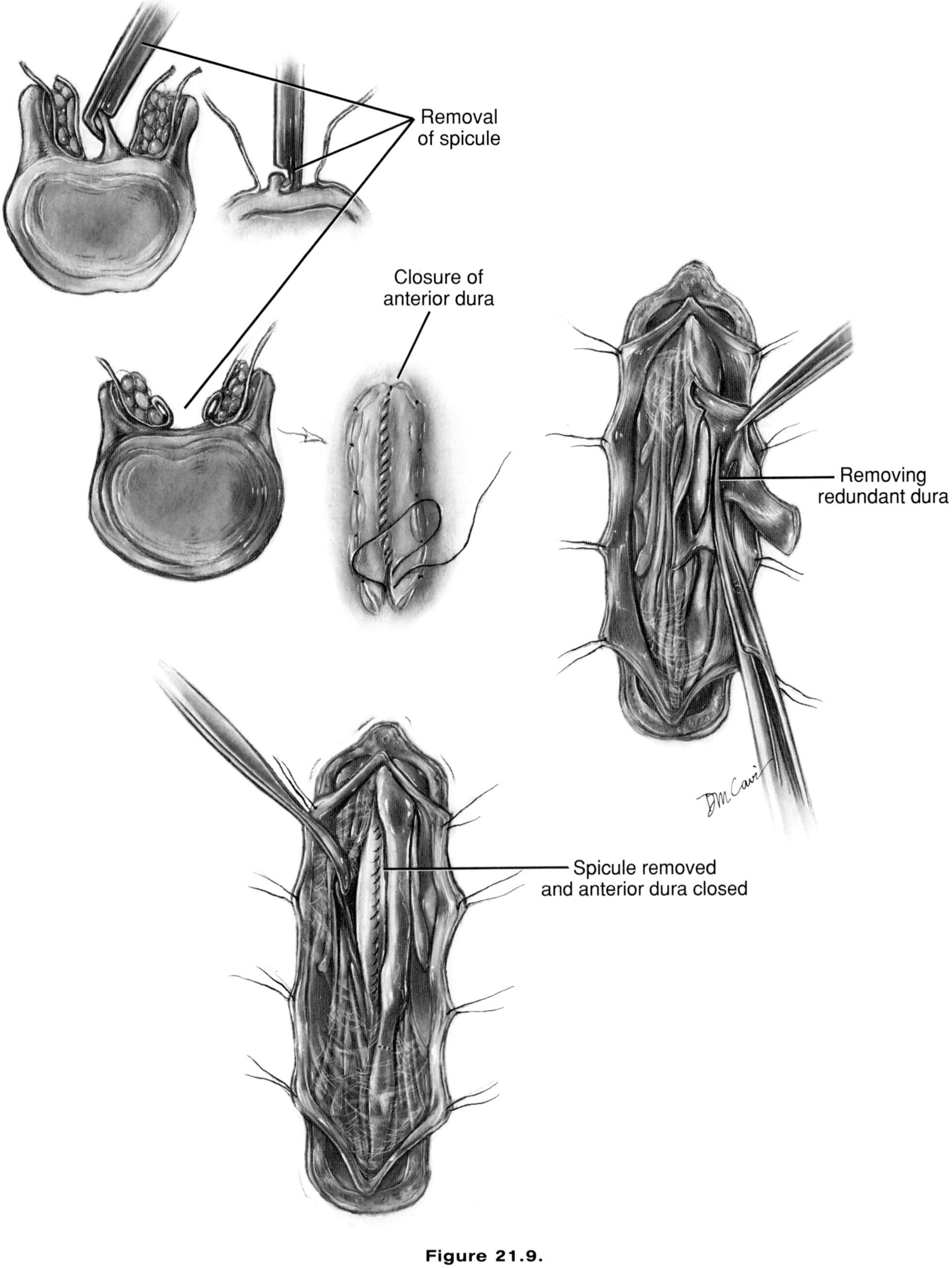
Removal
of spicule
Closure of
anterior dura
Removing
redundant dura
Spicule removed
and anterior dura closed

Figure 21.9.

nice handle for manipulation of the band. If the spicule is bony, the dissection should be done in the same way as described for the extradural lesion. Use of a sharp Rosen knife is an excellent way to break down the adhesions between the cord. These are extrapial lesions, and if the dissection is in the proper plane, the spinal cord should not be entered at any level. The spicule should be dissected free completely circumferentially down to the body and then gradually removed with sharp rongeurs. An experienced surgeon can remove the mass with a high-speed drill, but this is only for the surgeon who is a master of drilling techniques. The bone should be removed to the level of the body. It is not necessary to try to close the dura anteriorly. The dura should be closed posteriorly in a linear fashion or with a patch, if necessary, to provide adequate decompression. When the band is fibrous, it is much simpler to remove it. It should be dissected free; then it simply can be divided along the base with microscissors. There is no need to close the anterior dura. With these fibrous bands, there is rarely an anterior opening. The cord should be mobilized to make sure no adhesions continue to tether it to the abnormal area. The dura can then be closed in the midline or with a patch, as circumstances dictate.

Diastematomyelia with Lipoma

Lipomas will sometimes occur in association with a tethering transfixing band or bony mass. The basic approach to lipoma has been described in Chapter 22. With these lesions, when the lipoma has been mobilized posteriorly and laterally, there apparently still is a tethering effect, usually in the midline. A bony spicule will have been recognized on the CT scan or with MRI. This is not the case with the fibrous band, and the surgeon must be alerted to the possibility of fibrous connections within the lipoma by the lack of mobility of the mass. The dissection of the transfixing mass is much more difficult in the face of the lipoma, which obscures the posterior anatomy. Furthermore, the adhesions to the cord are much more difficult to free because of the abnormal fat. The dissection should be carried through the lipoma with coagulation and cutting or with the ultrasonic dissector, which is a handy way to remove the fat until the transfixing band or spicule is identified and removed. In the way described the closure then proceeds in standard fashion. A posterior dural patch is almost always required when a lipoma is present. Closure of muscle and skin requires no special precautions.

22

Myelomeningocele and Lipoma

Meningocele, Myelomeningocele, and Associated Anomalies

There are three basic types of these congenital malformations: the true meningocele without neural elements, the myelomeningocele, and the lipomyelomeningocele. Most are lumbar, at least in part. When repair is planned, the goals are elimination of the sac, coverage with healthy skin, preservation of neural elements, and restoration of normal relationships insofar as possible.

Operations are done with the patient under general anesthesia in the prone position, with thoracic rolls or a small frame used. Some extensions of the incision may be necessary to obtain adequate closure. The operative area should include the buttocks down to the beginning of the gluteal fold, laterally to the flanks, and superiorly to the scapulae. It is not likely that the extensive flap mobilizations that were once utilized to cover these defects now will be required, but it is still a good idea to have all of this area available. The skin, but not the sac, can be covered with adhesive drapes if desired.

Meningocele

Meningoceles are lesions that can be recognized by the fact that no neural elements are visualized in the sac. Sometimes, the skin coverage is quite good. Computed tomography (CT) scans should prove the nature of the abnormality and demonstrate the absence of neural elements within the sac. When the skin over

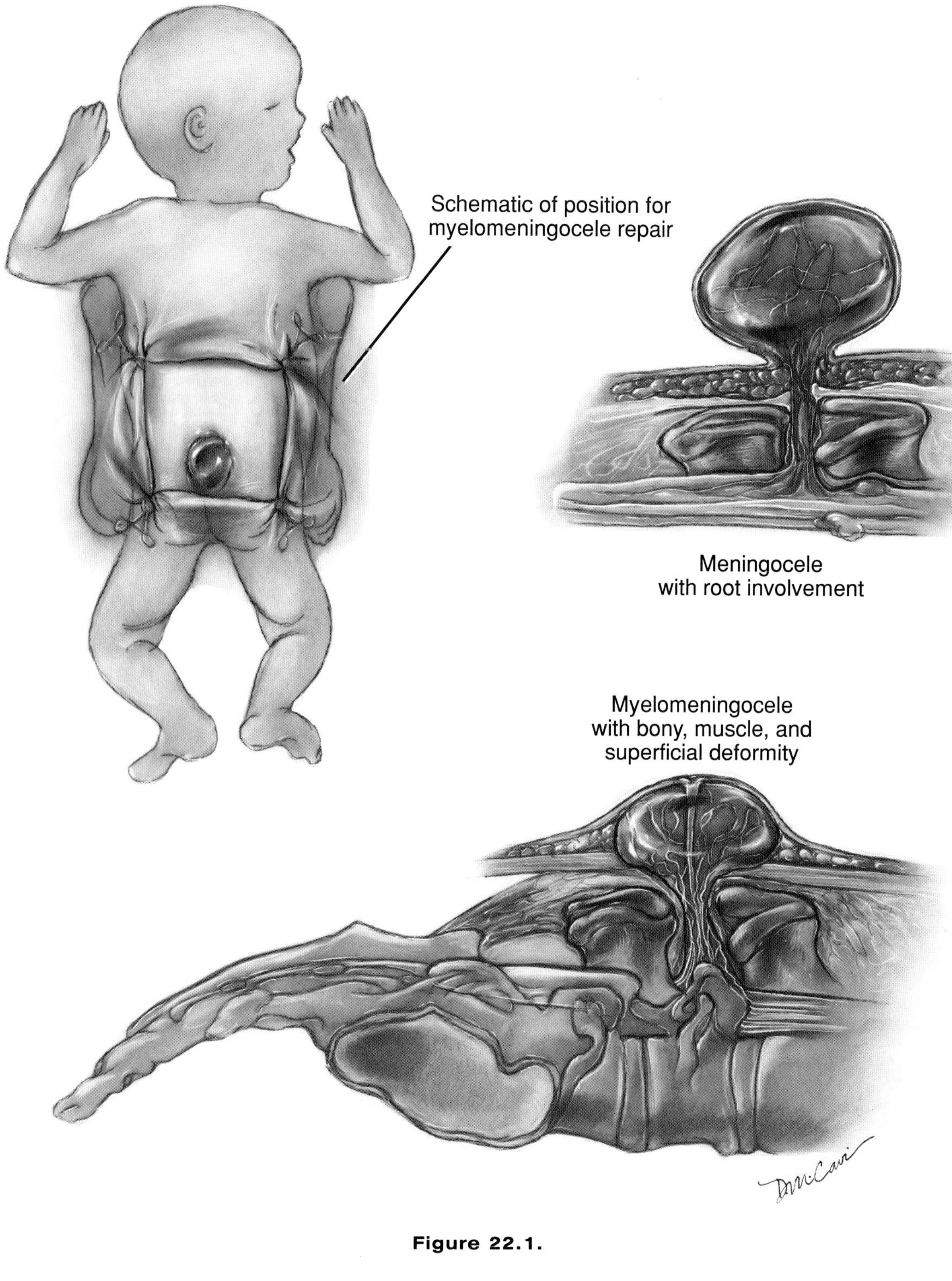
Schematic of position for
myelomeningocele repair
Meningocele
with root involvement
Myelomeningocele
with bony, muscle, and
superficial deformity

Figure 22.1.

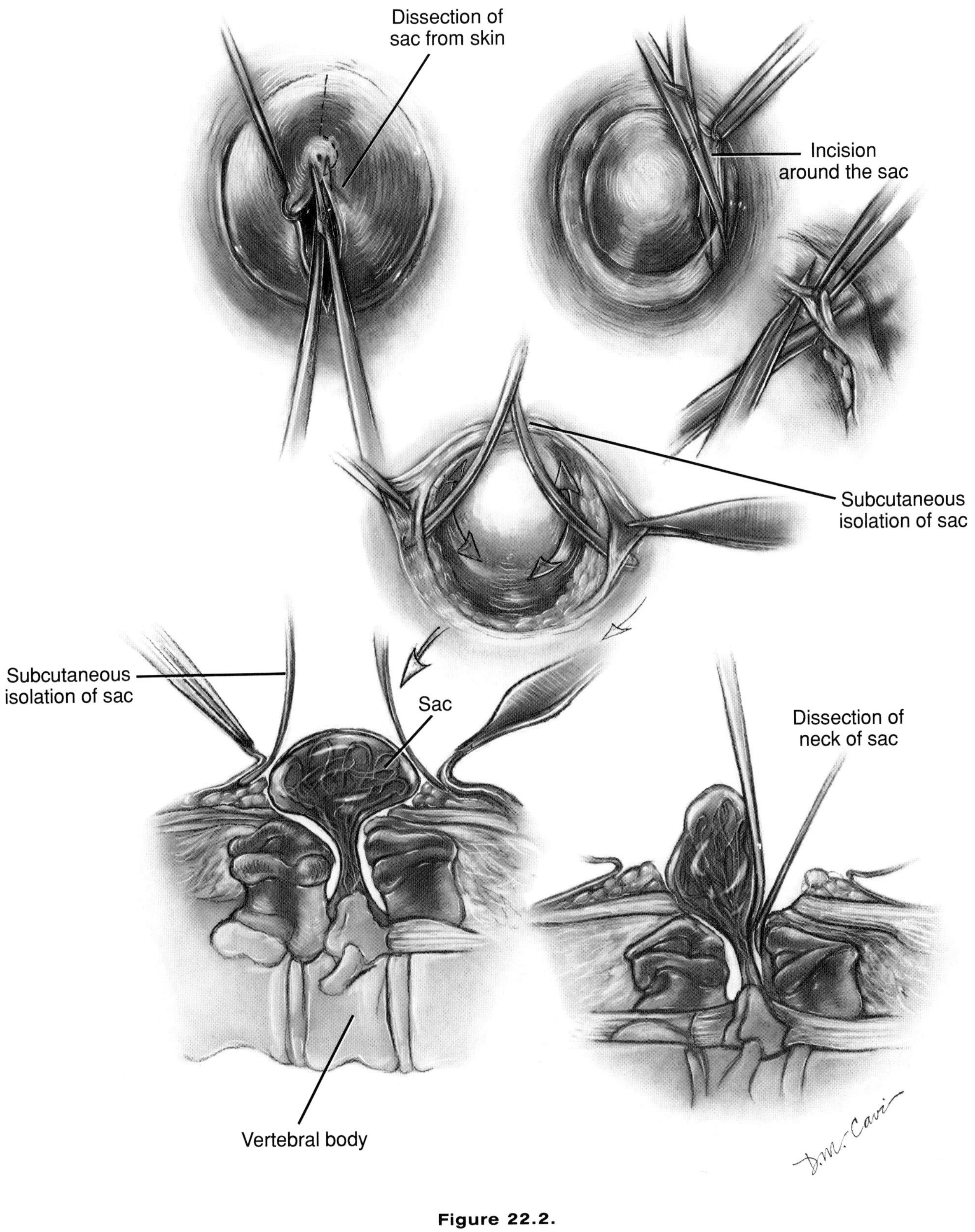
Dissection of
sac from skin
Incision
around the sac
Subcutaneous
isolation of sac
Subcutaneous
isolation of sac
Sac
Dissection of
neck of sac
Vertebral body
D.M. Cavi

Figure 22.2.

the sac is normal, the sac is best exposed by a midline skin incision. When the skin does not completely cover the sac and the meningocele is presenting with the meningeal sac actually exposed, then the approach is very much the same as that for a myelomeningocele. It is important to save all the skin possible and to dissect the neck of the meningocele free from surrounding tissue without rupturing it. The neck of the sac can be isolated by a skin incision that extends circumferentially around the sac at the junction of the meninges and skin. This is a time-honored method of exposing the sac. If it is utilized, the skin incision should be made carefully through skin to subcutaneous tissue at the margin of the sac, with all skin possible saved. Even when the skin is very thin and appears abnormal, it can be very useful in closure, and all should be saved. When this approach is used, the skin incision is made circumferentially around the sac to subcutaneous tissue. Then the space between the sac and the subcutaneous tissue is developed, first via sharp dissection with scissors and then via blunt dissection, freeing the sac from surrounding subcutaneous tissues. Next, the loose areolar plane that is always present following the neck down into the defect between the paravertebral muscles is developed, thereby exposing dura at the origin of the sac from the spinal dural tube.

An alternative method is simply to make a small vertical incision near the base of the sac and near its superior apex in the midline. A clamp can then be inserted and a blunt dissection carried out, separating the neck of the sac from surrounding tissue until the clamp exits at the incision above. The skin can then be dissected free from the sac wall by an incision that parallels the clamp and is made at the junction of the sac and the overlaying skin. The procedure is repeated on the opposite side, isolating the sac with maximum preservation of skin. This technique provides the greatest amount of skin for coverage. The neck of the sac should now be isolated completely by blunt dissection down to the level of the laminae.

The sac can then be opened in the midline, and the junction of the sac with a relatively normal dural tube identified. It is important to be certain that no neural elements are adherent. Then the sac should be excised, trimmed carefully to make certain there is enough sac wall to reconstitute the dura in its normal relationships. This opening should be closed with a single linear watertight suture in such a fashion that a normal-sized dural tube is constructed.

The paravertebral muscles should then be mobilized via small osteotomes from the spines and laminae above and laterally over the zygapophyseal joints. Excellent instruments for this purpose are the Adson periosteal elevator or a small Cobb elevator. This will allow mobilization of enough of the paravertebral muscle mass to close the lumbar fascia in the midline, providing adequate muscle coverage over the dural sac. The skin should be closed in the midline if at all possible. Adequate skin for midline closure without tension can usually be obtained by undercutting the skin between the subcutaneous tissue and the lumbar fascia. Undermining may be necessary laterally and superiorly to gain adequate relaxation to close the skin easily. The skin should not be under tension. If it is not possible to obtain a closure utilizing full-thickness skin, it may be feasible to tack the full-thickness skin down at a convenient location laterally to relieve tension on the midline closure and then allow the thin skin from the wall of the sac to cover the defect. This serves almost as a split-thickness graft and will take nicely as long as it is not closed with tension. Watertight dural closure is required for this maneuver.

Myelomeningocele

The basic approach to the repair of a myelomeningocele with neural involvement is the same as that for the repair of a meningocele. The principal difference is that the neural placode must be managed. The operation is done with the patient in the prone position, and all of the skin around the myelomeningocele itself is prepared. It is not necessary to put any chemicals on the sac itself. If the sac is not completely clean, it should be washed gently with saline, and then the skin around it should be prepared. The back should be widely draped from flank to flank and from gluteal fold to scapulae. Give some thought to closure before beginning the surgery. Small defects are likely to be closed without difficulty, and a vertical closure is desirable. A transverse closure is the next best alternative. Large defects may require ingenuity in closure and the rotation of flaps to achieve adequate skin closure. Preservation of all possible viable skin found on the wall of the sac is important to allow the least complicated skin closure.

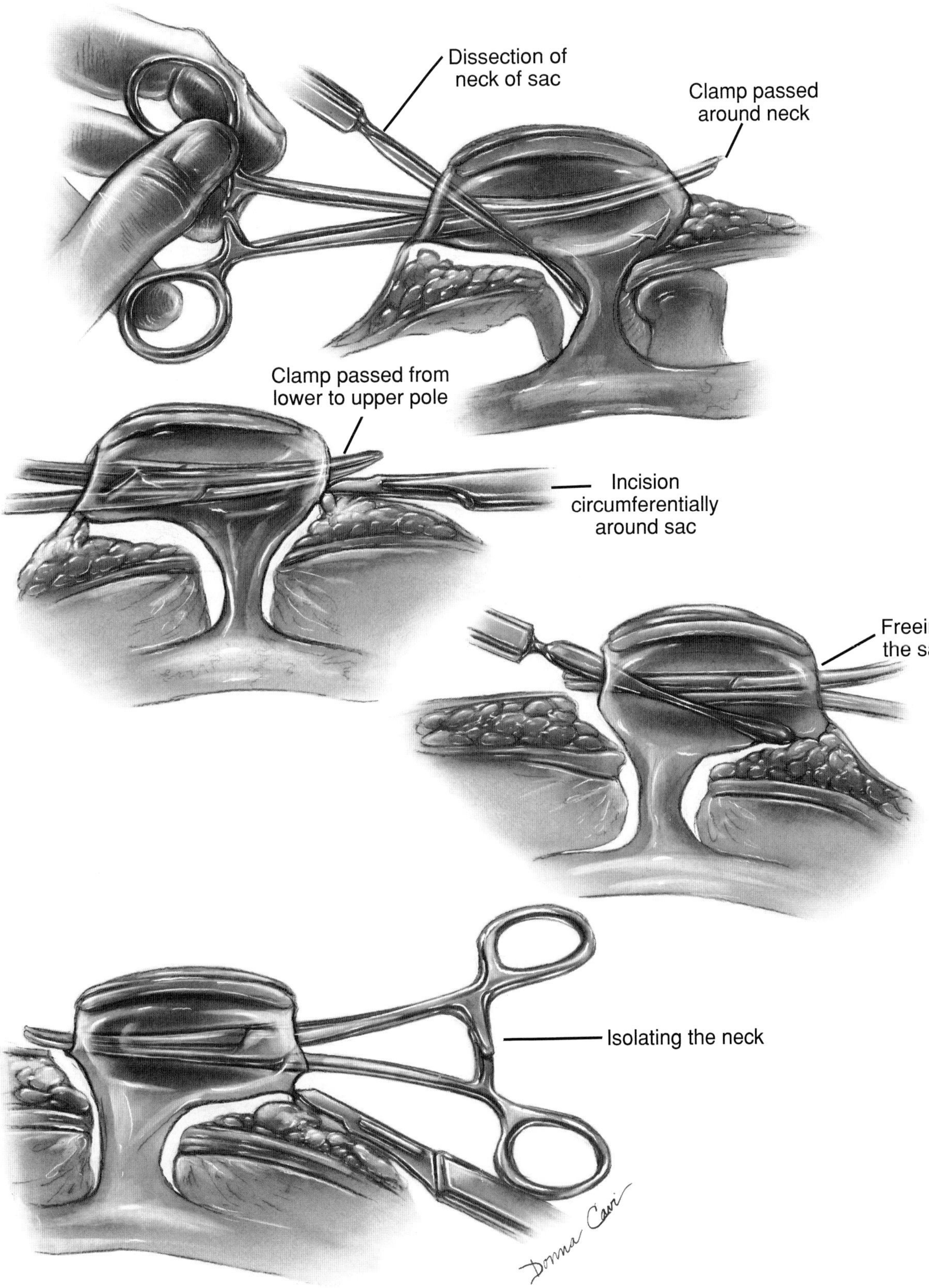
Dissection of neck of sac
Clamp passed around neck
Clamp passed from lower to upper pole
Incision circumferentially around sac
Freeing the sac
Isolating the neck
Donna Cavi

Figure 22.3.

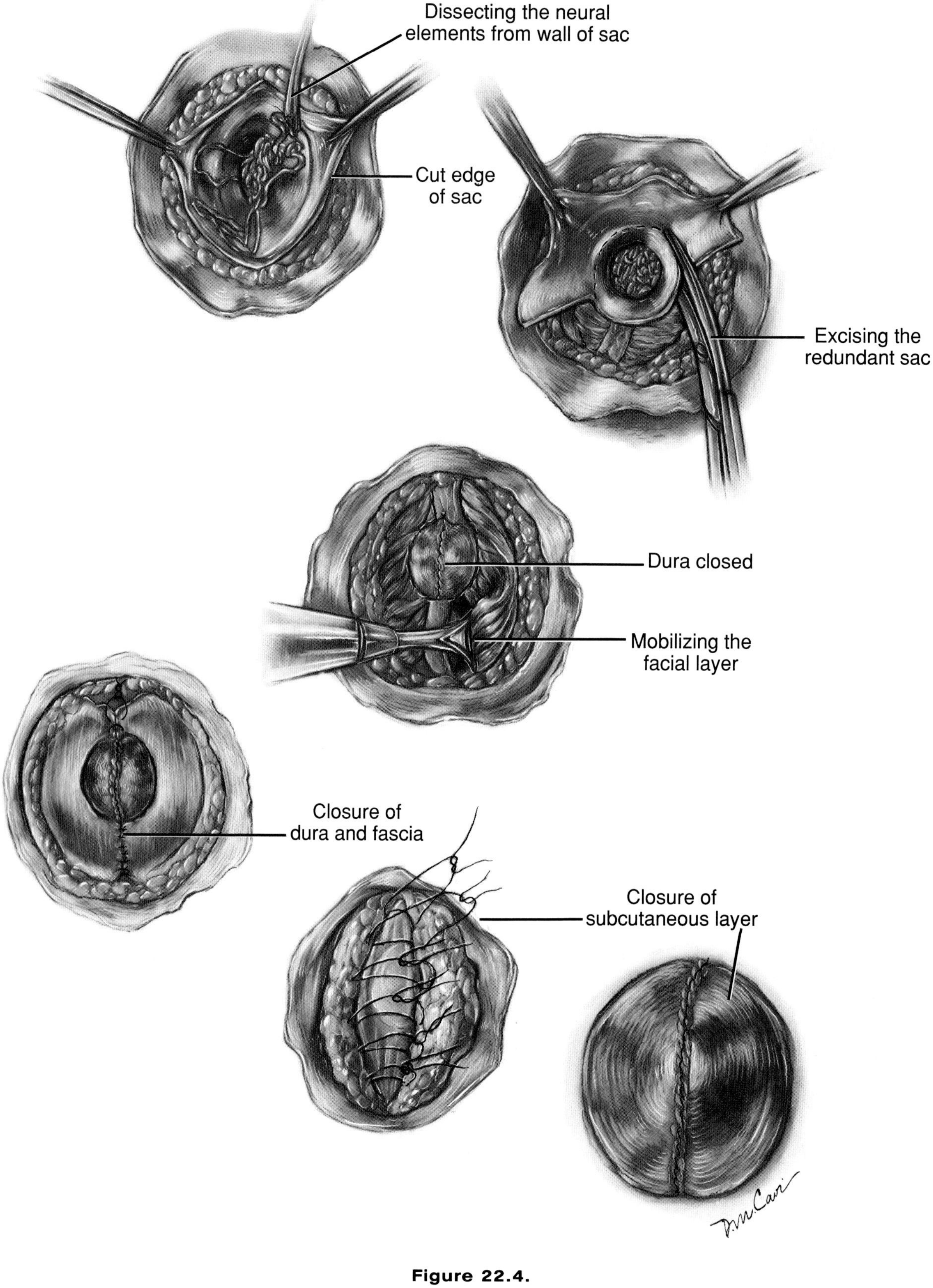

Dissecting the neural elements from wall of sac
Cut edge of sac
Excising the redundant sac
Dura closed
Mobilizing the facial layer
Closure of dura and fascia
Closure of subcutaneous layer

Figure 22.4.

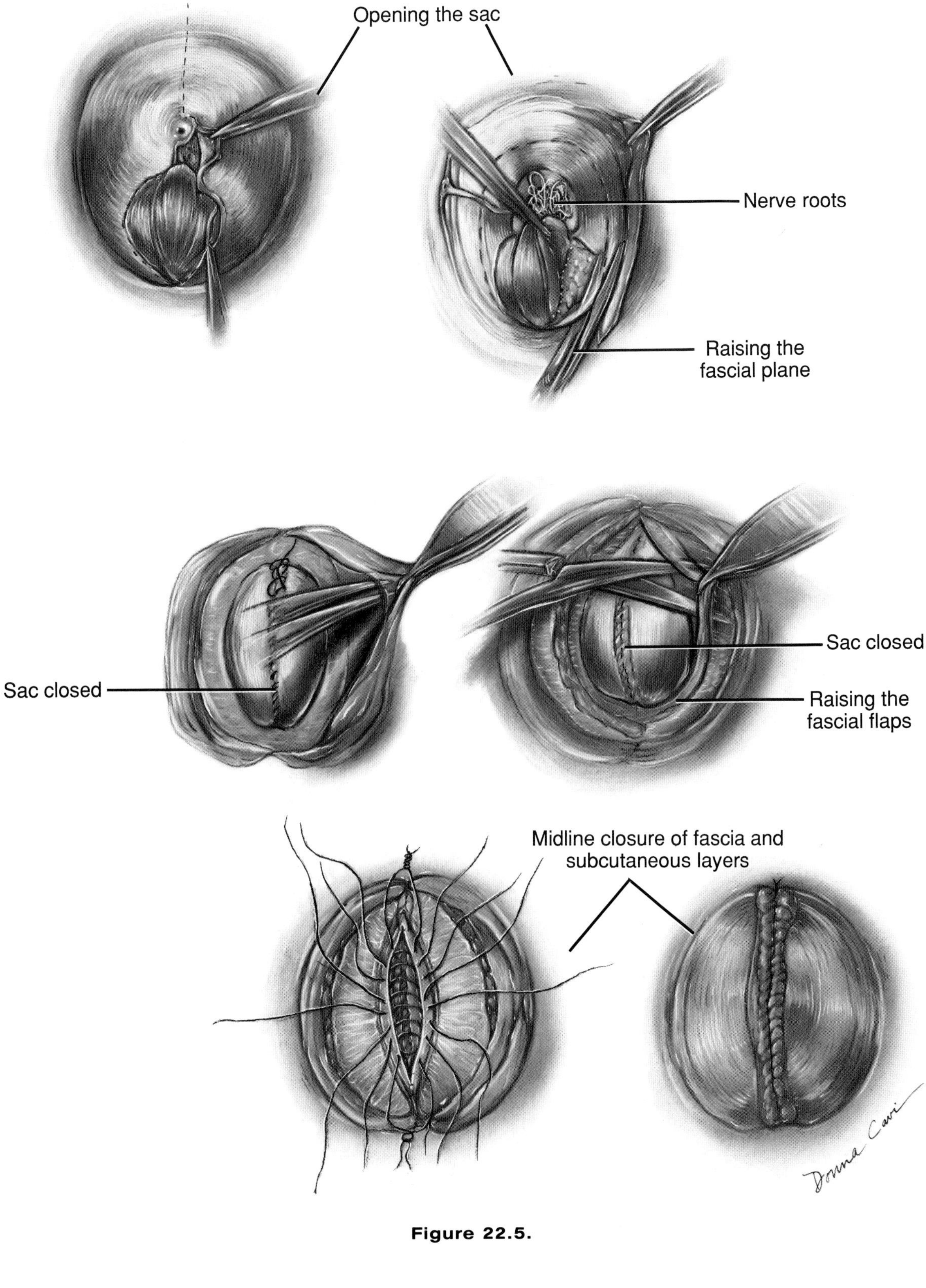
Opening the sac
Nerve roots
Raising the fascial plane
Sac closed
Sac closed
Raising the fascial flaps
Midline closure of fascia and subcutaneous layers
Donna Cavi

Figure 22.5.

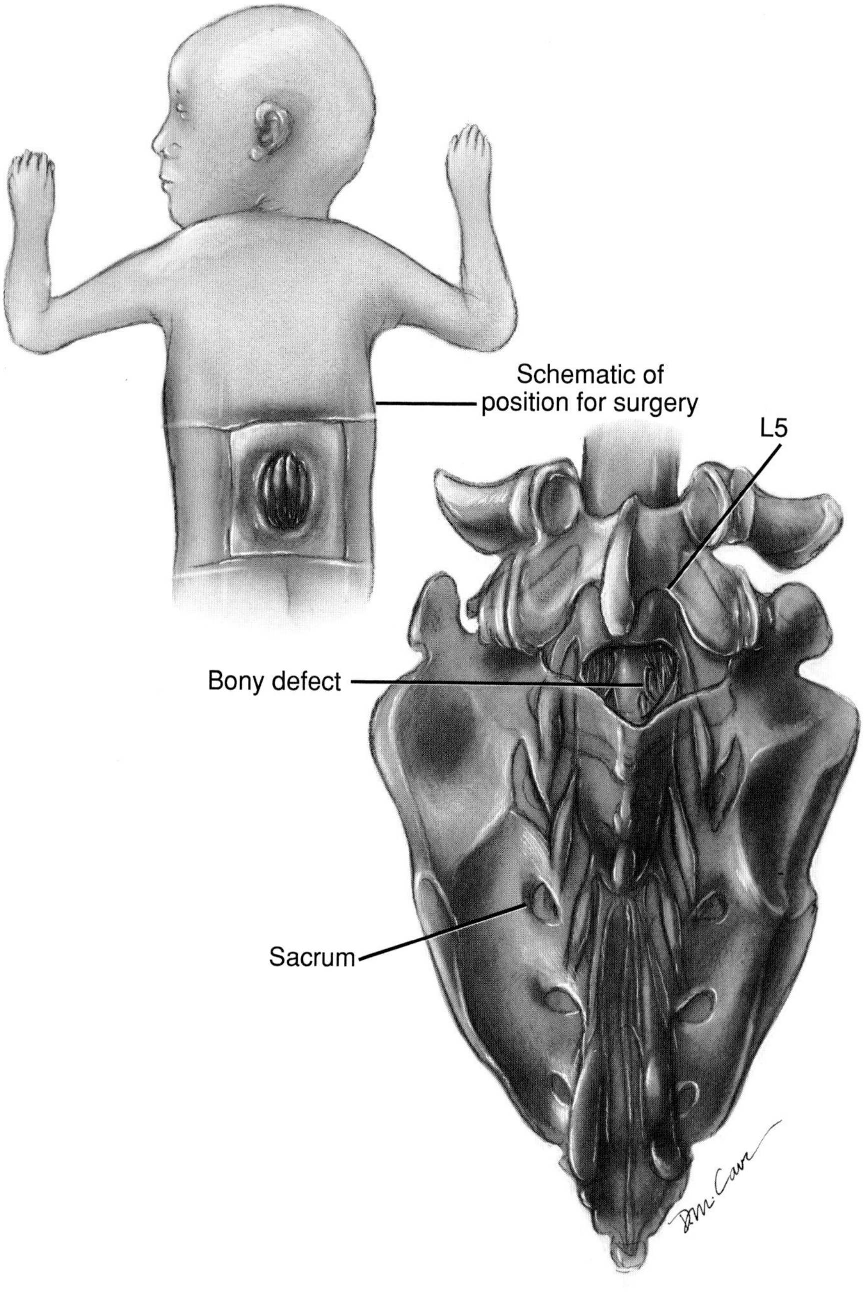

Figure 22.6.

The same incisions described for meningocele can be employed. One technique for the smaller defects is to make an incision circumferentially around the sac at the junction of the sac with skin. This incision is carried through subcutaneous tissue to isolate the neck of the sac from paravertebral muscles down to its exit through the bony and muscular defects. The technique described of carrying out the dissection of the neck bluntly through small superior and inferior incisions is also useful here. This technique has the advantage of freeing all possible viable skin from the sac, a technique that is useful in all but the smallest

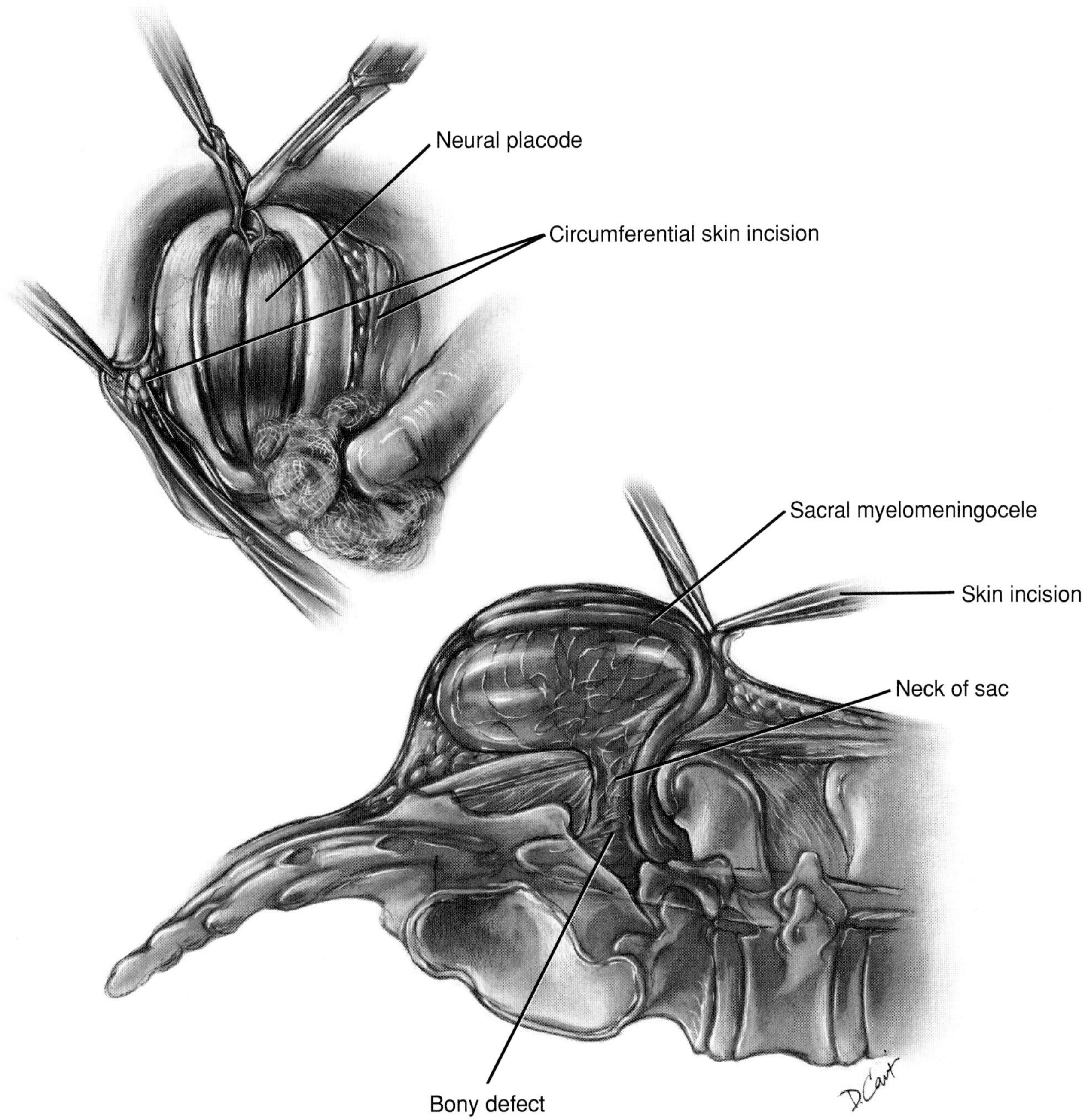

Figure 22.7.

of the abnormalities. Once this isolation is complete, the neural placode should be carefully identified, and the sac opened immediately beside it. The neural placode should be isolated by cutting the sac circumferentially around it. Remember the nerve roots are exiting from the margins of the placode and are usually in the wall of the sac. Magnification can be of help in their identification. They are dissected away from the wall in the sac by gentle blunt dissection. Finger pressure with cottonoid is usually adequate.

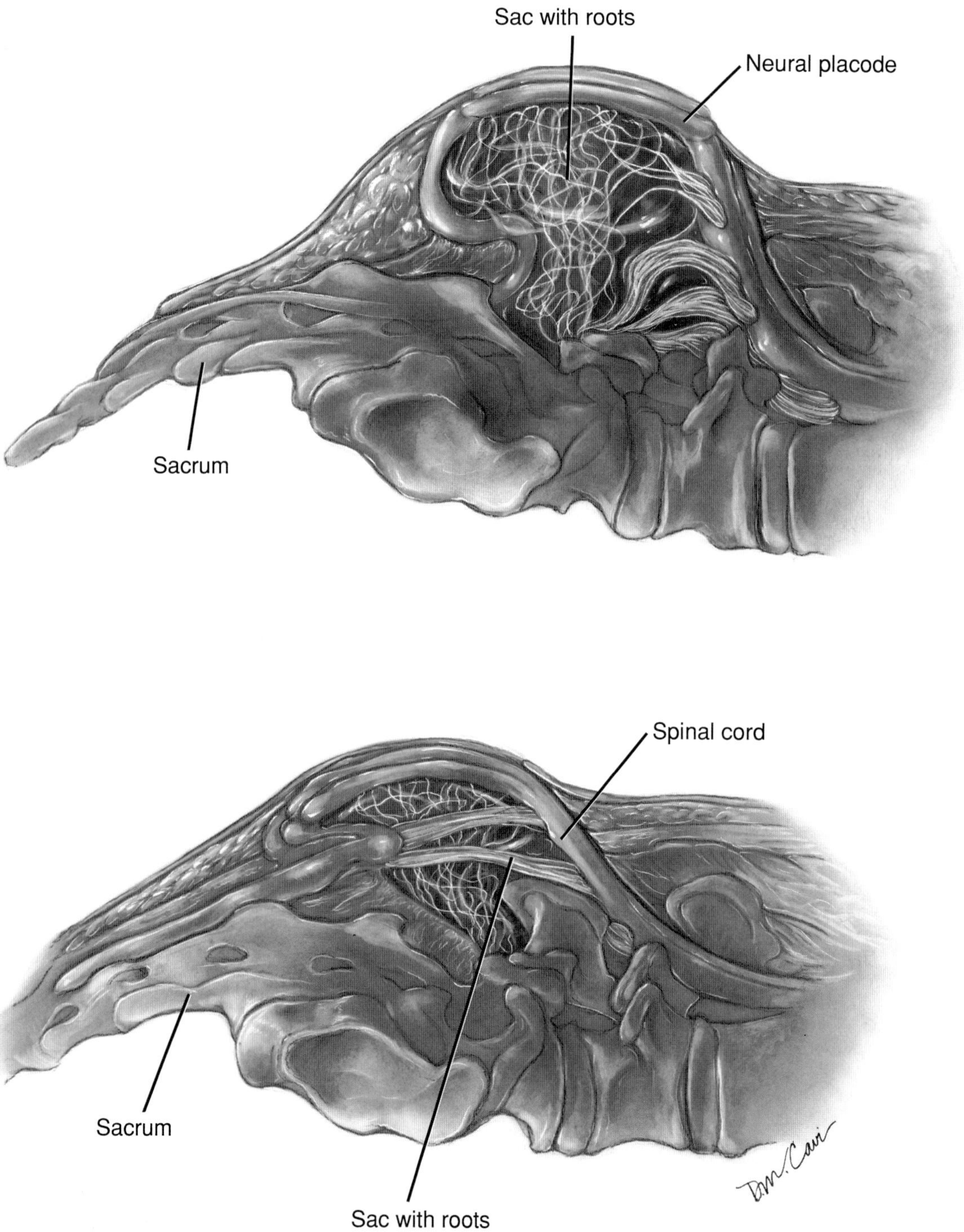

Figure 22.8. Two low-lying sacral myelomeningoceles.

Occasionally, more active dissection even with microscissors is required to free the nerve roots from the sac itself. This should be done circumferentially until all roots are free. It is usually easier to identify them if the dissection begins at the superior margin of the neural placode and extends downward. The smaller distal roots are more difficult to identify, and it is helpful to have the plane well started before they are reached. The placode with all attached nerve roots now free of all overlaying structures is ready for placement into the reconstituted dural tube. The dural sac into which the neural placode can be placed should also be completely isolated from skin; the neck should be identified as it exits from the defect in bone and muscle; and the skin should be completely separated from the sac but as yet untouched otherwise. Even the thinnest remnants of skin should be saved for the closure. There are two possibilities for managing the neural placode. It simply can be dropped within the canal, and the dural tube reconstituted above it. Some investigators have advocated that the opened cord be resutured into more normal anatomical position with fine sutures in the margins, which pull the opened dorsal plates together in the midline, more nearly reconstituting normal anatomy. There is no evidence as yet that this has any effect on function. Closure of the dura can also be carried out in several ways. The sac can be trimmed so that a midline closure is possible. The closure should be watertight with a continuous suture. This reconstitutes an almost normal dural sac. Frequently, particularly with low-placed lesions where it is hard to find good inferior margins, a plication technique can be employed for added strength. This is particularly desirable when skin coverage is questionable. In this technique the dural sac is trimmed so that the end of one wall can be sutured to the side of the second, leaving a large redundant flap of dura above the reconstituted tube. Then, the redundant flap is folded on itself and sutured as a living graft circumferentially to paravertebral muscles. This provides a dual closure that gives an extra layer of tissue, which is particularly valuable if the skin coverage is tenuous. No tethering should occur if the first reconstitution of the dural tube is generous. To provide this secondary closure, the skin must be undermined, exposing the lumbar fascia so that the circumferential suture can be watertight. This technique is usable only with larger sacs where there is adequate redundant dura.

The subcutaneous and skin closure is critical. If possible, the skin closure should be in the midline. This may require undermining the skin flaps even further to allow a vertical closure without tension. The subcutaneous stitches should be heavy enough to pull the skin margins together and release any possible tension on the skin sutures. If a vertical closure is not possible, then a horizontal closure or one that is slightly angled from the horizontal may be possible. With large defects, it is possible that skin flaps will have to be rotated to provide adequate coverage. There are many ways this can be done, and the types of skin incision extensions and flaps will depend on the configuration of the defect to be covered. The most common extension is to convert the skin defect into an exaggerated "S" by making one curvilinear incision upward at the upper outer lateral margin of the flap and one curvilinear incision downward at the lower outer margin on the opposite side. This will allow rotation of flaps to meet in the midline, and undermining of the newly created extensions will usually allow them to be closed without difficulty. The critical factor is the tension with which the flap is closed. If the tension is excessive, then necrosis can occur and the healing can be extremely prolonged. The presence of cerebrospinal fluid (CSF) leak in the face of such necrosis may be catastrophic. Saving all possible skin is the most important trick to good healing. Even when the skin remnants do not have a complete subcutaneous layer beneath them, they can serve as a full-thickness graft, and good healing can be obtained by suturing the viable portions of the skin and allowing the less normal portions to meet in the midline, covering the area that cannot be tightly sutured. In the absence of a CSF leak, this kind of closure will usually provide a satisfactory healing and cosmetically acceptable wound. The lateral relaxing incisions or enormous flap mobilizations that have been recommended in the past are rarely necessary with current techniques for repair.

Lipomyelomeningocele

The presence of a significant lipomatous mass complicates the dissection and repair significantly. Basically, the techniques involved require the combination of the principles used for the treatment of a lipoma, coupled with those utilized for treatment of myelomeningocele. Those myelomeningoceles that have a significant lipomatous component characteristically are

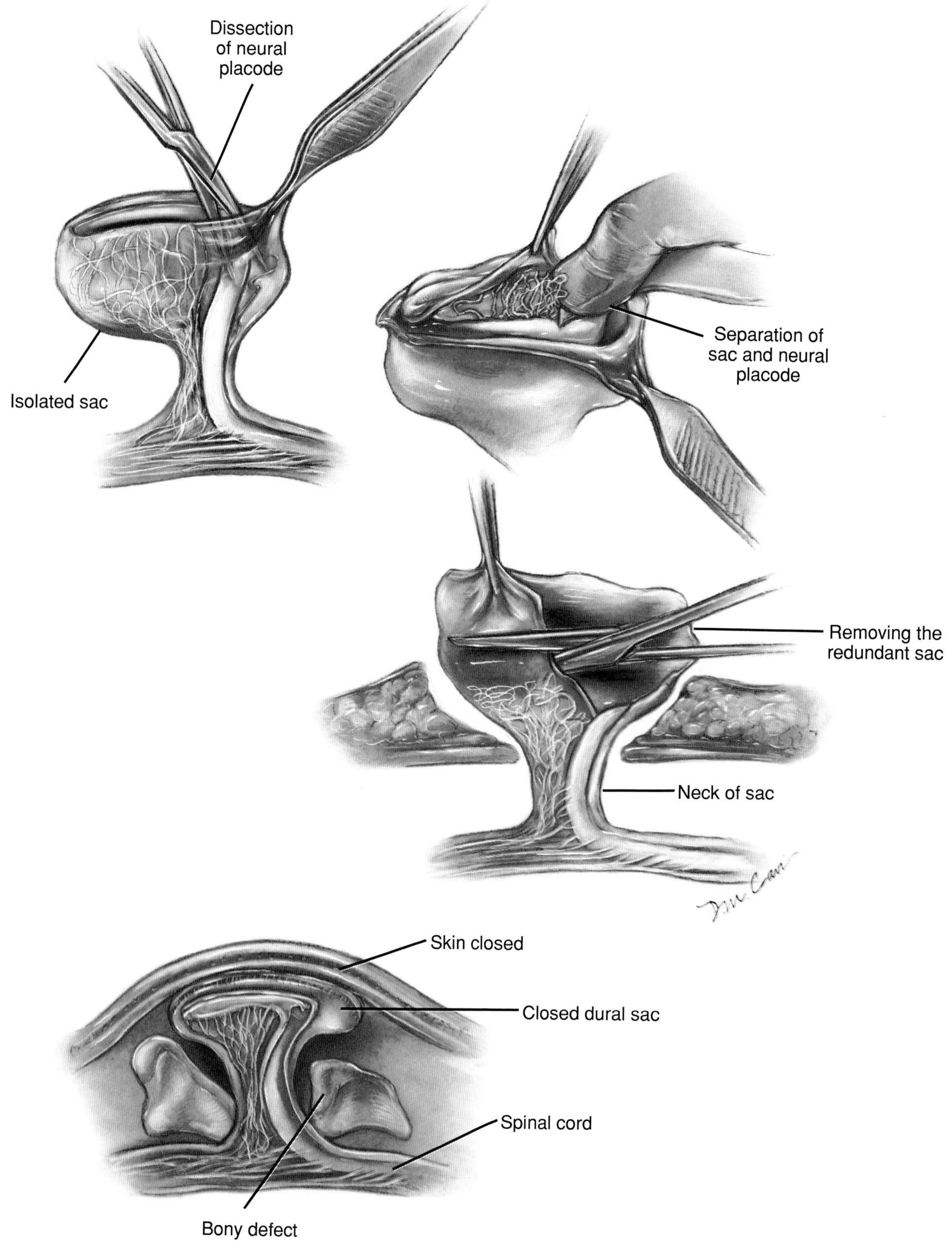
Dissection of neural placode
Isolated sac
Separation of sac and neural placode
Removing the redundant sac
Neck of sac
Skin closed
Closed dural sac
Spinal cord
Bony defect

Figure 22.9.

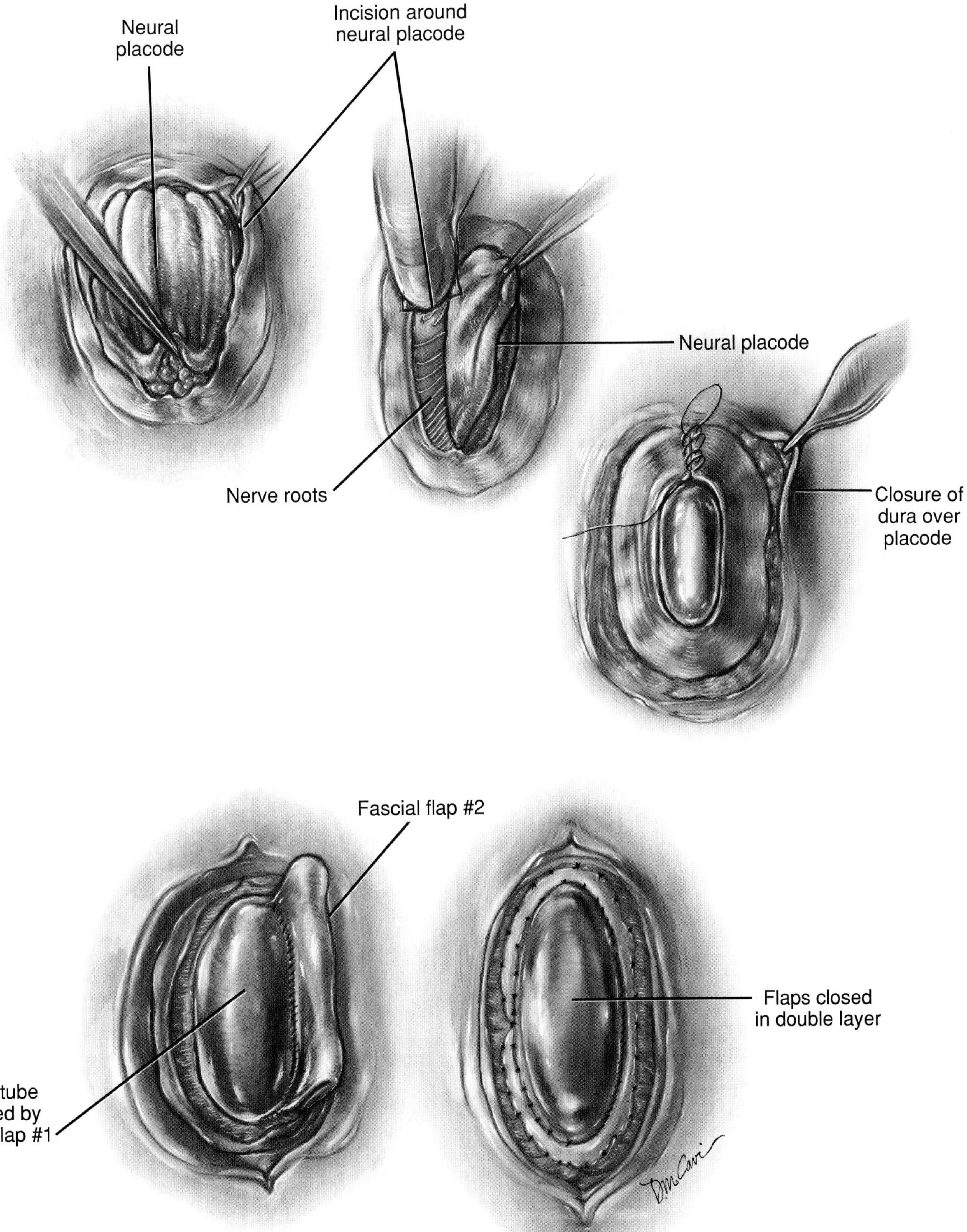
Neural placode
Incision around neural placode
Neural placode
Nerve roots
Closure of dura over placode
Fascial flap #2
Flaps closed in double layer
Dural tube covered by fascial flap #1

Figure 22.10.

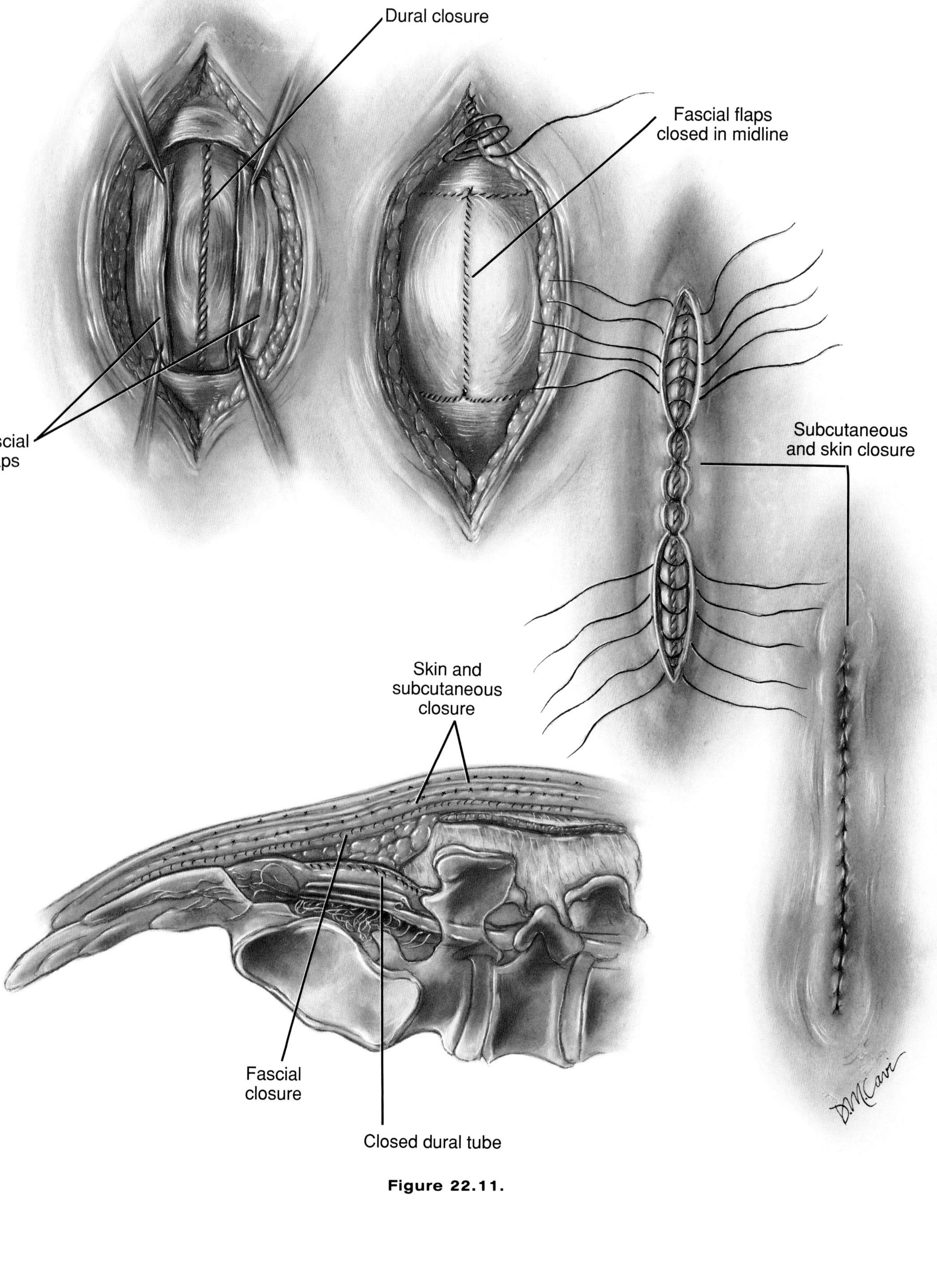
Dural closure
Fascial flaps closed in midline
Fascial flaps
Subcutaneous and skin closure
Skin and subcutaneous closure
Fascial closure
Closed dural tube

Figure 22.11.

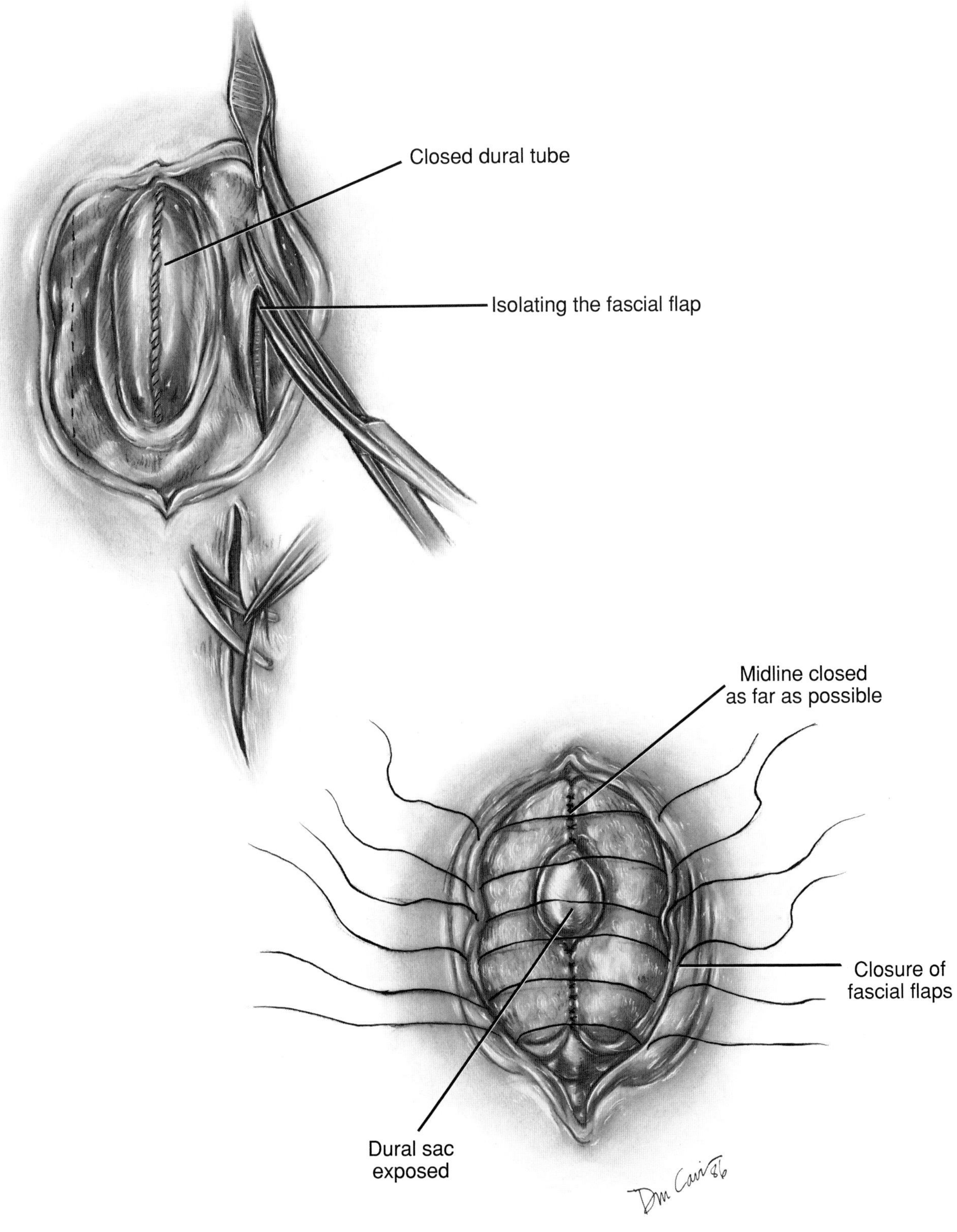
Closed dural tube
Isolating the fascial flap
Midline closed
as far as possible
Closure of
fascial flaps
Dural sac
exposed

Figure 22.12.

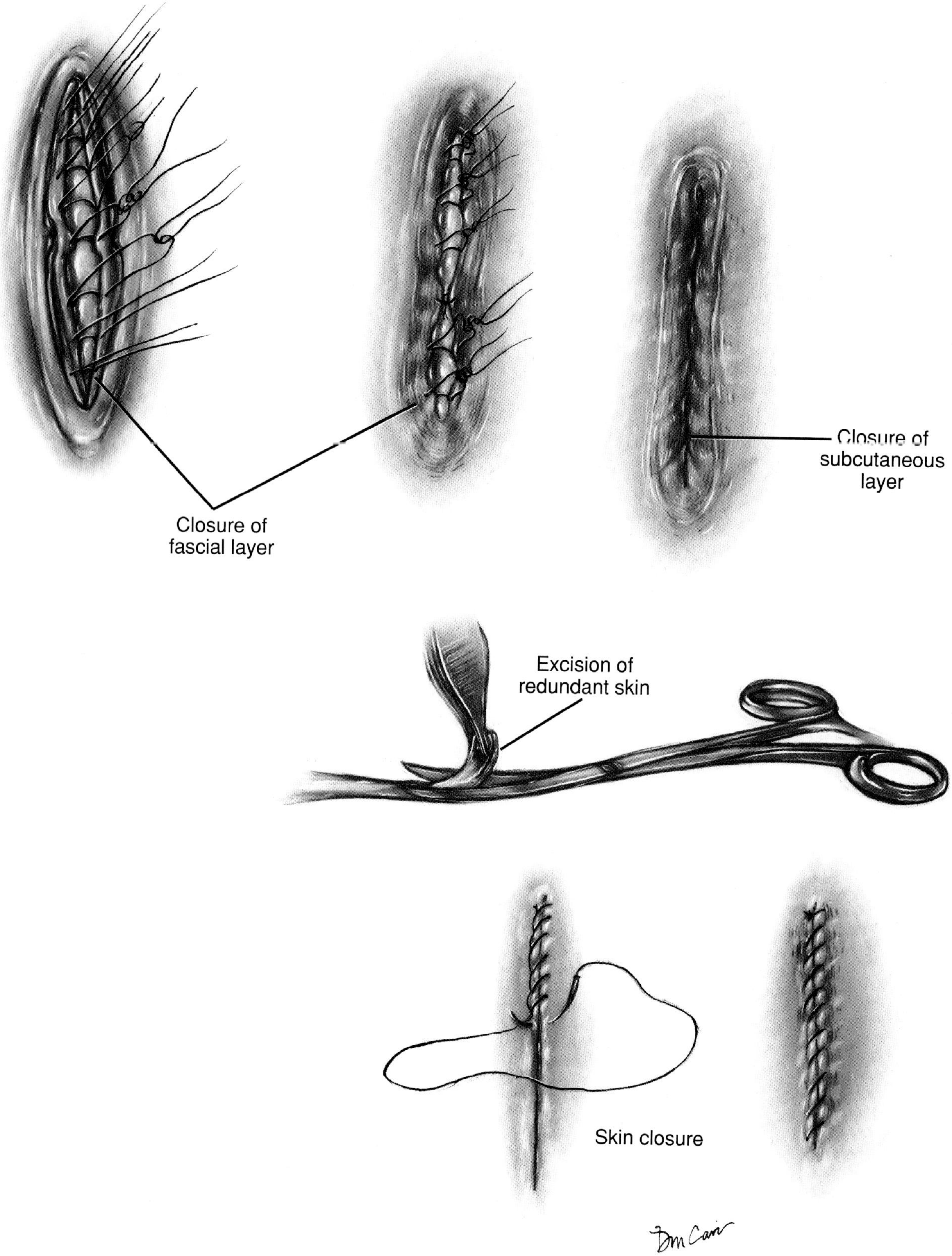
Closure of fascial layer
Closure of subcutaneous layer
Excision of redundant skin
Skin closure

Figure 22.13.

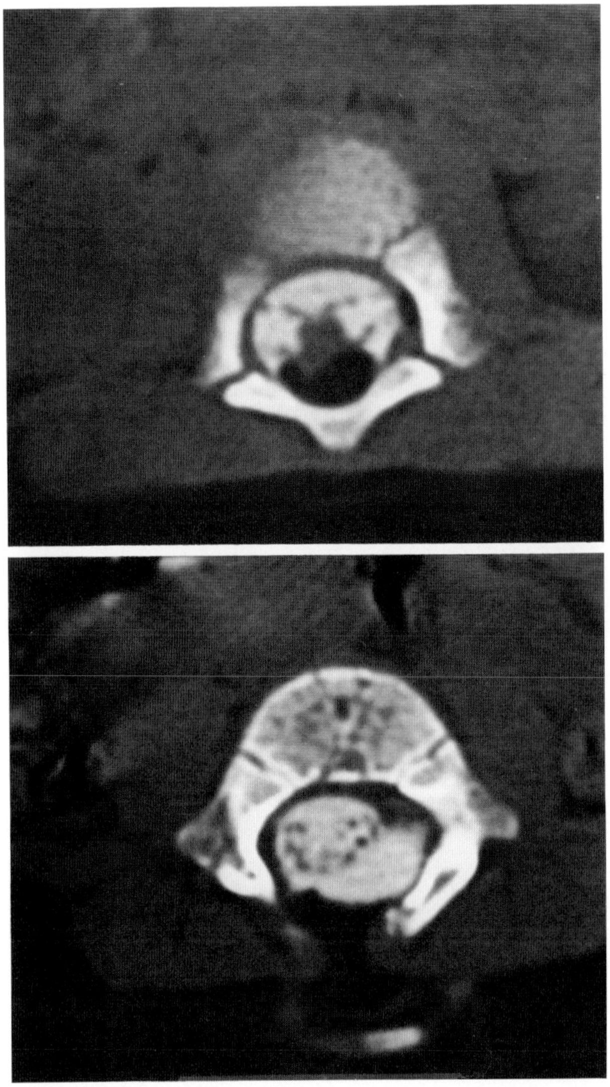

Figure 22.14. Small lipomyelomeningocele showing relationships of fat and roots. Detailed images aid in planning the lateral exposures and lysis of adhesions.

covered wholly or nearly so by normal skin. Skin closure is virtually never a problem with them. The operations are carried out with the patient in the same position, and a midline skin incision is made from well above to well below the lipomatous mass and myelomeningocele. When there is a skin defect, it usually is small with relationship to the entire mass, and the incision can simply approach the defect in the midline, extend circumferentially around it, and then extend to well below the lowermost margin of the lipomatous mass. These lesions often are quite low on the sacrum, so it may not be possible to extend far beyond the lower margins of the mass. Skin flaps are raised, immediately separating normal subcutaneous tissue from the lipoma; the lipoma should then be isolated down to the lumbar fascia. Various anomalies are associated with these lesions. The lipoma may have a significant angiomatous component to it. There may be dermoids within a thickened filum, there may be lipomas within the filum, or there may be additional lipoma within the conus. Each of these situations is quite different, and the surgeon must carefully identify all of the structures involved before resecting anything. The first material to be removed is usually the subcutaneous portion of the lipoma. Most commonly, the myelomeningocele is within the lipoma, so if the resection is injudicious, the sac may be entered and neural structures injured. It is important to remove redundant portions of the lipoma that are subcutaneous, all the while recognizing that neural structures may be encountered within the upper part of the mass, a situation quite different from the usual lipoma uncomplicated by myelomeningocele.

The dissection should be carried around the lipoma until its exit from the defect in muscles and bone is identified. CT scanning and magnetic resonance imaging (MRI) techniques will usually have demonstrated the nature of the lesion explicitly, so that the removal can be tailored to the expected abnormalities. The neural elements within the sac must be dissected free, but this is often very difficult to do completely, and it is probable that lipoma will be left attached. It is not important to obtain a total removal of the lipoma, but untethering the cord is important. In those situations where the neural elements are completely within the lipoma and obtaining a reasonable estimate of their location from external appearance is not possible, it is better to carry out a laminectomy one or two segments above the abnormality, exposing normal dura. The normal dura can be opened and the cord followed from above downward through the lipomatous mass. These abnormalities are so variable in their details that it is difficult to describe each possible variation. The basic principles are the same as those used both for myelomeningocele repair and for removal of congenital lipoma. Enough bone must be removed above that there is no tethering effect from the bone. Enough of the lipomatous mass must be

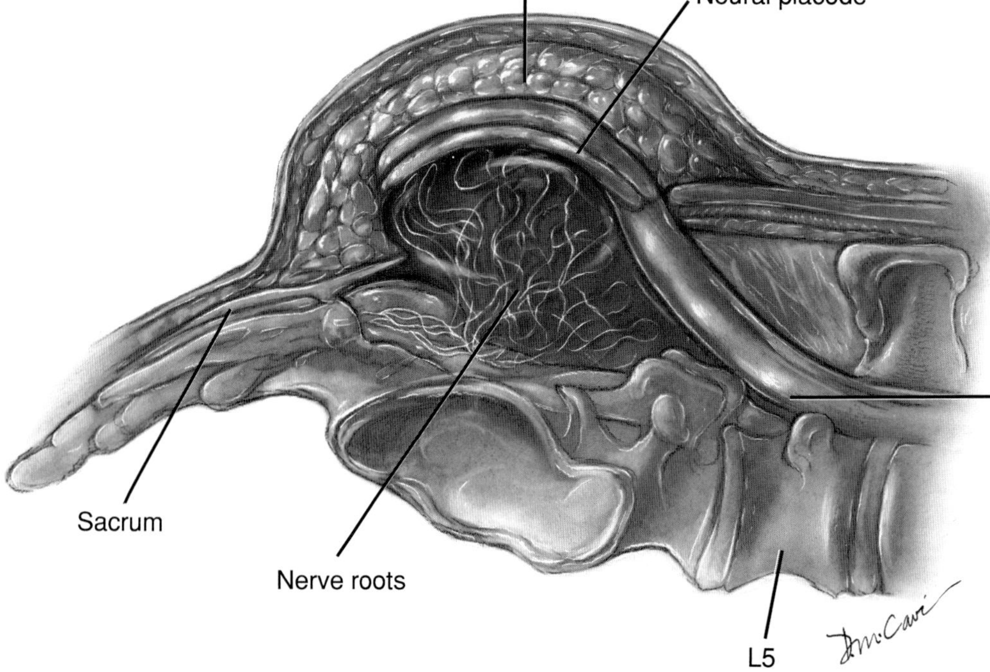

Figure 22.15. Typical sacral lipomyelomeningocele.

removed to provide a cosmetically acceptable result and to untether the spinal cord. This means that the mass must be dissected free circumferentially and cut across at the base while all viable or potentially viable nerve roots are preserved. Then the remainder of the mass should be replaced in a reconstructed dural tube. Accomplishing the first goal requires that the principles described for both anomalies separately are combined to achieve a satisfactory surgical result. Then, the dura must be closed. It is unlikely that there is enough sac to provide (1) a closure that does not compress the lipoma and (2) neural elements that must be replaced within it. Larger lipomyelomeningoceles may provide enough redundant dura for the closure, but most do not. One possibility is a flap of lumbar fascia. Subcutaneous skin flaps are lifted on one or both sides to allow exposure of enough lumbar fascia to close in the midline. When the midline defect is small, a single flap on one side can be fashioned. When the defect is large, bilateral flaps should be raised and brought together in the midline. These are obtained by measuring the appropriate distance to provide a flap that will cover all or half of the defect. Then this flap is incised with a knife, and the resultant graft is dissected free from underlying muscle. The base is left intact, but the flap is cut free superiorly, laterally, and inferiorly. One or both flaps are then brought across to cover the defect. If a single flap is used, it should be sutured circumferentially with interrupted stitches to the paravertebral muscle. Obtaining a watertight closure is important. When bilateral flaps are required, they are sutured together in the midline, and then the superior and inferior margins are carefully sutured down to obtain a watertight closure. In most situations, there is adequate skin to obtain a primary closure without tension. The subcutaneous tissue also should be closed in a watertight fashion, and then the skin closed with interrupted sutures without tension. Occasionally, significant undermining to obtain a closure will be necessary, and rarely, the rotation of flaps by extension of the incisions is required, but these are uncommon.

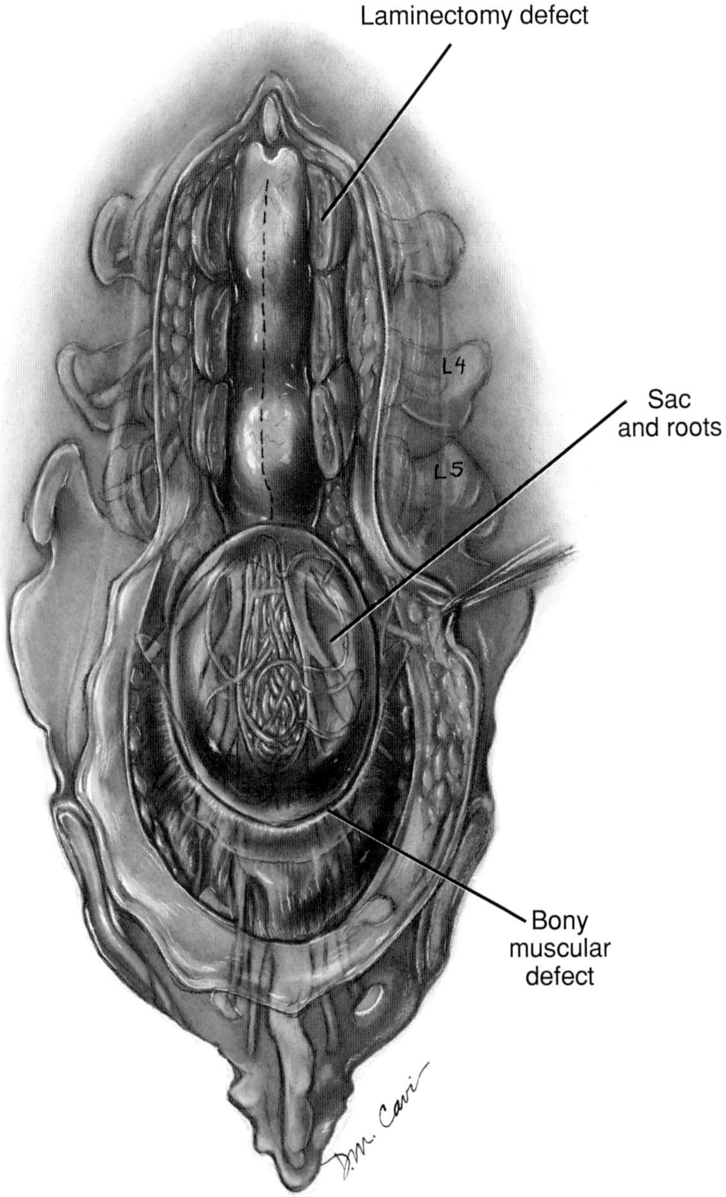

Figure 22.16.

Bony Anomalies and Their Treatment

Some children with bony anomalies will have kyphotic defects that are so severe that they clearly will compromise skin closure. Extensive repair of bony anomalies rarely should be undertaken with primary closure of the defect. Some investigators have recommended bony reconstitution of the spine at the time of the primary closure. Others have recommended delaying definitive spinal surgery until the child is older and the need is determined. Nevertheless, it is important to eliminate deformities that would complicate a satisfactory repair, particularly with regard to skin closure. The bony anomalies are apparent immediately under the skin, and when the skin flaps are raised, the protuberant bony masses are seen on

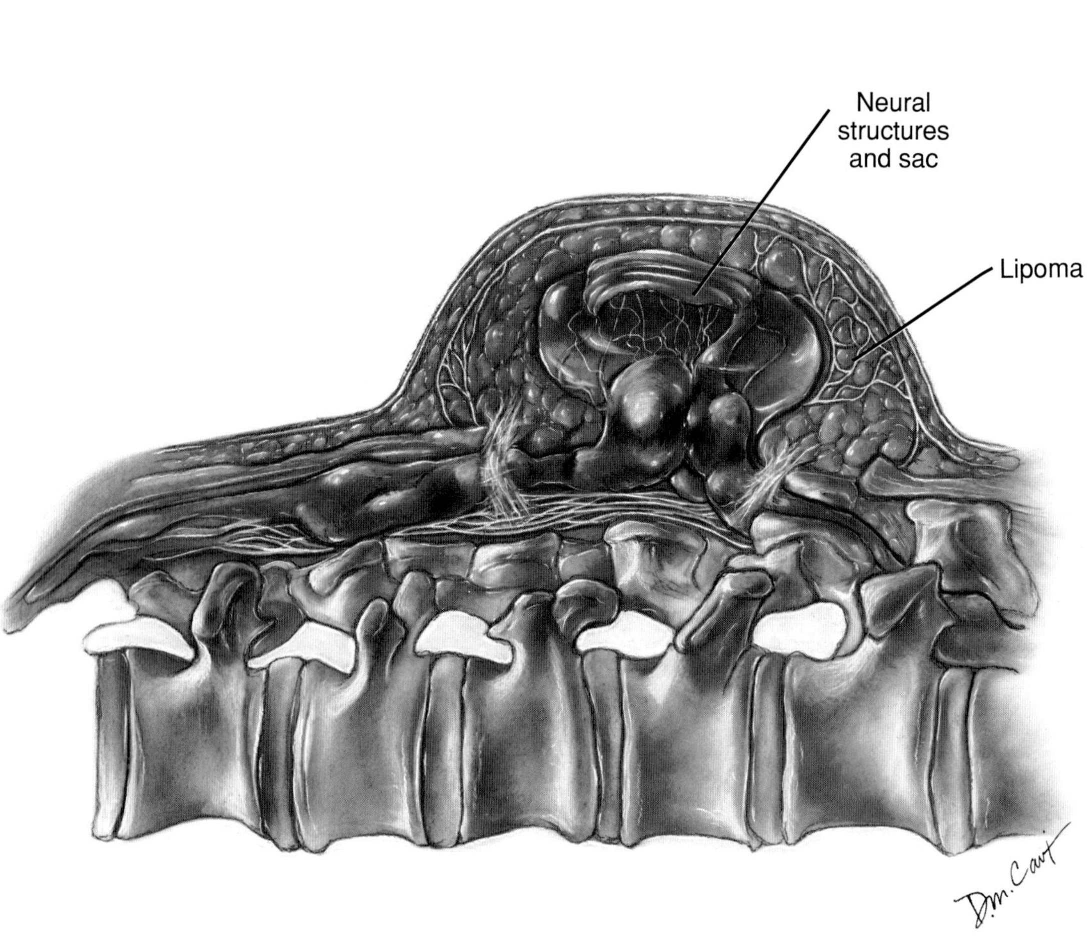

Figure 22.17. Thoracolumbar lipomyelomeningocele.

either side. They include deformed remnants of spine, laminae, and zygapophyseal joints with the pedicle beneath. The exposed portion usually consists of laminar remnants and the abnormal joints. These are managed by excision. A careful subperiosteal dissection of the paravertebral muscle mass from the bony area that is protuberant is accomplished first. The muscle mass should be displaced laterally. This will expose the deformed bone. Since the sac and its contents have been identified and the exiting nerve roots are also seen, bone can be rongeured away until the mass is reduced in size. This bone can bleed copiously, and the bleeding can be a real threat to these small children. As the procedure progresses, the bone should be waxed to minimize blood loss from the cancellous bone. Bone should be removed until the kyphosis is relieved and skin closure can proceed. Frequently, the paravertebral muscle masses can be brought together in the midline to augment the closure, and then the subcutaneous tissue and skin should be closed as carefully as with any other defect. These bony anomalies occur most commonly in paraplegic children with large myelomeningoceles, so that rotation of skin flaps is commonly necessary.

Repair of Bony Abnormalities Associated with Myelomeningocele

The need for repair of the bony anomalies associated with myelomeningocele is still an open question. The techniques advocated by experts in this area vary. Available clinical data concerning the need for any repair are inconclusive and experts argue about the desirability of early repair versus reconstruction of specific deformities at a later time. The patient with a marked kyphotic deformity that compromises skin closure during definitive repair clearly needs immediate attention. The usual procedure is to remove exposed bone. This bone is the deformed remnant of spinous process, laminae, splayed transverse process,

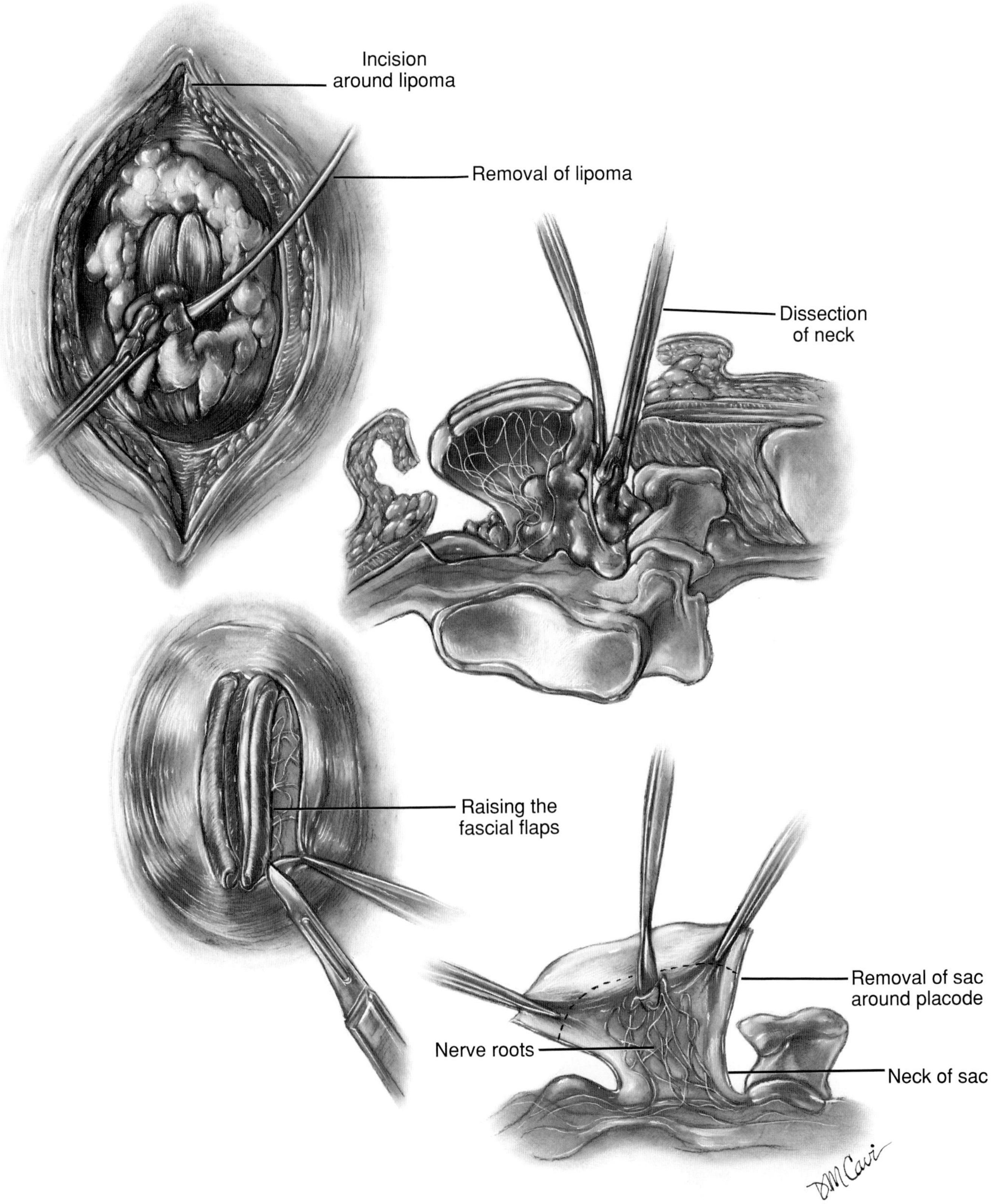

Incision
around lipoma
Removal of lipoma
Dissection
of neck
Raising the
fascial flaps
Removal of sac
around placode
Nerve roots
Neck of sac

Figure 22.18.

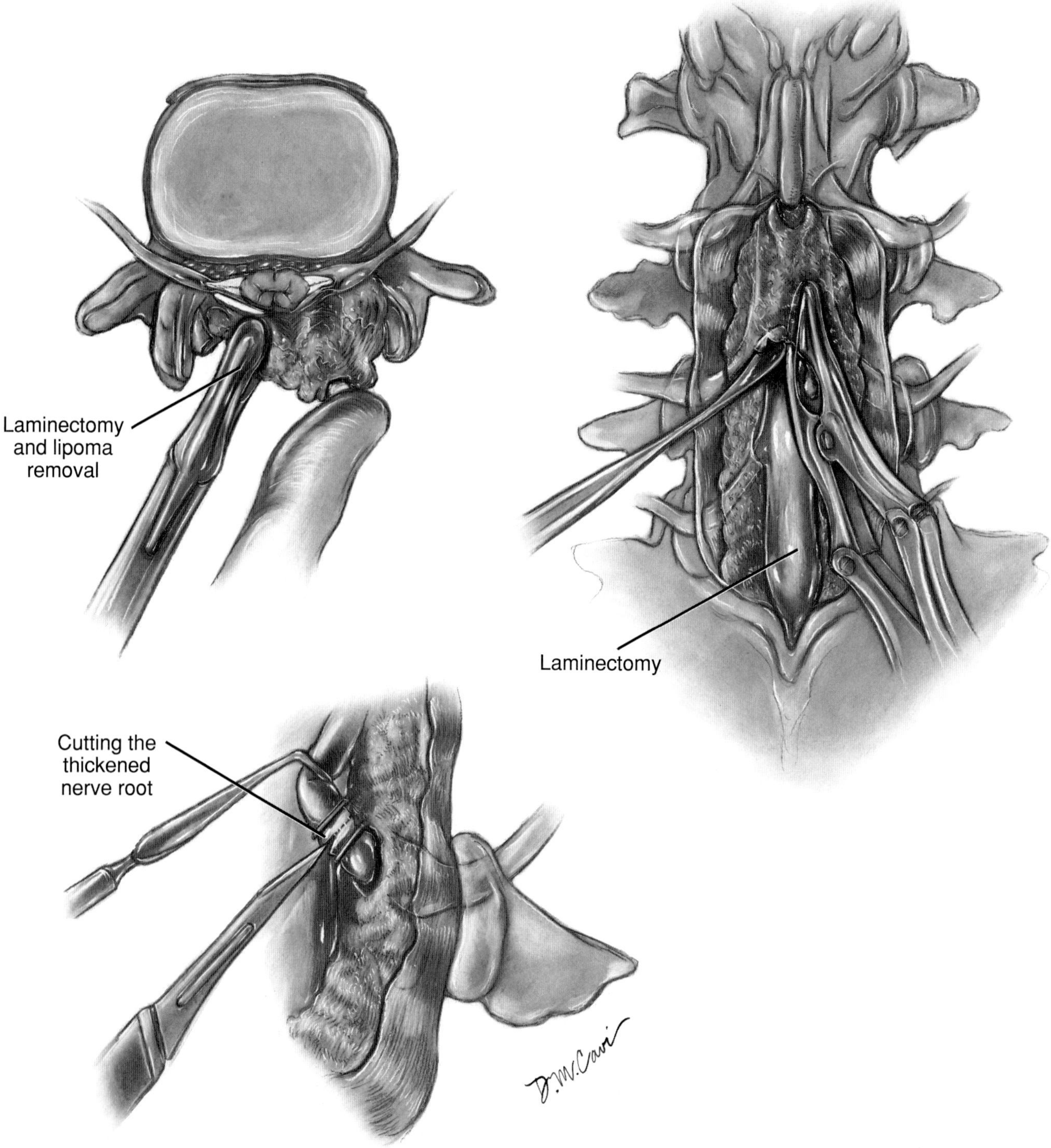
Laminectomy and lipoma removal
Laminectomy
Cutting the thickened nerve root

Figure 22.19.

and pedicle. These patients are virtually always paraplegic, so that reconstructive questions are usually unimportant. Enough bone is removed by standard technique to allow adequate wound enclosure.

Some surgeons advocate reconstruction of the spinal canal in most patients undergoing myelomeningocele repair. The technique advocated is to expose the bony elements on either side of the spinal defect, beginning with the last normal spine and working downward to the base of the defect. These lateral elements are cut through at the junction of transverse process and pedicle and folded toward the midline in an attempt to restore a more normal bony spinal anatomy. Currently available data do not prove that this is a necessary component of the early repair. This is still an area for investigation. Those interested in the possibility of this surgical technique should consult the relevant surgical literature where the matter is still being debated.

Postoperative Care

The postoperative care of these wounds is important. The children should be positioned face down with an abdominal support so that there is no undue tension on the wound. An impervious dressing should be utilized and changed regularly to keep urine and feces from the incision. The wound should be inspected regularly to be certain that CSF is not collecting under tension. If CSF does appear to compromise the incision, the regular taps may be necessary until the wound heals well. Usually, repeated collections suggest hydrocephalus that needs treatment. If a CSF leak does occur, it should be stopped promptly. Reenforcing stitches may have to be utilized in the incision, although multiple taps and a light compression dressing will sometimes suffice.

Lipoma and the Tethered Cord Syndrome

Solid lipomas not associated with myelomeningocele present in three age groups. They may be apparent in the newborn, and in this age group they are often operated on before they are obviously symptomatic. There is a second peak of presentation at the time of the growth spurt when previously asymptomatic lesions present with decreased function in the lower extremities and impairment of bladder control. There is a much smaller group that usually present in young adult life. Symptoms commonly occur in women during their first pregnancy. These patients may have been treated successfully as children, only to suffer an exacerbation of symptoms many years later. The principles of surgery are very much the same in all these groups, varying only in the size of the structures involved.

The goal of surgery is to untether the spinal cord and roots of the cauda equina. In doing so, it is necessary to remove at least some of the lipomatous mass, but the excision of the mass is not the primary goal. When the cord is untethered, further removal of lipoma at the risk of neural function is not necessary.

The operation is done with the patient under general anesthesia in the prone position. A midline skin incision should be made over the lipomatous mass if a posterior subcutaneous lipoma is present. If it is not, then a straightforward midline laminectomy approach is used. In most instances, however, there will be a subcutaneous lipoma. The incision is carried down to the lipomatous mass. The abnormal fat is identified by its consistency, since it is much more firm and septated than the surrounding normal fat. A plane should be developed and the subcutaneous lipomatous mass identified. If it is excessively large, amputating the superior surface of the mass down to the level of the lumbar fascia is worthwhile at this time. There will be no roots at this level. When the mass is smaller, it is better to leave it in place so that the planes simply can be extended toward the dura rather than new planes developed after the removal of the subcutaneous portion of the lipoma. The upper extent of the mass should be identified, and the first intact spinous processes exposed. Self-retaining retractors should then be employed to expose completely the mass, the sacrum below it, and two or three spinous processes above. A subperiosteal dissection of the muscles from the spines and laminae above is carried out. This dissection should be sharp because of the incidence of bony anomalies in the area. The upper retractor should be replaced, exposing at least three laminar segments above the upper extent of the lipoma. The planes around the lipomatous mass can then be developed down to the level of the laminae. This must be done carefully, and magnification is of help, but there is little chance roots will be encountered at this level. At least two spinous processes above are then removed, and a laminectomy is done. It is easier to enter the epidural space one level above the lipoma than at the junction of the bone with the lipoma.

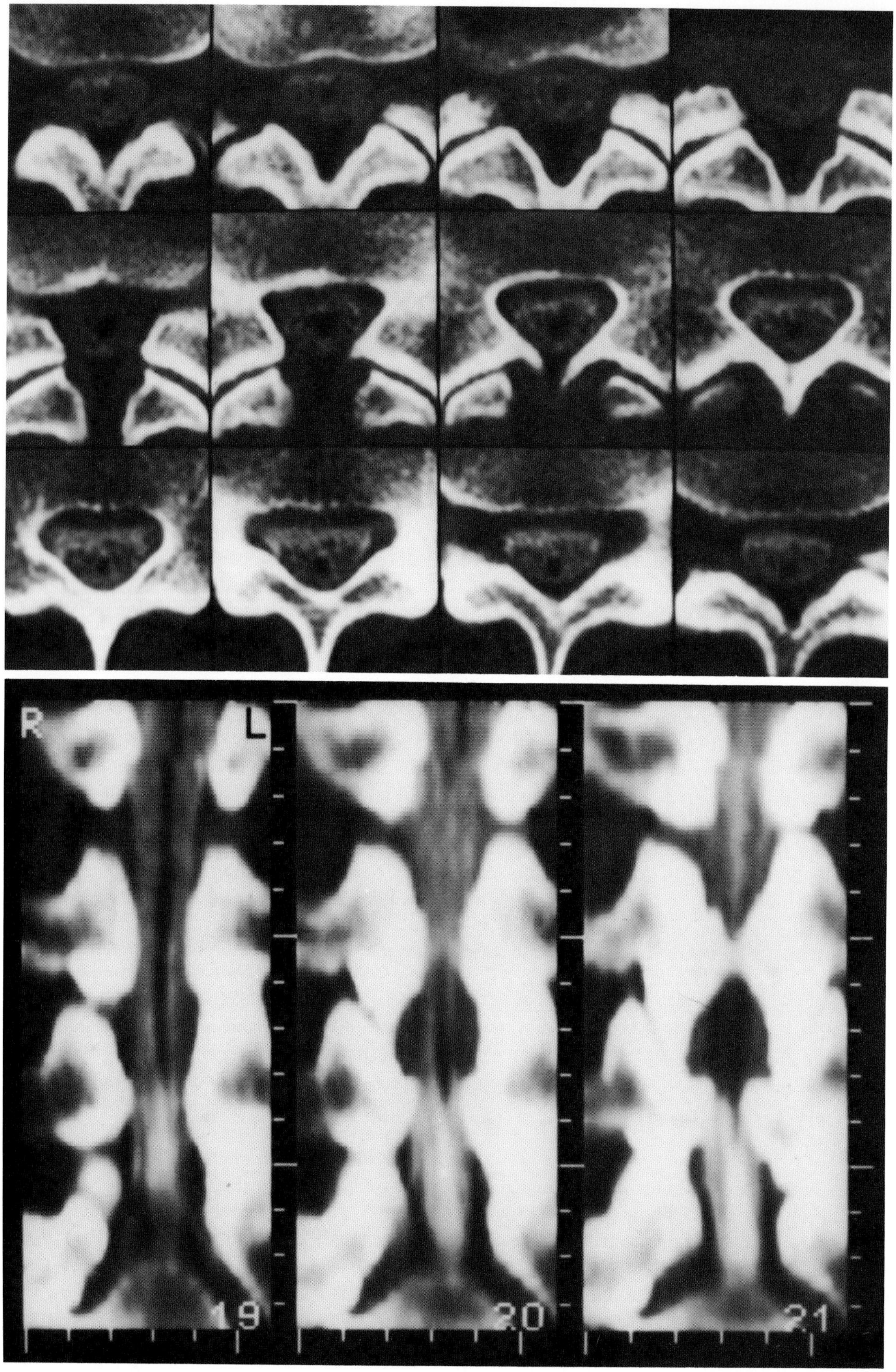

Figure 22.20. Typical picture of lipomyelomeningocele, with fat showing as a bright signal separate from dural sac and nerve roots. Reconstruction demonstrates the meningeal component and the fat.

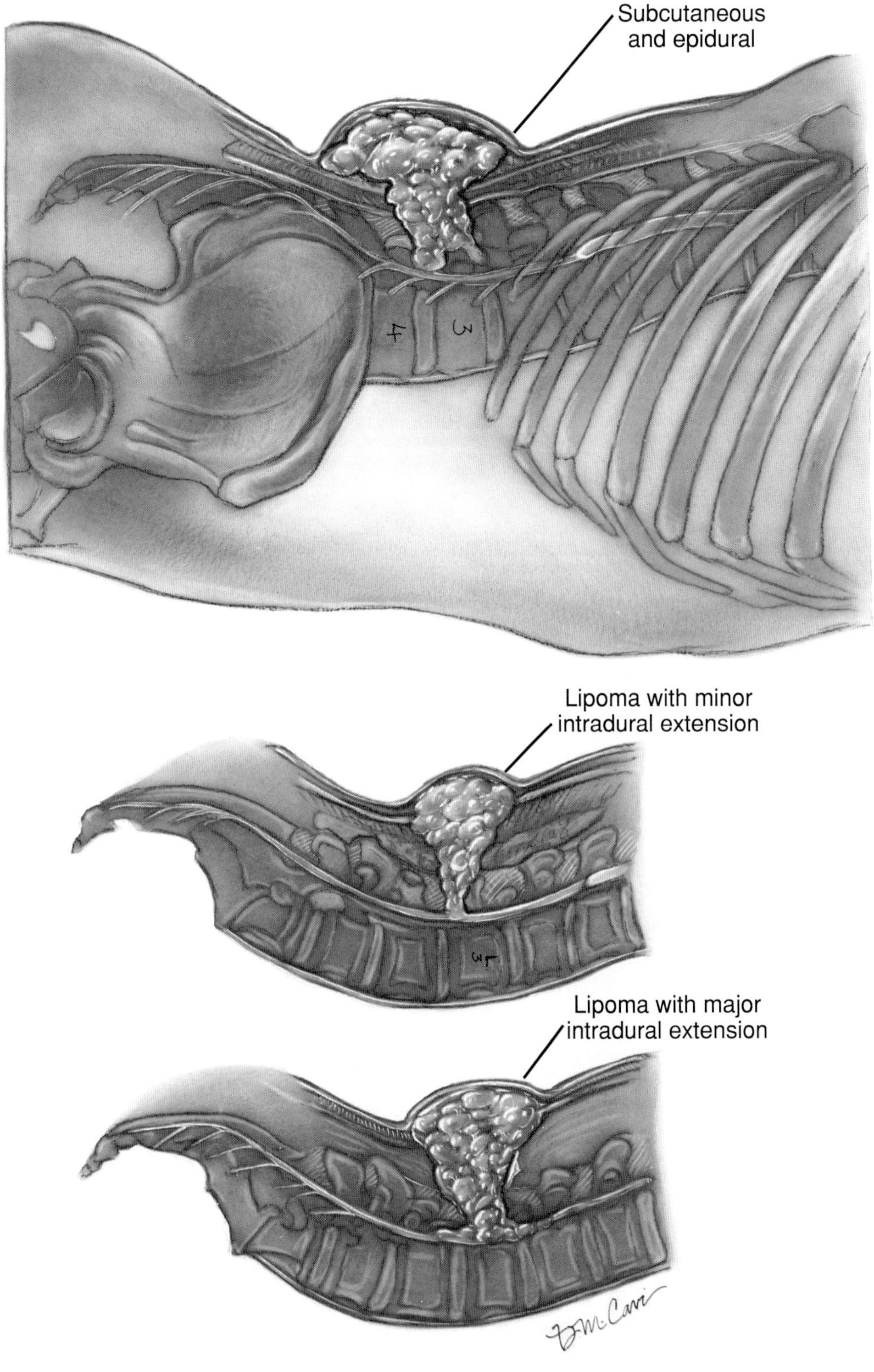

Figure 22.21. Lumbar lipomas.

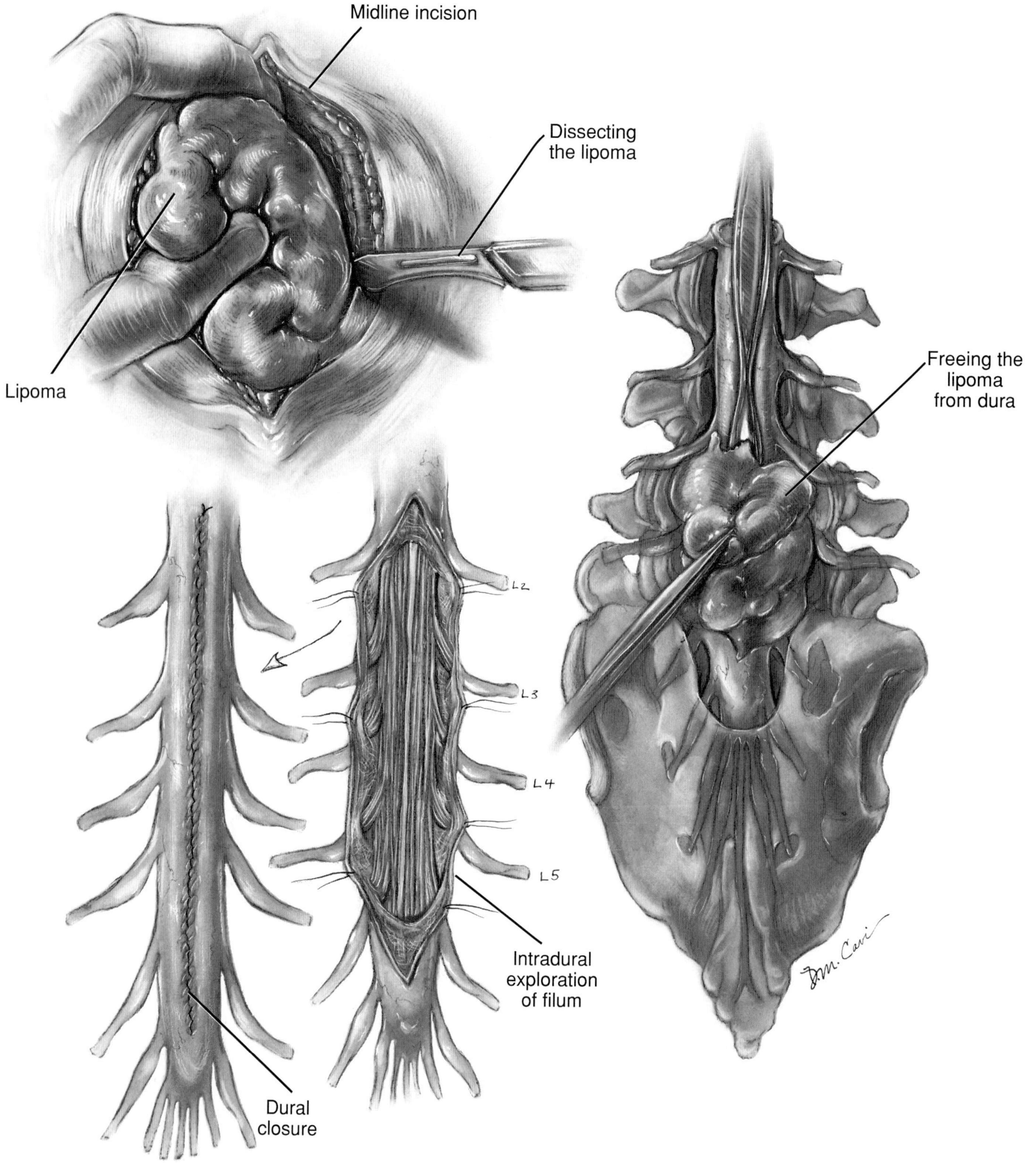
Midline incision
Dissecting the lipoma
Lipoma
Freeing the lipoma from dura
L2
L3
L4
L5
Intradural exploration of filum
Dural closure

Figure 22.22.

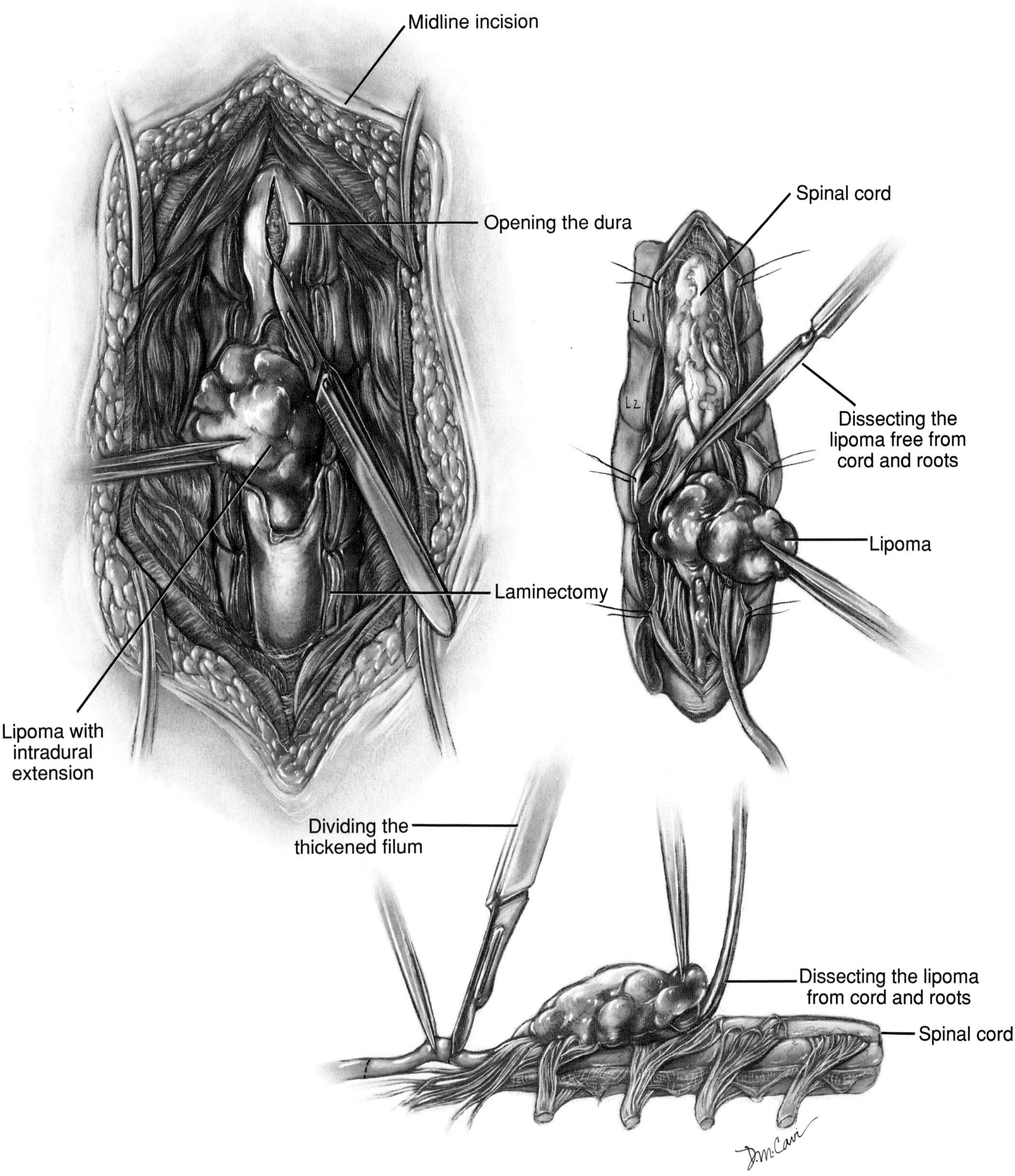
Midline incision
Opening the dura
Spinal cord
Dissecting the lipoma free from cord and roots
Lipoma
Laminectomy
Lipoma with intradural extension
Dividing the thickened filum
Dissecting the lipoma from cord and roots
Spinal cord

Figure 22.23.

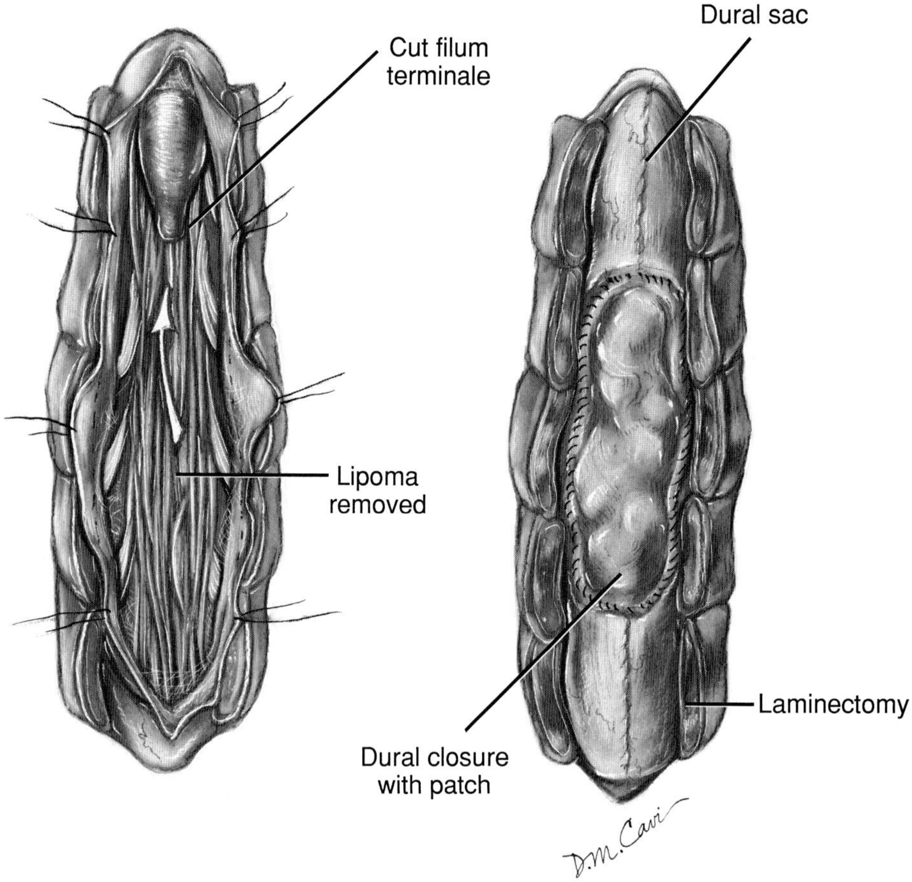

Figure 22.24.

These lipomas may present in several ways. Some simply end on the dura. In that situation, the lipomatous mass can be completely removed from the subcutaneous space and shaved off the dura, leaving that structure intact. After this is done, open the dura and make sure that there is no tethering effect on the roots. Often, there is an intradural component with involvement of the neural elements. One type of lipoma simply involves the roots locally at the level of the intradural extension. A second type of lipoma shows extension superiorly to involve the region of the conus that is nearly always encountered by an abnormally low lying position, and the third occurs when there is a true myelomeningocele involved with the lipoma. In this situation, the lipoma is usually attached to the open neural placode. The operation for this condition is described under myelomeningocele repair.

Once the dura is opened, the extent of intradural involvement can be demonstrated. Usually, the dural tube can be identified laterally at the margins of the lipomatous mass penetrating through it. When this is the case, the dural edges should be carefully separated from the lipoma and tagged back out of the operative field, exposing the lateral margins of the lipoma and the associated nerve root. By opening the dura two segments above, it will be possible to identify whether the spinal cord is abnormally low and if the lipomatous mass involves the conus. The goal of the surgery is not the total excision of the lipoma. The operation is designed to untether the cord. This is accomplished by removal of the subcutaneous mass, opening the dura, and removal of as much of the intradural mass as possible. However, nerve roots should not be sacrificed for the removal of lipoma. With use of high magnification, the next goal of surgery should be to

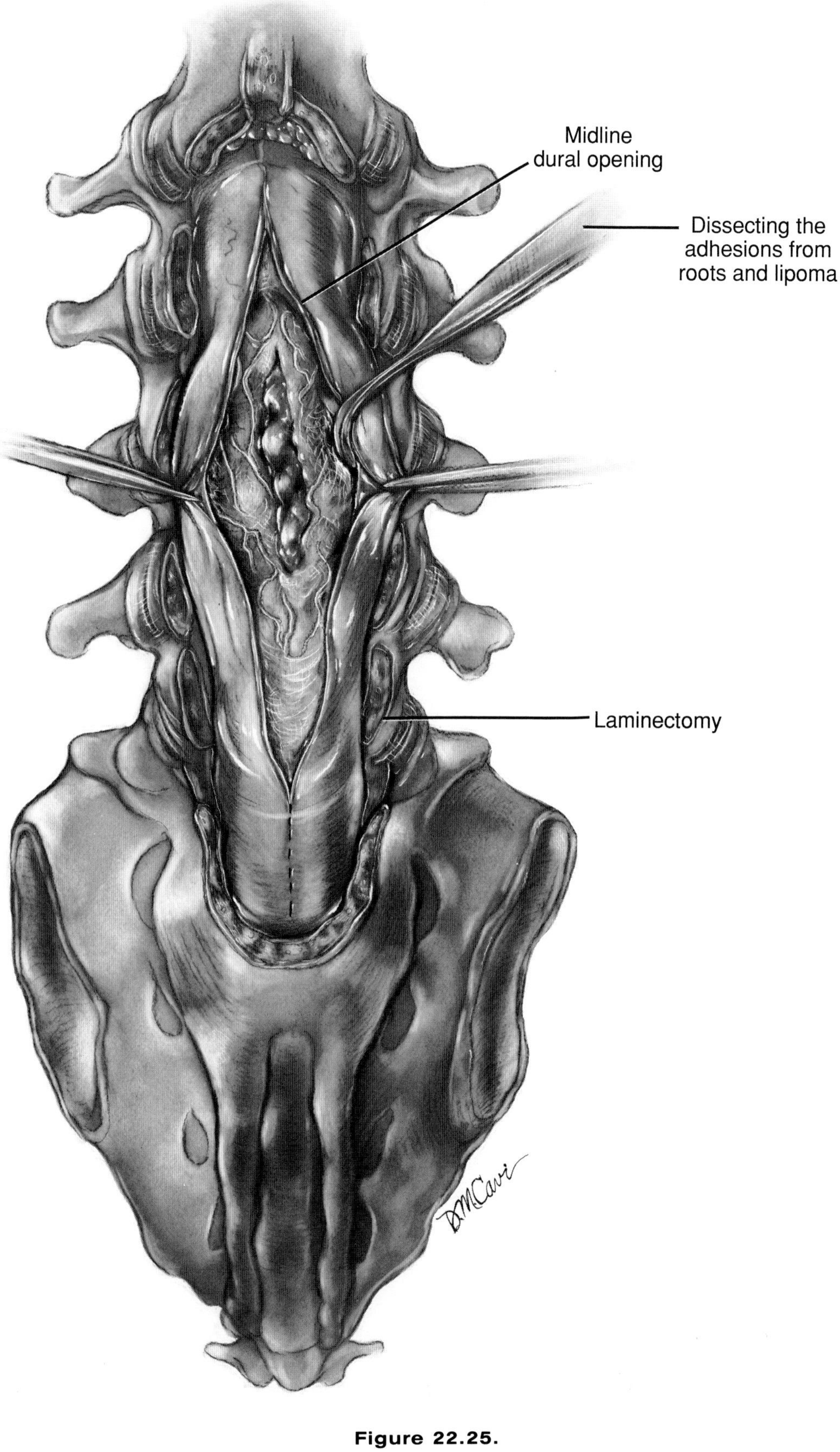
Midline
dural opening
Dissecting the
adhesions from
roots and lipoma
Laminectomy

Figure 22.25.

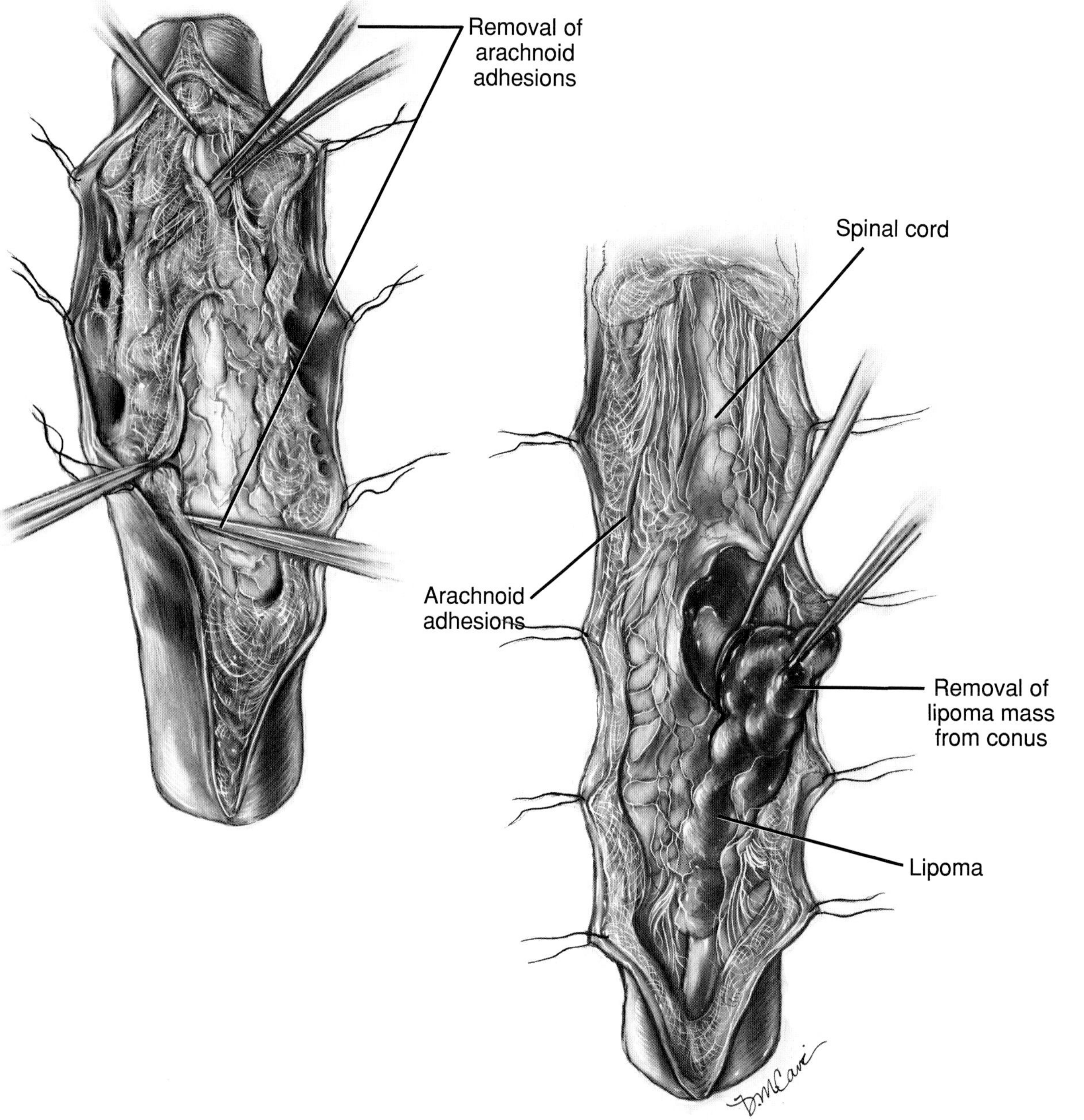

Figure 22.26.

identify the lateral margins of the lipoma carefully, freeing any dural or subcutaneous adhesions and identifying the roots at their exit zone. The roots should also be free. When this is done on both sides, from the superior to the inferior margin of the mass, it should be possible to identify all of the exiting roots. Those that leave the lowermost portion of the lipoma are the smallest and most difficult to dissect free. Sometimes, an enlarged filum terminale can be seen, and this may contribute to the tethering effect. When it is easily identified, it should be divided. Differentiating this from sacral nerve roots can be difficult but

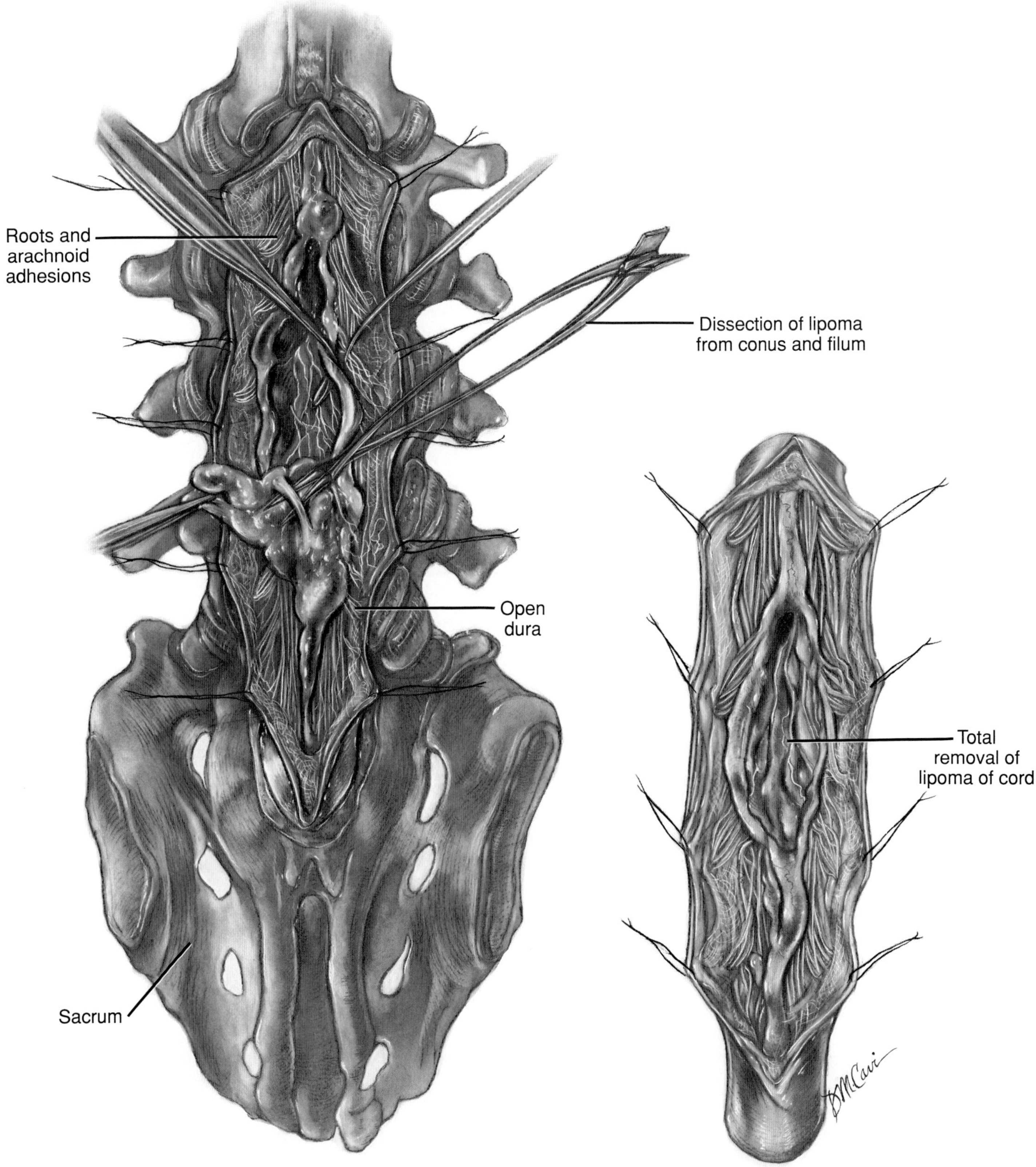
Roots and
arachnoid
adhesions
Dissection of lipoma
from conus and filum
Open
dura
Sacrum
Total
removal of
lipoma of cord

Figure 22.27.

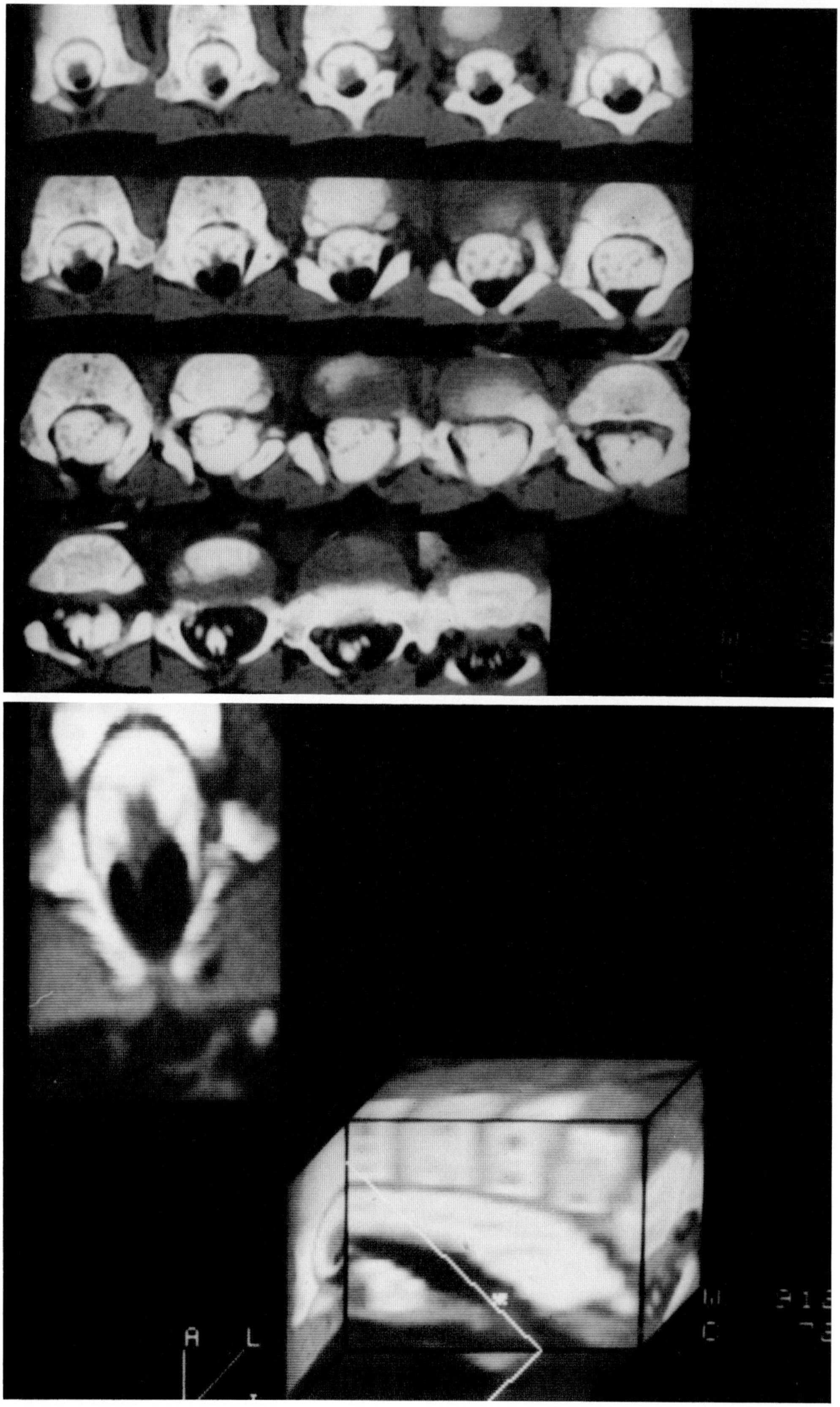

Figure 22.28. CT myelogram demonstrates a prominent filum terminale with attachment to the sacrum. Simple section of the filum resulted in relief of the tethered cord syndrome.

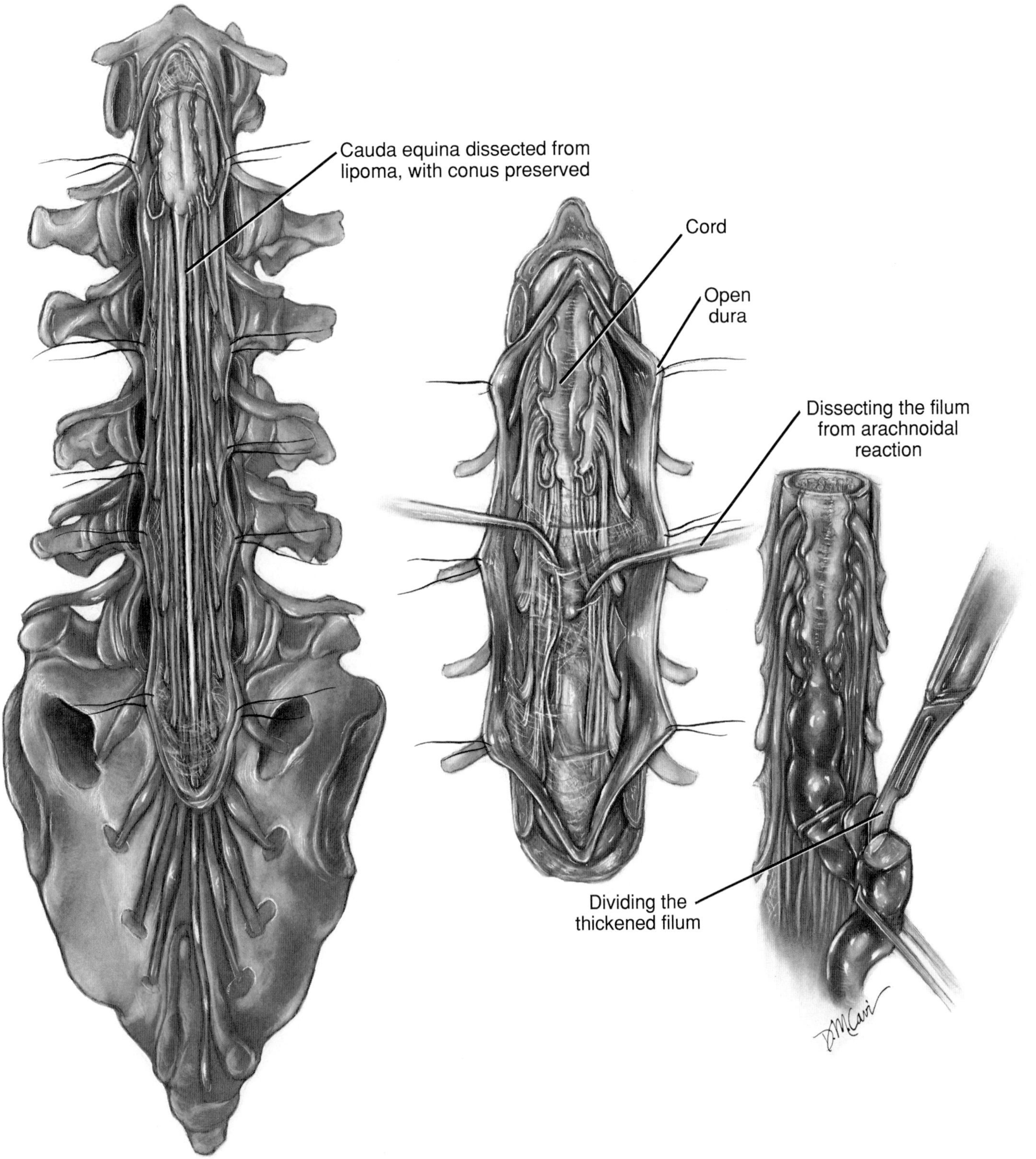

Cauda equina dissected from lipoma, with conus preserved
Cord
Open dura
Dissecting the filum from arachnoidal reaction
Dividing the thickened filum

Figure 22.29.

is a necessity if the filum is to be divided. A nerve stimulator can be of help in identifying neural elements. Since these are sacral roots, it may be helpful to have a catheter in place so that simple cystometrogram studies can be carried out. Once the lateral and inferior margins have been freed from surrounding tissue and all possible lipoma has been removed, it is unlikely that anything further can be done or needs to be accomplished. These maneuvers will untether the cord and provide the best chance for maintenance or restoration of function. A dural patch is used to achieve circumferential watertight closure. If the lipoma has terminated on the dura, then the dural opening simply can be closed with a linear suture. When there has been a significant intradural lipoma, it is unlikely that the dura can be closed without compromise of the intradural structures. A patch of lumbar fascia or artificial dural material can be applied in a watertight fashion. The dural patch should be tailored so that the dura is closed without creating a pseudomeningocele from flap redundancy. Closure of the incision is difficult. The collection of fluid beneath these large flaps required by the isolation of the lipoma can be a troublesome postoperative complication. The flap should be tacked down to lumbar fascia to obliterate dead space, and the midline incision closed so that the suture line can be as watertight as possible. Then the skin also should be closed to prevent CSF leak, and a lightly compressive bandage applied to try to keep the subcutaneous flaps in that position until healing occurs. The denervated skin in large lesions may interfere with wound healing, and major breakdown is not uncommon.

Tethered Cord and Diastematomyelia

There are situations in which the cord is tethered from an abnormally thickened filum without any associated myelomeningocele or lipoma. This is an unusual anomaly but does occur and can be treated effectively with surgery. Current imaging techniques allow the abnormal anatomy to be accurately localized. By using standard techniques the laminectomy should be carried out one or two segments below the demonstrated end of the spinal cord and at least one segment above. This allows the conus to be explored and means the filum can be identified with accuracy. Following standard exposure, the dura is opened in the midline, and the conus is identified. Anterior and posterior roots should be separated until the filum is seen. A midline approach between the posterior roots at the tip of the conus is best. The filum can be identified because it exits from the tip of the conus. Often, this filum is greatly widened and thickened, so it is very hard to tell where the conus ends. It should not be cut when there is any question of neural tissue remaining, and it may require extension of the incision to find a definite fibrous filum. Usually, an incision two segments below the conus is enough. Rarely are there blood vessels of any consequence, so it is possible simply to crush the filum at this level with a small clamp and divide it. Clips will obscure future imaging. The dura should be closed in a watertight fashion, and the wound needs no other special attention.

SECTION 7

Arteriovenous Malformations

23

Spinal Arteriovenous Malformations

It is now recognized that there are two major types of spinal arteriovenous malformations (AVMs), distinguished by whether the location of the vascular nidus of the AVM is dural or intradural. The intradural lesions are further classified into three distinct subtypes: juvenile and glomus AVMs, in which the nidus lies completely or partially within the cord parenchyma; and direct arteriovenous fistulae, in which the transition from artery to vein occurs without an intervening glomus of abnormal vessels.

Since the goals and the techniques of treatment of the discrete types differ, the first stage in successful treatment is delineation of the specific type of AVM with which an individual patient is afflicted. Preoperative radiographic studies should also demonstrate the presence and precise location of the vascular nidus of the AVM, permit determination of the operability of the malformation, and aid in the safe obliteration of the malformation by demonstrating the vascular anatomy of all feeding vessels of the AVM and the anatomy of the normal cord vasculature in the region of the AVM. This preoperative requisite information usually requires a combination of currently available diagnostic studies.

Most spinal AVMs are discovered by myelography, through which serpentine filling defects in the dye column merely indicate the presence of a process that increases vascularity. Digital vascular imaging (DVI) after intraaortic injection of contrast often confirms

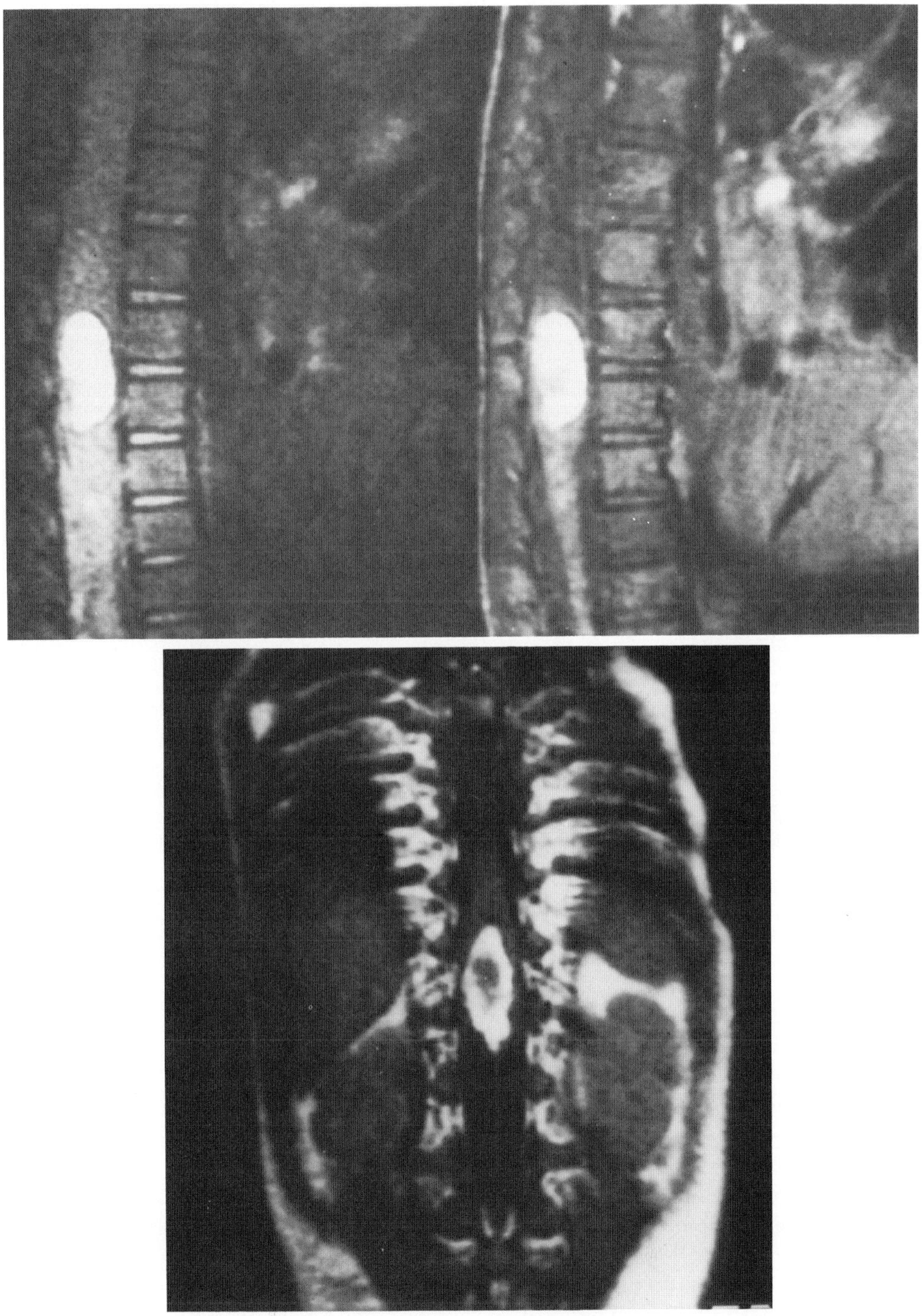

Figure 23.1. Typical high-flow AVM is demonstrated. The mass is almost totally within the spinal cord.

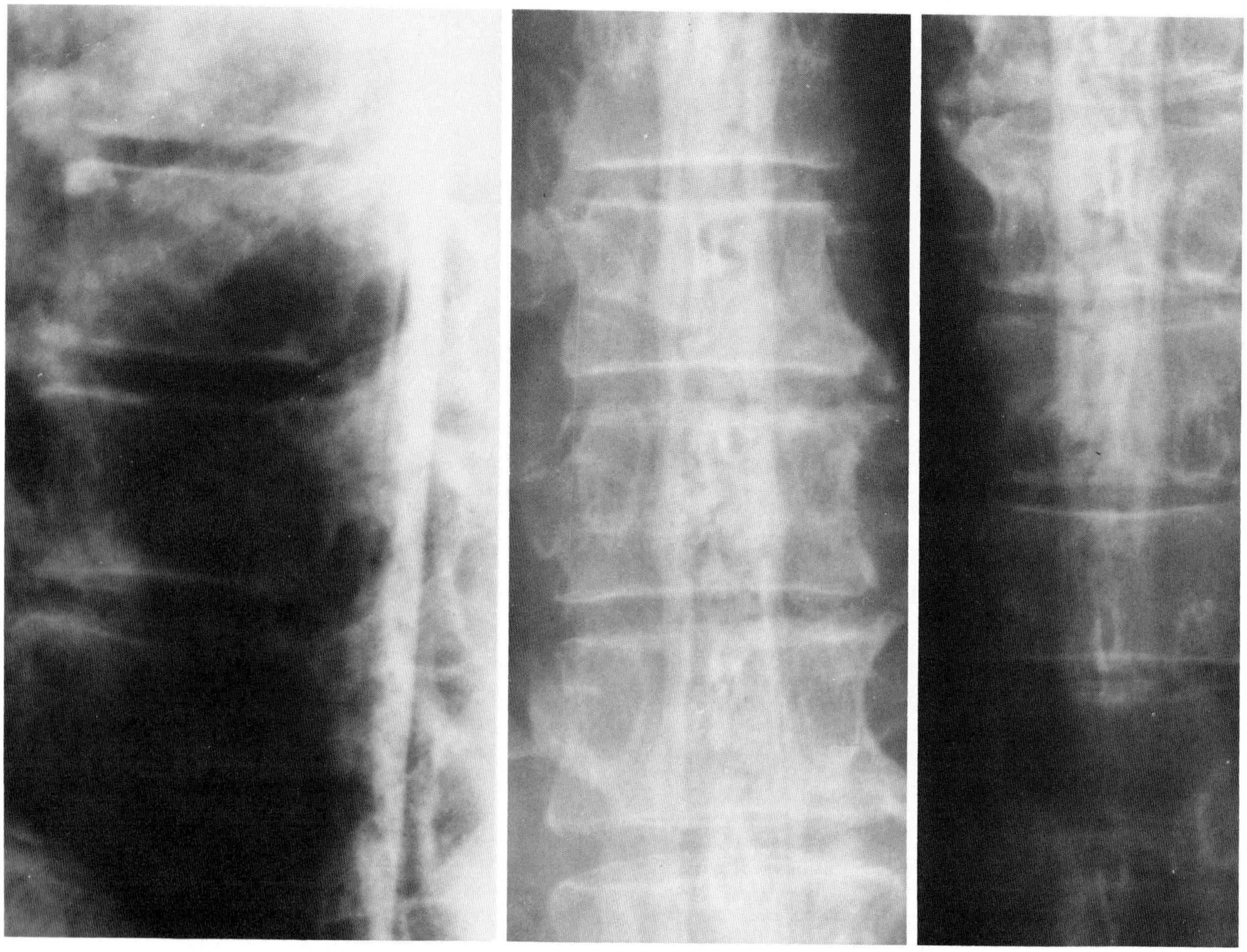

Figure 23.2. Myelographic appearance of low-flow dorsally placed AVM. The prominent vessel is the draining vein, which does not need to be removed.

the presence of an AVM, demonstrates the spinal level of involvement, and reveals the origin of feeding vessels. This limits the area of interest to a short segment of the spinal axis, so that selective spinal arteriography can be limited to the involved segment of the spine. Magnetic resonance imaging (MRI) demonstrates the intramedullary location of juvenile and glomus lesions and, in some instances, the extramedullary, lateral nidus of dural AVMs. Dynamic enhanced computed tomography (CT) scanning, i.e., the acquirement of a rapid series of CT images during a bolus injection of contrast media, detects the presence of spinal AVMs with sensitivity and, if performed at the level of the nidus of the AVM, demonstrates the relationship of the spinal cord and the vascular nidus in cross section.

However, the recent advances in clinical imaging have not eliminated the necessity of selective spinal angiography. Patients with vascular tumors with arteriovenous shunting, such as hemangioblastomas, occasionally appear to have AVMs by intraarterial DVI and by MRI. Patients with small spinal dural arteriovenous fistulae may have negative MRI and DVI, even after intraarterial injection of contrast. Furthermore, the arterial supply to the spinal cord in the region of the AVM must be identified preoperatively so that inadvertent occlusion of a medullary artery, such as the artery of Adamkiewicz, does not occur

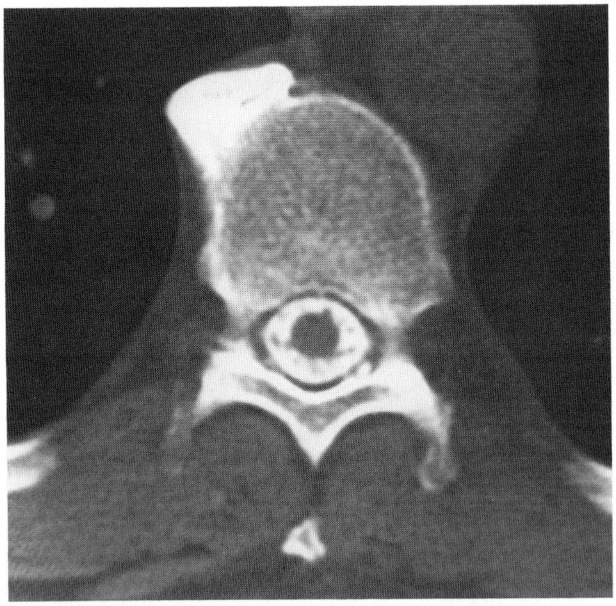

Figure 23.3. Thoracic AVM. CT myelogram demonstrates several filling defects on the posterior surface of the cord. These were proven at angiography to be a thoracic AVM of the low-flow variety. Obliteration of multilevel feeding vessels reversed the patient's rapidly progressive paraplegia.

during treatment. The resolution of DVI, even after selective intercostal injection of contrast, is not sufficient to reveal the anatomy of the normal cord blood supply. For these reasons, selective arteriography is required preoperatively in all patients. No other procedure reliably demonstrates the fine vessels that supply the spinal cord, or consistently distinguishes the different subtypes of AVMs.

When the decision to treat patients with spinal AVMs, which may involve considerable risks, is being made, the dismal natural history of these lesions must be considered. Once symptoms appear, outcome is predictable. Without treatment, most patients are confined to bed or to a wheelchair or are unable to walk unaided within 3 years of the onset of leg weakness or gait disturbance. Therefore, when the diagnosis is established, most patients with spinal AVMs merit treatment. Successful treatment depends on (1) diagnosing the distinct type of AVM, (2) recognizing that the mechanism of cord injury differs in the different types (as do the goals of surgery), and (3) successful implementation of planned surgery. In all types of AVMs the ideal treatment should permanently obliterate the nidus of the AVM without damaging cord tissue and without compromising the blood supply of the spinal cord.

Operative Technique

Normal Vascular Anatomy of Spinal Cord

Familiarity with the anatomy of the normal cord vasculature is imperative to treat patients with spinal AVMs safely and for understanding the different mechanisms of cord injury in the various subtypes of AVMs. At each segmental level the spinal ramus of each intercostal artery divides, after entering the intervertebral foramen, into radicular arteries, which penetrate the dura and supply the anterior and posterior nerve roots, and dural arteries, which provide arterial blood to the spinal dura and the root sleeve. In addition, at some levels and in a sporadic manner the spinal ramus of an intercostal artery is also the origin of a medullary artery, which enters the dura adjacent to the nerve root ganglion and joins the anterior or posterior spinal artery to supply the spinal cord. Spinal rami from the vertebral, subclavian, and aortic intercostal arteries supply 6–10 anterior medullary arteries that inosculate with the anterior spinal artery at intervals along its axis. This is especially notable with the artery of Adamkiewicz, which arises from an aortic intercostal between T8 and L4. The anterior spinal artery, which supplies the anterior two thirds of the cross-sectional area of the cord, including the corticospinal tracts, extends without interruption along the anterior surface of the spinal cord from the foramen magnum to the filum terminale. The posterior spinal arteries, two plexiform interconnecting channels running along the posterolateral surface of the cord, perfuse the posterior third of the spinal cord.

The cord tissue is initially drained by radial veins via centrifugal flow to the cord periphery where the blood enters the coronal venous plexus, a plexiform network of interconnecting veins on the cord surface. The venous blood flows from the intradural to the epidural veins by medullary veins that carry blood from the coronal venous plexus through the dura to the epidural venous plexus. The medullary veins penetrate the dura adjacent to, but separate from, the dural penetration of the nerve roots. The medullary veins, like the medullary arteries, are not present at every segmental level but have an inconstant occur-

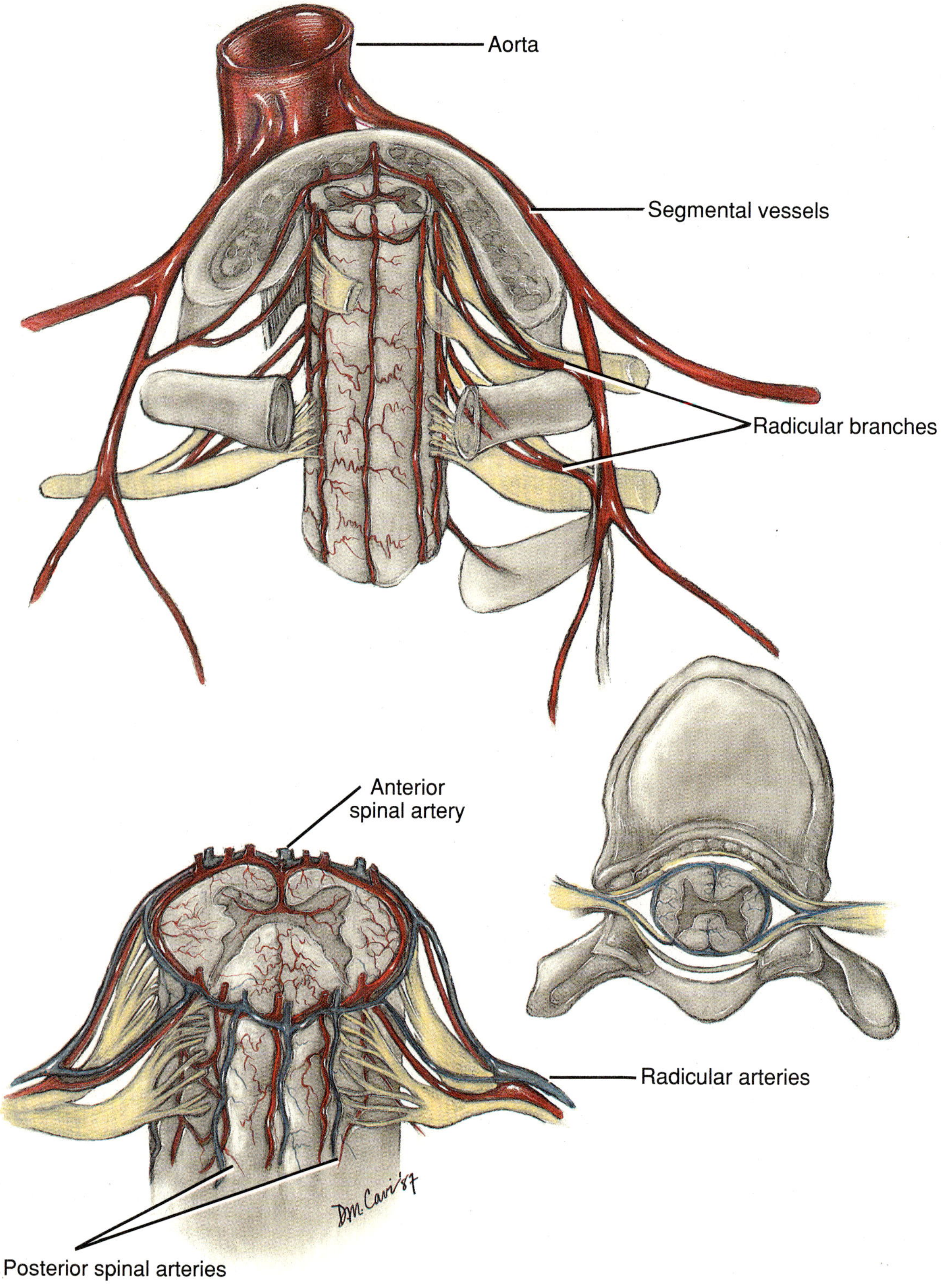
Aorta
Segmental vessels
Radicular branches
Anterior spinal artery
Radicular arteries
Posterior spinal arteries

Figure 23.4.

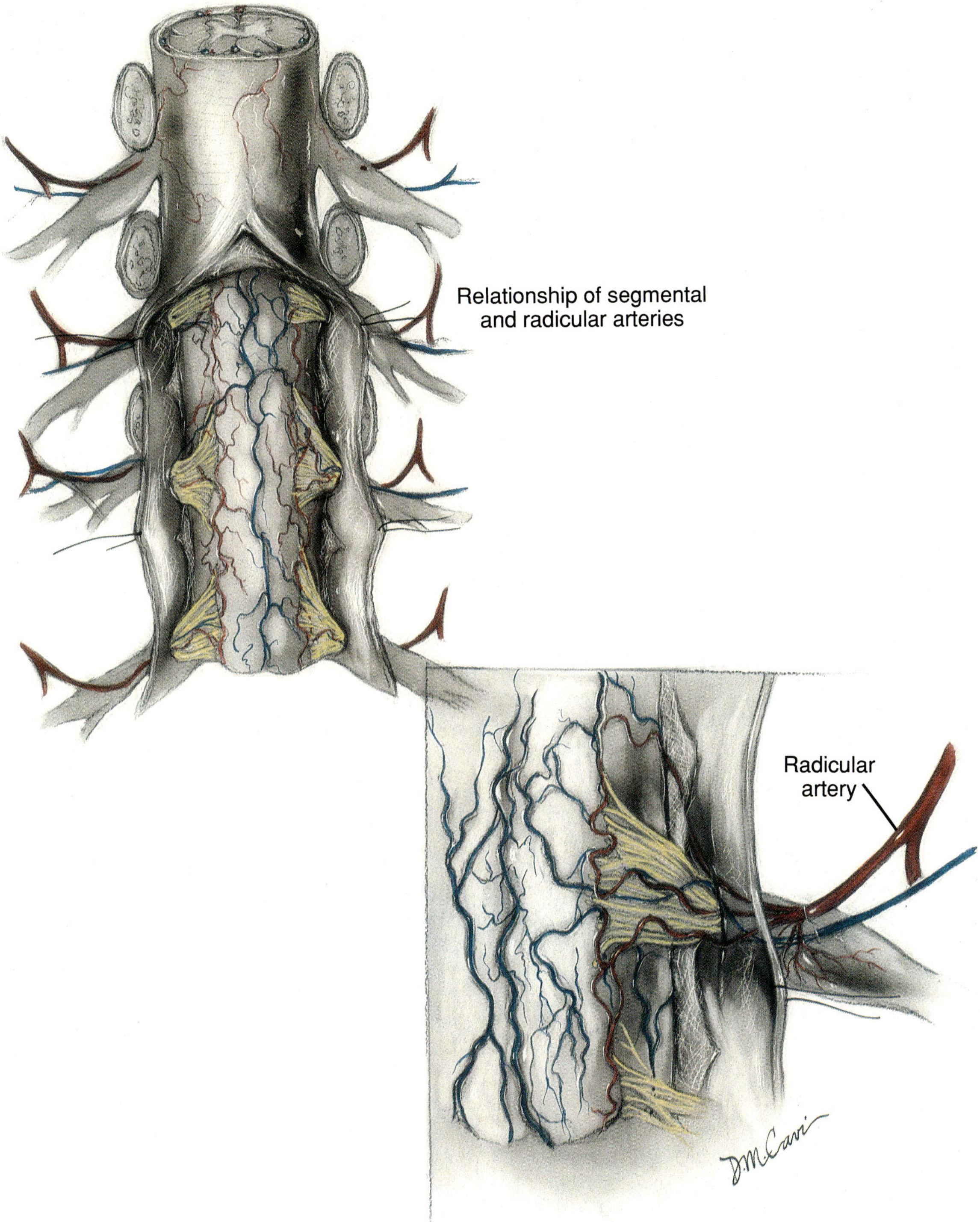
Relationship of segmental
and radicular arteries
Radicular
artery

Figure 23.5.

rence along the longitudinal axis of the spine. There are functional valves at the level of the dura so that substances injected into the epidural venous system do not reach the intradural venous system or the spinal cord. However, there are no valves in the intrathecal or intraparenchymal veins.

Dural Arteriovenous Malformations

Dural AVMs constitute 80–85% of spinal AVMs. Most patients are adults who experience gradual onset and progressive disturbance of cord function. This type was previously described as the single coiled vessel type of AVM of the spinal cord. Many small communicating vessels between the arterial plexus covering the cord surface and the veins of the coronal venous plexus were once considered likely shunting sites, but the site of arterial to venous transition, the nidus of the arteriovenous fistula, was not clearly identified. At surgery, the vessels covering the cord seemed to be the glomus of the AVM, and the patients were treated by surgical stripping of the engorged vessels from the cord surface.

It is now recognized that these lesions are actually spinal dural arteriovenous fistulae. They are routinely amenable to safe and curative treatment. Spinal angiography demonstrates an arteriovenous nidus of fine vessels in the lateral aspect of the spinal canal and within an intervertebral foramen. Contrast flows through the fistula and intradurally, with slow flow, into a single, tightly coiled continuous vessel on the cord surface. The nidus of the AVM is embedded in the dura covering the proximal nerve root and in the adjacent spinal dura. It is the dural branch of the spinal ramus of the intercostal artery that supplies the dural arteriovenous fistula. Blood flowing through the dural arteriovenous fistula is carried through the medullary vein in a retrograde manner to the coronal venous plexus, which becomes dilated, tortuous, and elongated by the reception of excess blood flow under increased pressure. The absence of valves between the coronal venous plexus and the radial veins permits transmission of high venous pressure to the cord tissue, which causes myelopathy.

The goal of treatment is to eliminate the transmission of venous hypertension to the spinal cord. Stripping the engorged coronal venous plexus from the spinal cord will accomplish this in some patients, but success depends on the vessel between the dural arteriovenous fistula and the engorged coronal venous plexus being included in the length of the specimen removed. It is the normal, but transfigured, veins that are stripped from the cord surface, and removing them may impair normal venous drainage from the cord and cause further cord injury. This procedure often requires an extensive laminectomy and an extended, tedious operation, which is unnecessary.

Simple interruption of the vein that carries blood from the dural arteriovenous fistula to the coronal venous plexus cures most patients by eliminating venous hypertension. Obliteration of the arteriovenous fistula, if it can be safely accomplished, should also be performed.

The lamina of the neural arches one level above and below the arteriovenous fistula is removed widely. The bone overlying the intervertebral foramen is removed by rongeurs or by drilling, and dissection of the epidural fat exposes the glomus of the arteriovenous fistula embedded in the dural covering of the nerve root. The spinal dura is then opened in the midline, and after separating the arachnoid from the underlying vessels and retracting the dura and arachnoid laterally, the site of intradural penetration of the vein draining the dural arteriovenous fistula is identified adjacent to the site of dural penetration of the nerve root. This vessel is divided as it enters the dura, and the glomus of the dural arteriovenous fistula is coagulated with bipolar forceps. In this instance, obliteration of the dural arteriovenous fistula cannot always be safely done, however, as in patients in whom the same intercostal artery that supplies the dural arteriovenous fistula also provides medullary supply to the spinal cord. The origin of these vessels is so close and intertwined that it is not possible to separate the medullary artery from the dural artery feeding the arteriovenous fistula. Obliteration by bipolar coagulation, or by excision, of the arteriovenous fistula risks cord infarction, and the surgeon may have to settle for simple interruption of the vein that drains the fistula intradurally into the coronal venous plexus.

Intradural Arteriovenous Malformations

In the AVMs of the spinal cord, the juvenile and glomus AVMs, the site of the arteriovenous fistula is within the tissue of the spinal cord. These AVMs cause myelopathy by repeated hemorrhage and, in some instances, by causing progressive ischemia by vascular steal from the normal arterial perfusion of the spinal cord. One of the feeding vessels of these AVMs is almost always an enlarged medullary artery that also supplies the spinal cord via the anterior

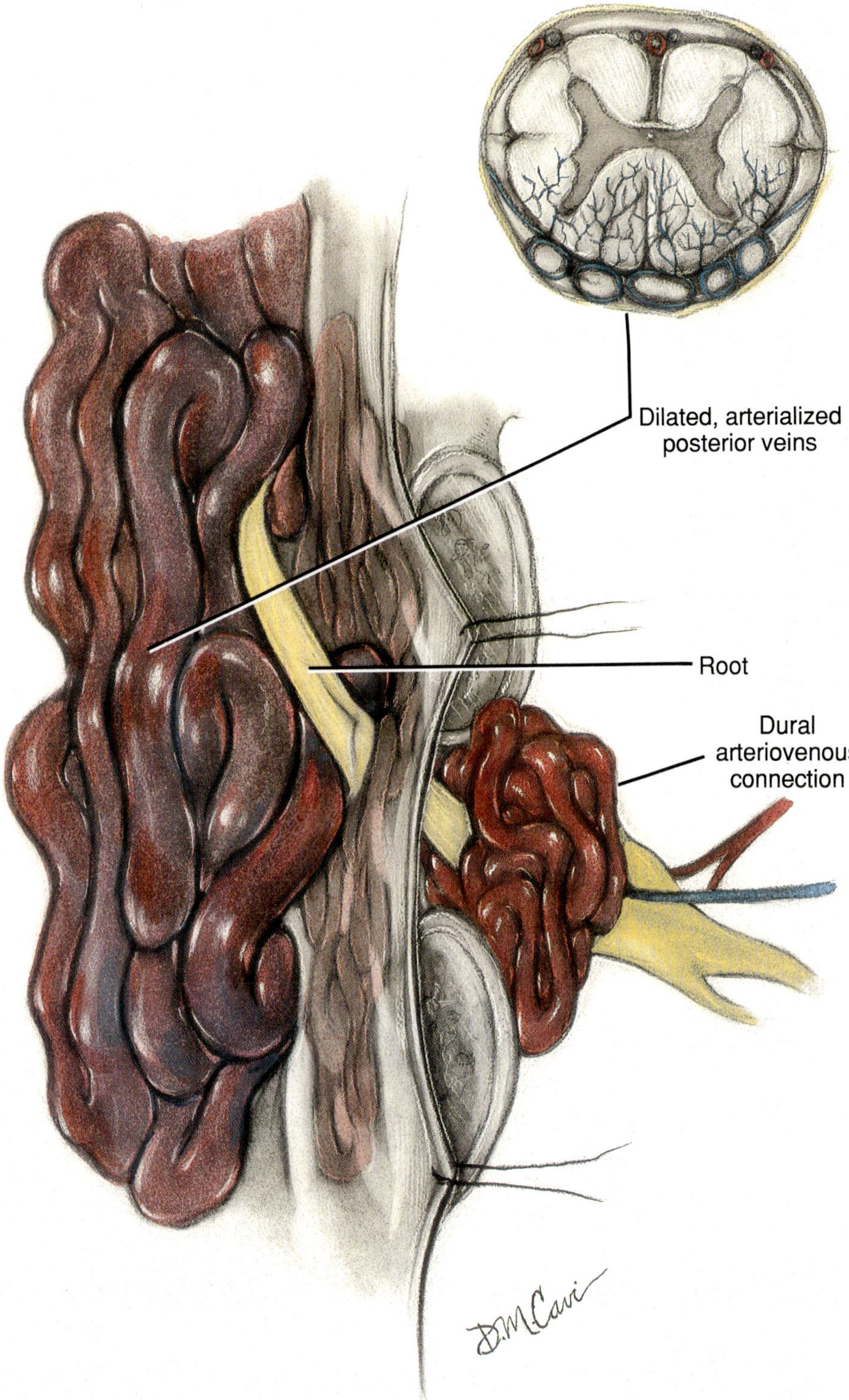
Dilated, arterialized
posterior veins
Root
Dural
arteriovenous
connection
D.McCavi

Figure 23.6.

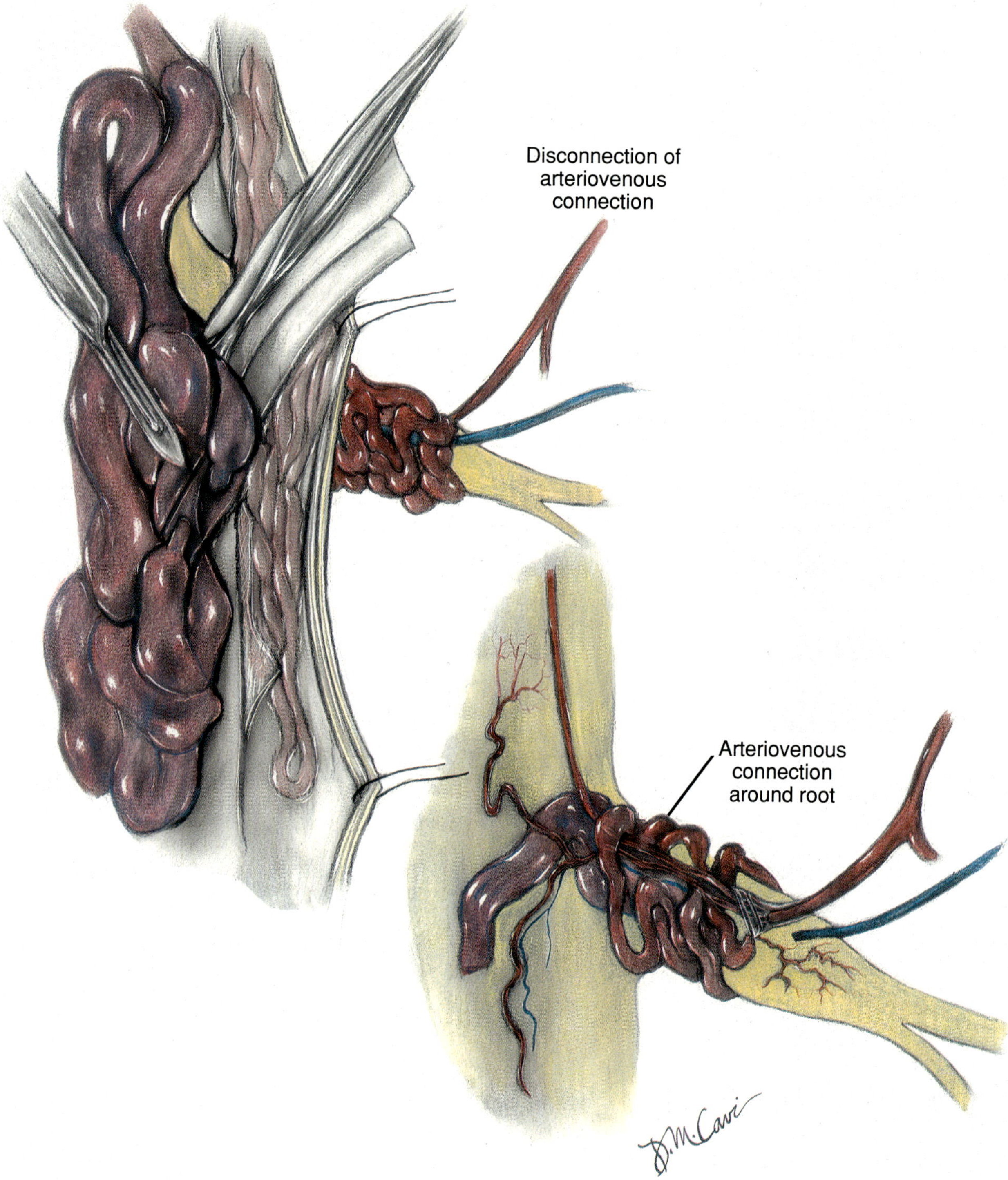
Disconnection of
arteriovenous
connection
Arteriovenous
connection
around root

Figure 23.7.

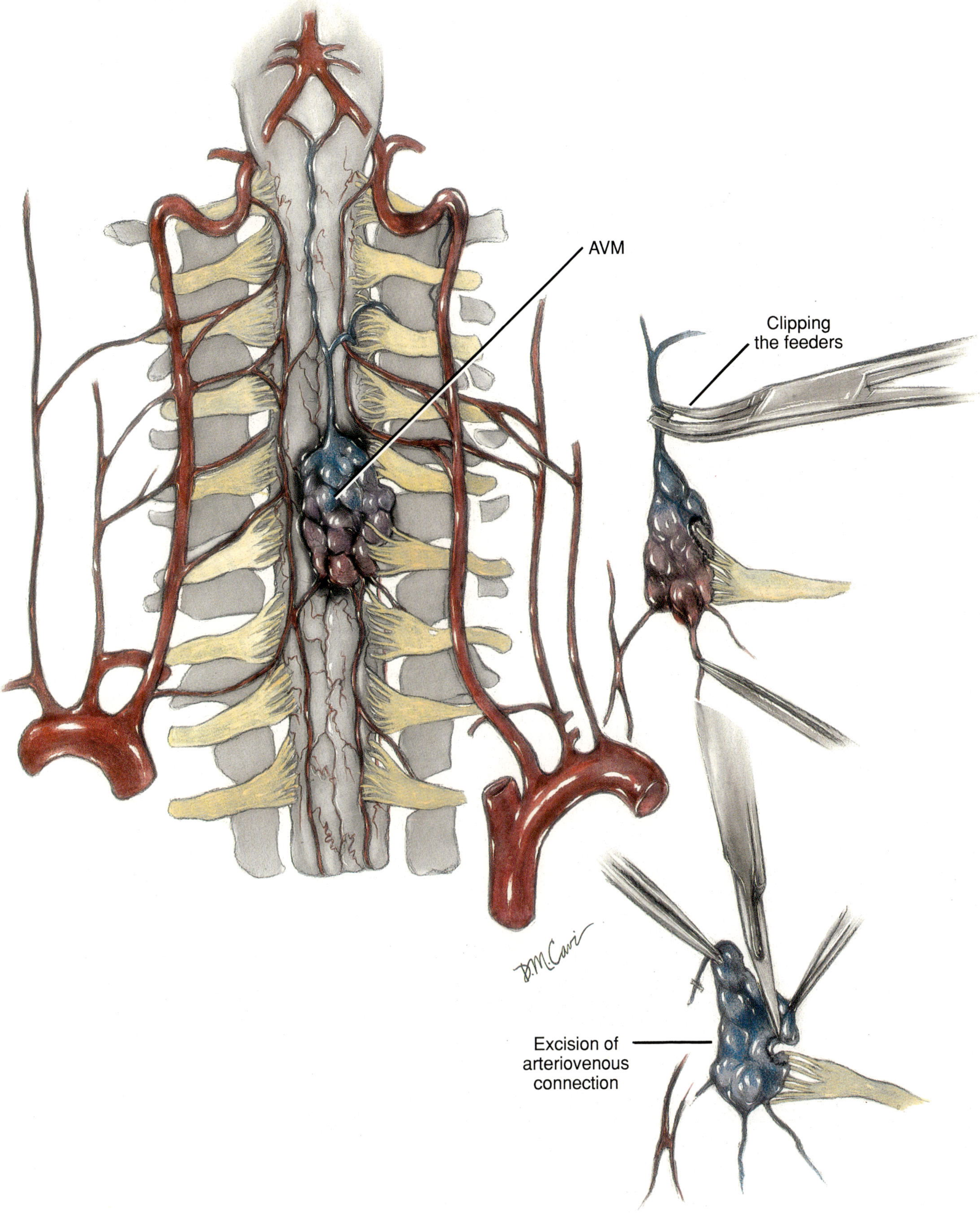
AVM
Clipping
the feeders
Excision of
arteriovenous
connection
D.M.Carr

Figure 23.8.

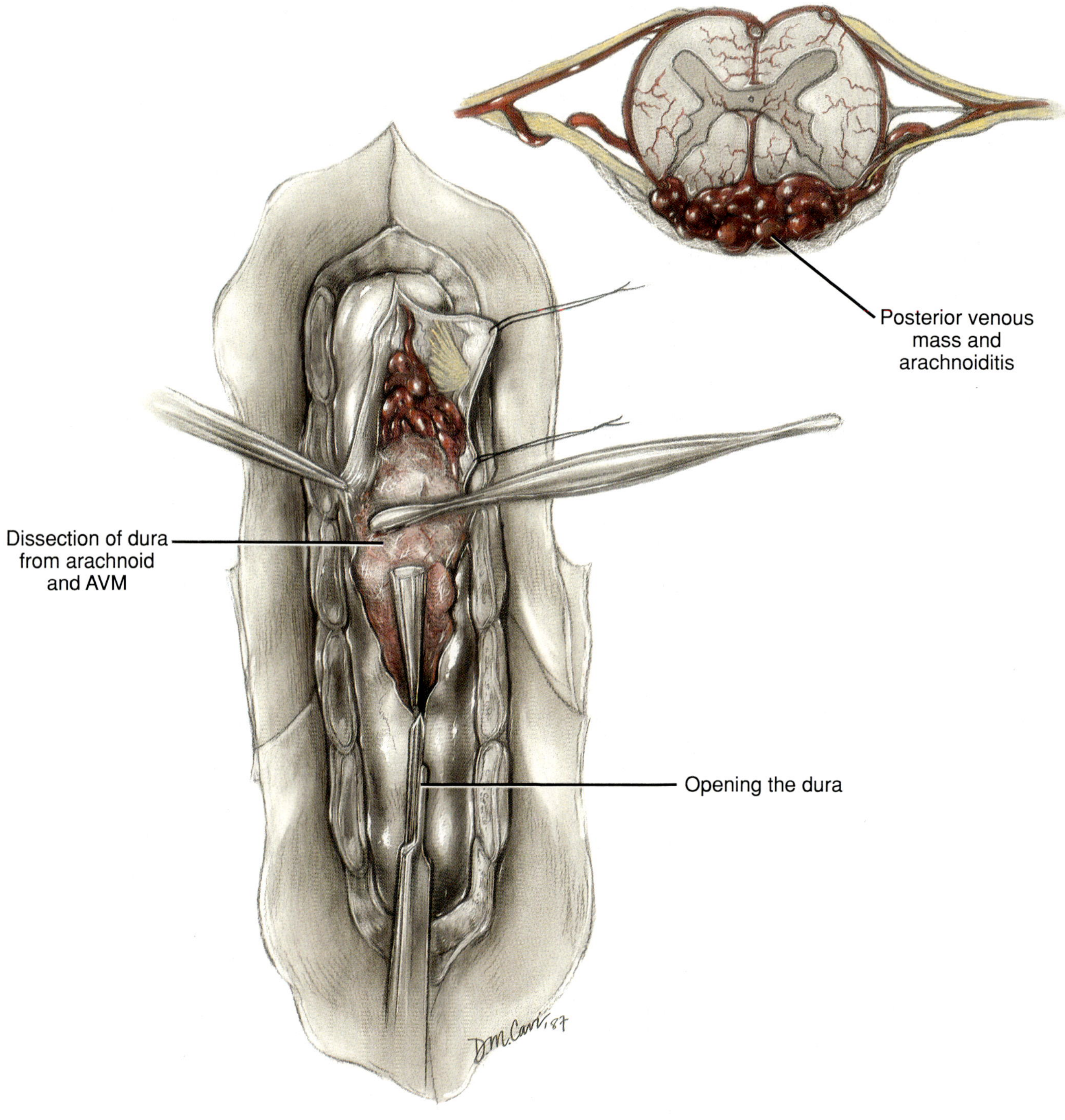
Posterior venous mass and arachnoiditis
Dissection of dura from arachnoid and AVM
Opening the dura
D.M.Carr '87

Figure 23.9.

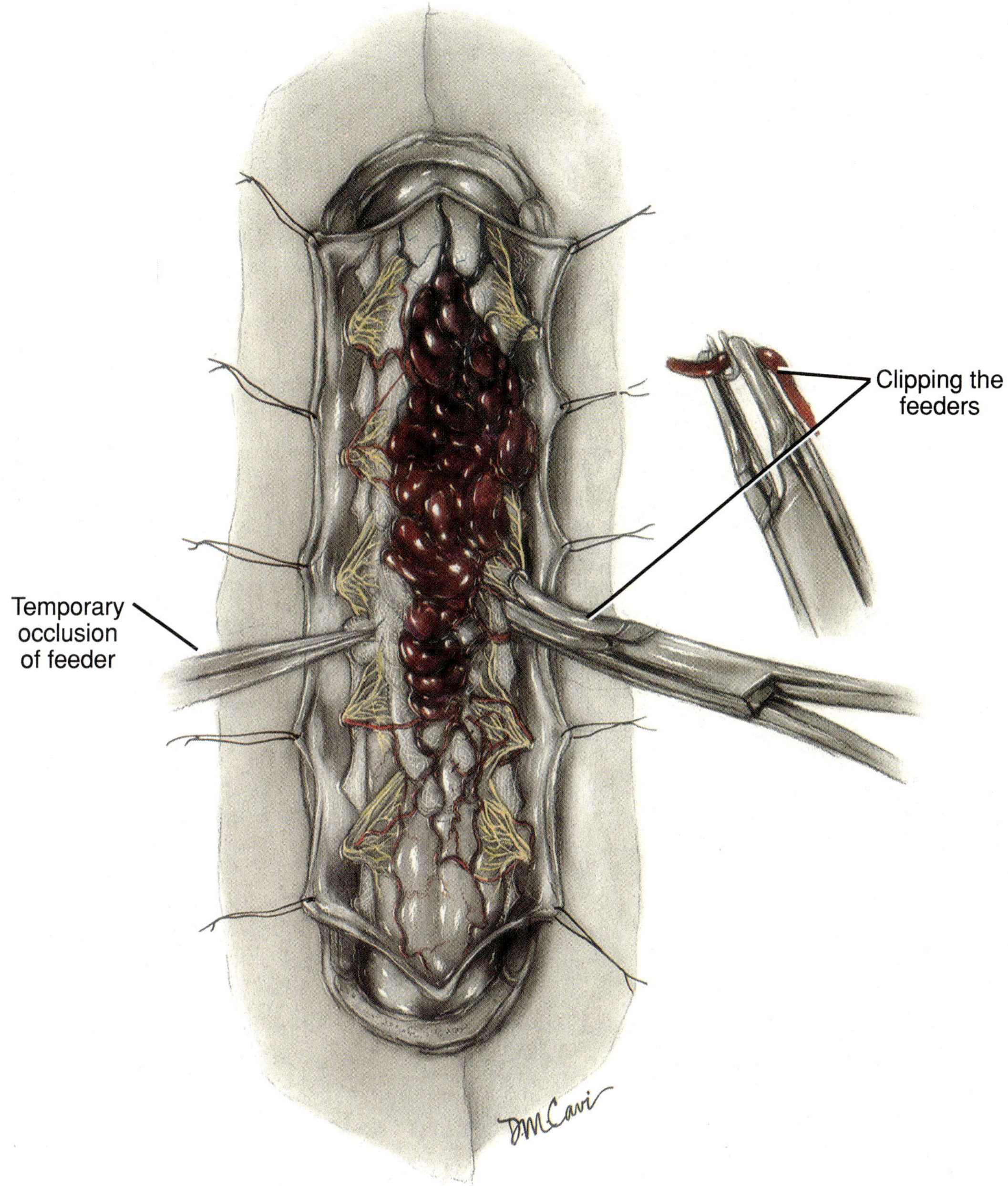

Figure 23.10.

spinal artery. The goal of treatment is total obliteration of the arteriovenous nidus.

Juvenile AVMs of the spinal cord occur almost exclusively in children and young adults (see Fig. 24.7). These spinal AVMs are analogous to cerebral AVMs with multiple large feeding vessels supplying a voluminous AVM. Rapid blood flow through the malformation may be associated with a spinal bruit. Unfortunately, most juvenile spinal AVMs fill the spinal canal and contain cord tissue within the interstices of the AVM and, therefore, are not amenable to excision. Since most of these lesions are supplied by vessels that also contribute blood supply to the spinal cord, they frequently cannot be safely occluded

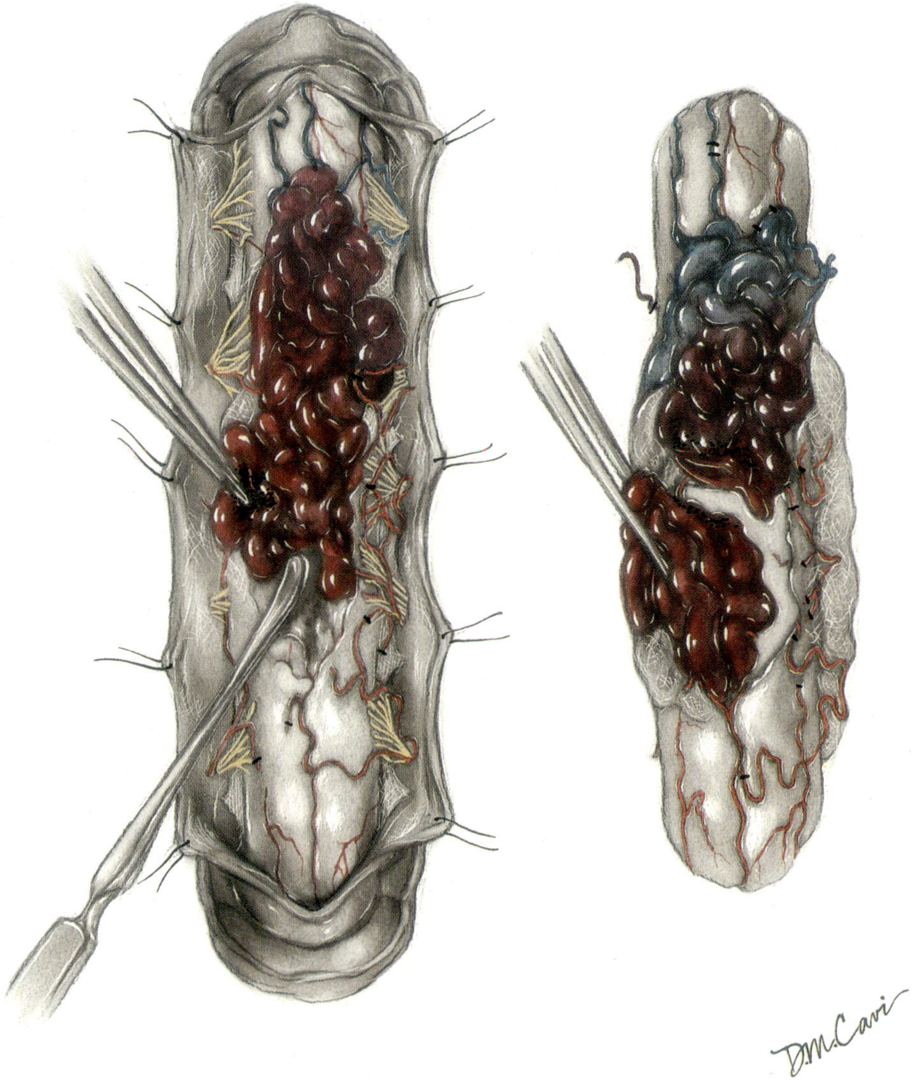

Figure 23.11. Dissection of posterior venous mass from cord.

by embolization either. Therefore, in these patients, treatment is only considered after it is apparent that major loss of neurological function is imminent. Embolic therapy reduces flow and may diminish the incidence of hemorrhage, but it usually does not provide curative treatment, and its efficacy remains unproven. Interruption of all feeding vessels by surgical ligation or by embolic therapy may permit temporary stabilization of the disease and occasionally allows temporary improvement.

The glomus AVM is a localized congeries of small blood vessels confined to a short segment of cord that generally occurs in adults. At angiography, there is usually a single feeding vessel with slow transit time of contrast through these lesions. With glomus AVMs, particularly those in the cervical cord where collateral flow in the anterior spinal artery can come from an inferior or superior direction, total excision is frequently possible. Surgical excision is more hazardous with lesions in the thoracic and lumbar segments of the spinal cord where collateral blood supply for the spinal cord is limited and frequently reaches the cord from a rostral to caudal direction only. Intraoperative interruption of the anterior spinal artery eliminates

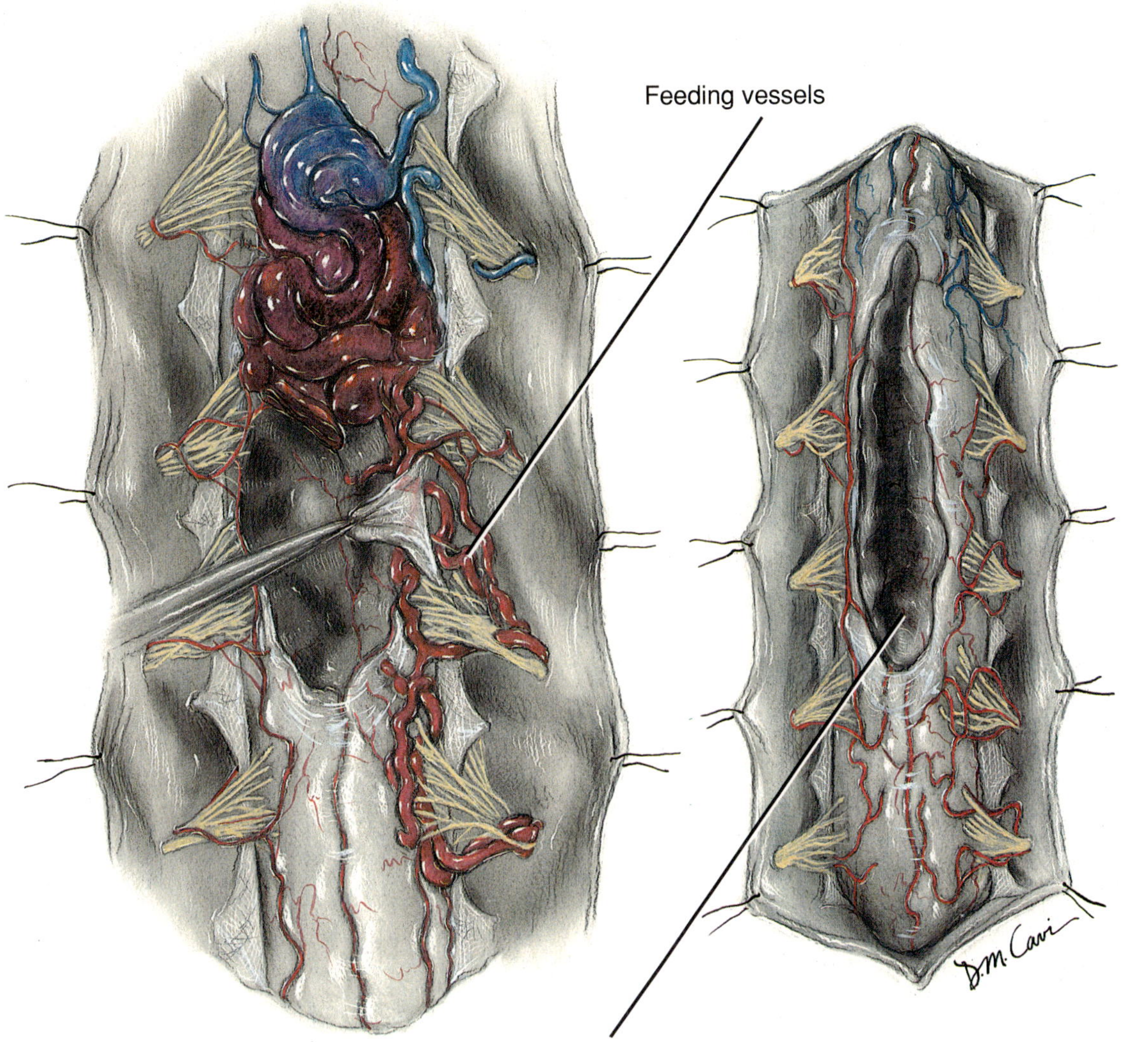

Figure 23.12.

arterial supply to the segments of cord below the level of the AVM. Embolic occlusion of the AVM with particulate occlusive material should be considered for glomus AVMs in the thoracic or lumbar cord segments.

Operative exposure of intramedullary spinal AVMs is performed with the patient in the prone position, with a complete laminectomy covering one segment above and below the glomus of the malformation. The dura is opened in the midline, with care taken to preserve the arachnoid intact so that tearing of the large, fragile underlying vessels is avoided. This is particularly important in patients with previous subarachnoid hemorrhage when the arachnoid may be quite adherent to underlying vessels of the malformation. In patients with recent hemorrhage into the subarachnoid space, surgery is postponed until enough time has passed for lysis of clots and absorption of blood products from the subarachnoid space. To improve visualization of the component vessels of the AVM, the arachnoid is then removed from the surface of the underlying malformation if it can be easily dissected away from these vessels. Sutures retract the dura and arachnoid laterally. Correlation of the vascular anatomy as seen on the preoperative diagnostic studies with that seen intraoperatively is performed so that all medullary arteries, particularly the artery of Adamkiewicz and the anterior spinal artery, are preserved during dissection and to aid the identification and interruption of major feeding arteries early as they enter the malformation. Throughout intradural dissection, meticulous hemostasis is essential, since blood-stained pia obscures anatomic details. Liberal irrigation during bipolar coagulation prevents coagulated vessel walls from adhering to the tips of the forceps, which can be bothersome at the wrong moment. Larger feeding vessels may require ligatures or clips, but most vessels can be managed with simple bipolar coagulation and interruption.

By microdissection with the tips of the bipolar forceps in the gliotic plane between the malformation and the adjacent cord tissue and by elevating the malformation as one works from one pole upward or downward, the malformation can be dissected from the surrounding cord. This permits exposure of vessels entering or leaving the malformation ventrally. As the margins of the malformation are dissected, gentle bipolar coagulation is used to shrink the AVM gradually and render the periphery of the lesion less friable to manipulation. Pial traction sutures are used to maintain adequate separation of the cord tissue from the AVM to permit room for dissection. Progressive shrinking of the AVM by gentle bipolar coagulation also reduces turgidity in the nidus as dissection proceeds. Hypotension is occasionally of help. Plans to exercise or obliterate the malformation completely may have to be abandoned intraoperatively if it becomes apparent that undue risk to cord function will occur with continued attempts at complete removal. At least one of the major draining veins is preserved patent until dissection around the periphery of the malformation has been completed and all arterial feeding vessels have been occluded.

If the juvenile or glomus AVM occupies a considerable portion of the parenchyma of the ventral half of the spinal cord, it may be impossible to remove it without eliciting unacceptable neurological deficit, and surgical excision should not be attempted. Reduction of flow in these lesions by embolization or by ligation of feeding arteries may diminish the incidence of subsequent hemorrhage and should reduce the degree of vascular steal and associated ischemia of the cord. However, in many instances benefits may be only temporary as reestablishment of flow to preexisting levels ultimately occurs.

The operating microscope and appropriate microsurgical instrumentation and technique are required for surgery for all spinal AVMs. Watertight dural closure is always performed. Continuous monitoring of spinal evoked potentials and continuous intraoperative assessment of tissue blood flow in the exposed cord may prove to be of help intraoperatively. The importance of these modalities remains to be demonstrated, however. Postoperative spinal arteriography is used routinely to assess the success of complete obliteration of the AVM.

24

Intradural and Parenchymal Arteriovenous Malformations

Spinal arteriovenous malformations have three basic intradural patterns. There is a high-flow variety composed of dilated vessels occupying the posterior and posterolateral surface of the cord. In these lesions the arterial shunts are large, and the mass may be significant, with extramedullary compression an important part of the syndrome. The flow of blood is high, and these lesions are much more like arteriovenous malformations of the brain in their risk of uncontrollable intraoperative hemorrhage. The second important group is the low-flow variety, with the arteriovenous shunts and most abnormal vssels outside the cord in the dura. These lesions have several variations. In some, the arteriovenous connection has a greater prominence, and there are more arterial connections. In others, the venous component is larger, and the arteriovenous connections are fewer. There may or may not be vessels exiting or entering the malformation through cord parenchyma. In these malformations the pressures are low, shunts are relatively small, and there is rarely a compressive effect. (See Oldfield, Chapter 23.) Malformations with a significant intramedullary portion associated sometimes with an hemangioma are the third major variety. Some of these are high flow, but most are low flow. Often, cord intrinsic vasculature is a part of the malformation.

Malformations of Cord

Surgical techniques for removal of malformations of the cord are quite different. The diagnosis is now made via computed tomography (CT) scanning or magnetic resonance imaging (MRI) most of the time. For the small lesions discernible on the back of the cord, spinal angiography is not absolutely mandatory and frequently will not demonstrate significant arterial feeding vessels. For larger masses, angiography is obligatory, and the angiographer should be prepared to embolize the largest feeding vessels at the time of the diagnostic angiography. In high-flow, large lesions, the obliteration of feeding vessels is an invaluable adjunct to surgical removal. An associated intramedullary tumor has high enough flow to be seen on angiography most of the time. Demonstration of the presence or absence of arterial feeders can be an important aspect of planning surgery for all these lesions. However, spinal angiography is both difficult and dangerous and is not a technique for the occasional angiographer.

High-Flow Arteriovenous Malformations Presenting as a Mass

Operations on high-flow arteriovenous malformations presenting as a mass are done with the patient under general anesthesia in the prone position. A laminectomy should be planned that will extend at least one level above and below the malformation as demonstrated. The dura must be opened carefully, and complete hemostasis obtained. Even a small amount of blood contaminating the operative field will destroy the definition of the malformation and make the dissections extremely difficult. Hemostatic agents can be placed in the gutters, and the dura sutured back to paravertebral muscles, which are then covered with cottonoid. Sump sections in the gutters may also be necessary. The dural opening should be carefully done with the aid of magnification; the blood vessels are often adherent to the posterior dura and can be inadvertently opened if the dural incision is attempted directly over them. The arachnoidal connections should be freed so the dura is separated from the frequently thickened arachnoid and from the vessels. Once the dura is opened, the entire malformation is visualized, and the location of the feeding vessels, which have previously been demonstrated by angiography, is verified. It is hoped that these will have been virtually occluded by embolization and much of the malformation will be thrombosed or carrying venous blood. It is important to remove all of the arachnoid from the surface of the malformation, but doing this may not be easy because sometimes the arachnoid is thickened and discolored from previous hemorrhages. Definition of the entire malformation makes total excision much easier, and it is worth spending time with the arachnoid to obtain a definitive removal. Once most feeding vessels are identified, removal of the mass can begin. Feeding vessels should be identified, in turn, in the gutters. Usually, they are intertwined in the roots. It is necessary to dissect them adequately to be sure they enter the malformation and do not supply normal cord. Smaller vessels can be coagulated and cut. Larger ones should be clipped and divided. Usually, it is easier to begin at one extremity. The blood vessel must be carefully dissected free from the surrounding arachnoid and from the spinal cord. It is not necessary to unravel all of the vessels, but as the mass detached from the cord becomes larger, it may be easier to coagulate and remove portions of the arterialized vessels. It is important not to try to do this while there remains a high flow through the vessels. Once devascularization has occurred, then bipolar coagulation will suffice to stop any bleeding from the malformation, and individual segments of vessels can be coagulated and removed. The high magnification required for this will show the intrinsic cord vasculature. Sometimes, careful separation of the malformation from cord vessels will be necessary. The cord vessels can occasionally run within the malformation, and it is then necessary to divide malformation vessels, coagulate and cut them, and then slide the remnant of vessels gently out from beneath the intertwined vessels that appear to be important for the cord. More commonly with these larger lesions the malformation itself is separate and extrapial. As an extramedullary tumor it can be removed virtually as a single piece. The dissection is carried up or down depending on where the surgeon elected to begin; all small feeding vessels are coagulated as they are encountered. Larger vessels should be clipped with microclips. If the flow is high, it is necessary to clip both sides. When the malformation has been nearly devascularized, it is usually sufficient to clip only the feeding side of the vessel. Coagulation will control bleed-

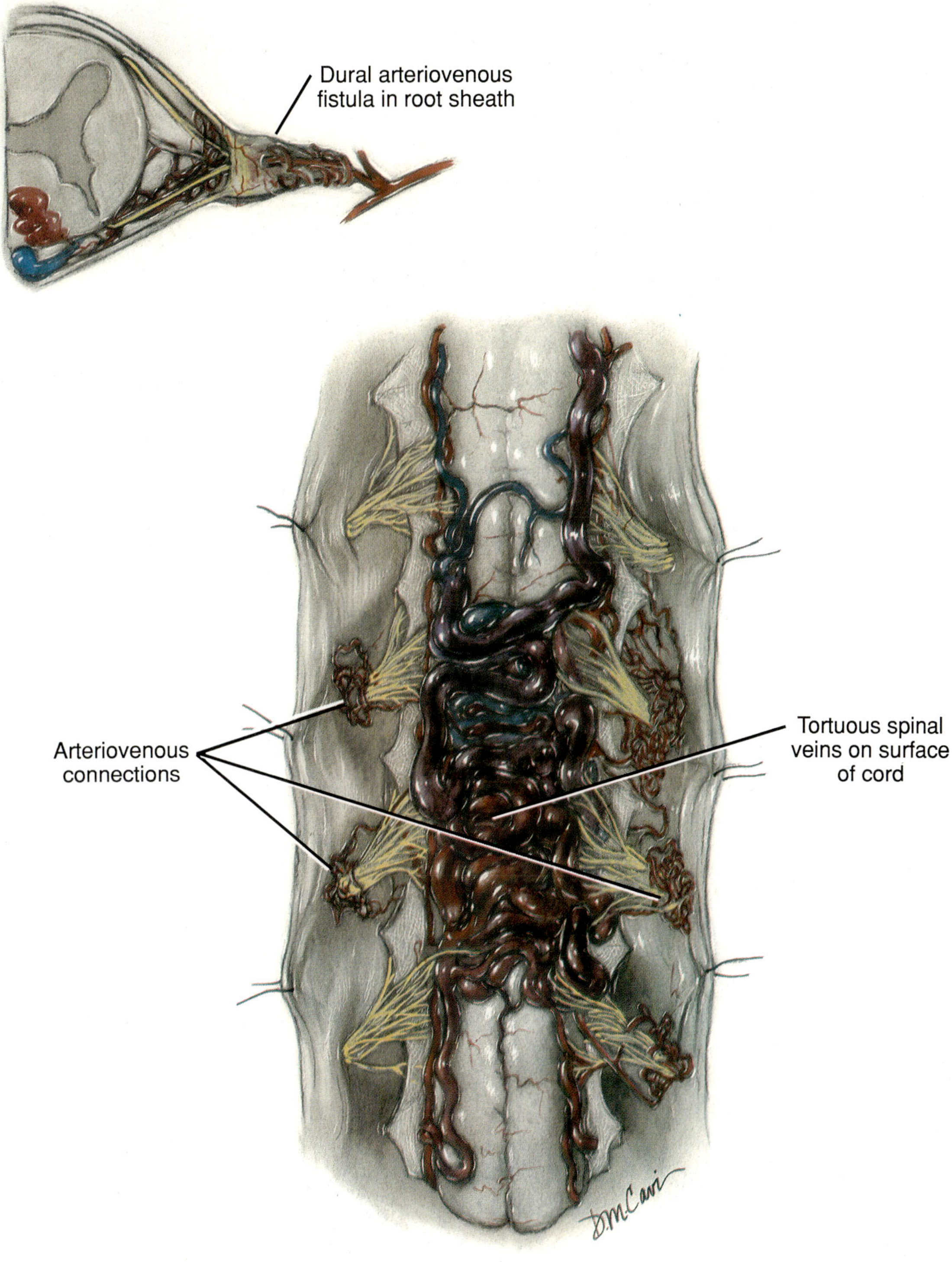
Dural arteriovenous
fistula in root sheath
Arteriovenous
connections
Tortuous spinal
veins on surface
of cord

Figure 24.1.

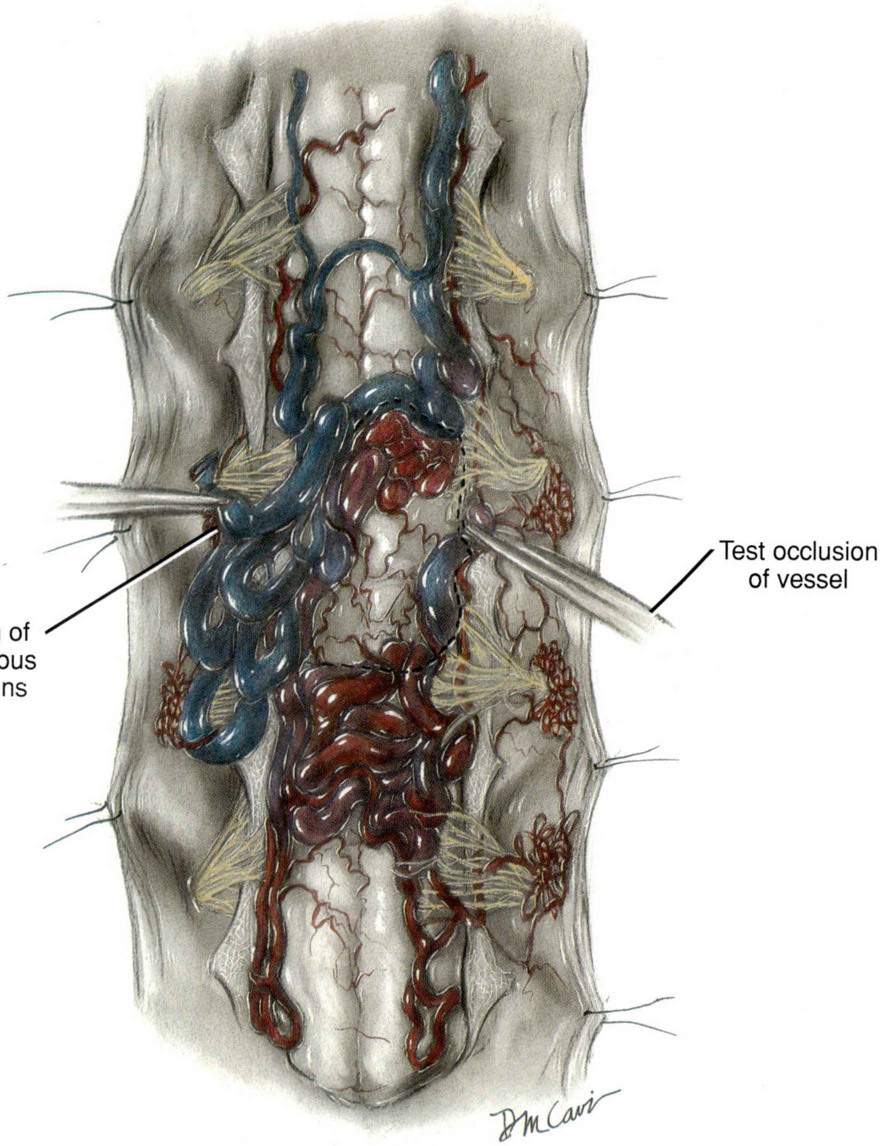

Figure 24.2.

ing on the malformation side. If any bleeding does occur, it should be promptly controlled with fine bipolar coagulation. To perform this delicate surgery while bleeding is ongoing is not possible. Once the malformation and its relationships are obscured by blood, the dissection becomes much more difficult. These maneuvers are continued until the mass has been isolated completely and can be removed from the back of the cord. The most difficult relationships occur around the dorsal roots. Often, there are sizable feeding vessels entering the malformation with the dorsal root, and these commonly are hidden anterior to the roots. The feeding vessels may also be obscured by large, tortuous, dilated draining veins exiting with the roots. As with any malformation, it is important to control the inflow before these large veins are sacrificed. The dissection is carried out level by level, with exploration done for each remaining feeding vessel bilaterally at each level before the effluent veins are occluded. Usually, it is wise to occlude the larger

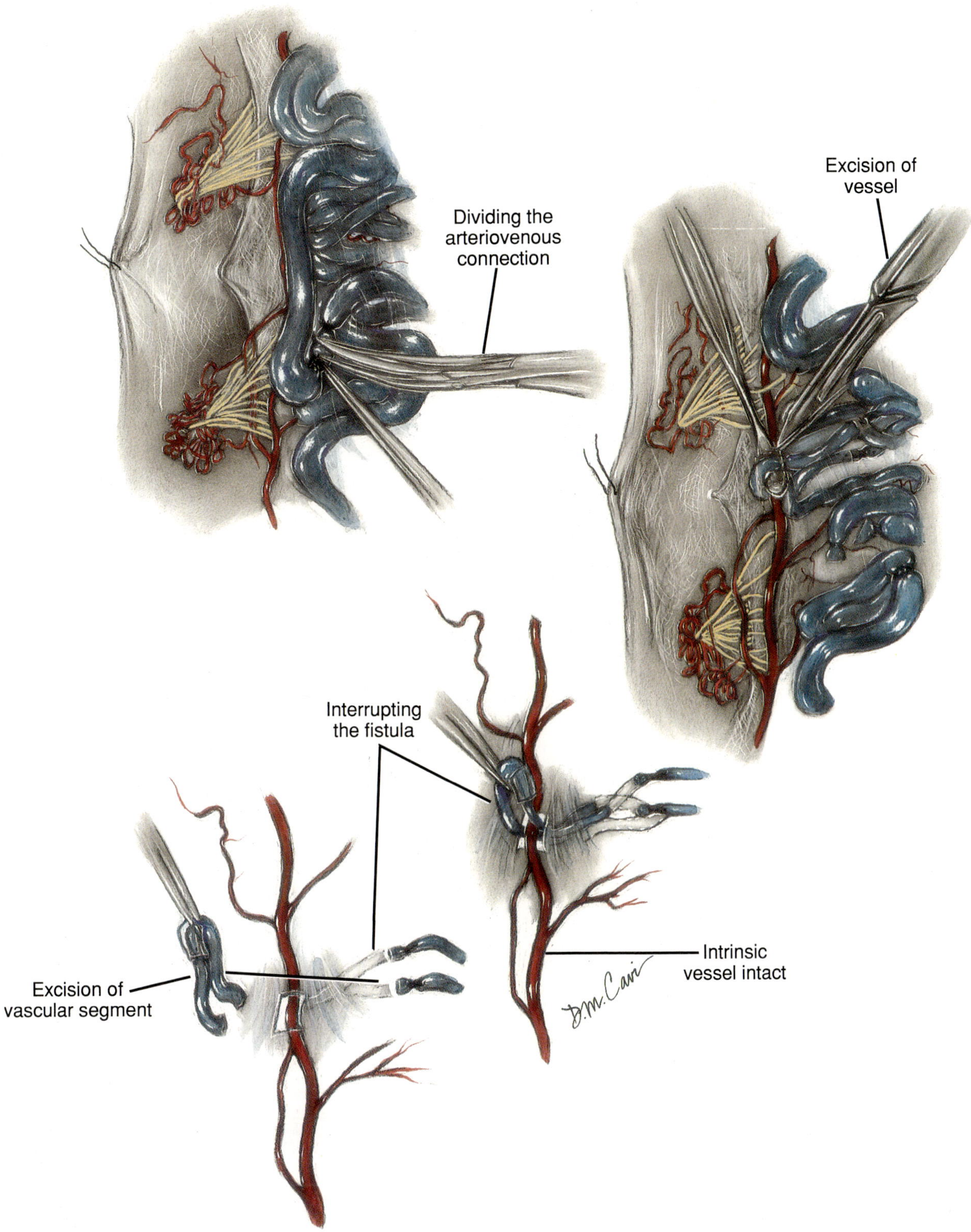
Excision of vessel
Dividing the arteriovenous connection
Interrupting the fistula
Intrinsic vessel intact
Excision of vascular segment
D.M. Cain

Figure 24.3.

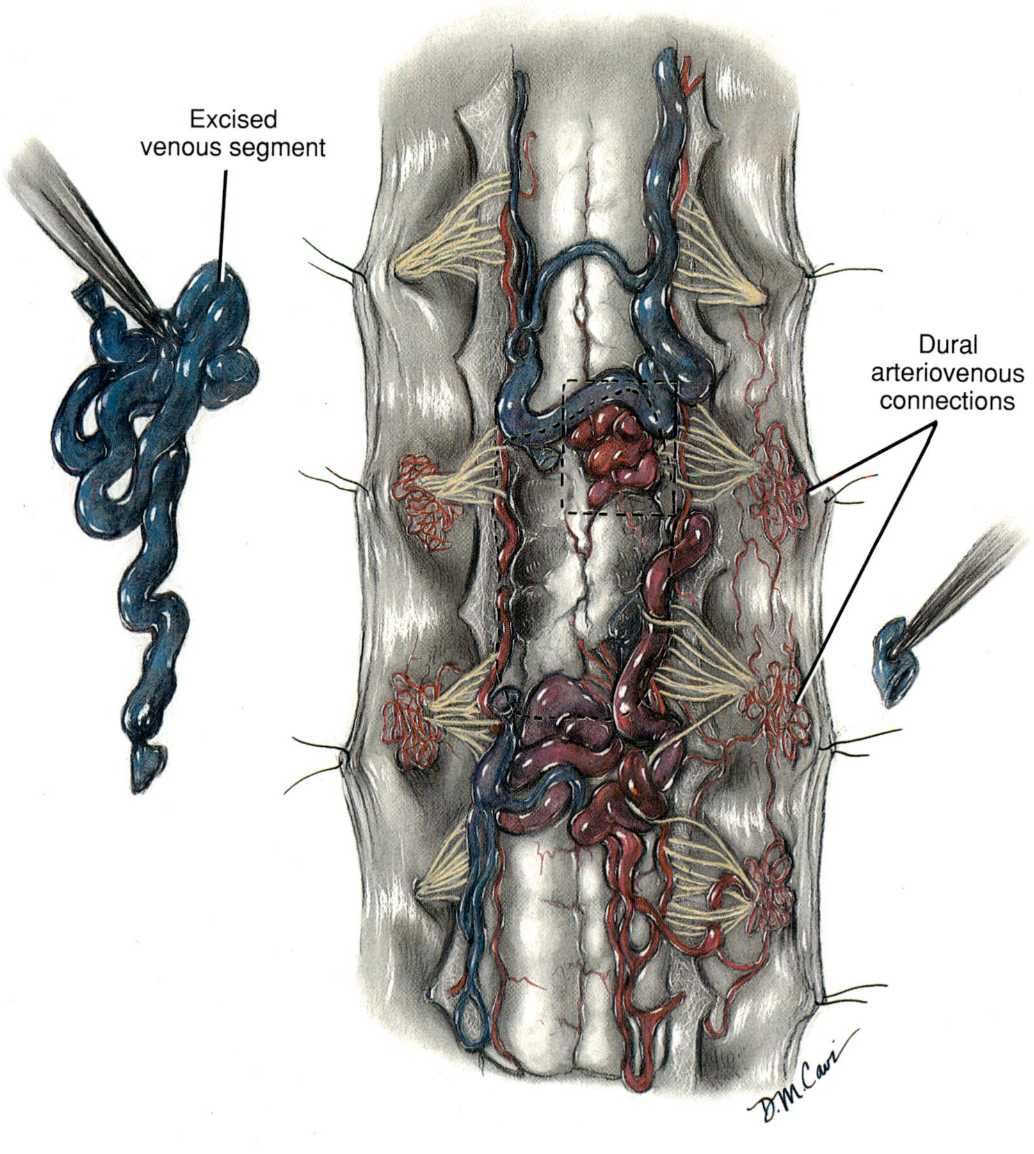

Figure 24.4.

veins temporarily for a few minutes before deciding to sacrifice them. Eventually, repetition of these maneuvers will lead to complete isolation of the malformation, which can then be removed entirely. Piecemeal removal is just as effective. Which approach is the better depends entirely on how easily the mass is mobilized. With these large malformations the pia is rarely opened, and when the procedure is complete, the cord should retain a relatively normal appearance. The dura should be closed in a watertight fashion, and the wound closed in the usual way without special precautions otherwise necessary.

Intramedullary Arteriovenous Malformation

The necessity to remove an intramedullary arteriovenous malformation is not frequent. Some malformations occur in conjunction with hemangiomas within the cord. In this circumstance the tumor should be

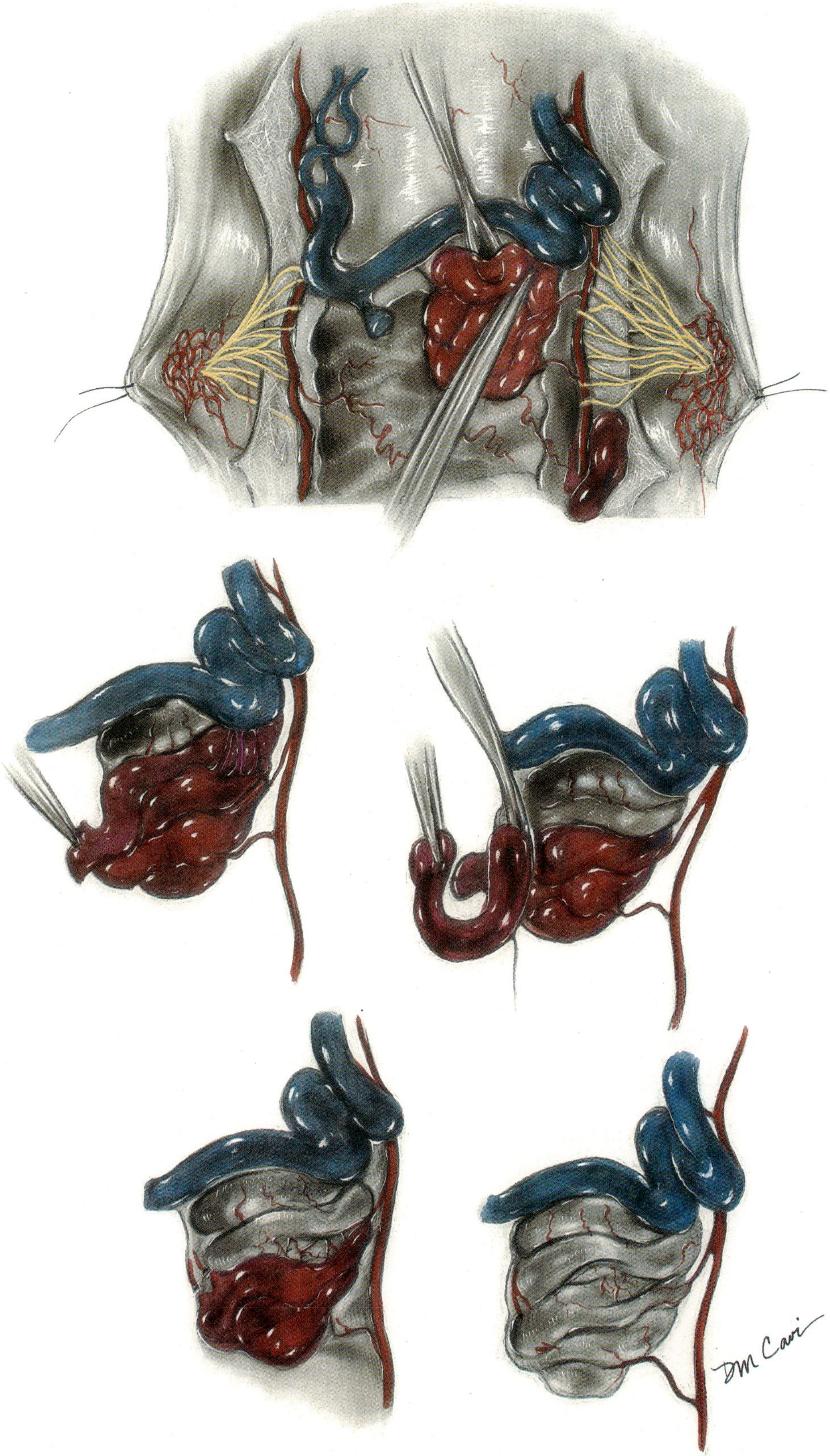

Figure 24.5. Removal of venous component.

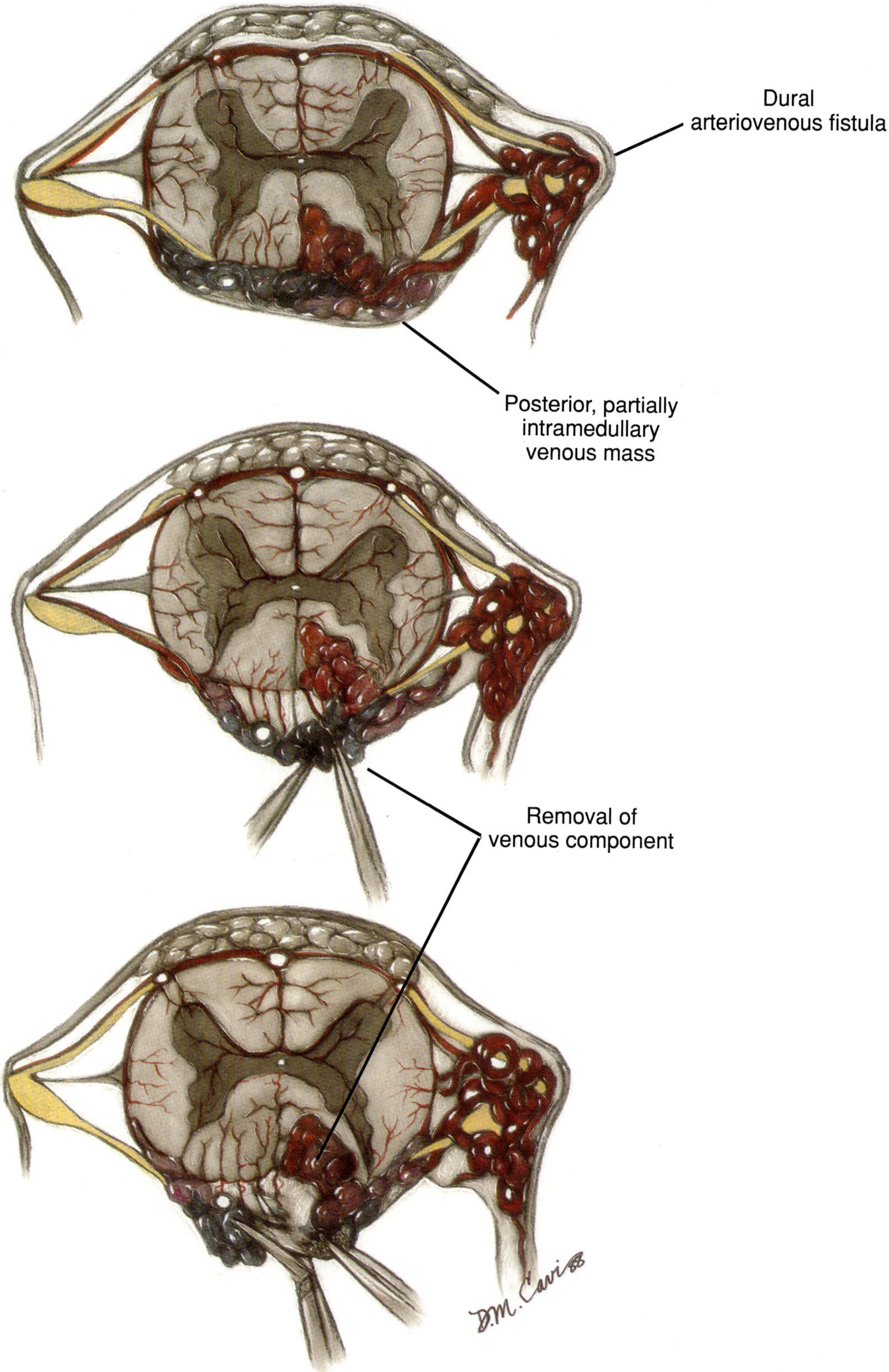
Dural
arteriovenous fistula
Posterior, partially
intramedullary
venous mass
Removal of
venous component
D.M. Cavi 88

Figure 24.6.

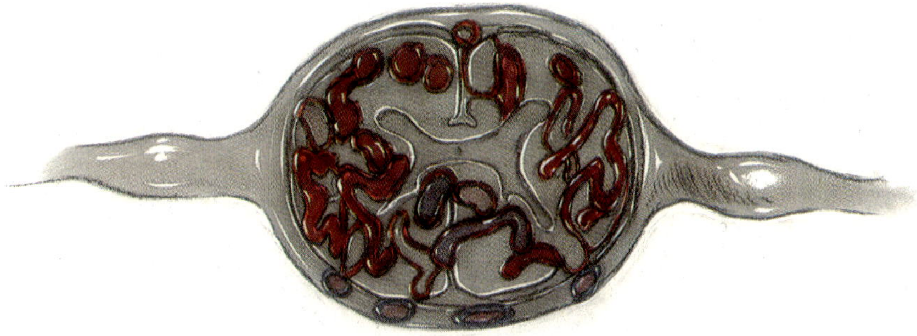

Unresectable
intramedullary arteriovenous
malformation (diffuse)

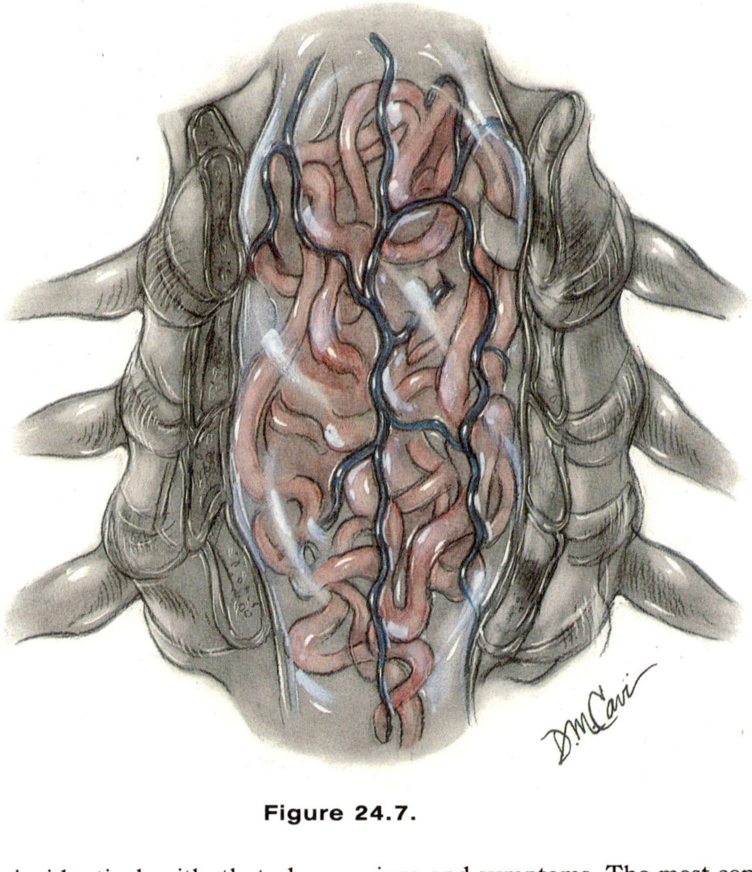

Figure 24.7.

removed. The dissection is identical with that described for the other kind of intramedullary tumors (see Chapter 28). The true arteriovenous malformation within the cord is a much more formidable lesion. The current state of surgical technique is such that removal of the intramedullary arteriovenous malformation must be warranted by the occurrence of grave signs and symptoms. The most common will be recurrent hemorrhage and progressive, serious neurological loss. The surgical procedure is planned as for any other malformation. The configuration of the vasculature will be known by a combination of the imaging techniques that will show the cord itself and angiography. Major feeders should be embolized whenever

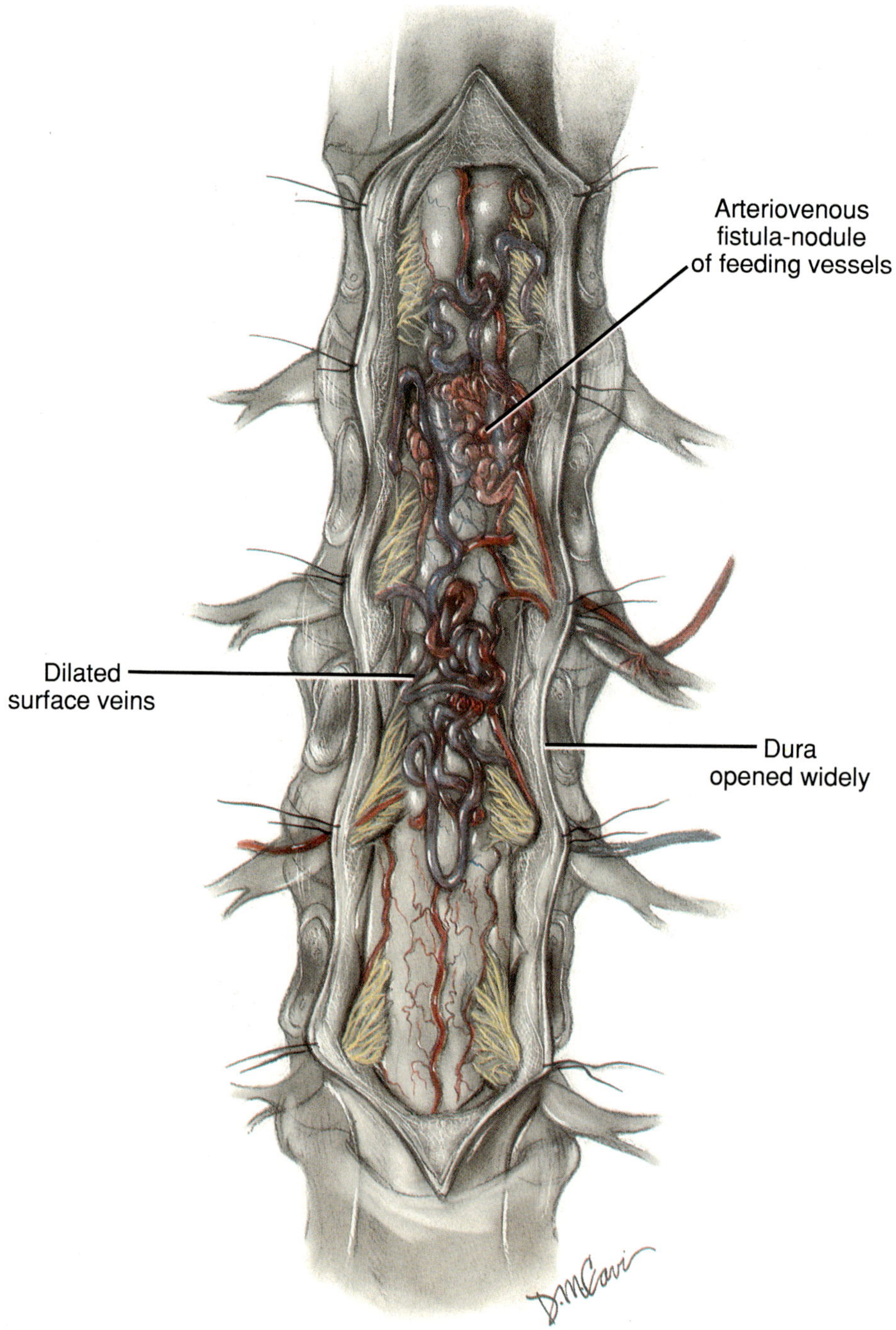

Figure 24.8.

possible. It may be that embolization alone will reduce flow enough to prevent hemorrhage or reverse a neurological trend. When obliteration of feeding vessels is not satisfactory alone, the mass may have to be removed.

Following exposure of the abnormal cord, the areas where the feeding vessels are expected to be found should be explored; each root should be viewed in turn. Major vessels that are obviously destined for the malformation should be obliterated immediately.

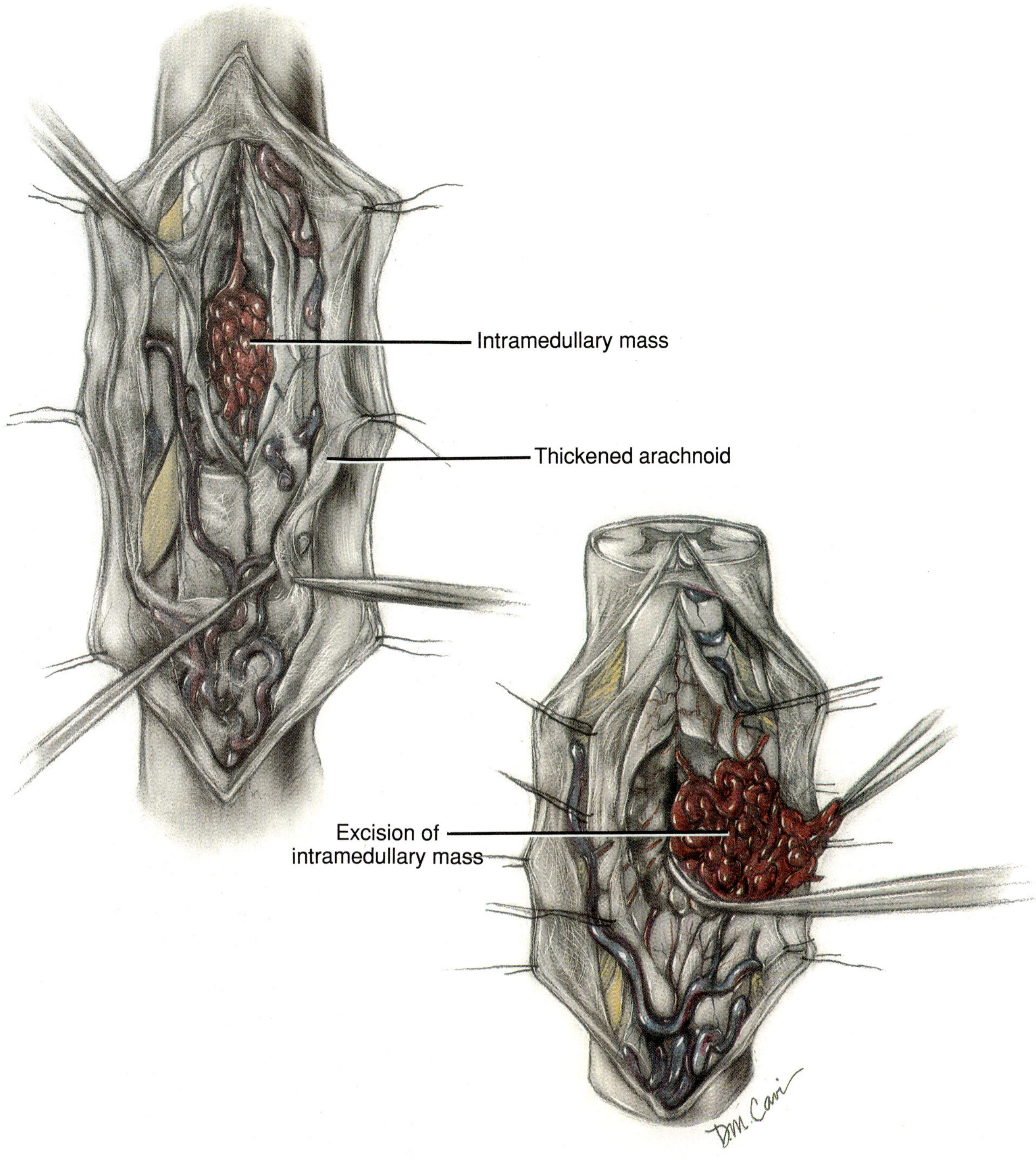

Figure 24.9.

Ligation and division or clipping with division will be required for large vessels. Smaller vessels can usually be coagulated with the bipolar coagulator and cut. The techniques of surgery of the malformation itself will be dependent on location; some lesions will be partially extramedullary and partially intramedullary. These are best approached by beginning with the obliteration of the extramedullary portion and then

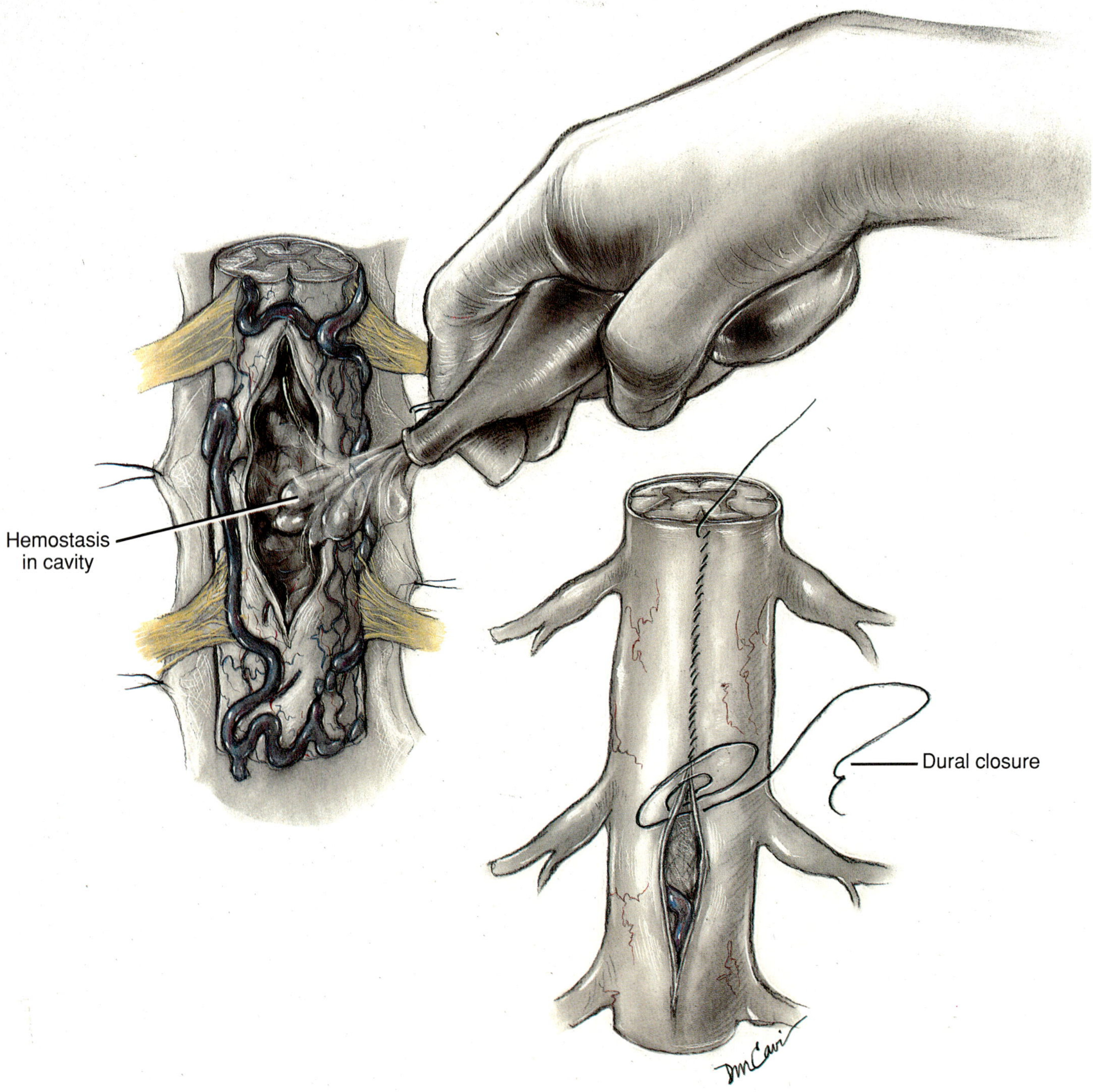

Figure 24.10.

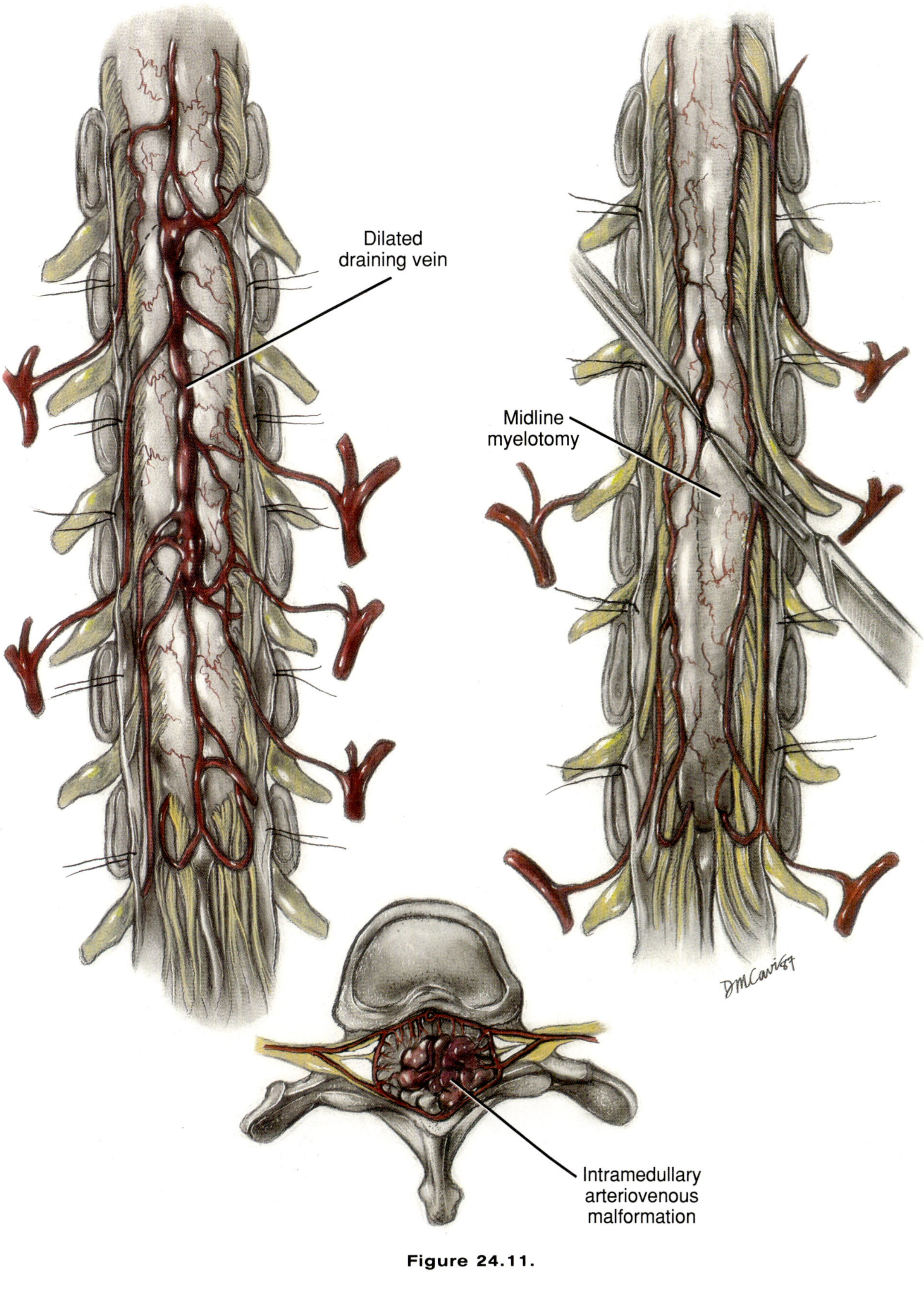
Dilated
draining vein
Midline
myelotomy
DMCavis87
Intramedullary
arteriovenous
malformation

Figure 24.11.

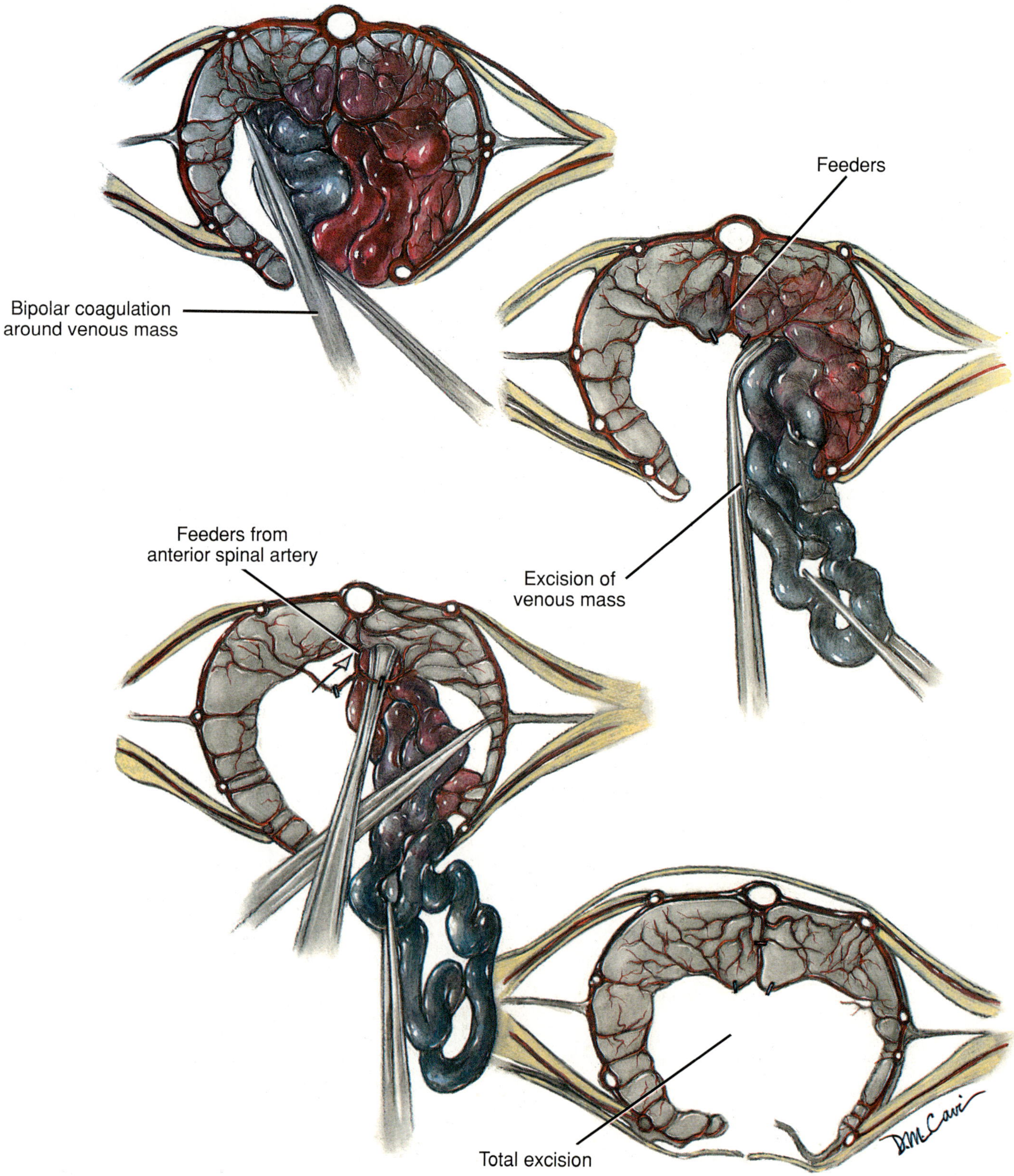
Feeders
Bipolar coagulation around venous mass
Feeders from anterior spinal artery
Excision of venous mass
Total excision
D.M. Cavi

Figure 24.12.

carefully dissecting the intramedullary portion free from the underlying cord wherever it is encountered. In this situation, the large vessels inside the cord are isolated by a combination of blunt dissection, with coagulation of feeding vessels, *and* division by sharp dissection wherever necessary. The malformation can gradually be devascularized and usually removed as a mass. The more common situation is one in which the malformation is virtually entirely within the cord. Only a few nodular excrescences bulging the spinal cord give a clue to the underlying abnormality. When this is the case, the cord is usually opened in the midline as for any other intramedullary tumor. The dissection should be carried down bluntly in the midline until the posterior aspect of the malformation is discovered. Then the dissection is extended around the malformation, with coagulation of all feeding vessels that remain. The large external vessels have already been obliterated by embolization so that only intramedullary shunts and vessels directly arising from the anterior spinal artery will be encountered. In these situations, the anterior spinal artery is often very large, and there are frequently large central tegmental arteries that feed into the malformation itself. These are hard to reach because of their anterior location. For this reason dissection laterally around the malformation is better done first, and then beginning either at the upper or lower pole, the dissection can be carried downward, isolating the anterior surface of malformation from cord. As the large central feeding vessels are encountered, they can be dissected free and coagulated or clipped near the anterior spinal artery. The use of small clips is better because it reduces the risk of an injury to the anterior spinal artery and also reduces the risk that one of the coagulated vessels will open, leaving a defect in the wall of the parent vessel. The malformation is peeled out of its bed while each of these feeding vessels is coagulated as encountered. Eventually, by these techniques the entire malformation can be delivered as a single piece. The lateral feeders present little problems, since they usually can be identified extraaxially and obliterated. The real difficulty is finding and interrupting the feeders from the anterior spinal artery without injury to that vessel. The principles of the dissection are the same as for any other intramedullary mass. The dissection on the cord must be done gently with blunt techniques, as suction removal of additional spinal cord tissue surrounding the malformation may lead to an unnecessary deficit. Since the dissection must be on the walls of the malformation, it is important to obliterate all possible feeding vessels before extrication of the mass begins. Fortunately, these malformations are not as high flow as those in the brain, where such a dissection carried out exactly on the malformation itself would be extremely dangerous. Once the malformation is removed, the bed should be carefully inspected for any potential vessel that might open, and all such vessels thoroughly coagulated. If there is adequate room, the dura should be closed in a watertight fashion. If there is not enough room, the dura can be patched, though the time-honored technique of simply leaving the dura opened is acceptable. The closure does not require special maneuvers otherwise.

SECTION 8

Spinal Cord Tumors

25

Intradural-Extramedullary Tumors

Intradural-extramedullary tumors are identified via computed tomography (CT) scanning, CT myelography, or magnetic resonance imaging (MRI). The location and extent of the tumor should be completely known in order to choose the appropriate operation. Posterior and anterolateral tumors are exposed by wide laminectomy. Anterior tumors may require a costotransverse or, rarely, an anterior approach. Removal of zygapophyseal joints laterally may be necessary to reach large anterior tumors, so preoperative plans for stabilization are required (see Chapters 6 and 16). No stereotyped approach is desirable.

Meningioma

Meningiomas characteristically occur in the thoracic region and, to a lesser extent, in the cervical area and are extremely rare in the lumbar area. They most commonly arise anterolaterally. Fewer meningiomas arise directly anterior to the cord. Posteriorly placed meningiomas are extremely rare, as are those that are truly extradural. The goal of surgery in all instances is total removal.

Operations are generally carried out with the patient in the prone position, though meningiomas in the high cervical region can also be approached with the patient in the sitting position. A midline incision should be planned to extend at least one segment above and below the expected tumor. Two segments

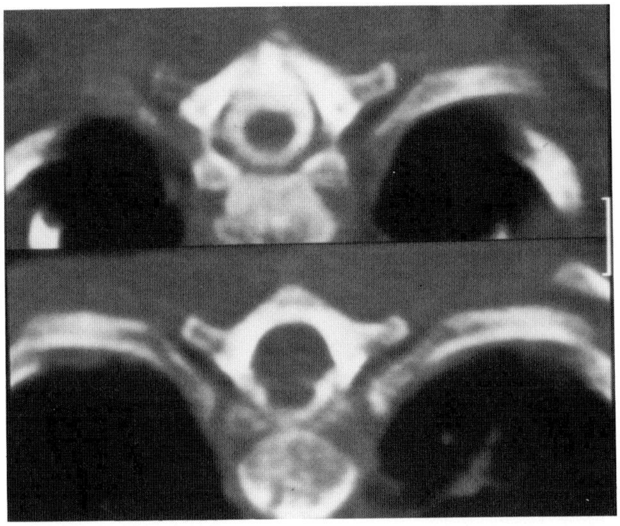

Figure 25.1. Posteriorly placed meningioma pressing the thoracic spinal cord from the posterior.

may make the manipulation of the cord easier with large tumors. Physiological monitoring of cord function is a helpful adjunct during tumor removal. A standard laminectomy should be carried out to expose the dura one or two segments above and below the lesion. The dura is then opened in the midline, via magnification, and once the dura is opened, the microscope is used throughout. Hemostatic materials in the gutter will be of help, and the opened dura should be sutured back against the muscle or held against the cut margins of the bone with retention sutures. Immaculate hemostasis in the epidural space is required before the dura is opened. The muscle edges should be covered with cottonoid, and sump suction may be of help in eliminating epidural ooze. Opening the dura usually exposes the tumor unless it is directly anterior. The arachnoid should then be opened around the tumor, exposing the superior and inferior margins and the whole posterior aspect. The tumor will usually present laterally as a purplish-brown soft mass with the posterior roots on the posterior aspect and the anterior roots in the tumor mass. Arachnoid should be freed from tumor, and the cord-tumor margin defined. Most of these intradural tumors are soft enough to be removed with suction or with the Cavitron ultrasonic dissector. The latter tool is desirable for the preciseness of the dissection. The laser is also of help for the same reason. A point on the tumor between roots should be identified posterolaterally, and the tumor mass entered with suction or the ultrasonic dissector. A laser is also useful, but for an intracapsular dissection the ultrasonic dissector is faster. The contents of the tumor mass are then removed, leaving the capsule intact to be gradually manipulated out from under the cord. This begins by removing tumor in the gutter laterally and by mobilizing the tumor from lateral to medial to allow it to be removed by suction or by the laser. This technique means the spinal cord does not have to be retracted. The dentate ligaments can be divided at their attachments to the dura, and the spinal cord can be rotated gently by the dentate ligaments with small clamps or forceps. Physiological monitoring is critical during this maneuver. The tumor is gradually mobilized laterally, and the capsule medially is dissected free from the spinal cord. The attachments of the tumor are most adherent in the anterolateral gutter. This is where tumor removal should be concentrated, so that the tumor is delivered from under the cord into the field rather than retracting the cord to expose the tumor. Via this intracapsular dissection, the tumor usually can gradually be teased from under the cord without retraction on the cord at all. The keys to safe tumor removal are the original definition of the tumor with removal of arachnoid from the true tumor capsule, the definition of the cord-tumor margin medially, and the beginning of tumor removal in the gutter, well away from spinal cord. Once the tumor mass is completely removed, a decision must be made about excision of dura. If the dura is involved, the involved portion should be completely excised. This may mean sacrifice of a root in the thoracic region, but roots must be preserved in the lumbar or cervical region if sparing is at all possible. Important roots must be followed through the tumor by using microtechniques and be preserved, and tumor fragments must be removed from them. If any must be cut, primary or graft repair should be accomplished.

Sometimes, the tumor is directly anterior to the cord. In this situation, some manipulation of the cord is required. Three dentate ligaments (or as many as necessary) should be divided to expose the tumor completely. The dentate ligaments can be used for lateral retraction, and the cord gently mobilized and rotated to expose the tumor. The laser or Cavitron can then be used to remove the tumor. Bilateral section of the dentate ligaments and rotation of the cord from side to side may be necessary. Physiological

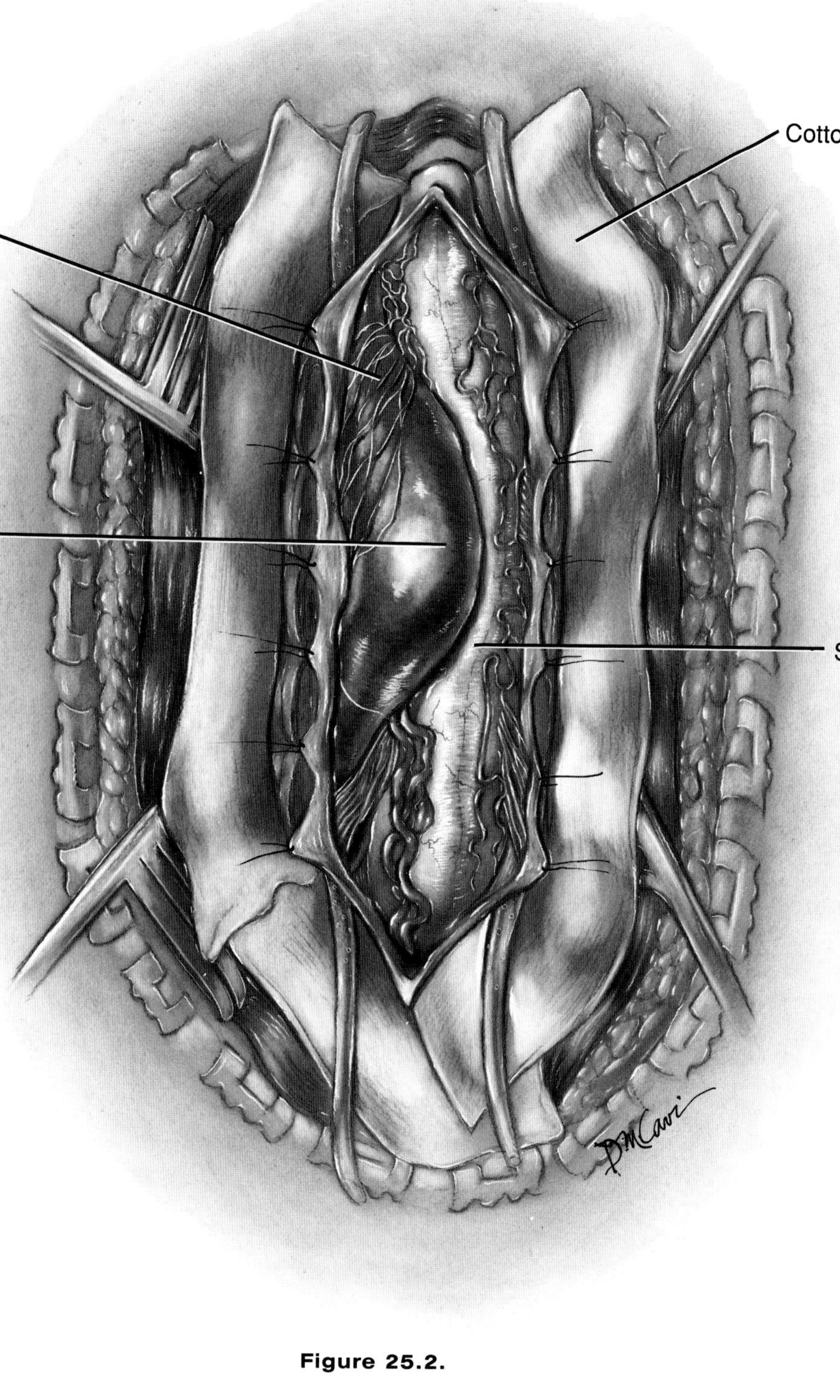

Figure 25.2.

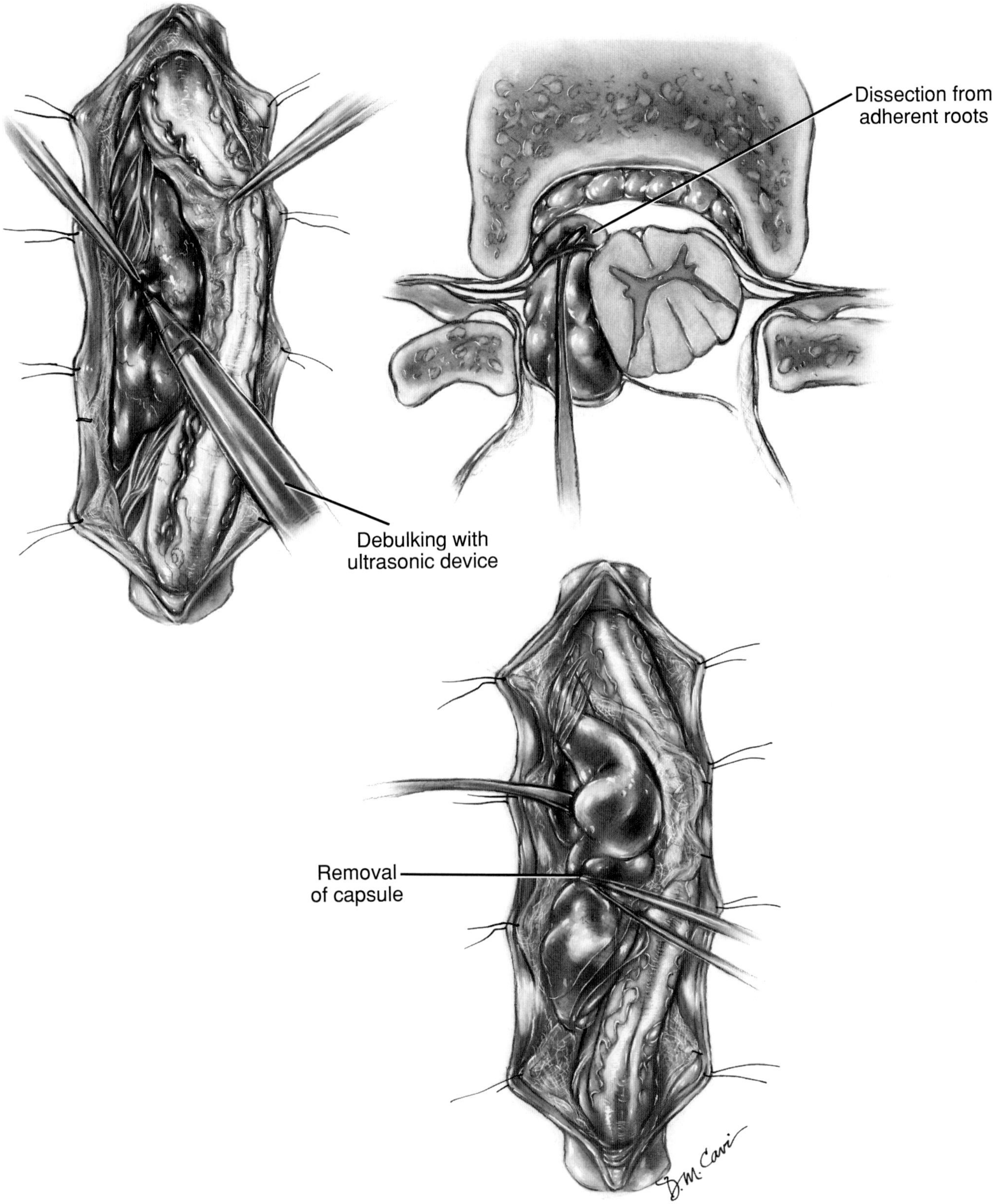
Dissection from adherent roots
Debulking with ultrasonic device
Removal of capsule

Figure 25.3.

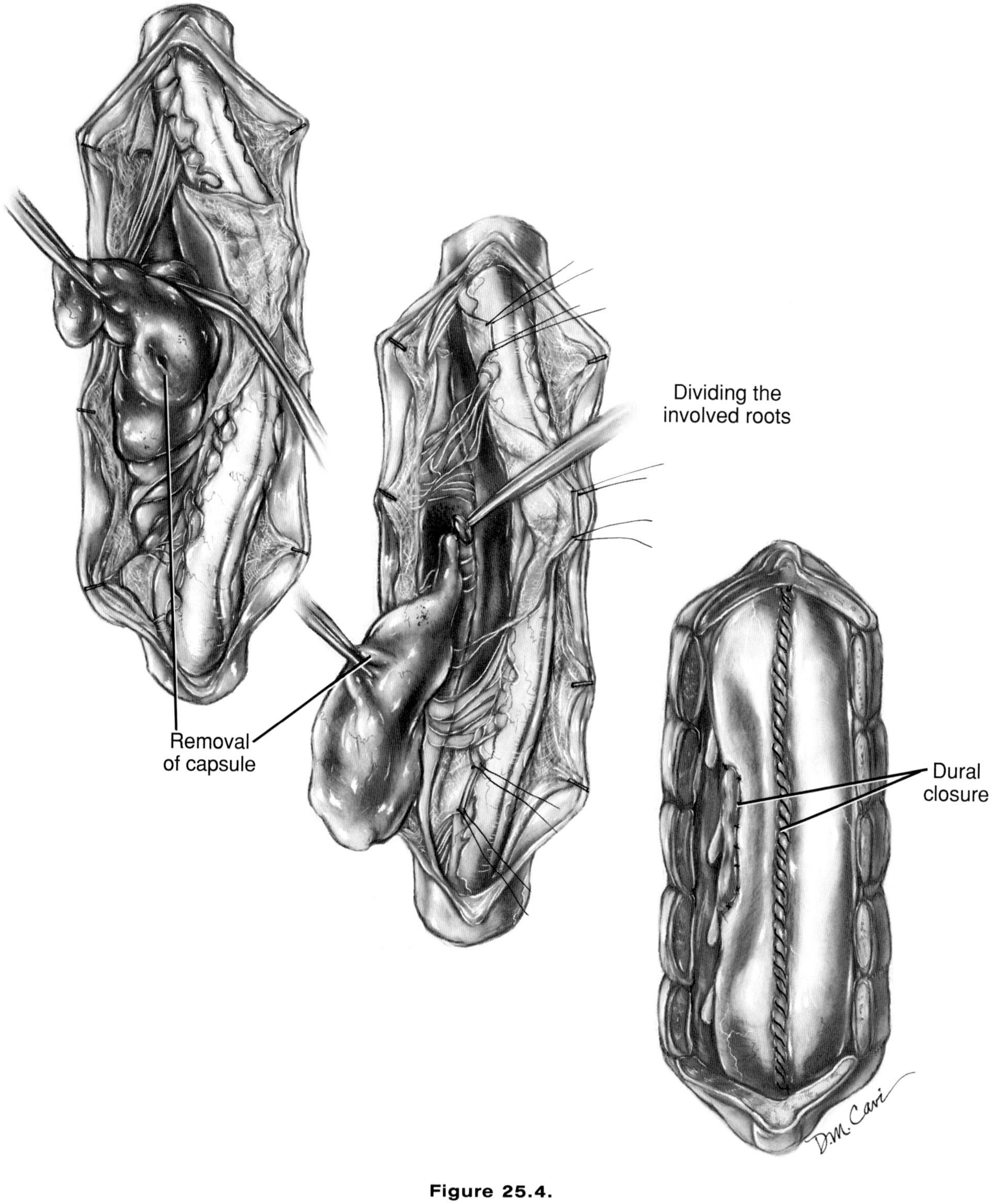
Dividing the
involved roots
Removal
of capsule
Dural
closure
D.M. Cavi

Figure 25.4.

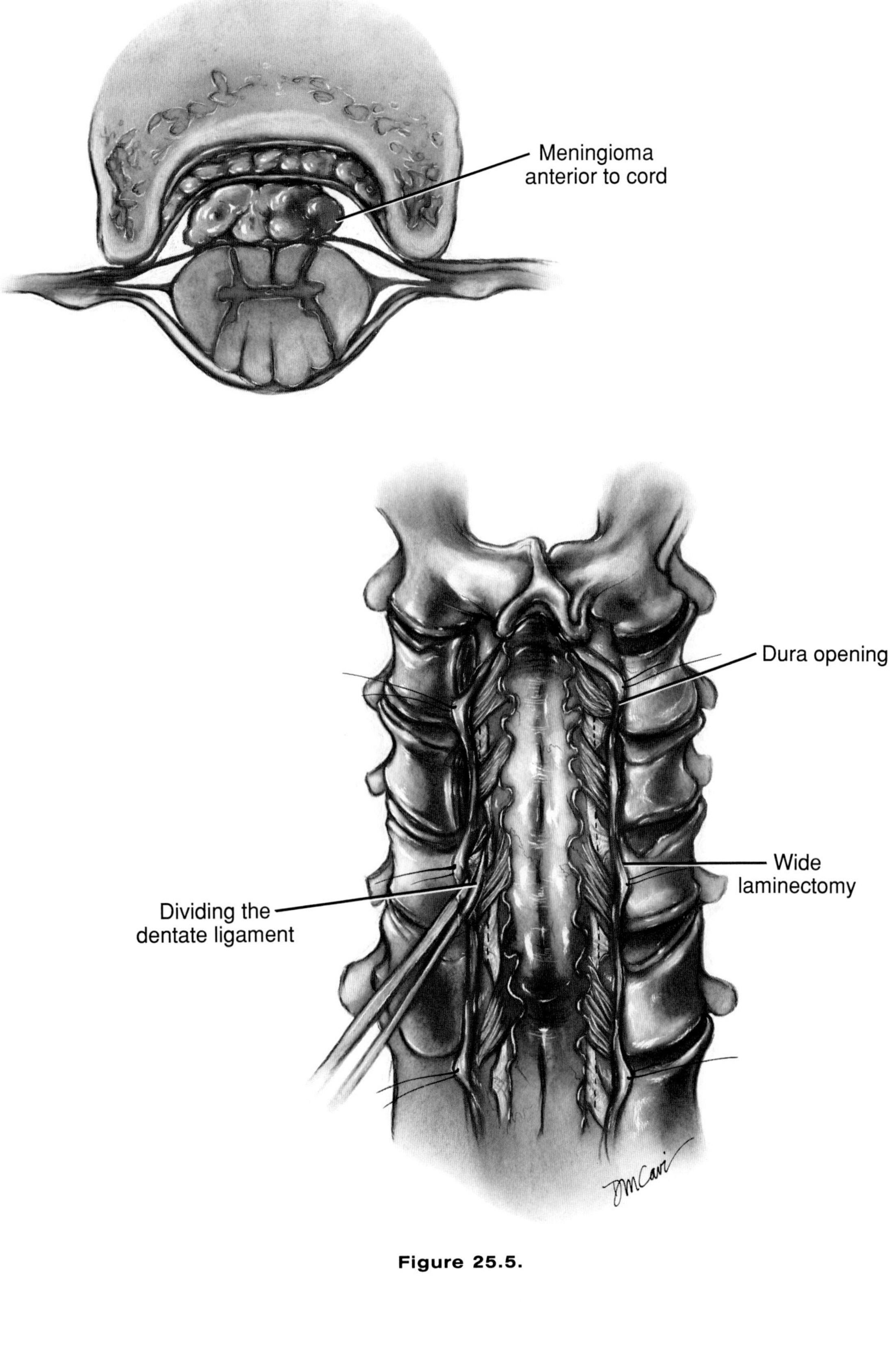
Meningioma
anterior to cord
Dura opening
Wide
laminectomy
Dividing the
dentate ligament

Figure 25.5.

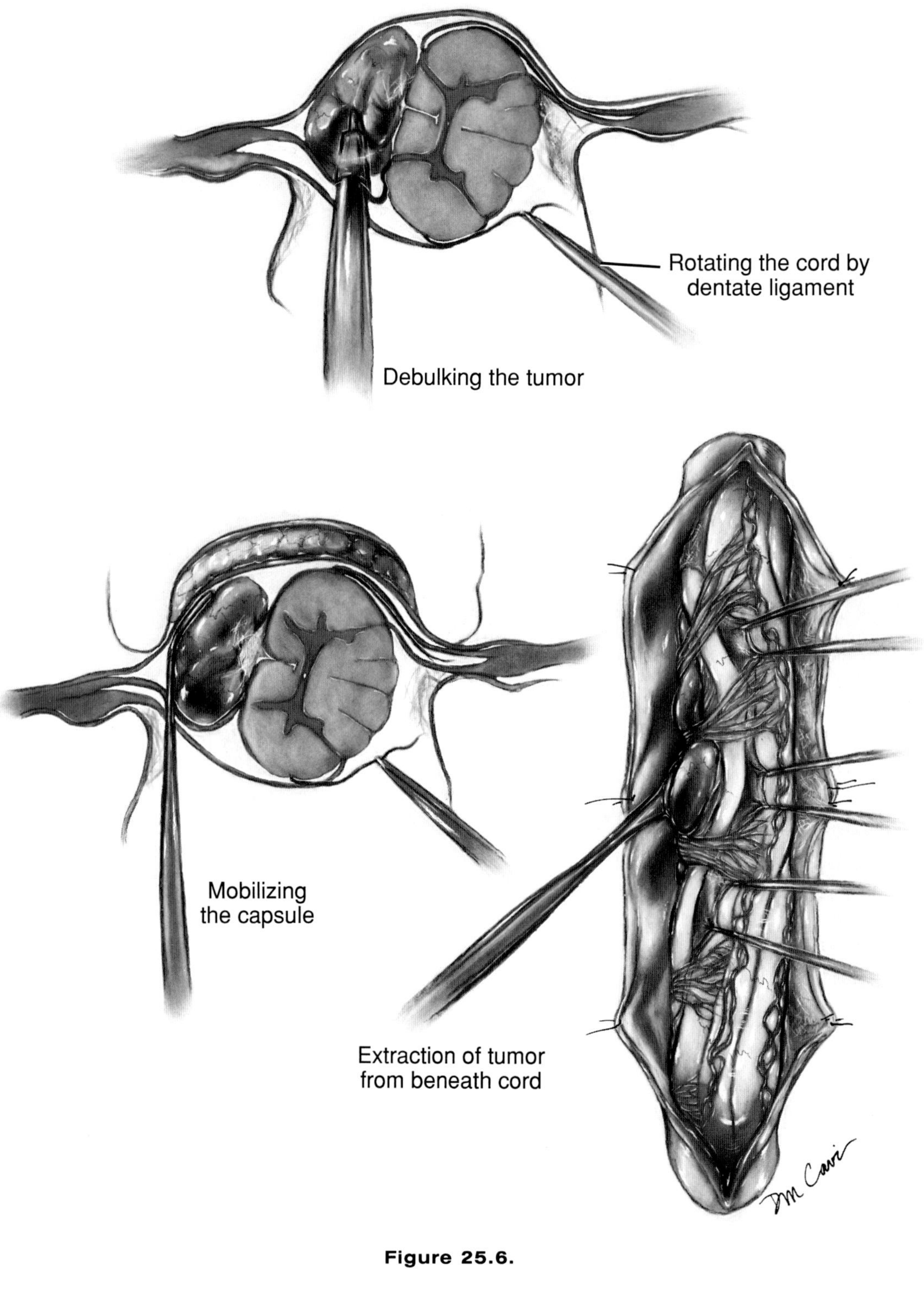
Rotating the cord by dentate ligament
Debulking the tumor
Mobilizing the capsule
Extraction of tumor from beneath cord

Figure 25.6.

monitoring during this maneuver is protective. If manipulation causes a change in spinal evoked potentials, the technique can be modified so that manipulation is less vigorous. If exposure of the anterior tumor is not adequate, bone is removed laterally, converting the approach to a modified costotransverse (transpedicular) exposure. This much removal of bone may require stabilization. The dissection should be at the junction of the tumor anteriorly with dura, not where the tumor impinges on the cord. Carrying the dissection across the base of the tumor by removing the attachment to the dura anteriorly and debulking the tumor internally, leaving the capsule intact, makes it possible to decompress the cord gradually and remove the tumor without dissecting the cord at all. Finally, the greatly thinned capsule and tumor mass can be dissected free from cord. The adhesions are usually not major, and the tumor can usually be delivered by gentle traction or blunt dissection under direct vision and high magnification. Care must be taken, while capsular vessels are being coagulated, to avoid any that also supply the cord. Major radicular vessels must also be preserved. If there is tumor involvement of the anterior dura, it should be excised. This may cause some bleeding, but the defect does not have to be closed. Once the tumor is out and hemostasis is satisfactory, the posterior dura should be closed in a watertight fashion. If a significant lateral portion has to be removed, then a patch is desirable but not mandatory. The defect can be covered with Gelfoam or fascia. The paravertebral muscles should be closed with a single layer of sutures in the fascia; the subcutaneous tissue and skin require no special precaution.

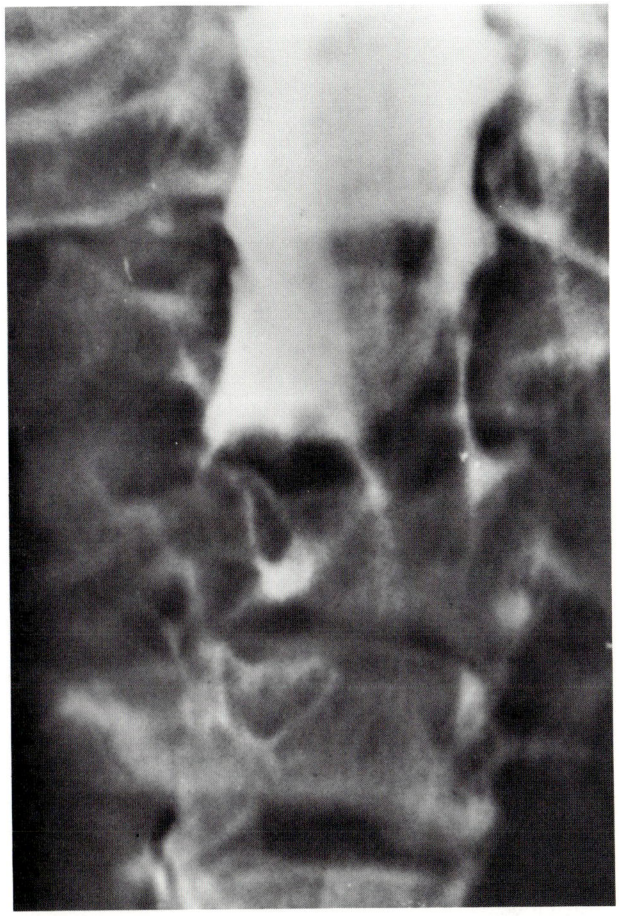

Figure 25.7. Typical myelographic picture of an extramedullary neurofibroma arising from the posterior root and displacing the spinal cord.

Neurofibroma

Operations on neurofibromas are very similar to those required for meningiomas, and the same general principles apply. The goal is operative cure. The neurofibroma also may have a significant extradural extension, and this must be considered in planning the operation. The first decision to be made is whether the operation will be in one or two stages. If the extradural extraspinal component is extremely large or located in a body cavity difficult to reach by the midline posterior approach, then a two-stage operation in which the intraspinal portion is removed first and the extraspinal portion is removed later may be desirable. This decision must be based on tumor size and the expected difficulty with the extradural approach and tumor removal.

For most tumors a midline incision with the patient under general anesthesia in the prone position is utilized. The incision should extend at least one or two segments above and below the margins of the tumor. A standard laminectomy is carried out, and the tumor is exposed by opening the dura in the midline. Neurofibromas generally arise from posterior roots and are found posterolateral to the spinal cord. The microscope is brought in to open the dura and is used throughout the operation. The first step must be removal of the intradural portion of the tumor. The arachnoid should be removed until the tumor margins are seen laterally, superiorly, and inferiorly. The relationship of dorsal roots should be identified. Some-

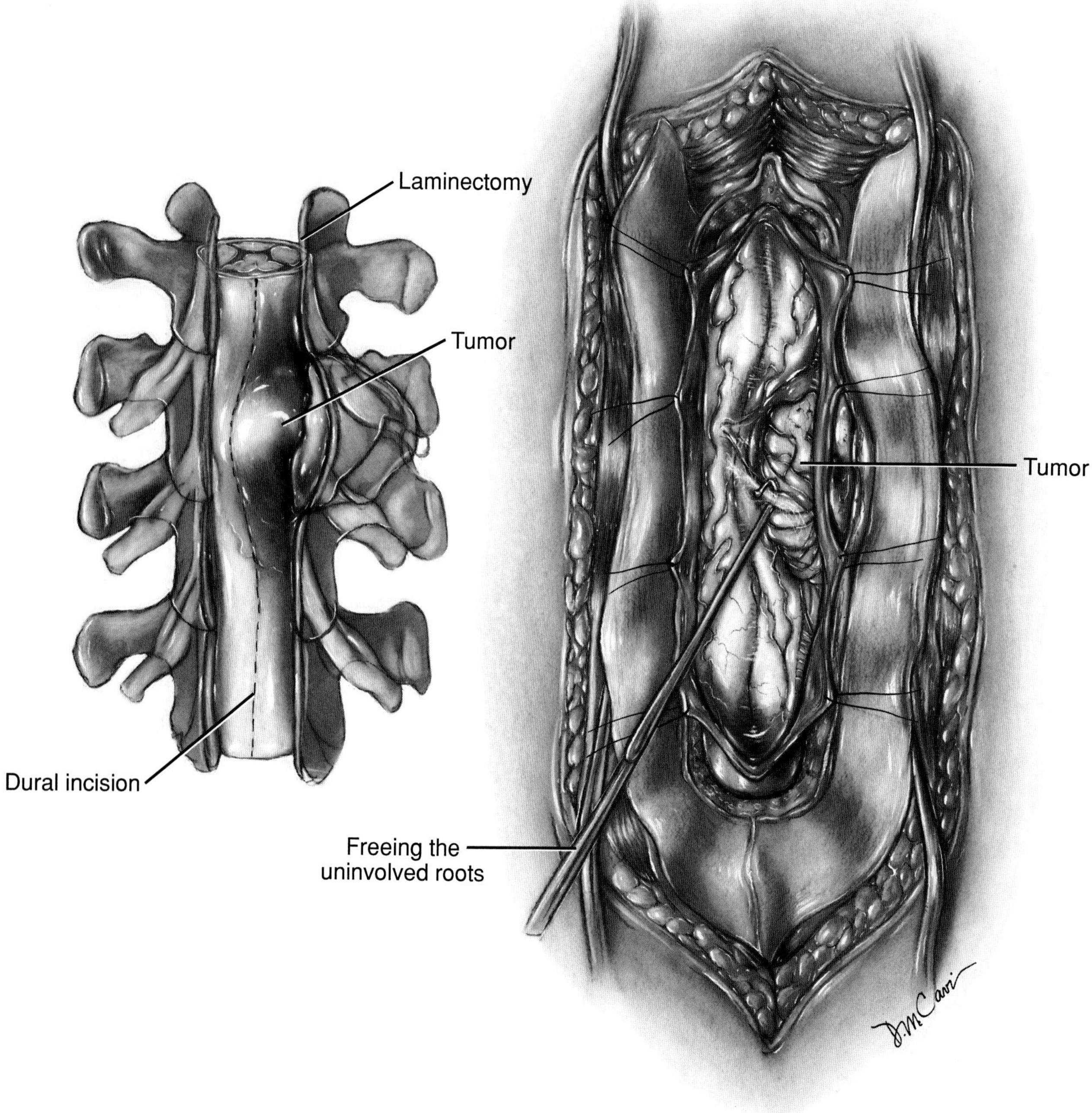

Figure 25.8.

times, some or all enter the tumor, and complete removal of the tumor without sacrifice of the roots is impossible. Frequently, only a few filaments are involved, and many of the dorsal roots can be saved. In the thoracic region, it may be simpler to sacrifice the root involved. In other areas, careful dissection of the filaments from the tumor is possible, and any neural elements that can be saved should be. Anterior roots are much more likely to be displaced by tumor than have tumor involvement and can routinely be

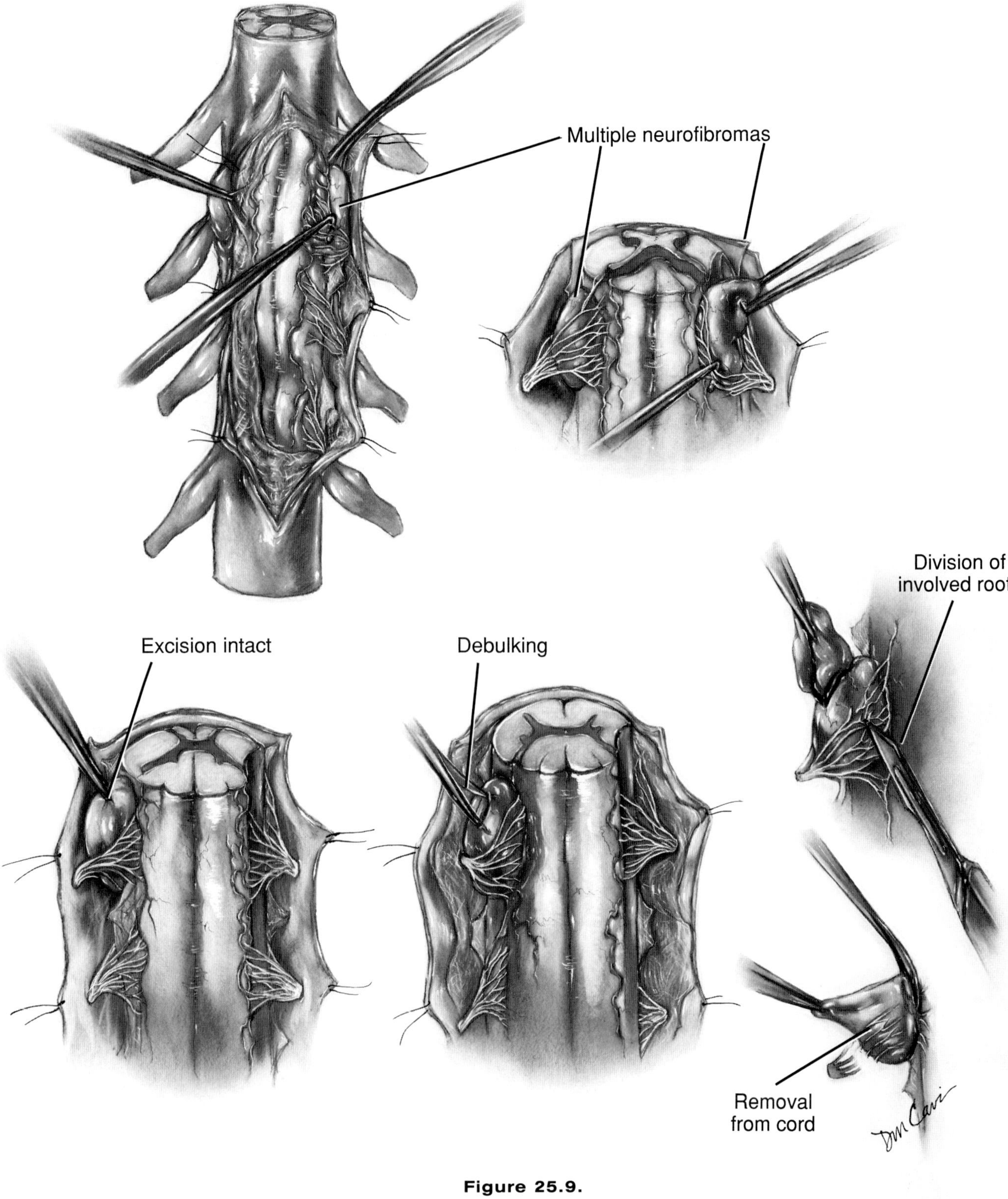
Multiple neurofibromas
Division of
involved roots
Excision intact
Debulking
Removal
from cord

Figure 25.9.

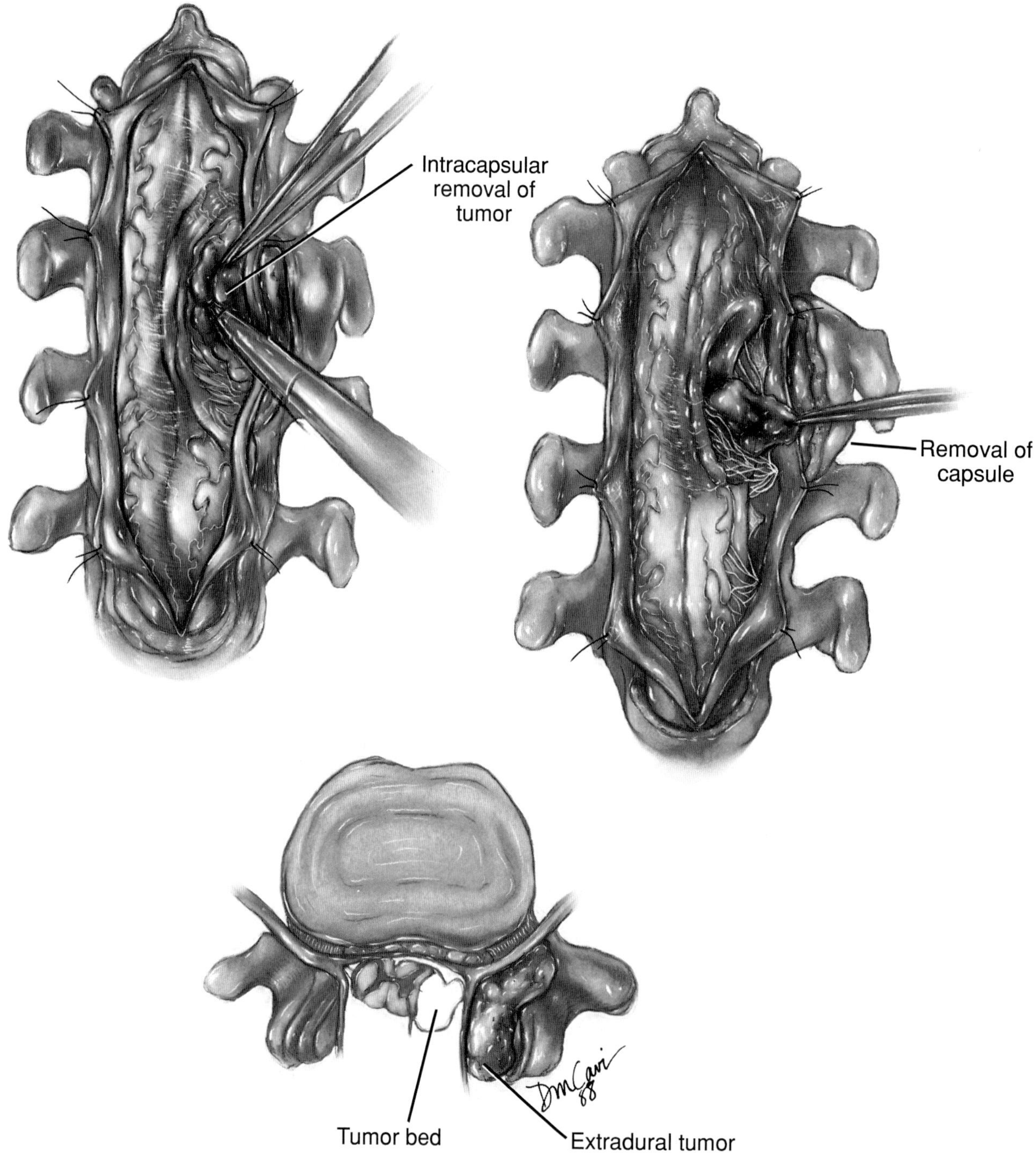
Intracapsular removal of tumor
Removal of capsule
Tumor bed
Extradural tumor

Figure 25.10.

saved. Once the posterior roots are separated from tumor insofar as possible, those inextricable are cut and tumor removal can begin. The laser or ultrasonic dissector is used to open the tumor and carry out an intracapsular removal. This should begin laterally, well away from the spinal cord; the tumor bulk should be replaced until the remaining capsule can be dissected free from cord and adherent roots anteriorly. The anterior roots are likely to be displaced and splayed out on tumor capsule. They should be dissected free after the cord dissection is complete. In the thoracic region their sacrifice is inconsequential, but in the lumbar and cervical area it is obviously important to preserve them, and the tedious dissection that may be required is well worth the effort for the patient. As the tumor is debulked, gentle blunt dissection will free the capsule from cord to which it is rarely adherent. There may be sizable vessels in the tumor capsule, but for these to traverse to cord is distinctly unusual. All important radicular vessels on the capsule must be separated. With small tumors an intracapsular removal is not necessary. A circumferential dissection freeing nerve roots and cord from tumor capsule is carried out, and then the nerve roots, which are an intimate part of the tumor, are divided medially and laterally to allow the tumor to be totally removed.

Once the neural elements are free of tumor and the intraspinal portion is removed, the extraspinal procedure can begin. When the tumor is moderate in size and its removal is feasible from the single posterior incision, excision continues with the dura open. If the tumor is large and a second procedure is going to be required, the tumor should be removed well out into the expanded neural foramen, and the operation terminated when the extraspinal portion of the tumor has been isolated and entrance to the dura will no longer be necessary at the second operation. The tumor should be removed well beyond the lateral margins of the dura. The defect in the foramen left by tumor removal should be packed with a hemostatic agent to make certain no intradural bleeding will occur, and then a small patch of dura is fashioned from fascia sutured in place over the defect. This will seal and effectively isolate the tumor from the subarachnoid space. At the second operation, it will be possible to remove the tumor without encountering cerebrospinal fluid.

The next step is to ensure adequate exposure of the extradural mass. The spinal dissection is carried laterally, exposing the zygapophyseal joints, and then is extended beyond, exposing transverse processes or ribs. In the lumbar and thoracic region, where there is no artery to worry about, the only requirement for continued tumor removal is excision of bone from the posterior margin of the enlarged foramen until the tumor can be dissected free circumferentially. The exposure should be continued laterally, with muscle retracted, until the lateral margin of the tumor is exposed. Small extensions can be dissected by grasping the capsule and slowly mobilizing the tumor back through the expanded foramen by blunt dissection, coagulating and cutting adhesions and blood vessels wherever they are encountered. With larger extensions, it is better to carry out an intracapsular removal, via the laser or Cavitron, gradually shrinking the tumor until the capsule can be separated from surrounding tissue. Only those nerve roots that are inextricably incorporated into the tumor should be sacrificed. The others can usually be dissected free. In the thoracic area, the entire nerve can be sacrificed. In the lumbar region, a careful dissection may be required to prevent an important neurological deficit, and some demonstrable loss may be unavoidable. If there is a major extension into the lumbosacral plexus, it is better to extend the incision to allow a retroperitoneal exposure. Brachial plexus extensions are better managed by a planned second stage.

In the cervical region, the dissection is complicated by the presence of the vertebral artery. The artery should be visualized by angiography, or its location estimated on the CT scan. Unless the extraspinal portion of the mass is very small, it is better to carry out a subtotal intracapsular removal before the capsular dissection is begun. This will minimize the chance of injuring the vertebral artery that is usually anterior and lateral to the tumor. The dissection should utilize blunt or semisharp dissectors whenever possible and should be carried out on the tumor capsule rather than on the soft tissue or bony side. Often, there are small feeding vessels leaving the vertebral artery to enter the capsule where it adheres. These should be coagulated on the tumor side and cut rather than torn by dissection. If they are not thoroughly coagulated or if they are inadvertently torn during the dissection, they may cause a small hole in the vertebral wall, which can be very troublesome. Rather than coagulating such a small opening or attempting to suture it

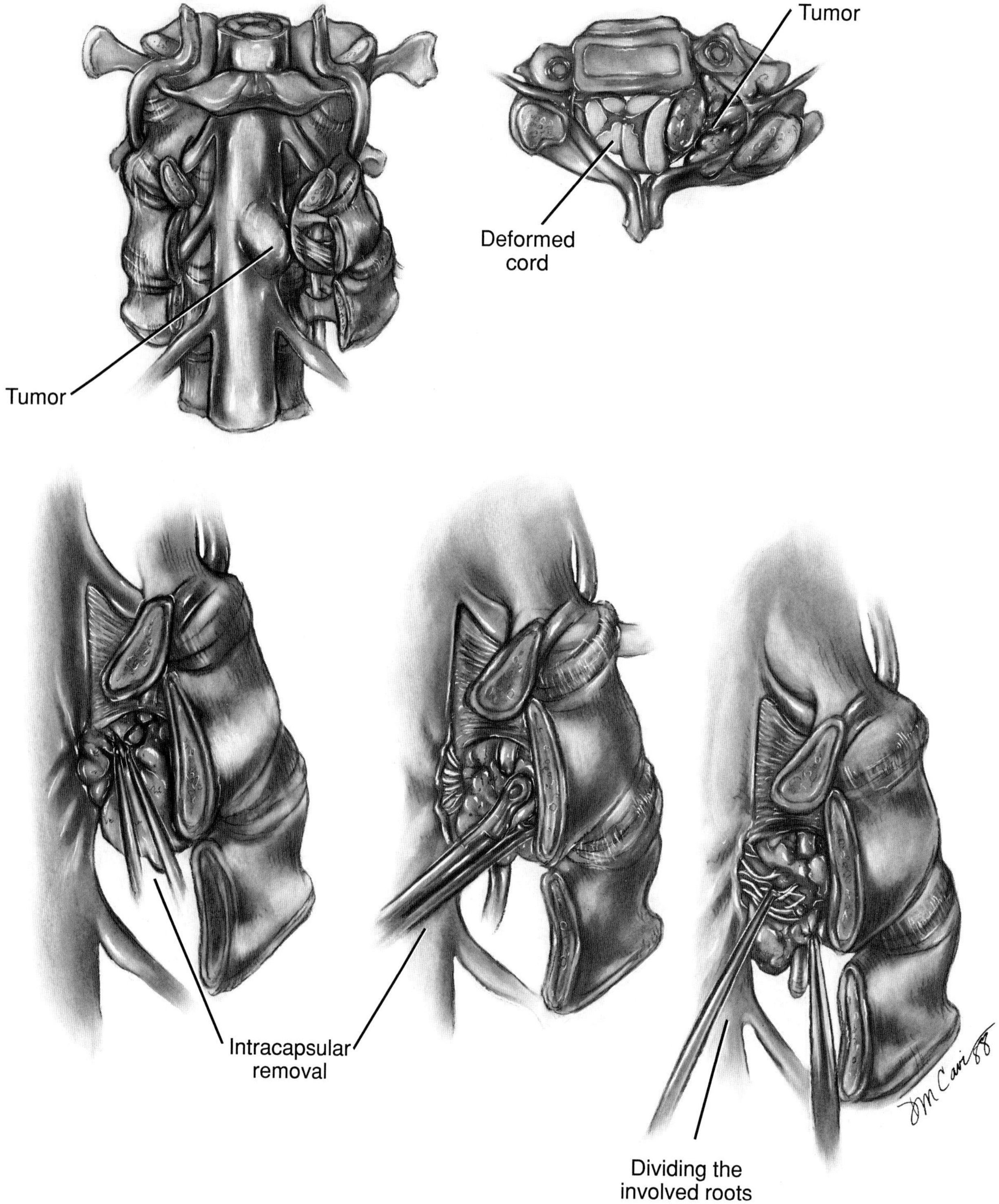
Tumor
Deformed cord
Tumor
Intracapsular removal
Dividing the involved roots

Figure 25.11.

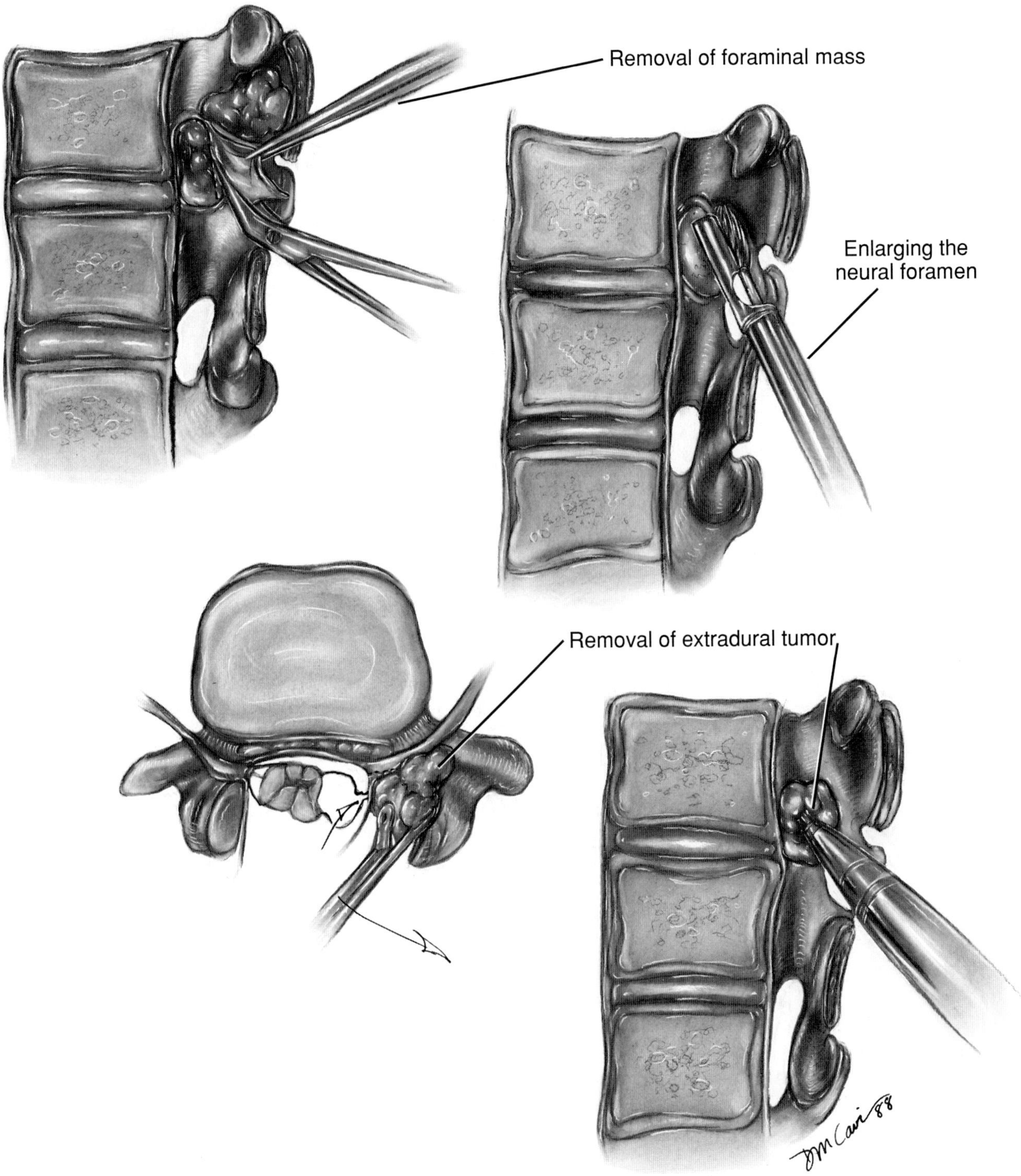
Removal of foraminal mass
Enlarging the neural foramen
Removal of extradural tumor

Figure 25.12.

directly, the application of a small amount of hemostatic material or small muscle pledgets to the wall will usually provide adequate hemostasis without running the risk of enlarging the vascular defect. Attention to these details allows the tumor to be dissected free from the vertebral artery, and even if the vertebral artery is not seen, these techniques will protect it so that total tumor removal is possible. The vertebral artery is often found only after tumor removal when its pulsations can be clearly identified. Frequently, total tumor removal leaving the dura intact is possible, since the tumor has expanded the root sheath. In this situation, nothing needs to be done except to close the midline dural incision. If there is a large lateral dural defect, it may be patched with pressure patch only. An appropriately sized piece of cervical fascia is harvested and placed over the defect. A slit should be cut in an appropriate place to allow it to be slid around the root and in front of the cord. The dura is then closed in the midline. A watertight dural seal with protection of the cord from adhesions at the bare extradural surgical site is obtained. The cervical muscles are closed with a single layer of sutures in the fascia; the wound needs no other special closure technique.

26 Foramen Magnum Meningioma

The removal of the foramen magnum meningioma varies to some extent from the removal of other meningiomas of the base of the skull and those of the upper cervical area. These tumors are notorious for the peculiarities of their clinical presentation. Computed tomography (CT) scanning and magnetic resonance imaging (MRI) now delineate them exactly so that the time-honored exploration of the posterior fossa is never necessary. Furthermore, surgery can be planned according to the exact location and configuration of the tumor. Those directly anterior to the cord are better approached by a transoral or lateral transcervical route.

The operations may be carried out with the patient in the sitting or prone position under general anesthesia. A midline skin incision is made from the inion to the midcervical spine, approximately at C4. Muscles are removed from the occipital bone and upper cervical spine by the subperiosteal techniques described in Chapter 11. A limited posterior fossa craniectomy is first done. The standard technique is to drill one or more burr holes in the occipital bone and then connect them by rongeuring away the remainder of the bone including the rim of the foramen magnum. The high-speed drill is also a convenient way to remove this bone. The arch of C1 and the posterior elements of C2 are then removed. The dura is opened in a Y-shaped fashion, with the foot of the Y extending

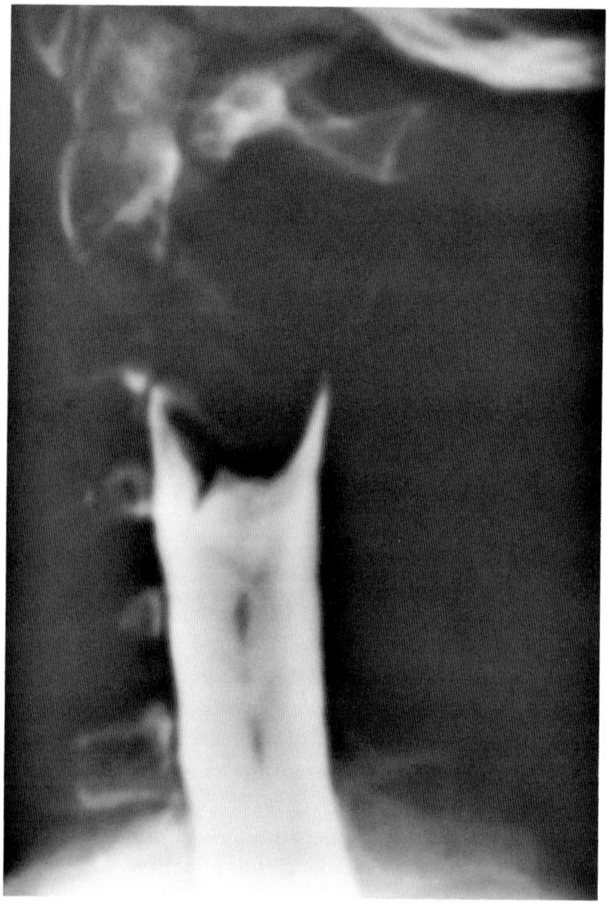

Figure 26.1. Typical myelographic picture of intradural-extramedullary meningioma of the foramen magnum and upper cervical spine.

from the margin of the foramen magnum to the lower exposure and with the arms of the Y extending toward the lateral superior margins of the bony removal. The dural edges are coagulated as necessary and retracted out of the field with retention sutures. If there is any epidural bleeding, it should be controlled with hemostatic packing before the dural sutures are placed. The dura should be opened from well below the lower extent of the tumor. Magnification makes the dural opening safer when the cord is tightly against the posterior surface of the dura. The imaging techniques currently available make it obvious when this is the situation, so the dural opening can be tailored to the exact anatomical configuration expected. Once the dura is opened, the arachnoid can be opened and cerebrospinal fluid drained. Usually, this will provide adequate relaxation. The tumors are nearly always seen immediately, for most are located laterally at the rim of the foramen magnum, often involving C1-C2 roots and the proximal intradural portion of the vertebral artery. The cervicomedullary junction is usually displaced to the opposite side. The tumor is visible lateral to the brain stem and upper cervical cord. Physiological monitoring of cord function throughout removal is desirable. Should any changes occur, the techniques or retractor position should be modified, and time allowed for recovery of the evoked potentials before proceeding. The ultrasonic dissector or the laser is ideal for the removal of these tumors. A lateral portion of the tumor should be identified where the tumor can be easily entered near the lateral dura. The tumor attachment is most common laterally near the exit of the upper cervical nerves. These nerves can be preserved if this seems easy, but their loss is of no great consequence to the patient, and it is better to sacrifice them in the interest of total tumor removal than to run any risk of leaving tumor behind or injuring the cord in the attempt to preserve them. If the nerves are to be sacrificed, they should be coagulated near the surface of the tumor and cut. Be certain that no major vessels destined for the cord are associated with these nerves. Any sizable radicular branch at this level should be preserved if it enters the cord. The Cavitron or laser should then be used to resect the lateralmost portion of the tumor; gradually the tumor mass can be debulked, and the tumor removed from beneath the cord. This is safer than attempting to dissect the cord tumor plane before the tumor is debulked. Remember that the vertebral artery may be encircled by tumor. The upper portion of the tumor should not be removed until the vertebral artery can be identified. As adequate debulking is obtained, it is then possible to grasp the capsule of the tumor and gently remove it from the cord. There may be blood vessels that are intimately adherent to the surface of the tumor and cord. Those that are clearly within tumor can be coagulated. If there is any question, they should be left and dissected free by gentle blunt techniques. A combination of these techniques will usually remove the tumor completely. At the upper margin, the intracranial portion of the vertebral should be identified, and tumor dissected from it by blunt dissection if possible. These tumors rarely

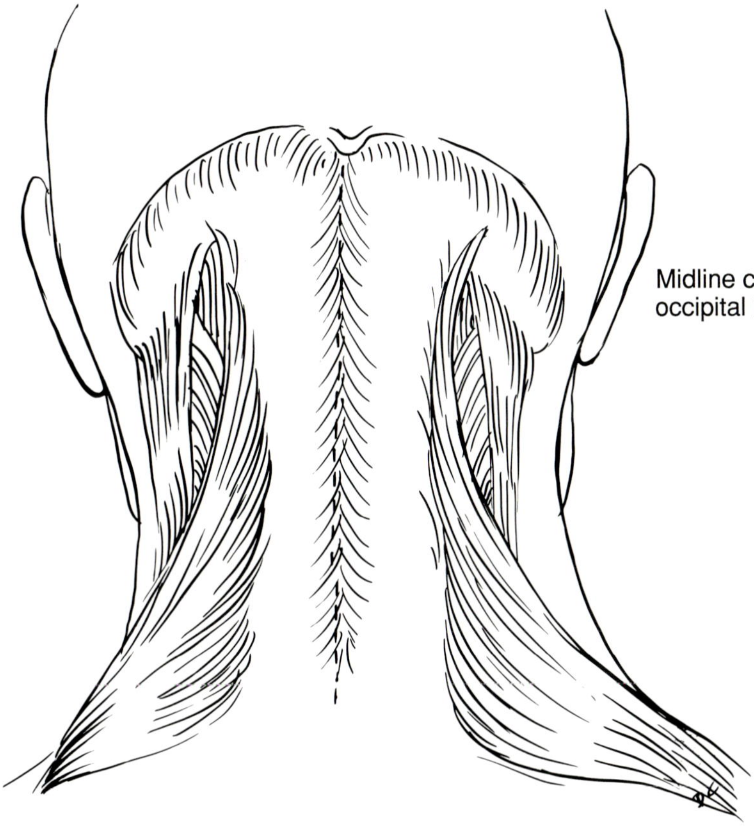

Figure 26.2.

have invaded the vessel wall and can be stripped from it. The Rosen knife is an excellent tool for this purpose. Once the extent of involvement of the vessel is identified, either Cavitron or laser can be used, provided an adequate margin of tumor is preserved on the vessel wall to be removed by blunt dissection later. Total removal of these tumors is the rule. Involved dura should be resected wherever possible. Around the vertebral artery where it is not possible to remove it, thorough coagulation will usually suffice to prevent tumor recurrence. Anterior dura that is resected should be replaced by a small pledget of cervical fascia. The dura should be closed posteriorly in a watertight fashion. Stitches are used in the deep cervical musculature to obliterate dead space and provide hemostasis. The main strength sutures are in the ligamentum nuchae. Subcutaneous layers and skin require no special techniques. To reduce the risk of cerebrospinal fluid leak, a seal should be obtained with these sutures.

Anteriorly Placed Foramen Magnum Tumors

Meningiomas or lower clival chordomas sometimes are located directly anterior to the cord and medulla in a location that makes it virtually impossible to reach the tumor from the side, without undue retraction. This rare situation can be appreciated by the scans and requires planning a different operative approach. A midline transpalatopharyngeal route provides the best exposure for small tumors. For larger tumors the lateral C1-C2 approach is better (see Chapter 14).

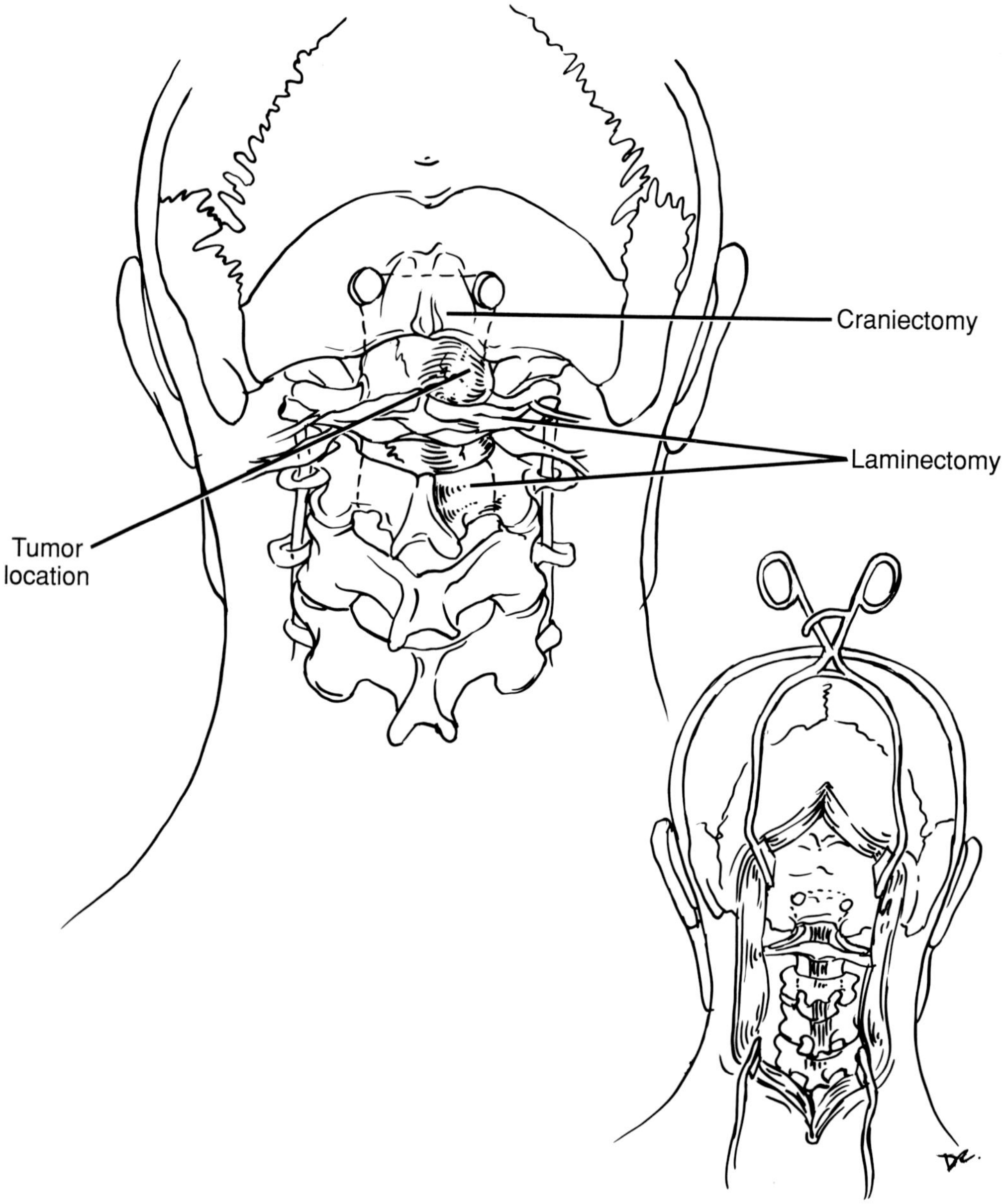

Figure 26.3.

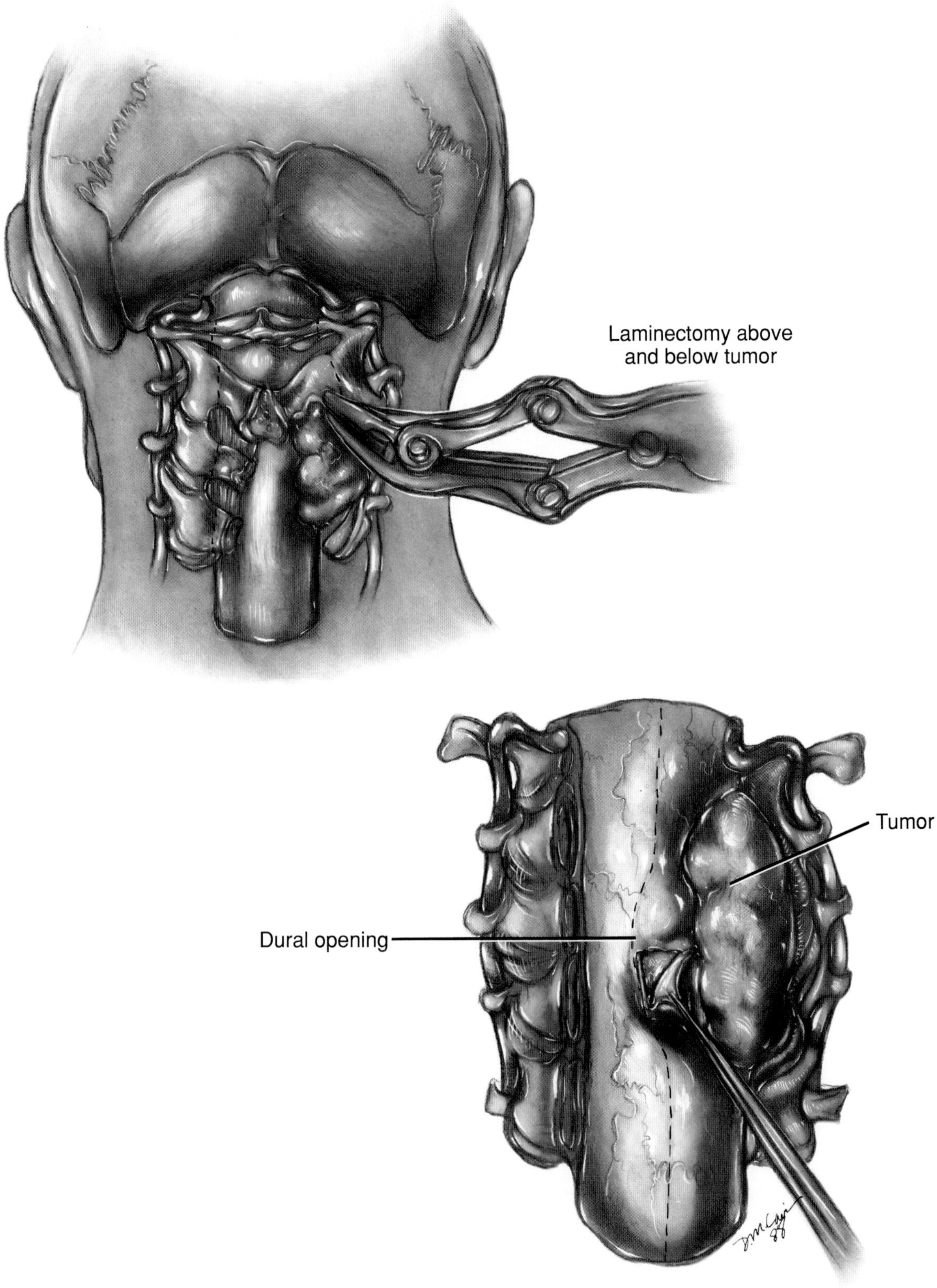

Figure 26.4.

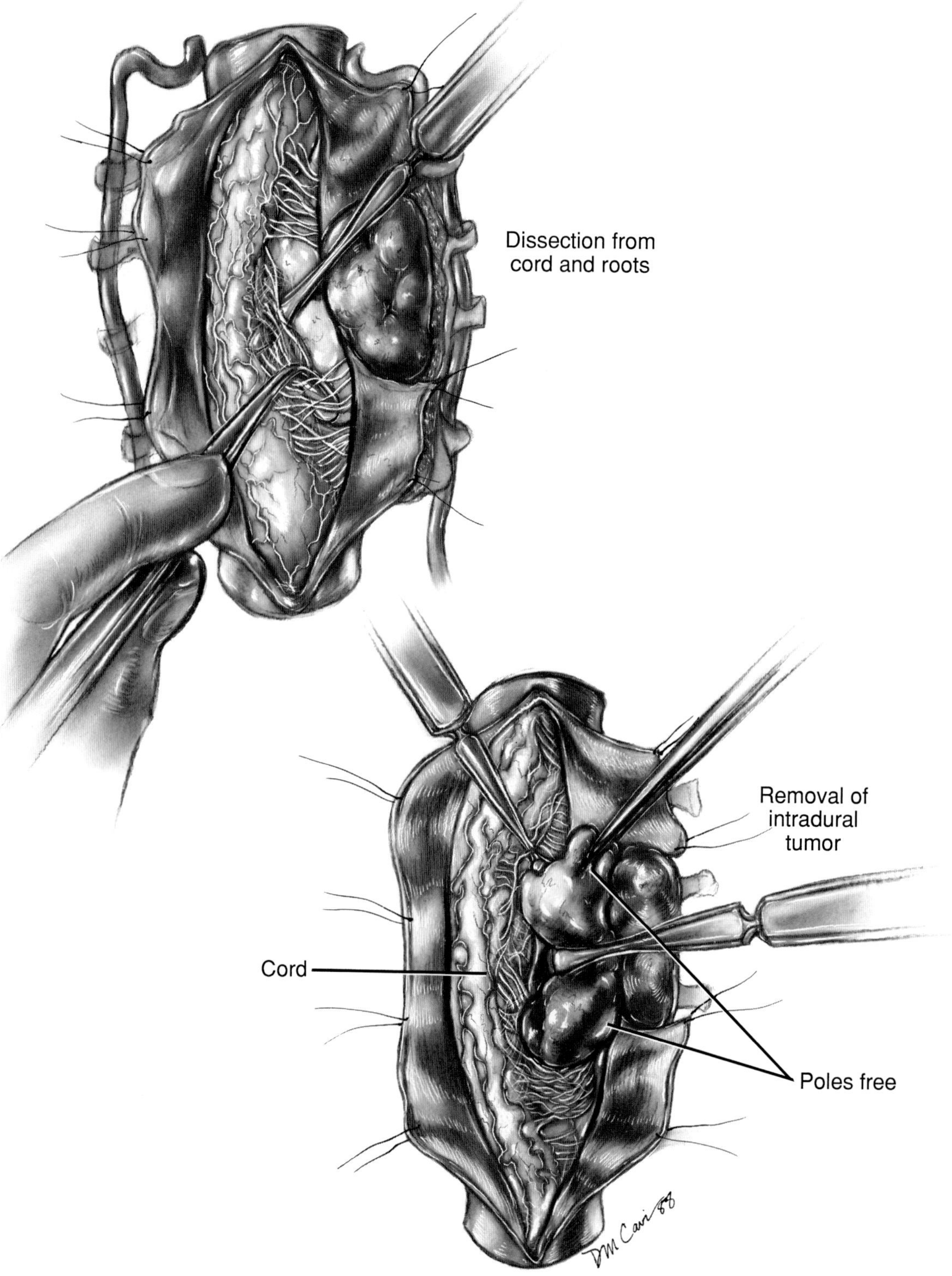
Dissection from cord and roots
Removal of intradural tumor
Cord
Poles free

Figure 26.5.

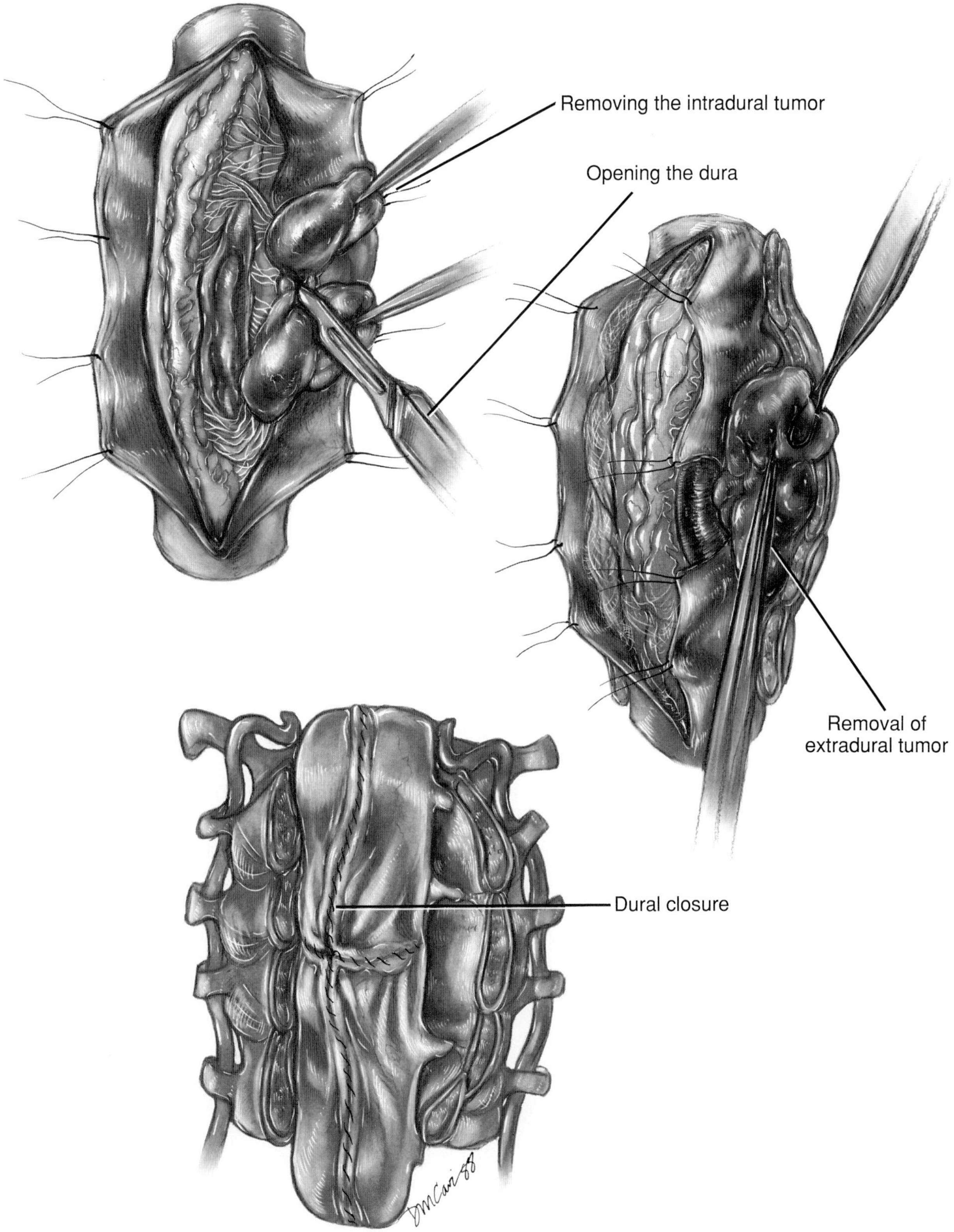
Removing the intradural tumor
Opening the dura
Removal of extradural tumor
Dural closure

Figure 26.6.

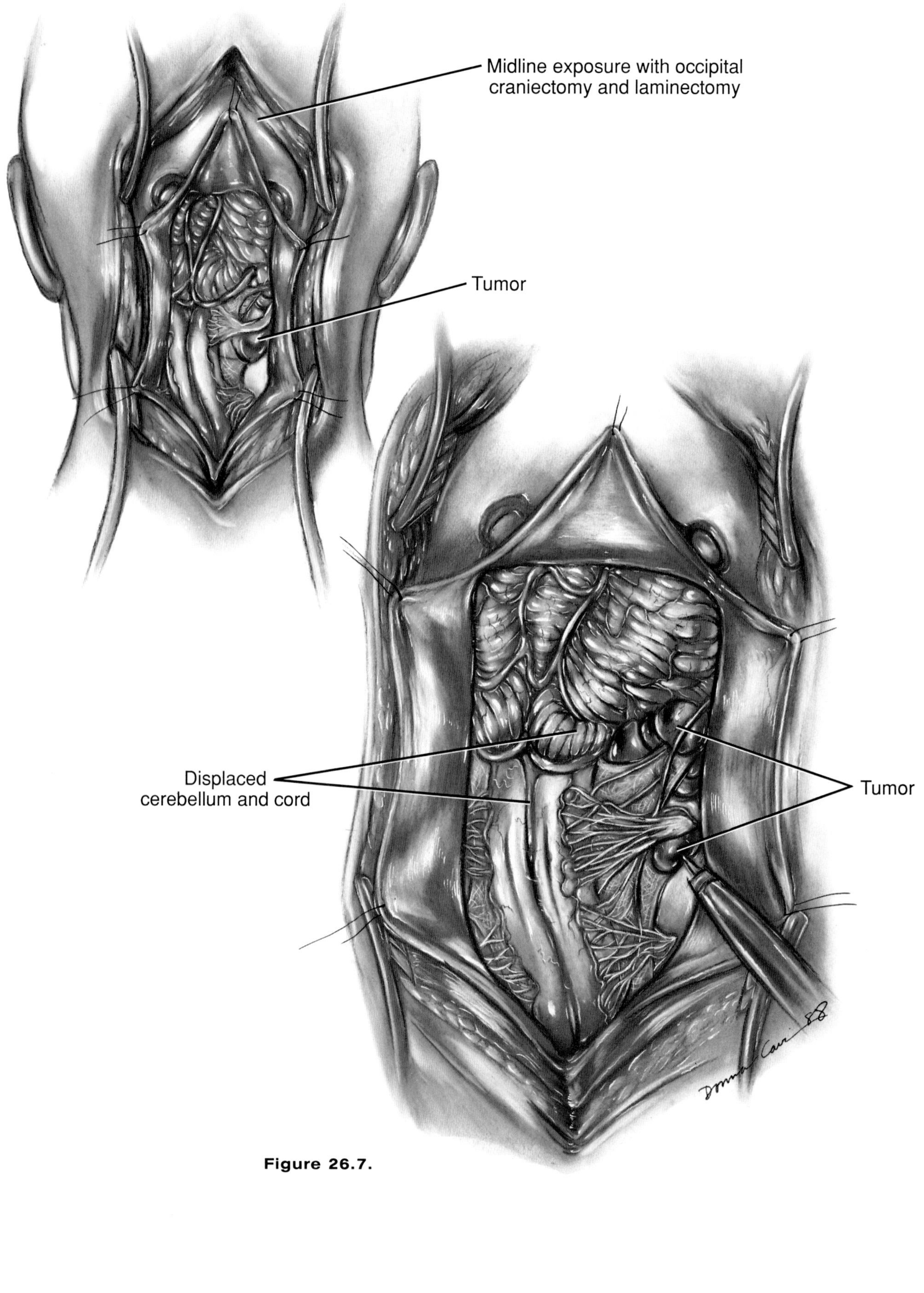
Midline exposure with occipital craniectomy and laminectomy
Tumor
Displaced cerebellum and cord
Tumor

Figure 26.7.

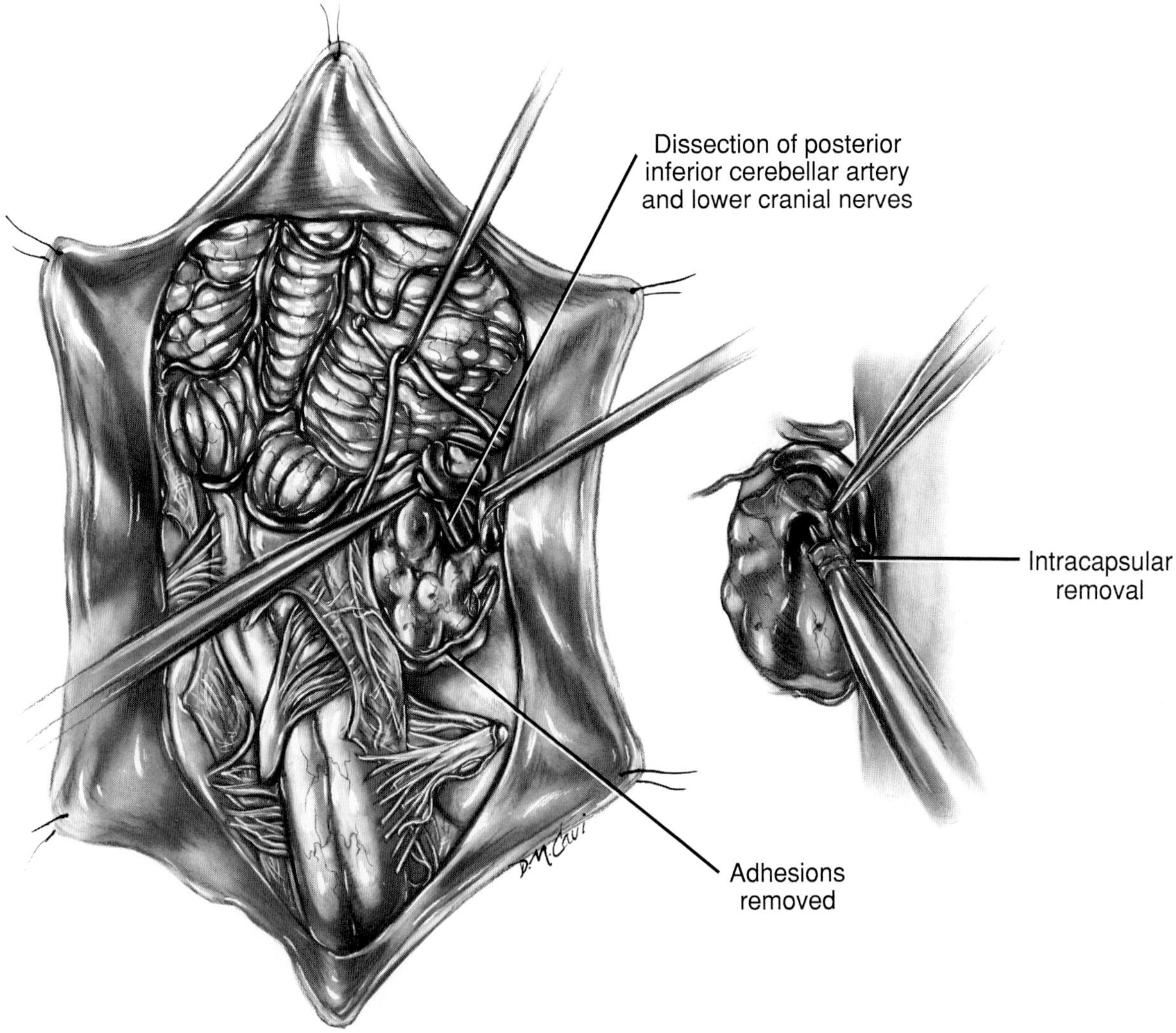
Dissection of posterior inferior cerebellar artery and lower cranial nerves
Intracapsular removal
Adhesions removed
D.M.Chui

Figure 26.8.

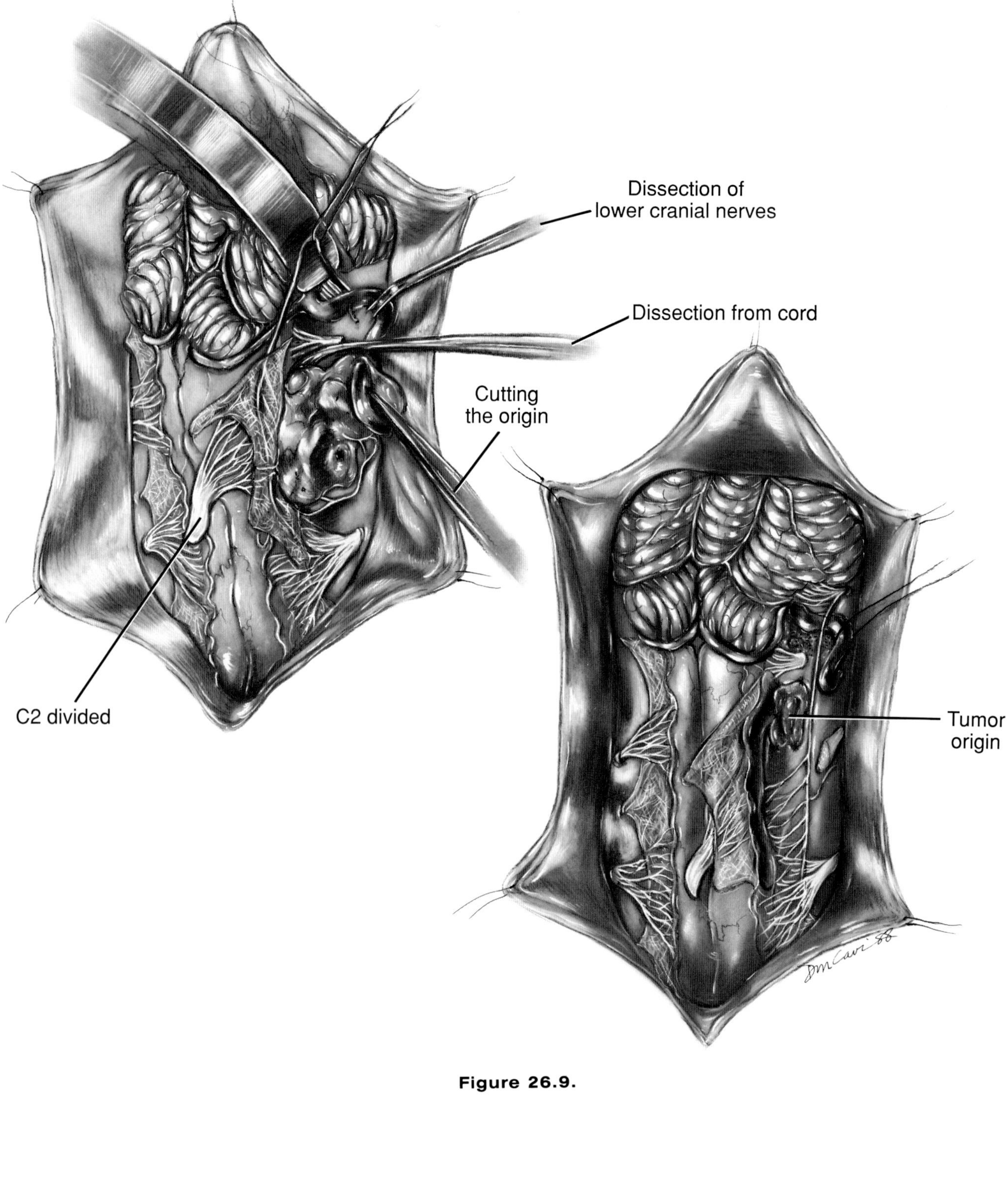
Dissection of
lower cranial nerves
Dissection from cord
Cutting
the origin
C2 divided
Tumor
origin

Figure 26.9.

27

Metastatic Spinal Extradural Tumors

The usual reasons for surgery with spinal metastatic disease are pain, progressive neurological deficit that is unlikely to be reversed by other therapy, and spinal reconstruction for progressive or impending neurological deficit. Before an operation is undertaken, however, it is necessary to define the compression and to tailor the operation to correct it. When the principal tumor mass or compression is posterolaterally located, laminectomy is the proper procedure. When the compression is anteriorly located, whether from tumor or from collapse and bony deformity, a lateral or even an anterior approach (see Chapter 12) is more appropriate. Accurate imaging of the deformity with assessment of the superior and inferior limits of cord compression is necessary to plan the appropriate operation.

Laminectomy for Metastatic Disease

Decompression by laminectomy is indicated when the compression is posterolaterally located. Usually, this will be the result of an epidural metastasis that requires removal. The extent of the mass must be determined so surgery can be planned. A midline skin incision is made to extend above and below the limits of the compressing mass. The skin incision should be taken to the spinous processes in the midline, and self-retaining retractors put in place to expose the bone. The laminectomy technique must differ from that employed with the intact spine. Tumor involvement may have weakened the bone, and the use of the heavy osteotomes that are appropriate for use in other diseases carries with it the risk of perforation of the bone and injury to the spinal cord. A subperiosteal dissection should be carried out, but it should be done sharply with an electric knife or a knife and sharp osteotome. The incision is likely to bleed, and it is important to coagulate bleeding points throughout so that blood loss is not excessive at this stage. The laminectomy should not begin until hemostasis is satisfactory. The appropriate levels should be identified. If, because of lack of conventional bony landmarks, this cannot be done with certainty, then it is preferable to take an x-ray than to make a major error in localization. The spinous processes can be removed with a large bone-cutting instrument, and bone wax applied to the base to reduce blood loss. The laminectomy should begin at least a segment below the identified mass. The laminectomy should be carried upward until the tumor is identified. Some of these tumors are extremely vascular, and a great deal of blood can be lost if attempts at hemostasis are protracted without total tumor removal. Unless the blood loss is excessive, it is better to complete the laminectomy quickly, removing the entire bulk of the epidural tumor. Hemostasis will be much easier to obtain when the tumor is out and venous compression is eliminated. The tumors are not adherent to the dura except in unusual circumstances and generally can be stripped away easily with bites of the rongeur. If this is not possible, then a sharp periosteal elevator, such as the Adson, can be used to strip away the tumor mass from the dura and remove it. Generally, the tumor comes with the laminectomy. The bone of the laminae is commonly infiltrated with tumor at multiple levels. The goal of this surgery is decompression of the spinal cord, not radical tumor removal. All soft tumor that can be removed should be excised, but excessive bony removal should be avoided. With the extensive laminectomies required, it is unlikely that any stabilizing procedure will be possible via this route. If radicular pain is a prominent part of the presentation, the clinically involved nerve roots should be carefully decompressed. If the root can be sacrificed, an extradural rhizotomy between metal clips is reasonable if adequate decompression is not possible. The rhizotomy should be carried out proximal to the dorsal root ganglion. The isolated root is crushed by two clips and divided. Be certain no cerebrospinal fluid leak occurs around the proximal clip. When tumor removal from the extradural space is complete, the dura will usually pulsate. Before closure, the adequacy of the decompression must be verified in all directions. Hemostasis is often difficult. Thrombin-soaked Gelfoam or other hemostatics, such as Avitene, are very useful. If there is any question concerning the quality of the hemostasis, a drain is desirable. The muscle should be closed with a single layer of sutures in the fascia, and the subcutaneous tissue and skin closed in the usual fashion.

Such patients must be carefully monitored for the development of instability. Bracing appropriate to the area involved may be required. Patients must be ambulated slowly, with attention given to providing stability.

28 Intramedullary Spinal Cord Tumors

The approach to the intramedullary tumor is virtually the same wherever it occurs in the spinal cord. The newer imaging studies will generally delineate the extent of the tumor, and magnetic resonance imaging (MRI) studies will define syrinx cavities within the cord also. A tumor nodule within such a cavity is usually well localized. These studies make it far easier to plan surgery for an intramedullary tumor, since both extent and nature of tumor are known in advance. The surgery is done with the patient in the prone position, and physiological monitoring is important. The use of spinal evoked potential monitoring offers a constant reminder of the effect of the surgical manipulation on the spinal cord.

The laminectomy should be at least one or two segments beyond the extent of the tumor or the syrinx that is to be opened. Remember that the pressure of the expanding mass may have greatly thinned the laminae, especially in children, so that the usual use of osteotomes could cut through the bone. The subperiosteal dissection of the muscles from spines and laminae must be done gently, and if the bones are thin, a sharp dissection is preferable. The electric knife is a good technique. The laminectomy should be as wide as possible without encroaching on the zygapophyseal joint, and even this is acceptable if necessary. Immaculate hemostasis is obtained, and the gutters should be packed with hemostatic agents

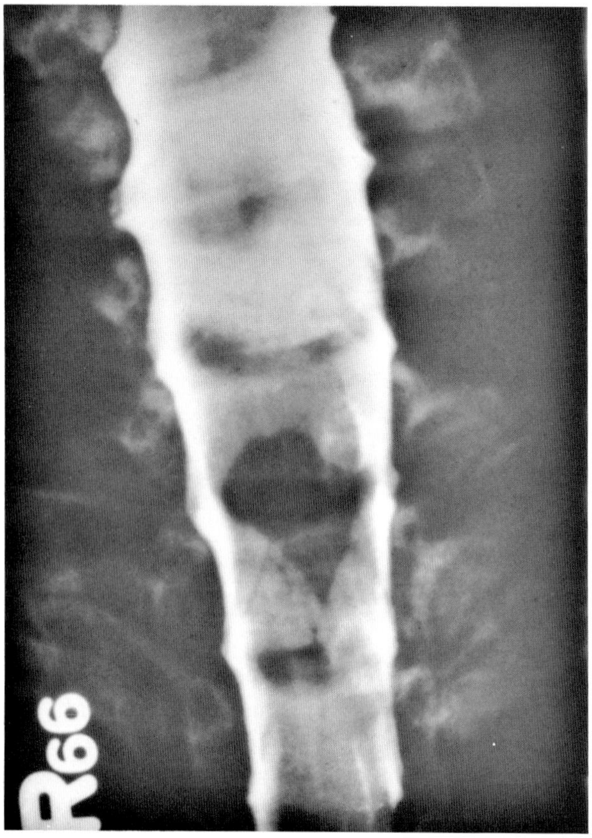

Figure 28.1. Cervical myelogram that demonstrates the widened cord typical of an intramedullary tumor.

unless the hemostasis is complete. Sump drains in the gutters will help keep the field dry. The operating microscope is brought into the field, and the dura is opened in the midline, leaving the arachnoid intact. Retention sutures are either sewn to the paravertebral muscles or brought out of the wound, weighted with clamps to ensure adequate dural retraction. The paravertebral muscle should be covered with strips of cottonoid to reduce the possibility of annoying bleeding into the operative site. The area should then be inspected, and the location of the tumor identified. Ultrasound techniques are useful in identifying the syrinx and tumor nodule with certainty before the dura is opened. With magnification it is usually possible to determine the location of a syrinx, if there is one, and the mass simply by observing the cord. Gentle palpation is also of help. The syrinx is ballottable, while the tumor mass itself will be quite firm. The area over the tumor is often devoid of blood vessels and appears swollen, but enlarged veins carrying arterial blood can occasionally be seen. It is rare that actual tumor is visible on the surface. Usually, it is necessary to open the cord in order to find the tumor. Beginning in the most likely area identified by all the techniques employed, the spinal cord should be opened in the midline. It may be necessary to coagulate crossing dorsal veins, but often these are very sparse over the tumor. Spinal cord should be opened over the entire extent of the expected tumor if the mass is localized. When the cord is diffusely involved, it may be possible only to obtain a biopsy, and in this situation, an extensive division of the cord may not be warranted. A limited opening of about one segment will allow you to judge whether the extensive myelotomy is indicated. Intramedullary spinal cord tumors are of three basic kinds. The most favorable tumors, usually ependymomas, will be well encapsulated and separable from surrounding compressed spinal cord. The capsules tend to fade into spinal cord at the extremities of the tumor, but in general, the tumors can be separated from spinal cord by gentle blunt dissection with coagulation of a few crossing vessels. Some tumors are not as well encapsulated but are nodular, usually associated with a sizable cyst, and can be separated from surrounding brain with the ultrasonic dissector or laser. Some tumors are simply diffusely spread throughout the spinal cord, and no real tumor removal or differentiation or separation is possible. Often, a biopsy is all that can be accomplished. The three tumors all offer different surgical challenges and require different techniques.

The well-encapsulated tumor should be exposed by midline myelotomy to its extremities. The myelotomy is best carried out by a sharp dissector; an appropriately sized Rosen knife is ideal. The myelotomy is actually carried down the posterior surface of the tumor from superiorly to inferiorly; then the dissection is extended to and around the tumor. If the operation is done with the patient in the sitting position, it is preferable to begin at the upper margin of the tumor and allow the tumor weight and gravity to assist in rolling the tumor out of its bed. If the operation is carried out with the patient in the prone position, then a few retention sutures through the tumor placed in gentle traction will help extract the tumor from its bed. Most of the dissection can be carried out bluntly

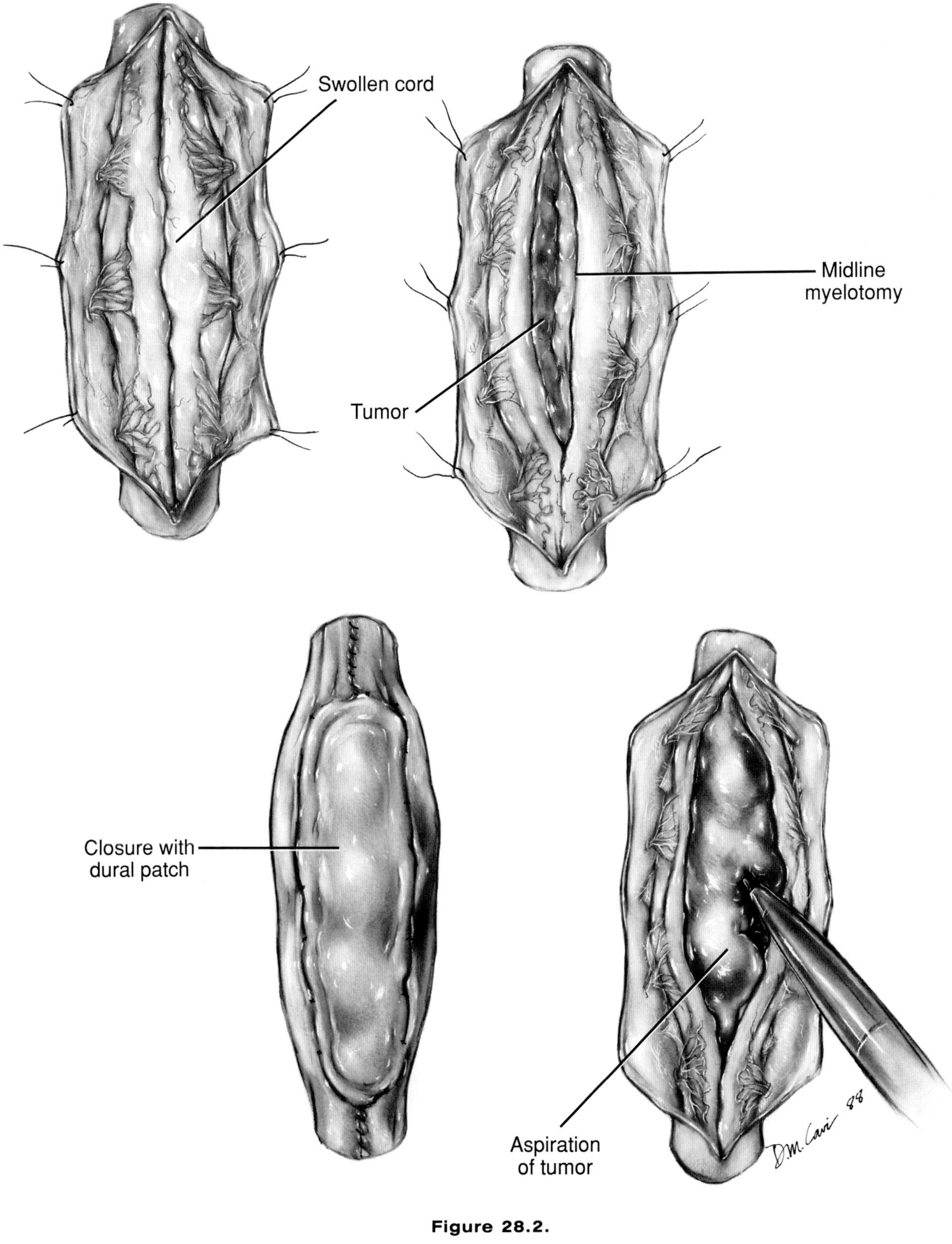
Swollen cord
Midline
myelotomy
Tumor
Closure with
dural patch
Aspiration
of tumor
D.M. Cavi 88

Figure 28.2.

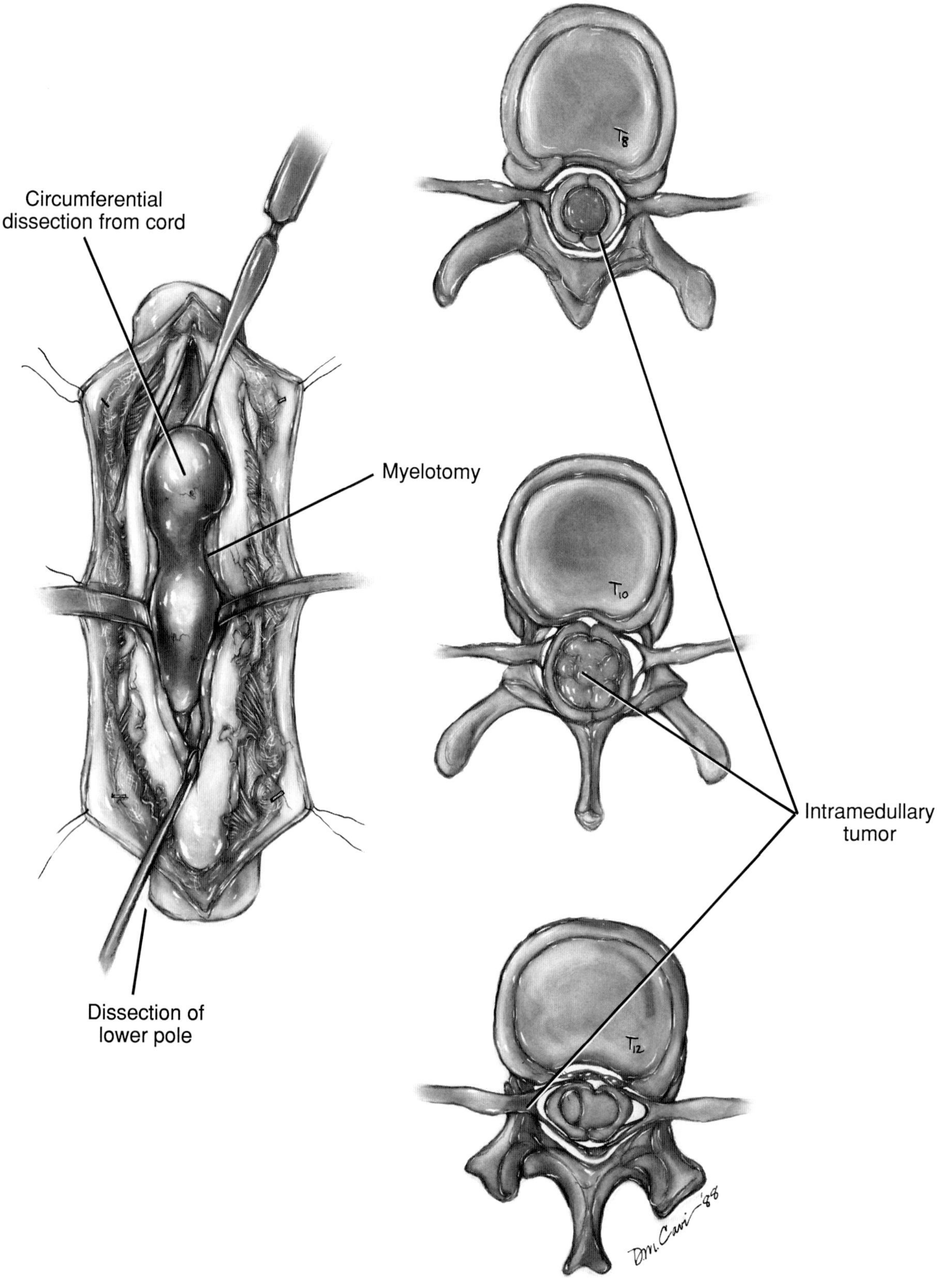
Circumferential
dissection from cord
Myelotomy
Dissection of
lower pole
T8
T10
T12
Intramedullary
tumor

Figure 28.3.

or via a sharp dissector such as the Rosen knife. Dissection and instruments should be kept on the tumor capsule side so that minimum disruption of the cord occurs. Physiological monitoring of evoked potentials throughout the procedure is of help in assessing whether or not injury to the cord is occurring during the dissection. If a change in the evoked potentials occurs, then it is possible to stop the maneuver responsible and use another technique. If the tumor is extremely large, it may be necessary to open the capsule and partially debulk the contents before carrying out the capsular dissection. It is important not to lose the capsular plane, however, and the dissection should be carried out with the laser or Cavitron in such a way as to maintain the capsule in position. Small blood vessels are often seen crossing between cord and capsule. These should be coagulated on the capsular side before they are cut. Keep bipolar coagulation on the cord itself at an absolute minimum. Small bleeders are best managed by temporary packing with cotton balls or application of hemostatic agents.

Tumor-Syrinx Combination

More diffusely invasive tumors are often associated with a large cyst, particularly in children. The newer imaging techniques will usually demonstrate the tumor mass and the extent of the syrinx. Sometimes, the cyst is within an extensive tumor, but it is quite common for there to be a relatively well circumscribed mass of invasive tumor with a cyst extending superiorly and inferiorly from the tumor nodule. The laminectomy should be carried out to expose all of the tumor, but it is not necessary to expose the entire cyst until it is proven necessary. Ultrasound localization of the tumor mass and syrinx at the time of surgery is a valuable technique to be certain of the localization. The laminectomy should be one or two segments above the mass to be removed and can be extended if necessary. The dural opening must be sufficient to expose the tumor completely without compromise of cord during the removal. Once the dura and the arachnoid are opened, the spinal cord and the tumor mass can be demonstrated. Ultrasound will be of help in delineating the tumor accurately. A midline myelotomy is then carried out to the extremities of the tumor, with the cyst entered above and below for a distance sufficient to demonstrate the extent of the tumor nodule. It may be difficult to separate the mural nodule completely from surrounding cord. The margins often will blend imperceptibly, so that an extracapsular removal is impossible. Nevertheless, a complete gross removal is feasible. The ultrasonic dissector and the laser are excellent instruments for this purpose. The tumors themselves are usually quite different in appearance from surrounding cord. Constant monitoring of a patient's spinal evoked potentials is an important adjunct during tumor removal. The Cavitron is used to remove all visible tumor; the laser can be employed in the same way. It is difficult to say that a total tumor removal is ever possible in this situation, and these techniques are too new to have allowed the long-term assessment that will be required to prove long-term outcome. The current short-term results are better than anything that has been accomplished in the past, so that an attempt at radical removal is feasible.

The cavity should be left open when tumor removal is complete. If the myelotomy is relatively small, it is wise to shunt the syrinx cavities on either end. This is done by placing ventricular hydrocephalus catheters into the cavities above and below and then suturing them to the dentate ligament or dura on one side to ensure that they stay in position and continue draining. Cutting a few extra holes in the portion to be left in the subarachnoid space is important. Be sure that the catheter tips are subarachnoid and not subdural.

Intramedullary Spinal Cord Tumors with Significant Cystic Component

Some intramedullary spinal cord tumors have a relatively discrete tumor nodule that has a sizable cystic cavity that usually extends above and below the tumor mass. The tumor mass may present as a neural nodule lying in the cystic cavity, or the cyst may extend above and below a solid tumor without any connection between the two compartments. In such a situation, the surgery is carried out in exactly the same way described as for a solid tumor, except that the initial incision needs only to be planned to be one segment above and below the solid tumor initially. The skin must be prepared and draped so that the incision can be extended beyond the limits of the cyst, if necessary. The initial incision is made and the laminectomy is carried out to expose the solid tumor and a small amount of the cyst. The dura is opened throughout

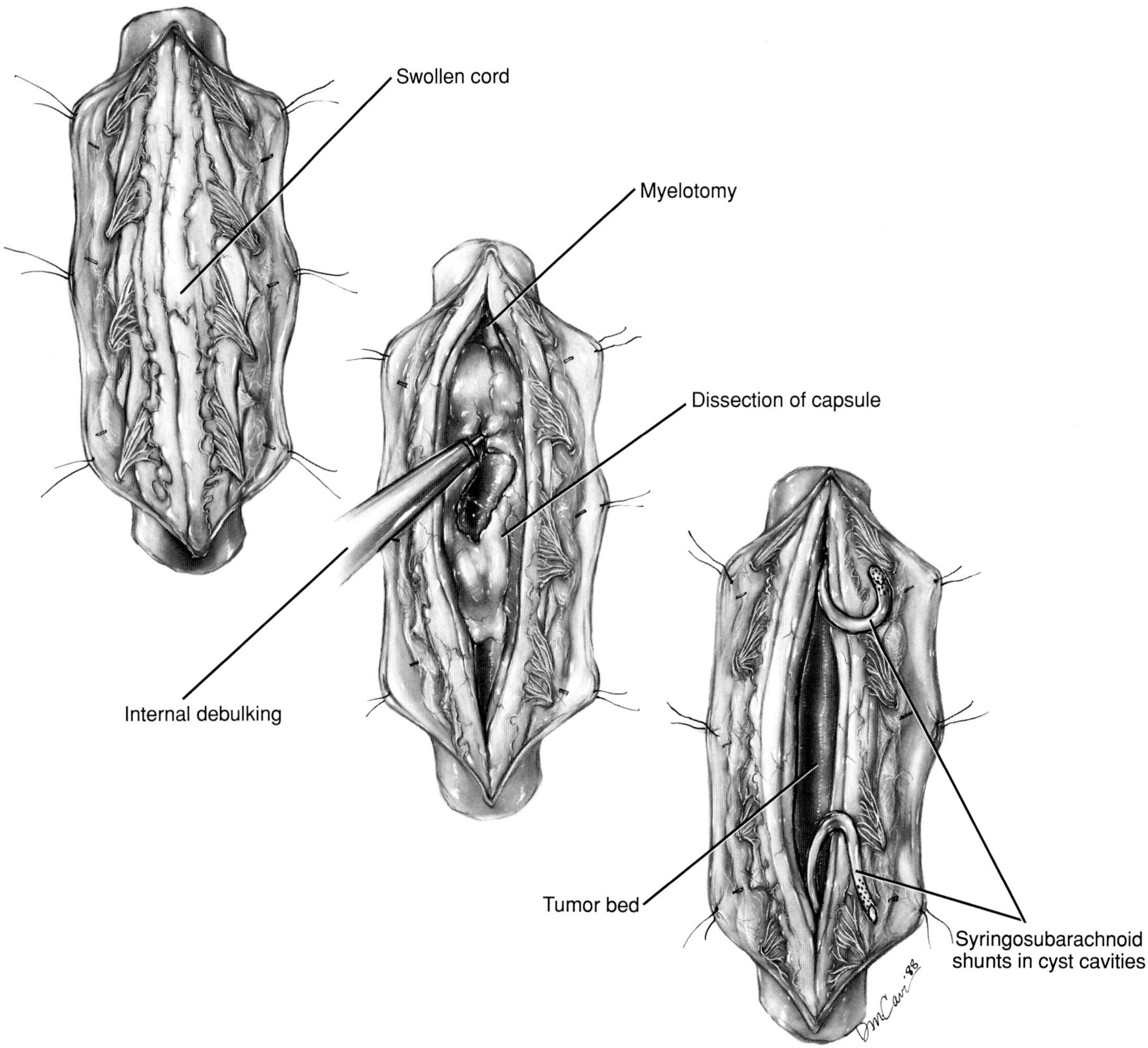
Swollen cord
Myelotomy
Dissection of capsule
Internal debulking
Tumor bed
Syringosubarachnoid
shunts in cyst cavities

Figure 28.4.

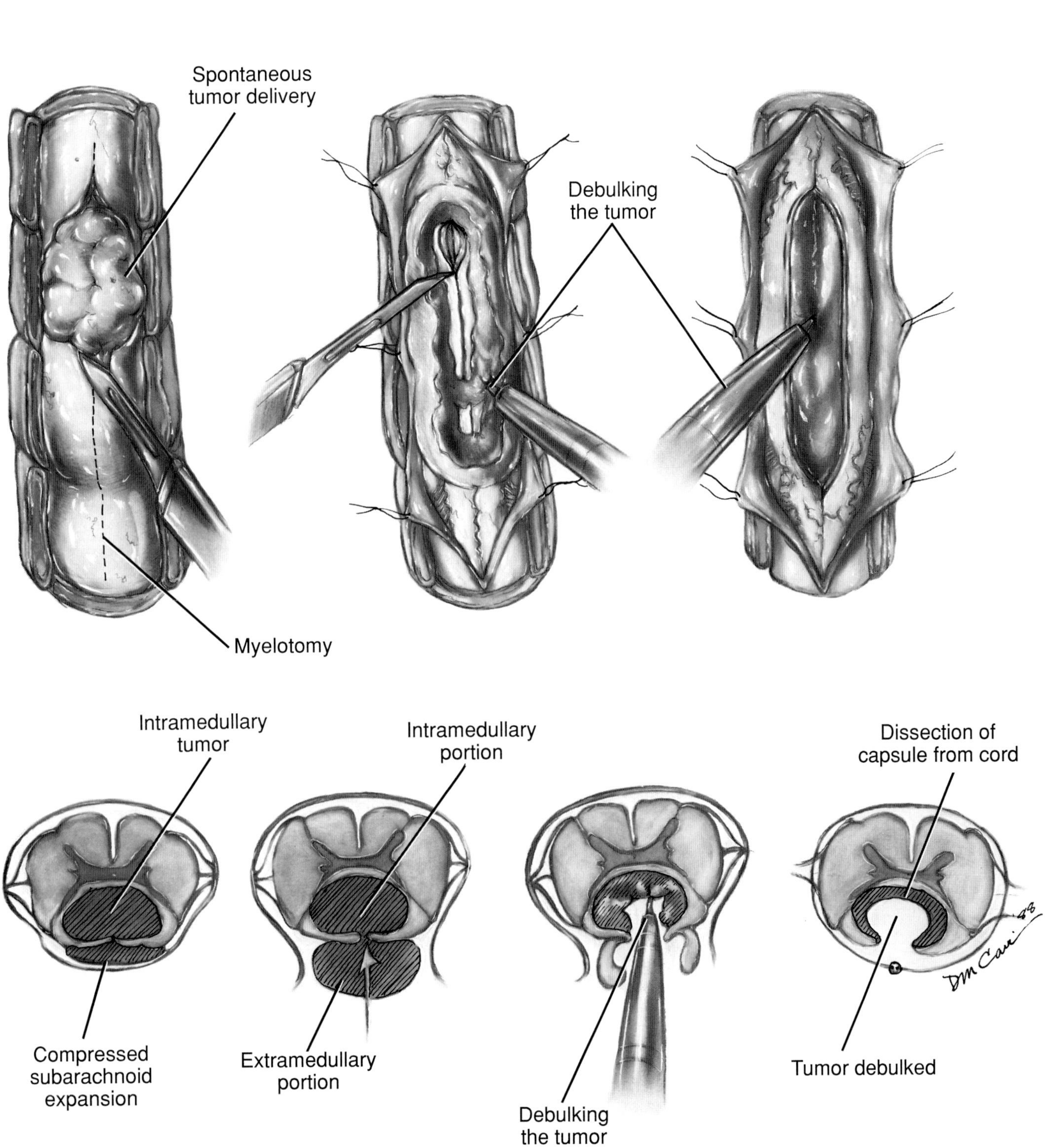
Spontaneous
tumor delivery
Debulking
the tumor
Myelotomy
Intramedullary
tumor
Intramedullary
portion
Dissection of
capsule from cord
Compressed
subarachnoid
expansion
Extramedullary
portion
Debulking
the tumor
Tumor debulked

Figure 28.5.

the length of the incision and held back with retention sutures either sewn to the muscle or retracted by hanging clamps. Thrombin-soaked Gelfoam in the gutters will help maintain the immaculate hemostasis required for this kind of surgery. Ultrasound can be useful to find tumors before the dura is opened. The combination of this technique with palpation will usually define the solid mass of the tumor very accurately. A myelotomy is then carried out, preferably in the midline between the right and left posterior columns to expose the tumor. The myelotomy should extend at least 5–10 mm into the cyst. With the tumor exposed, a decision for or against removal must be made. Virtually all tumors with major cystic components have reasonably definable margins and can be excised. Most are almost mural nodules, and a total removal is possible. In some, the tumor involvement is more diffuse. When this is the case, the tumor can be removed by laser or ultrasonic dissector. If the tumor is well circumscribed, then gentle blunt dissection with microdissectors will frequently free the mass. The choice of techniques will be dictated by the configuration of the tumor, not its histopathology. Evoked potential monitoring, while not mandatory, adds a degree of control. As long as the surgical maneuvers do not change the evoked potentials, it is our experience that the removals are usually safe. When the evoked potentials change, the surgeon is able to stop, hopefully allow them to recover, and then use other techniques that do not change the potentials. Physiological monitoring certainly does not guarantee the absence of a neurological deficit following this delicate surgery, but it does provide some protection. When the solid component of the tumor either is totally removed or cannot be differentiated further at its lateral margins, the cyst must be examined. Biopsies of the cyst wall near the tumor and well away from it are the next step. Usually the cyst wall simply is compressed cord. In this circumstance, the cyst does not have to be excised. Sometimes, the cyst wall is separable from compressed cord and is greatly elongated thin tumor capsule. In such a situation the incision in the cord must be extended to the extremities of the cyst, and the tumorous lining totally stripped away. Fortunately, this removal of the lining can be done by blunt dissection and is usually the easiest portion of the tumor removal. If a myelotomy is long, it is reasonable just to leave the tumor bed open and do nothing more. If the myelotomy is short, a shunt is advisable. A ventricular shunt catheter with a few additional holes cut in the end that will be in the subarachnoid space is inserted into the cavity. If there is enough room, it is better to have one tube going up to the top of the cyst and one tube going down. The ends of the catheters are brought out, placed in the subarachnoid space, and sutured to the dura laterally around the insertion of the dentate ligament. This will ensure that they will not migrate out of the cyst. The dura is then closed in a watertight fashion. If there is not adequate dura to allow a loose closure without compression of the cord, a dural substitute should be used to obtain the closure. There are no other special considerations in wound closure.

Intramedullary Tumors with Diffuse Cord Involvement

Some intramedullary tumors are so diffusely involved in spinal cord that any thought of total removal is facetious. There are no margins, and it is very difficult to identify the abnormality except by the gross appearance of the cord. In this situation, none of the imaging techniques or ultrasound will have shown a discrete tumor or cyst. When the dura is opened, the cord is seen to be diffusely enlarged, often nodular with microcysts, and frequently with decreased vascularity. If there is excrescence that can be biopsied easily, an answer may be obtained about the nature of the tumor. Most commonly, midline myelotomy is required through the most advantageous avascular place for incision. When the cord is diffusely involved, the myelotomy often does not disclose a discrete mass or any evidence of capsule. As the dissection is carried deeper in the cord, it is apparent that the cord is unusually firm, frequently white or yellow in appearance, and avascular. Frozen section of small pieces may be difficult to interpret. Often, the surgeon is a better judge of the presence of tumor, and the pathologist can only describe gliosis. There is little that can be accomplished surgically in this situation, except to verify the nature of the tumor and provide adequate bony decompression. The limits of the bony removal should be well beyond the tumor, for any swelling may cause acute compression at the upper or lower level of the laminectomy. Extensive midline myelotomy the entire length of the apparent tumor mass has been advocated, with a second-stage operation proposed for 10–14 days later. At this point some

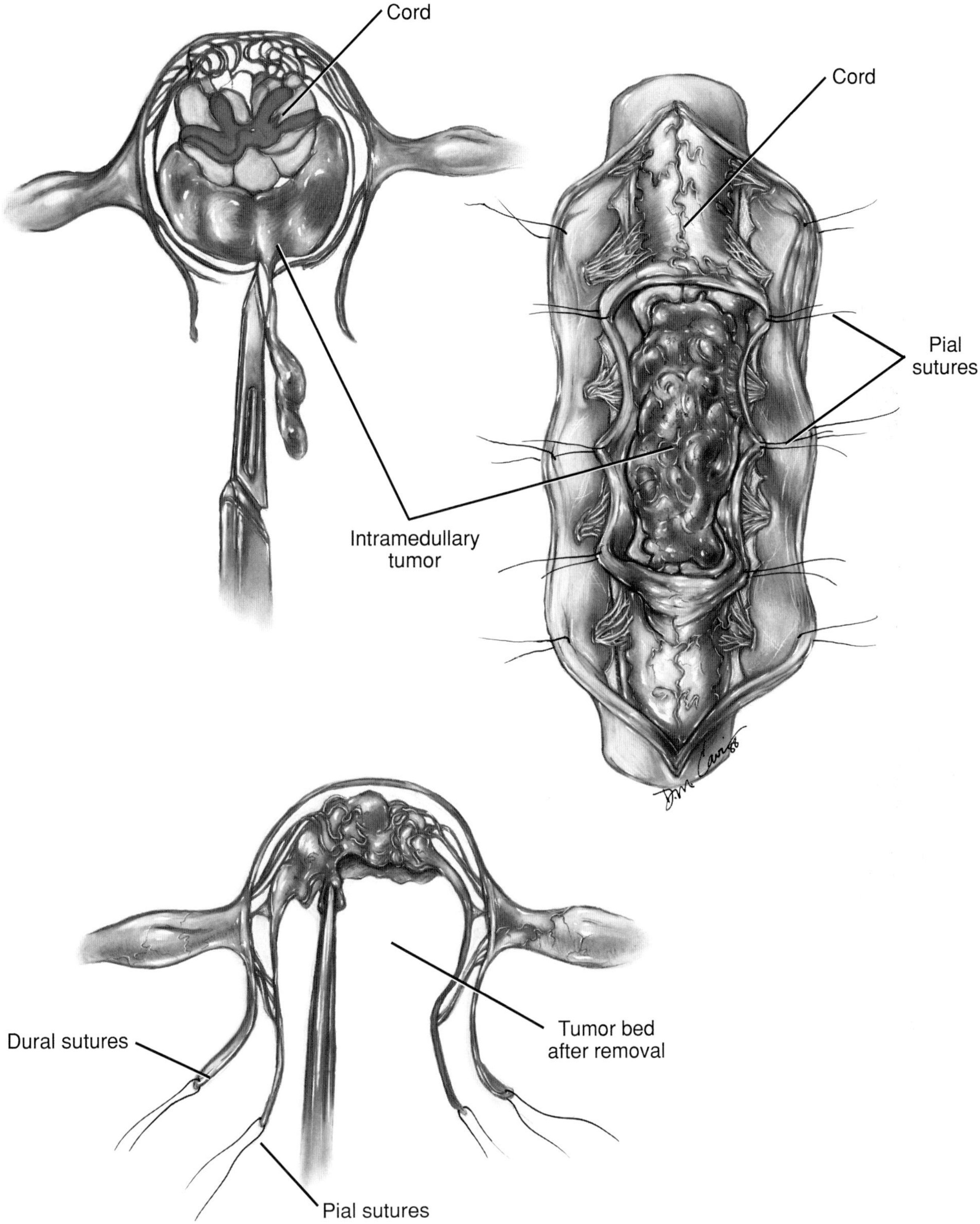
Cord
Cord
Pial
sutures
Intramedullary
tumor
Dural sutures
Tumor bed
after removal
Pial sutures

Figure 28.6.

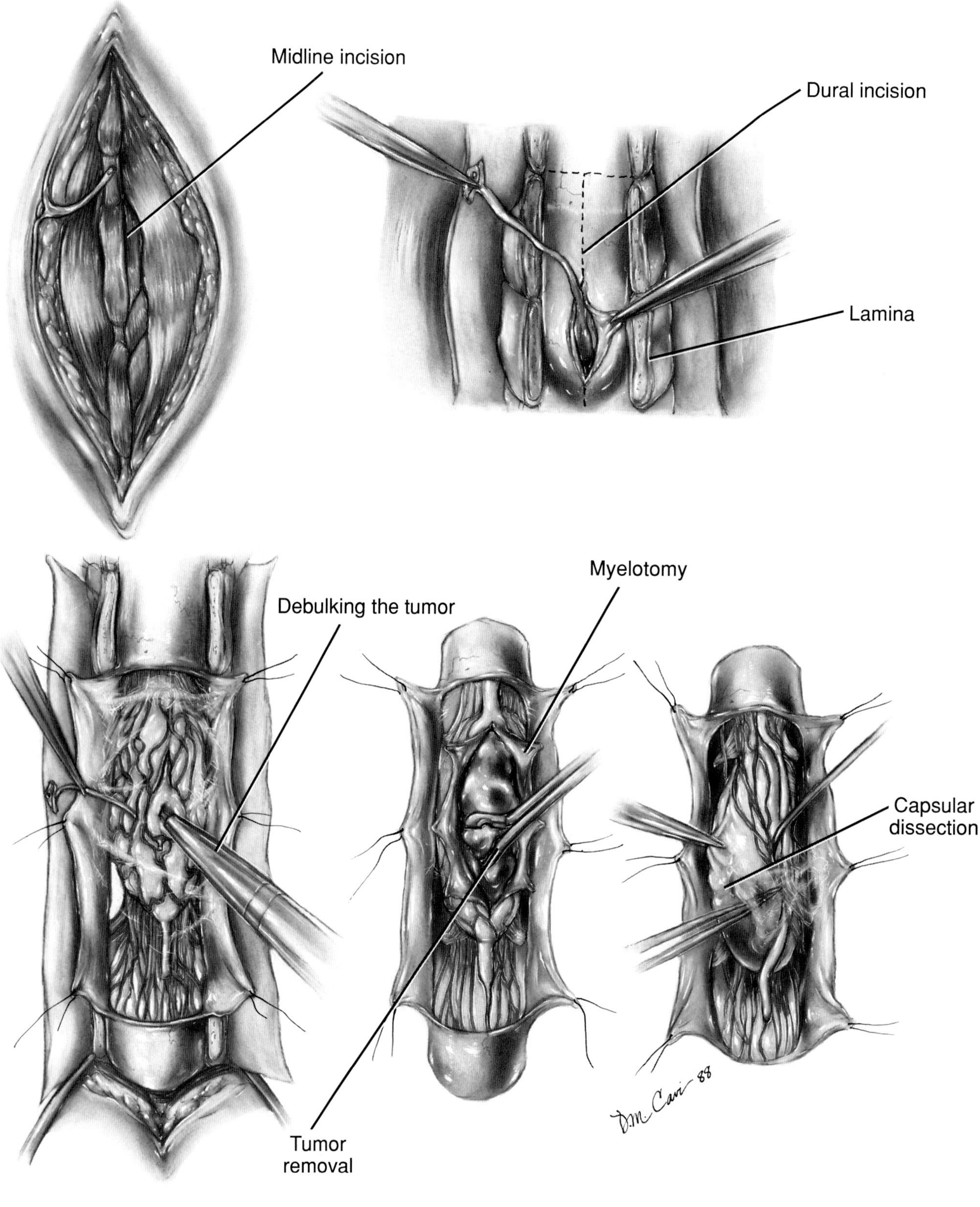

Midline incision
Dural incision
Lamina
Debulking the tumor
Myelotomy
Capsular dissection
Tumor removal
D.M. Carr 88

Figure 28.7.

of the tumor mass may have herniated out of the spinal cord and be amenable to removal. With very low grade diffuse tumors this technique has limited value. When the solid tumor is less diffuse and better demarcated, however, a second stage may be very useful. When the tumor is discrete and yet does not have any reasonably definable margin with spinal cord, it is possible to carry out the myelotomy over the entire length of the tumor, radically removing the part that can be safely removed via laser or Cavitron. With evoked potential monitoring as a guide, it is possible to be much more radical than was thought possible in the past. Virtually total removals can be obtained with tumors previously judged to be hopeless. The trick is gradual removal of the firm abnormal tissue with Cavitron or laser, with constant assessment of cord function. This is a technique for the expert in the management of these rare tumors and not for the surgeon who deals with one rarely. Returning for the second stage when the tumor has had the opportunity to herniate posteriorly out through the myelotomy site can result in a great deal more tumor, which can be removed by the Cavitron or the laser. MRI can then be used to estimate the value to be gained from reoperation. If this approach is to be utilized, it is important to patch the dura. Closing the dura primarily is difficult because so doing may constrict the spinal cord. A dural patch provides a reasonable operative site for return later. If a longer wait is contemplated, the subsequent scarring will make it extremely difficult to expose the spinal cord, and a dural patch is a better alternative. The decision as to whether to settle for decompression and biopsy, subtotal removal at one operation, or subtotal removal in two stages will depend on the anatomy of each tumor and cannot be generalized. The surgeon must judge each tumor individually.

Cordectomy for Malignant Spinal Tumors

Low-grade spinal tumors usually are better palliated than treated by radical removal. Simple decompression may provide relief of symptoms, and the time course of the disease is variable. Many patients do well for years. High-grade tumors behave much differently. Those that are truly glioblastomatous have a very poor prognosis. Highly malignant tumors that occur at the thoracic and lumbar regions can be totally removed for the price of paraplegia, and this alternative must be considered. It is preferable not to make the decision at the first operation, even though a second procedure does present some increased risk of subarachnoid spread of tumor. It is important to have absolute pathological confirmation of the malignant character of the tumor and to have the appropriate discussions with the patient and family members concerning alternatives for treatment. At the time of reoperation the laminectomy should be extended up well above possible tumor infiltration—at least five segments is desirable. The dura is opened to expose the cord above, and the spinal cord is then divided sharply at a convenient location between nerve roots. The anterior spinal artery is exposed last and should be coagulated and divided; clips are usually not necessary. It is important to be certain that radicular arteries entering at the level of cord section that appear to be important to cord nutrition above are preserved. The cord is then lifted out of its bed, and the anterior and posterior roots are divided sequentially by crushing them with a small blunt clamp and cutting them. Larger radicular vessels can be coagulated, but this is an unusual necessity. The cord should be removed beyond the tumor for at least several segments. If possible, the conus should be left intact because this will help establish an automatic bowel and bladder control system. Careful frozen section study of the extremities of the removed cord is important, and time must be taken to examine multiple sections above and below to be certain that there is no visible tumor near the cordectomy margin. Serial section of the cord to determine the extremities of the tumor is required on the permanent specimen. If the tumor has not been totally removed with wide margins, further cord removal can be accomplished promptly. Frozen sections are reliable, however, and reoperations for additional cord removal are not likely as long as the original decision for cord removal has included frozen section analysis of a number of normal segments above and below the obvious tumor. Even the radical step of cordectomy cannot be a guaranteed cure for patients with these tumors, and recurrence of tumor higher in the cord above the cordectomy limit can occur in spite of negative serial sections near this limit.

Following removal of the cord, the dura is closed in a watertight fashion. The closure requires no special techniques.

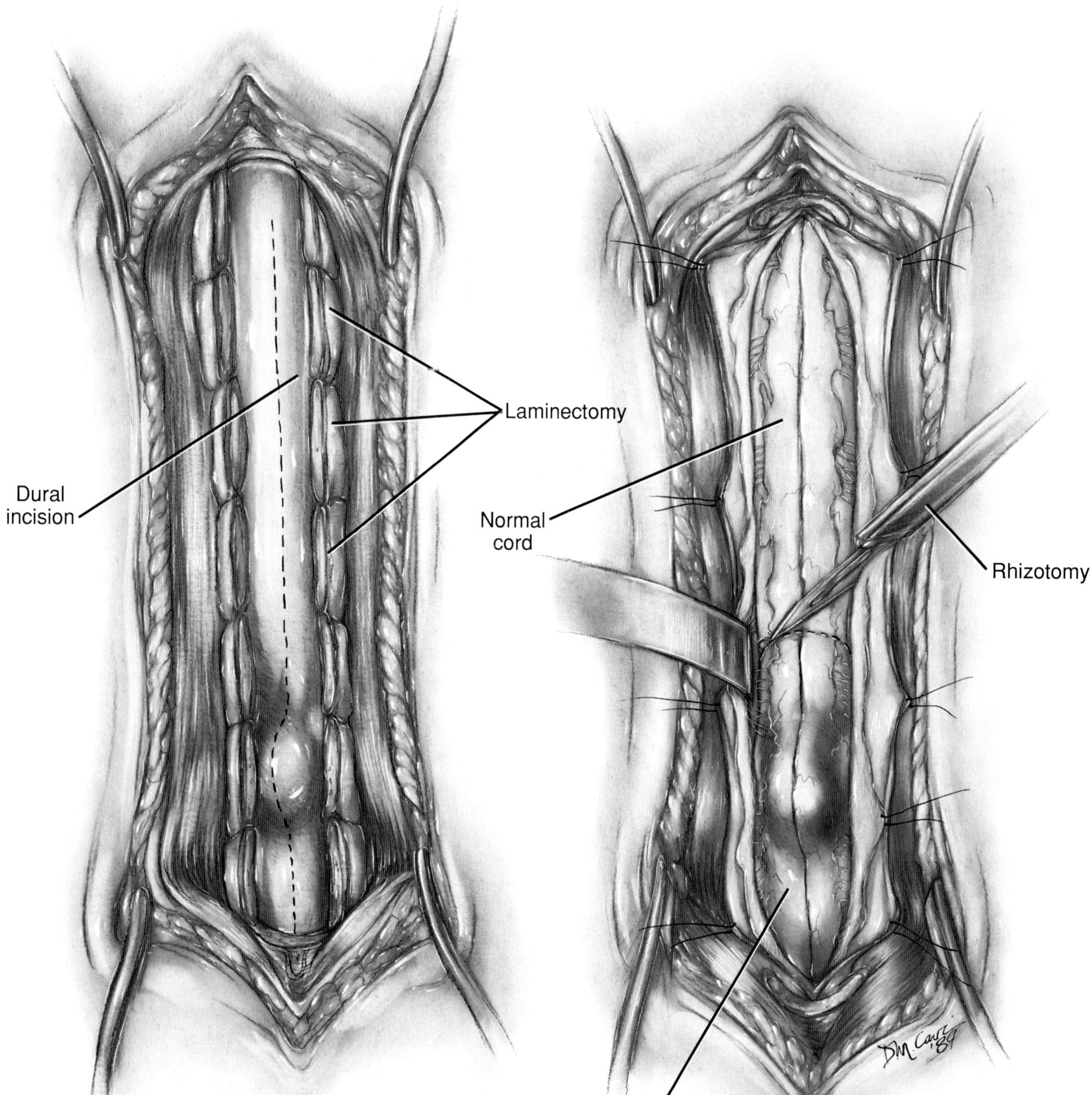
Laminectomy
Dural incision
Normal cord
Rhizotomy
Tumor-filled cord

Figure 28.8.

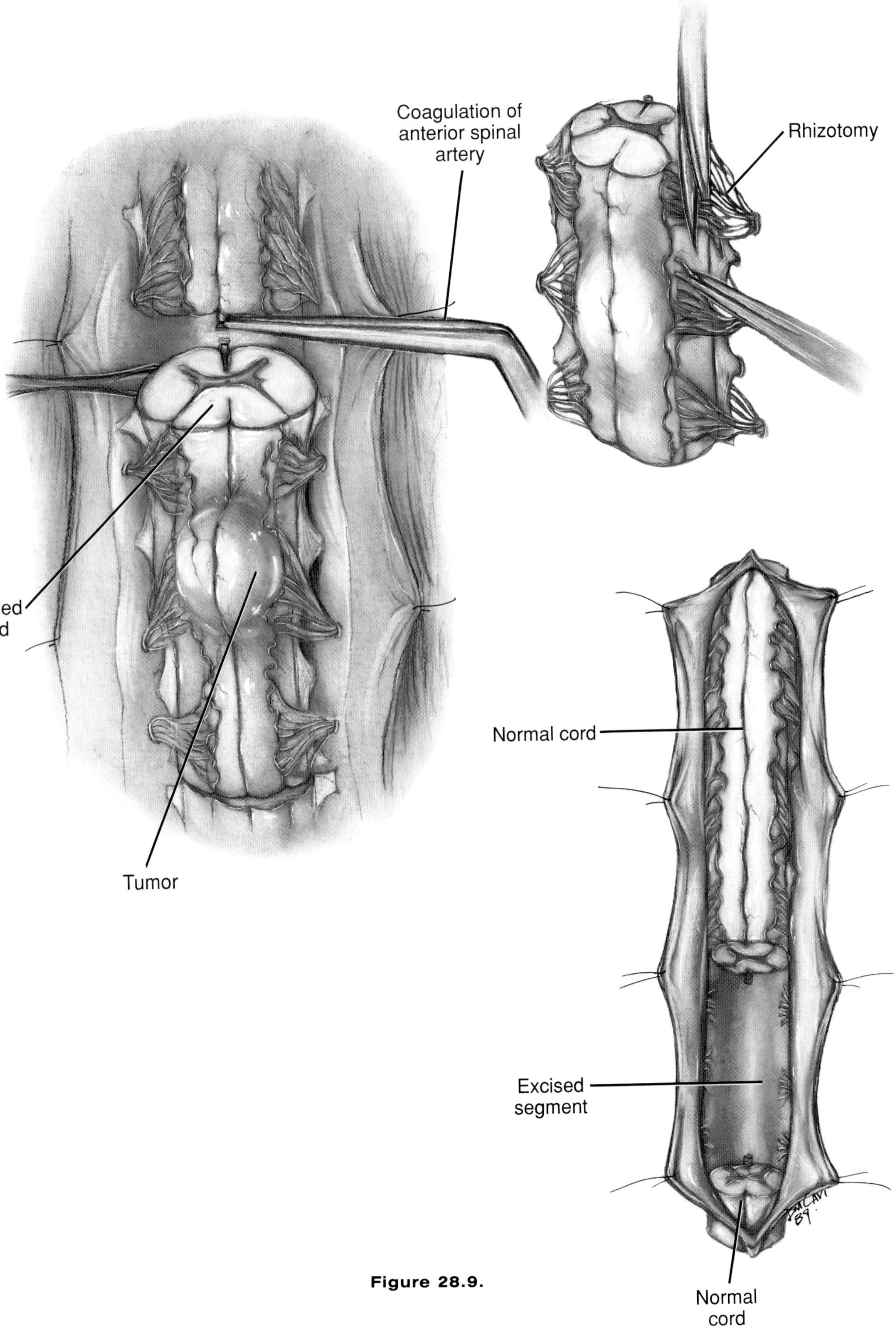

Coagulation of anterior spinal artery
Rhizotomy
Divided cord
Tumor
Normal cord
Excised segment
Normal cord

Figure 28.9.

Surgery for Filum Ependymoma

The diagnosis of the filum ependymoma is now virtually certain from MRI or computed tomography (CT) scanning with intrathecal contrast. The extent of these tumors is well defined by either technique. The exposure of the tumor is by standard lumbar or lumbar thoracic laminectomy with the patient in the prone position under general anesthesia. The laminectomy should be as wide as possible to allow adequate exposure of the tumor and at least one segment above and below. The dura is then opened in the midline, leaving the arachnoid intact if possible. Before the dura is opened, it is very important to have absolute hemostasis, and packing the gutters with a hemostatic material may be a useful technique. The exposed muscle should be covered with saline-soaked cottonoid or some similar material to reduce the possibility of any blood spilling into the spinal canal. Once the dura is opened, the dural margins should be tacked back to muscle. Clamps should be attached to these sutures to pull the dural margins out of the way and give the widest possible exposure. A sump suction in the gutters bilaterally is a useful technique to reduce the troublesome bleeding that can obscure the surgical field. Most surgeons prefer to open the dura with the operating microscope, but if it has not been used, it should be brought into the field at this point. Laminectomy was planned to allow exposure of the tumor at least one segment above and below its extensions. If the tumor is large, an exposure two segments above and below is preferable to allow adequate manipulation of the nerve roots around it. The next step is to open the arachnoid, which should be done in the midline with dissection of the arachnoid adhesions from all roots and the tumor. This will expose the tumor, which is usually a well-encapsulated mass with a mat of nerve roots adherent to it. The nerve roots have to be dissected free from the capsule, and if possible, the tumor should be removed as a single mass to reduce the possibility of seeding the subarachnoid space. The next step is to free the nerve roots from the length of the tumor. This is usually best done by identifying the nerve roots inferiorly, beginning in the midline, and carefully dissecting them free, moving from inferior to superior. Only the anatomical relationships should dictate whether to begin the dissection above or below. It is best to begin where the nerve roots are best visualized. Since the tumor is often more densely adherent at the conus, dissection is usually begun with the inferior pole of the tumor and carried superiorly. As the nerve roots are freed, they are retracted gently laterally until all of the posterior roots will be freed from the tumor. Freed roots can be contained by a soft blood vessel loop for ease of handling. With relatively small tumors the mass can be manipulated within the spinal canal to free the anterior roots in the same way. With a small tumor these two maneuvers result in a tumor mass attached to the conus or filum, separated circumferentially from all of the surrounding nerve roots. The filum should then be divided as far above the tumor as possible without invading the conus and should be cut below. The tumor can be removed as a single mass. When the tumor is larger, it may not be possible

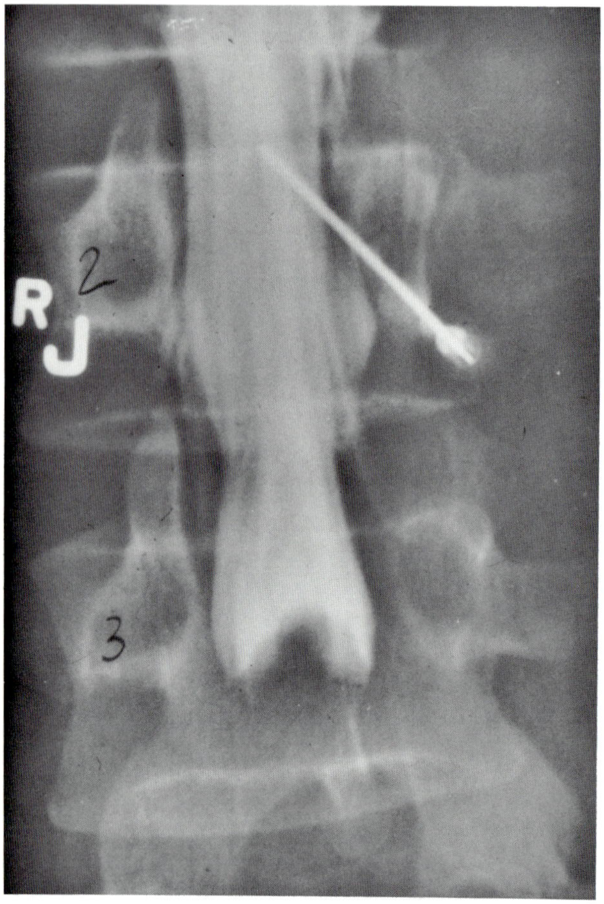

Figure 28.10. Typical myelographic picture of intradural ependymoma of filum. Note that the entire spinal canal is filled with tumor. All of the roots are expected to be involved in the tumor mass.

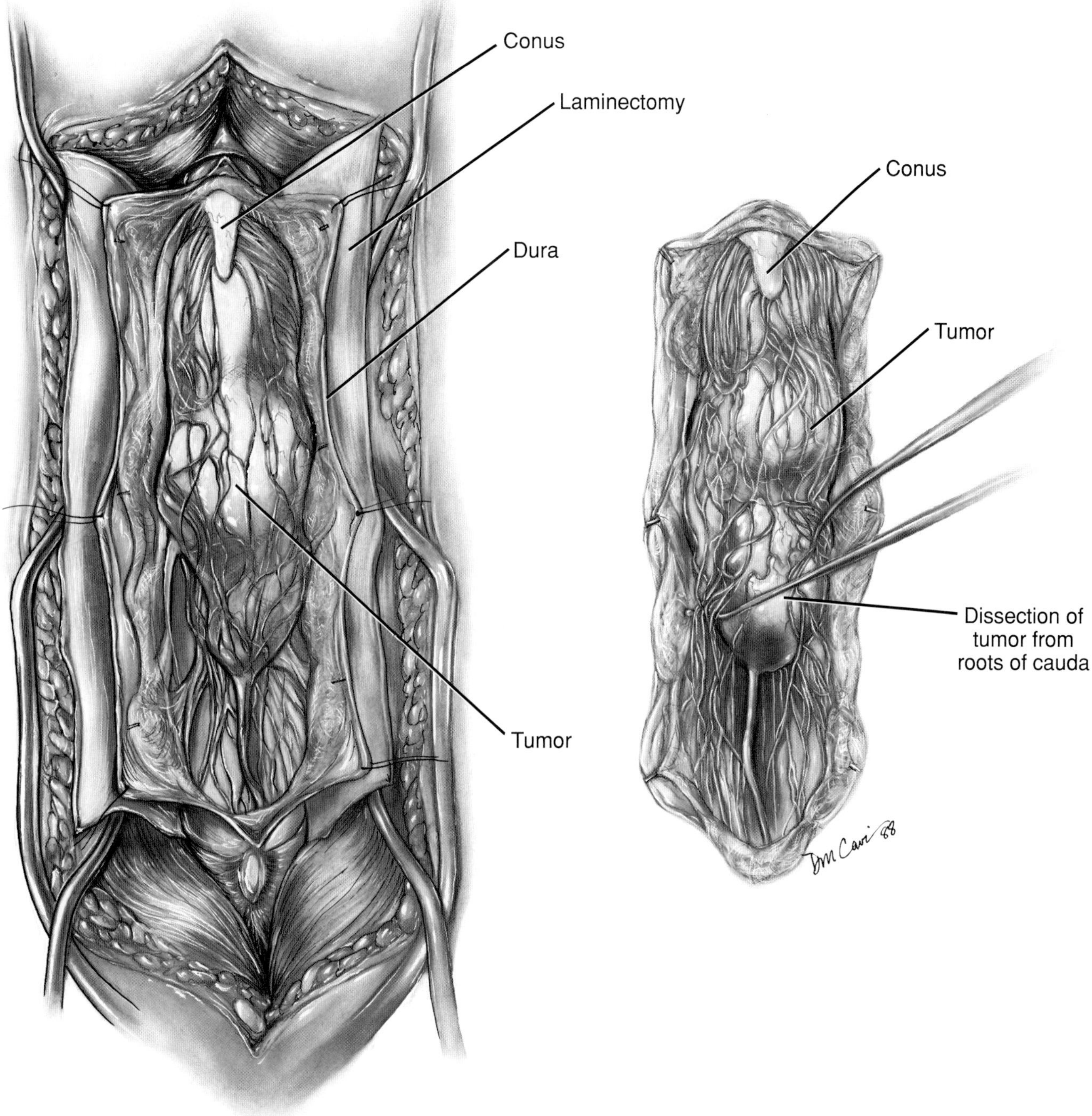
Conus
Laminectomy
Dura
Tumor
Conus
Tumor
Dissection of tumor from roots of cauda

Figure 28.11.

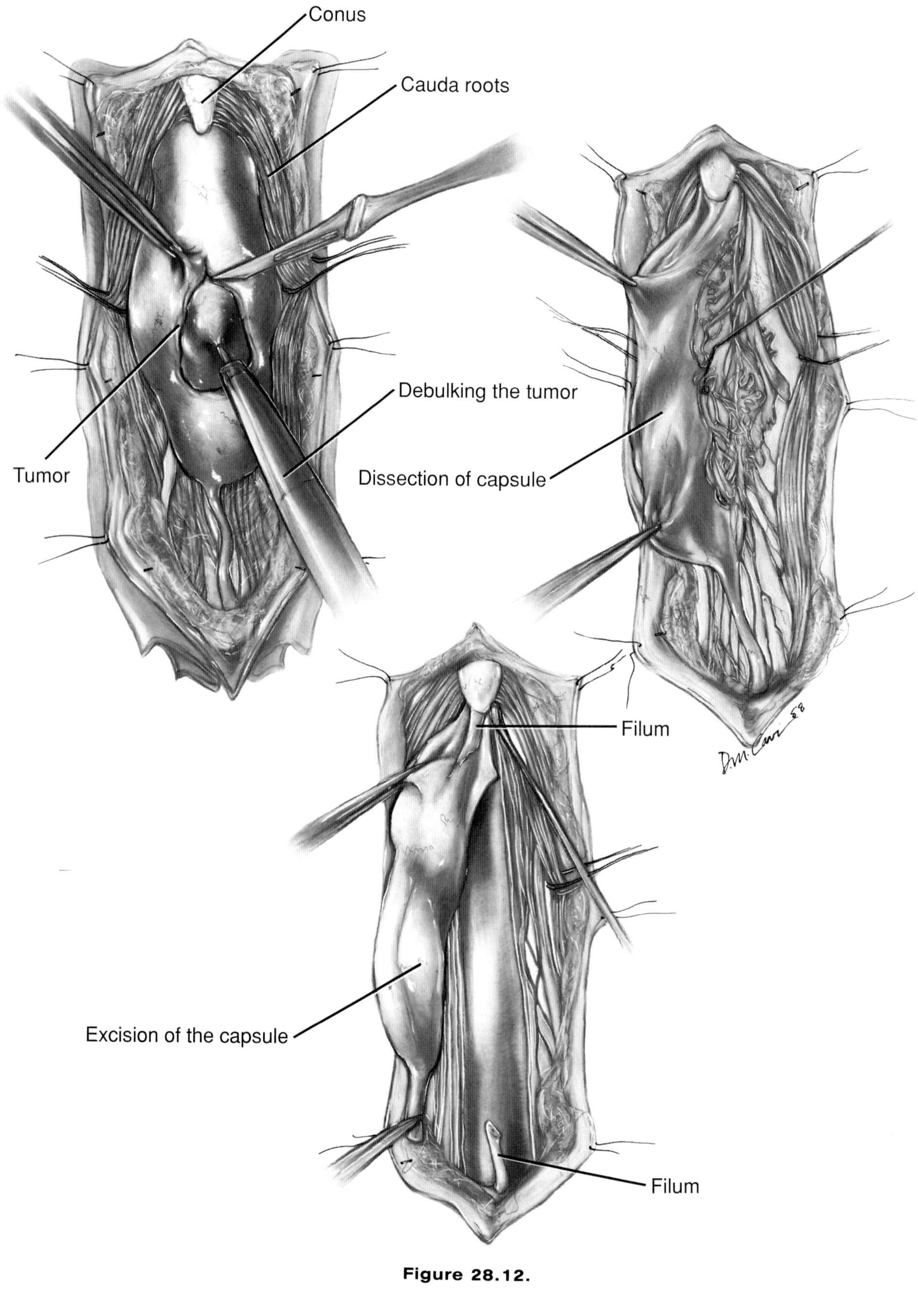
Conus
Cauda roots
Tumor
Debulking the tumor
Dissection of capsule
Filum
Excision of the capsule
Filum

Figure 28.12.

to carry out the entire dissection, for manipulation of the intact tumor within the canal might injure the nerve roots. In such a case, the canal should be carefully packed away with cottonoid, and the tumor capsule opened in the midline after posterior roots are free. The laser or Cavitron should then be used to carry out an intracapsular removal of the tumor, leaving the capsule intact. Once the bulk of the tumor is removed, the nerve roots can be dissected from the capsule as with smaller tumors. They are frequently quite adherent and must be removed by sharp dissection. The differentiation between nerve roots and tumor is obvious enough in most cases that it is possible to identify and separate them without injury. Some of these tumors are so adherent that nerve roots are virtually surrounded. Often, such tumors are soft and removable by suction, but the desirable extracapsular dissection is not possible. Some are firm and so adherent that total tumor removal cannot be obtained without the risk of major neurological deficit. A few roots, the loss of which would result in acceptable neurological deficit, may be sacrificed, but if paraplegia or loss of bowel and bladder function is likely to be the result of surgery, it is probably better to settle for subtotal removal and postoperative radiation. This is a decision that must be made with the patient prior to surgery. Once the tumor is completely removed, the area should be irrigated vigorously to wash all blood and debris out of the wound. The dura should then be closed in a watertight fashion, and the wound closed as with any other laminectomy. A single layer of sutures in the muscle and the subcutaneous layers is satisfactory, but closure of both the muscle and the subcutaneous layers should be made as watertight as possible. In the event it is not feasible to obtain watertight dural closure, it is acceptable to leave the dura opened widely, although it is preferable to obtain a dural closure with a patch.

29

Spinal Cord Lipoma

Spinal cord lipomas represent a special situation because it is not necessary to carry out total removal in order to obtain a long-lasting resolution of symptoms. The management of lipomas that involve the spinal cord is quite different from management of those that involve the conus and cauda equina (see Chapter 22). These spinal cord masses are usually both intramedullary and extramedullary. Total removal can be a goal, but subtotal removal and decompression of the cord are also commensurate with permanent relief of symptoms. The tumor may have more than one extramedullary excrescence, so that thorough myelography and computed tomography scanning that covers all areas that can be involved are extremely important. Careful neurological examination will usually give the appropriate clues for the areas that need to be covered.

Surgical Technique

The laminectomy is done in the same way required for other intradural tumors. Physiological monitoring is protective. Exposure should extend over all of the cord demonstrated to be involved by the imaging studies. The dura should be opened for the entire extent of the tumor. The usual situation is to find the cord expanded by an intramedullary component with a posteriorly placed excrescence of tumor that obscures a portion of the posterior columns. Often, this mass is tightly packed in the dura and will expand greatly when the dura is opened. The nature of the tumor is immediately apparent, for they are white, avascular, and smooth in appearance. The extramedullary portion should be defined and, if large, can be removed by removing the fat down to the level of the cord. This is possible if the posterior roots are not involved. If the posterior roots are included in the mass, their dissection from the fat becomes almost impossible. The extramedullary lipomatous mass is removed first. If it cannot be removed effectively because the posterior roots are involved, the extramedullary mass is debulked. The next step is to enter the intramedullary portion in the midline. The tumor virtually always exits from the spinal cord in the midline. Occasionally, such a tumor may be asymmetrically placed. In this situation, the tumor should be entered wherever it is exiting from the cord. The laser or Cavitron makes the removal of the lipomatous material within the cord easier. As the mass is debulked, it may be possible to find a plane that allows separation of the intramedullary portion from cord. More commonly, no plane exists, and the spinal cord will be injured if total removal is attempted. Because this is a benign lesion, not a true neoplasm, the cord should not be unnecessarily endangered by attempting a total removal. It is better to leave the material within the cord, having provided adequate decompression. In the event there is more than one lipomatous mass, the procedure should be repeated at each level where extramedullary mass can be demonstrated. The dura should be closed with a patch to provide adequate decompression; closure does not require special care otherwise.

30

Intraspinal Dermoid

Surgical Technique

The removal of the intraspinal dermoid is very similar to total removal of myxopapillary ependymoma (see Chapter 28). Only minor variations and techniques are important to describe.

The skin incision may need to be modified according to the presence of a dermal sinus. When such a sinus is present, its excision should be included in the skin incision by means of a small ellipse. The sinus should be left intact and should be followed to the laminae and dura. Magnification is of help in doing this. The laminectomy should be carried out around the sinus tract, exposing its entrance into the dura. When no sinus is present, routine exposure and laminectomy over the tumor mass are all that is required. The sinus must be excised in its entirety in order to prevent the development of subsequent tumors along it. If sinus is present, the dura should be opened above and below it, and the sinus entrance into the dura removed by a small ellipse. The widely opened dura is retracted by suturing it to the muscle or by using traction clamps or sutures. Cottonoid is placed to absorb any blood that may run down from the exposed muscle mass. The tumor is lying in the subarachnoid space with the nerve roots intimately adherent. Sometimes, the transdural tract will extend throughout the subarachnoid space to the conus and may even have multiple small tumors along its course. It is much more common for there to be a single tumor that is intradural without any external tract. The tumor may lie anywhere in the subarachnoid space up to and including the conus. The nerve roots may be extremely adherent to the capsule. When there is a tract, it is conceivable that the contents are infected also. Every remnant of capsule must be removed, or the tumor has the potential to recur. A meticulous total removal is required. With smaller tumors this is done by careful microdissection of every nerve filament from the tumor capsule. This should be done without opening the capsule and under direct vision so that every remnant of capsule is stripped from the nerve roots. The dissection should be attempted first with small blunt dissectors. Various-sized Rhoton dissectors are ideal for this purpose. If the adherence is too great for blunt dissection, then small Rosen knives are a useful adjunct. If even these are not sharp enough, then microscissors should be used. As individual nerve roots are removed they can be gathered into a soft vessel loop to be retracted gently out of the way. This "trick" will keep them out of the operative field and make it easier to dissect the remaining roots without the freed roots sliding back into the plane of dissection. It makes little difference whether the roots are dissected free from above downward or from below upward. This decision can be made based on the relationships of the tumor to the conus. If the tumor mass is free from the conus, then it is usually easier to carry the dissection from above down. If the tumor mass reaches the conus and blends with it, then it is easier to begin at the lower extremity and proceed upward, freeing the root and gradually freeing the conus. Once the nerve roots are completely freed circumferentially, the filum should be cut above and below the tumor, and the tumor removed as a single piece.

With large tumors it is probable that the mass cannot be removed without evacuating at least some of the contents. Before doing this the subarachnoid space should be damned above and below to make certain that the contents of the tumor do not gain access to the subarachnoid space. Enough nerve roots should then be freed from the posterior aspect of the tumor mass to gain free access into it. The tumor should then be opened over one third to one half of its length, preserving capsule posteriorly. The tumor contents are soft and can easily be evacuated with suction until the mass is adequately decompressed. It is not necessary to remove all of the contents, and in fact, the dissection of the capsule may be more difficult if this is attempted. Be careful to avoid spillage into the subarachnoid space. If manipulation of the capsule appears to express material into the subarachnoid space continuously, it is better to remove nearly all of the contents so that this does not occur. Once the mass is decompressed, the dissection can continue, stripping the entire capsule from the nerve roots. If recurrence is to be avoided, it is mandatory to remove all of the capsule. Sometimes, marked thickening of the arachnoid surrounding the tumor can make separation of tumor from thickened arachnoid very difficult. Fortunately, the dissection from the nerve roots is not as difficult, and it is usually possible to distinguish nerve roots from the thickened arachnoid and reactive capsule. Unfortunately, the very nerves that most need to be preserved are those most difficult to distinguish from the sacral roots. It is better to leave tumor capsule than to sacrifice a significant number of nerve roots, but the tedious dissection required to obtain a total removal is well worth it for the patient. Complete removal means cure. Failure to obtain total removal condemns the patient to recurrent symptoms. When the tumor is completely removed, the operative site should be irrigated with large quantities of saline until the irrigant is completely clear and none of the fatty bubbles are obtained. The dura should then be closed in a watertight fashion, and the wound closed in the usual way. Occasionally, one of these tumors will virtually be extra-arachnoidal, and a total removal is not possible. In this situation, it is better to leave the dura open, when there is no cerebrospinal fluid visible in the wound. This is because recurrence of what is then essentially an epidural tumor is much easier to treat and much less likely to be symptomatic than if the dura is closed over it. This situation exists almost only with enormous tumors that fill the entire lumbar space and compartmentalize the nerve roots on one side with the tumor on the other. Converting them to extradural tumors means that reoperation for evacuation of the tumor contents is much less dangerous. This maneuver is desirable only when complete excision of tumor capsule is impossible. Closures require no special care.

31

Arachnoid Cyst and Arachnoiditis of Spinal Cord

Arachnoid Cyst

Two kinds of arachnoid cysts may be symptomatic. The first kind occurs as intradural-extramedullary tumors. These tumors are extremely rare, usually not diagnosed in advance by myelography, but easily recognized via magnetic resonance imaging (MRI) or computed tomography (CT) scanning with intrathecal contrast. Surgical therapy consists of limited laminectomy and excision of the cyst. The second type is also rare and presents more difficulties in diagnosis. These arachnoid cysts are sacral, usually connect with the subarachnoid space through pinhole lesions or not at all, and present as a tumor with bone erosion (Fig. 31.1). Characteristically, such patients have pain in the back. Plain films demonstrate erosion of the sacrum and portions of L5. The erosion has a sclerotic margin. Typical radicular deficits may accompany this lesion. The syndrome is usually slowly progressive. Diagnosis with CT or MRI is simplified because of the cerebrospinal fluid density of the mass. The goal of surgery is obliteration of the cyst.

Surgical Technique

Operations are carried out with the patient in the prone position, and exposure is as for any lumbosacral laminectomy. It is important not to use heavy osteotomes over the cyst, since the bone is often extremely thin and the osteotomes may enter the cyst. Occasion-

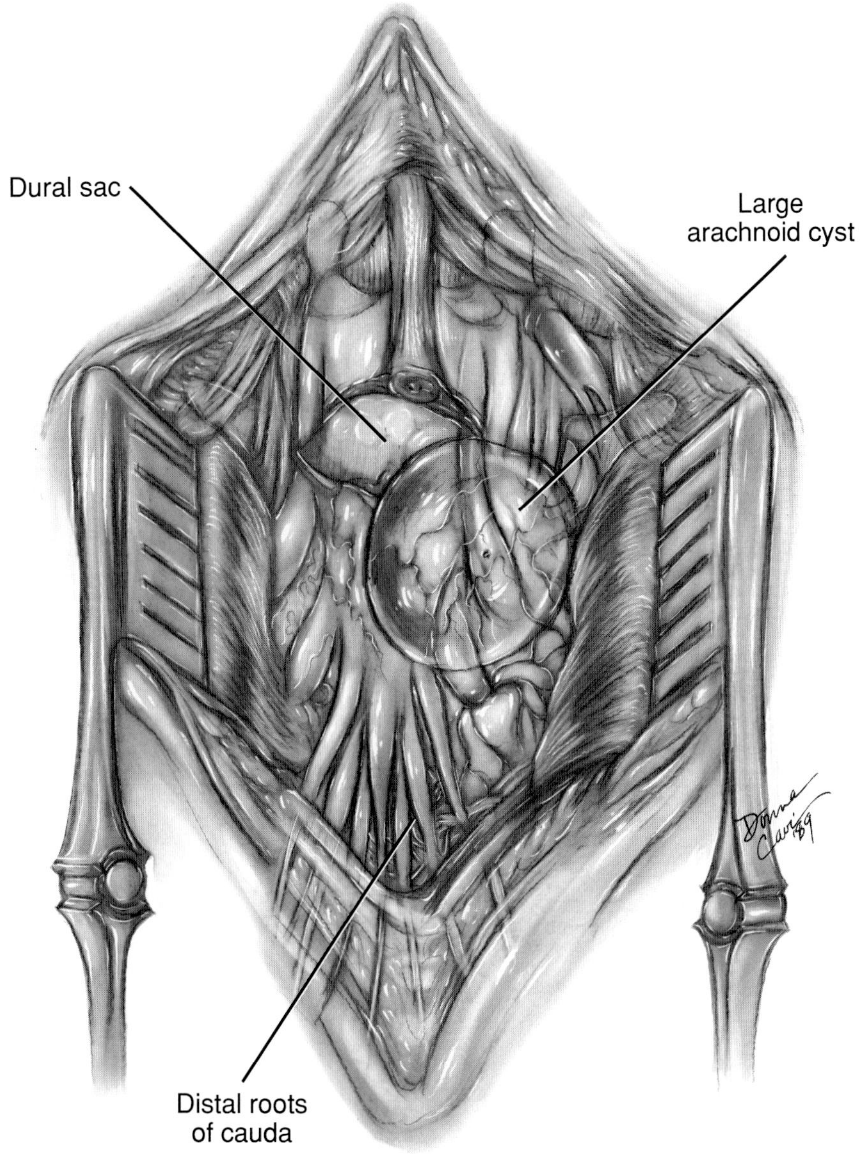

Figure 31.1.

ally, nerve roots will be incorporated in the cyst and might be injured by an osteotome. It is better to use sharp dissection to expose the eroded portion of the bone. The incision is extended down onto the sacrum until the extremity of the cyst is identified. The subperiosteal dissection of muscle from bone from the sacrum should be to the lateral margin and should expose the cyst inferiorly (Fig. 31.2). Self-retaining retractors are put in place, and the entire area of the cyst is exposed. The bone should then be removed with rongeurs, exposing the cyst beneath. The wall of these cysts is usually quite thin, and the cysts may be entered during the bony removal. Two basic configurations will be encountered. There may be a very small opening from the L5 or S1 root sheath, with the cyst ballooned out over the root, obscuring it completely (Fig. 31.3). This opening is usually seen immediately after the cyst is opened. The other circum-

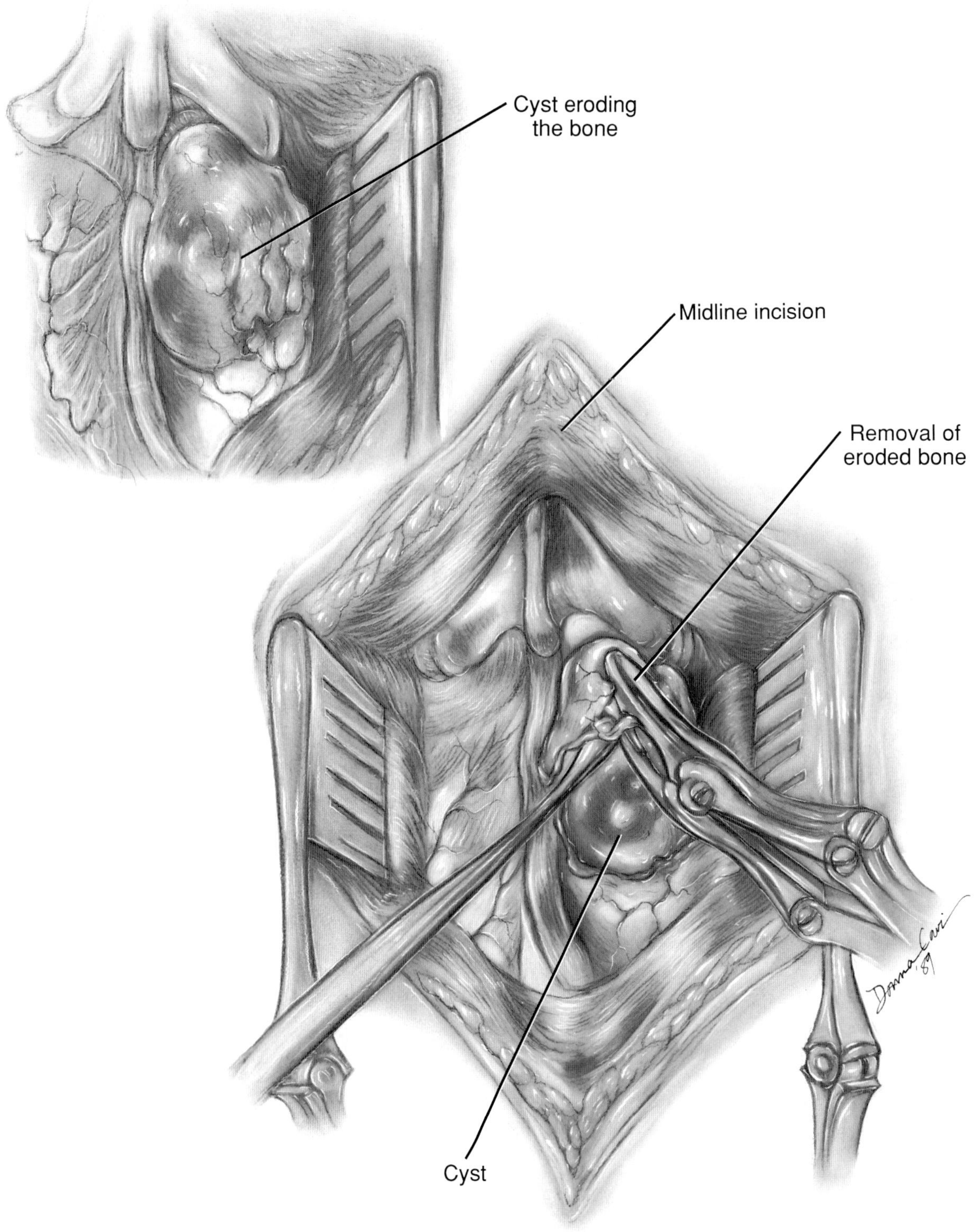
Cyst eroding
the bone
Midline incision
Removal of
eroded bone
Cyst

Figure 31.2.

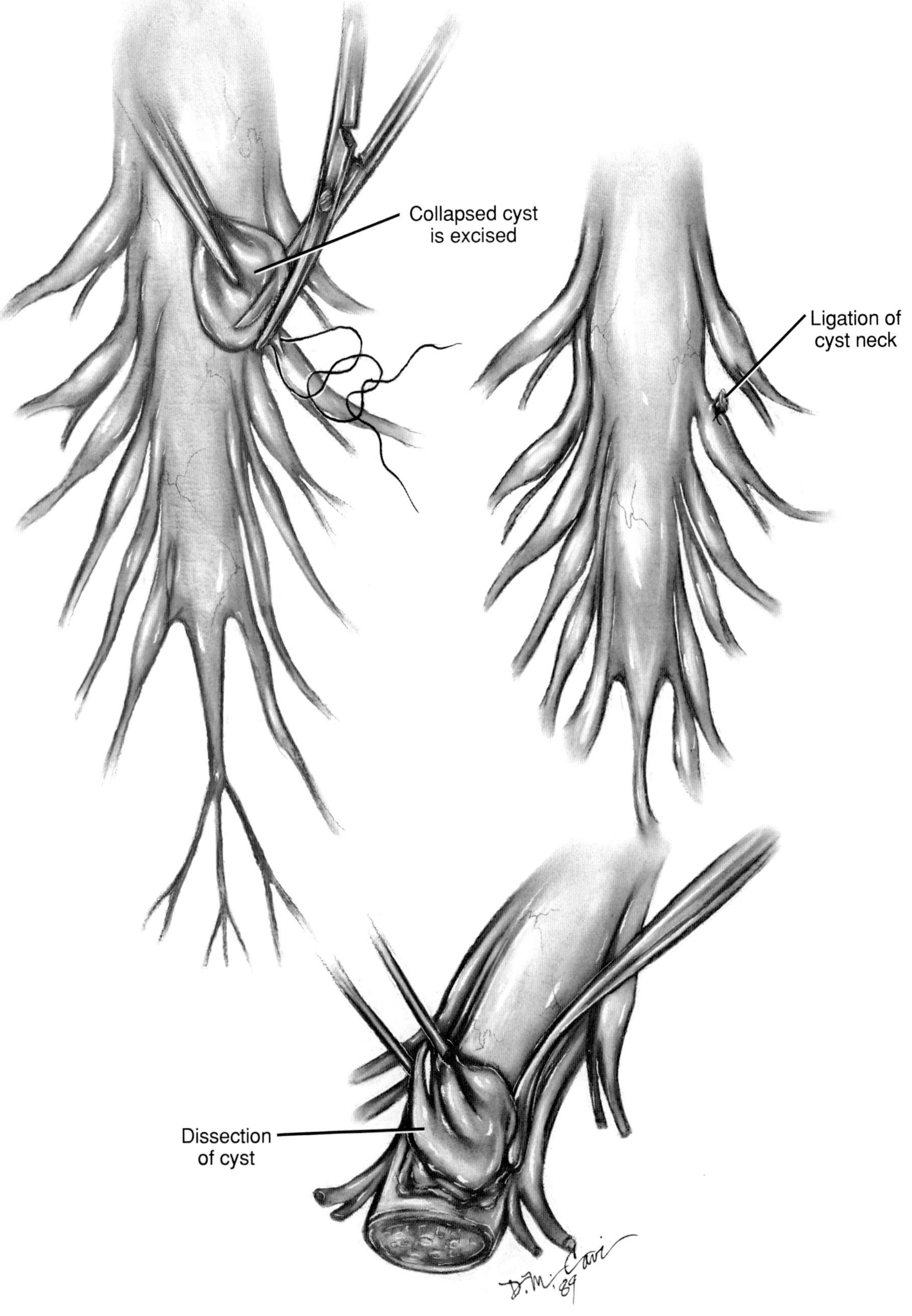
Collapsed cyst
is excised
Ligation of
cyst neck
Dissection
of cyst

Figure 31.3.

stance is a closed cyst in which no apparent opening from the root or dural sac is seen. These symptomatic cysts present with pain and obvious bone erosion and are usually quite large, often measuring 5 or 6 cm. These are quite different from the usual normal variations, which are asymptomatic, the so-called "Tarlov cysts." The wall of the cyst should be bluntly dissected free from bone, and if there is an orifice, it should be ligated with a nonabsorbable suture. If no orifice is found, it is sufficient simply to remove the cyst. The resulting cavity should be packed with fat, and the wound can then be closed routinely.

Arachnoiditis of Spinal Cord

Arachnoiditis calcificans is a rare constrictive problem that produces a progressive myelopathy. The surgery is difficult and dangerous, but the results are good, and the disease is well worth identifying and treating. The common causes are trauma, probably associated with extensive intraspinal hemorrhage, surgery and Pantopaque myelography, and infection. The process tends to be in the thoracic region. This localization is likely because the patients who develop this process are frequently quite ill and are bedfast for a long time. Because the thoracic area is dependent, the disease process focuses there. The length of spinal cord involved is variable, but the compression tends to be extensive. The usual story is a progressive myelopathy beginning after the original disease process and often becoming evident only several years following the initiating event. The diagnosis is made by standard imaging techniques. Rarely, arteriovenous malformations or tumors will be obscured by an arachnoiditis process, and this possibility must be kept in mind. The MRI techniques greatly reduce the possibility that an obscure lesion will be missed. The upper and lower margins of the block must be identified accurately because one of the principal goals of surgery is restoration of spinal fluid flow. The laminectomy must be extensive and should be at least one level above and below the block.

Surgical Technique

The operation is carried out with the patient under general anesthesia in the prone position in whatever frame the surgeon chooses. A standard laminectomy is carried out throughout the length of the block. The laminectomy must be wide but must avoid destabilizing the spine. Fortunately, this is not a real consideration in the thoracic region. Epidural bleeding is often profuse until the block is relieved. The epidural space should be packed with hemostatics. The dura is opened with the operating microscope. The dura is often densely adherent to the spinal cord, and opening the dura and dissecting it from the spinal cord may be the most difficult part of the operation. The dural opening can begin above or below the block and then proceed upward. As the dura is opened it is dissected free from the spinal cord and sutured back to expose the lateral margins of the arachnoid tube and the cord. Removal of the thickened, often calcified arach-

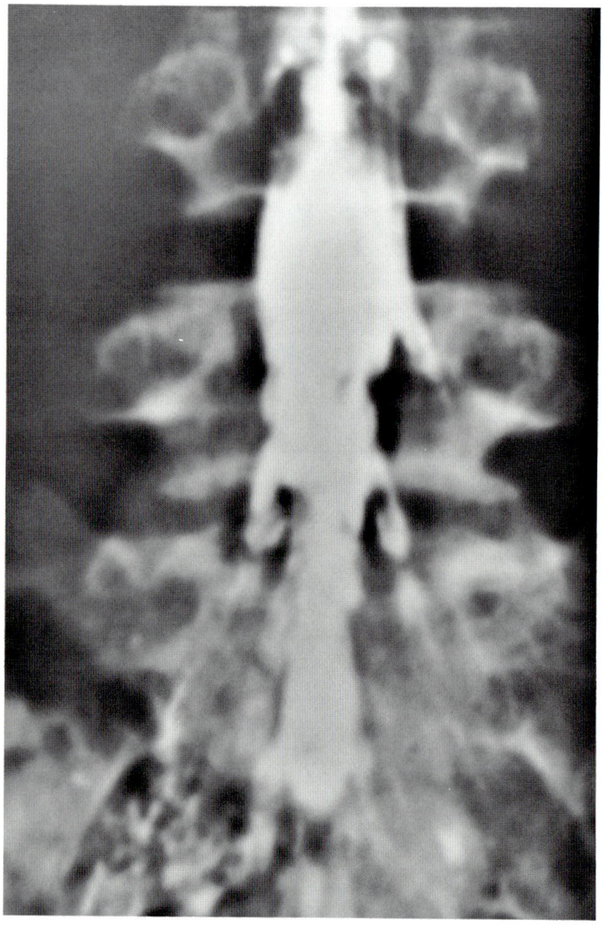

Figure 31.4. A myelographic demonstration of severe arachnoiditis with loss of definition of cauda equina within distal subarachnoid space, narrowing of contrast column, and trapped Pantopaque around roots.

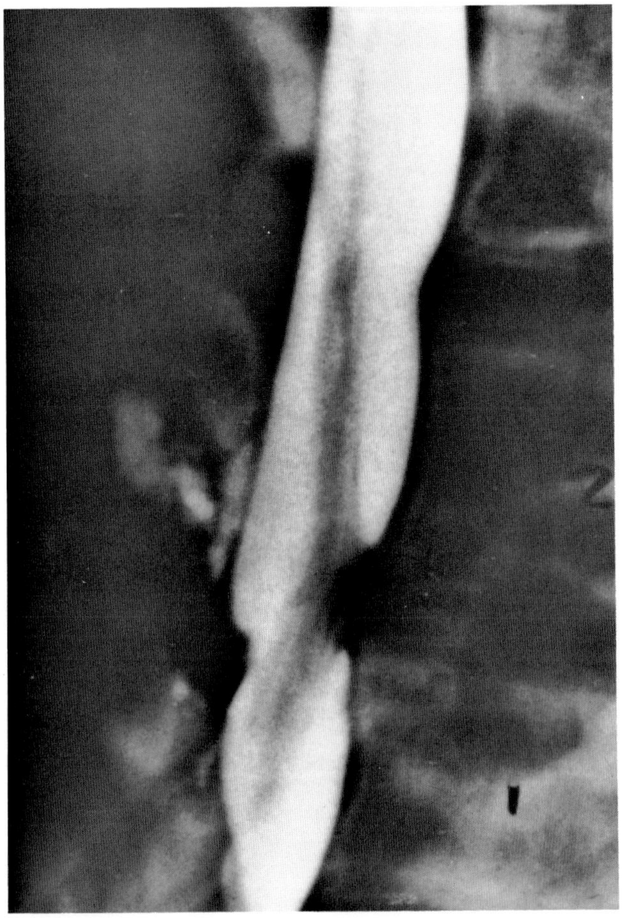

Figure 31.5. A myelographic demonstration of clumping of roots of cauda equina, typical of adhesive arachnoiditis.

noid then proceeds (see Fig. 2.22). This is one of the most difficult maneuvers in neurosurgery and very dangerous. The arachnoid is often so thick that it can scarcely be cut with microscissors. Frequently, small rongeurs must be used to remove the calcified plaque. At the same time, it is densely adherent to the surface of the cord and vessels. Remember the posterior arachnoidal compartment attaches in the midline, over the dorsolateral sulci, and again around the dentate ligaments. This process is almost always posterior, and the anterior subarachnoid space will be relatively open. The attachments will conform to the usual anatomical septae. Unfortunately, one of these, the midline septation, means that the arachnoiditis is particularly adherent over the ectatic dorsal vein. Dissection of this area, although preserving the dorsal vein, is the most difficult part of the removal. The ensheathing arachnoiditis should be totally removed from gutter to gutter, thus decompressing the spinal cord. At either end, normal subarachnoid space should be entered, and the anterior space, usually relatively free of adhesions, should be opened between the dentate ligaments at every level. This ensures normal circulation of cerebrospinal fluid. It is better to leave patches of arachnoid on the cord than to risk injury. The principal goals are to remove the encircling compressive sheath and the masses of calcium and to establish normal cerebrospinal fluid circulation, not to remove every last scrap of arachnoiditis. When these goals are met, the dura should be closed, usually with a patch. It is extremely difficult to close the dura primarily without constricting the spinal cord in most situations. Human dural substitute makes a good watertight patch. In the past, many surgeons would have left the dura opened, but now that there are reasonable dural substitutes, it seems better to close it (see Fig. 2.20). The time-honored method of leaving the dura widely open is acceptable, however. The wound is closed in layers without special considerations.

SECTION 9

Missile Wounds

32 Gunshot Wounds of Spine

Gunshot Wound of Spinal Canal

When injury to the spinal cord is partial or the bullet fragments lie within the spinal canal, prompt exploration may be necessary. Whenever possible, the exploration should include the wound of entrance, so that it can be thoroughly explored and debrided. When this is not possible, the spinal column is exposed by an incision placed to allow access to the bullet fragment with a margin of at least one level above and below. When the wound of entrance is in the general area of the injury but cannot be encompassed by one incision, it is better to explore and debride the bullet track down to bone and then return to the bullet fragment through a separate incision.

The exposure of the bullet fragments and the laminectomy do not differ from a laminectomy required for any other purpose. Remember that a fracture often has occurred and sharp dissection, preferably with an electric knife, may be necessary to avoid further injury to the cord. The preoperative computed tomography (CT) scan will define the extent of bony injury and so guide the exposure. Once the area of injury is identified, self-retaining retractors are put in place to expose one segment above and below, and the laminectomy is carried out. The degree of injury always seems to be much worse than one imagines from looking at the film. Often, the dura is lacerated, there is extradural as well as intradural hemorrhage, disrupted neural elements are adherent to surrounding structures, and it may be very difficult to reconstitute

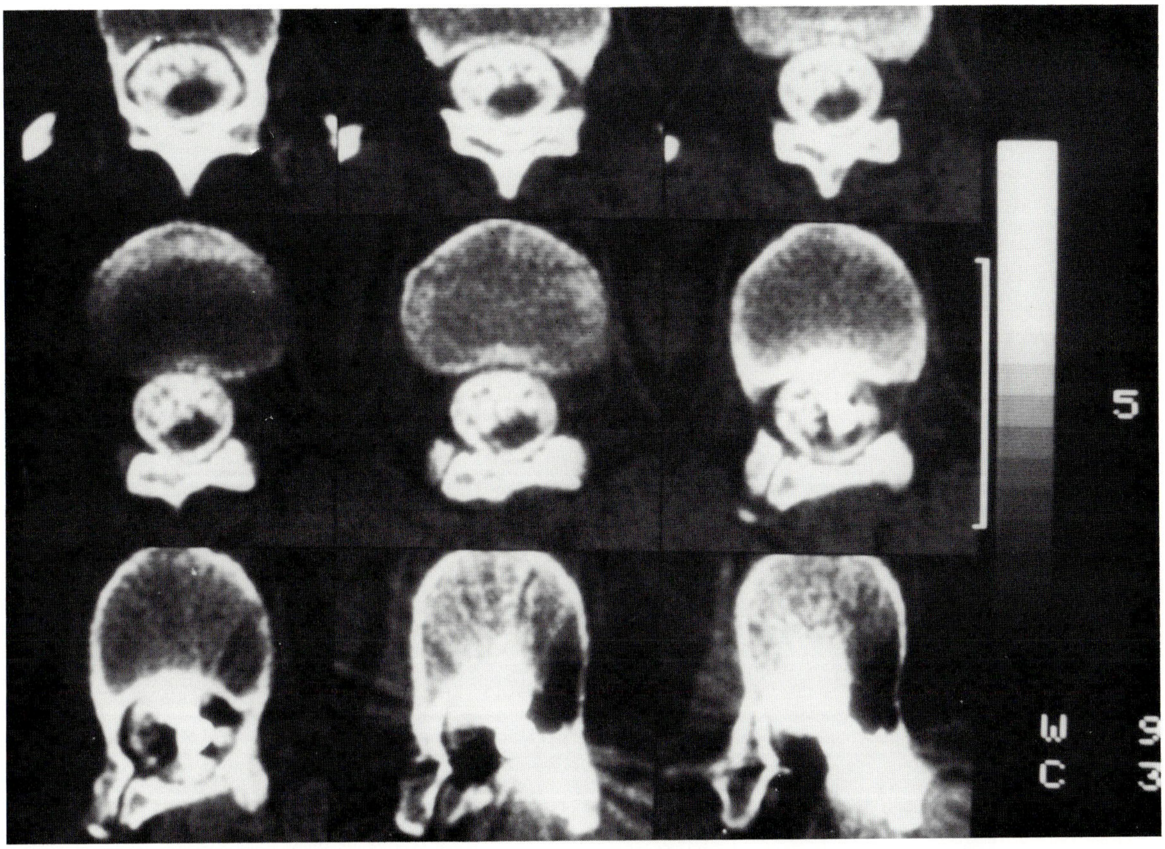

Figure 32.1. Gunshot wound. CT myelogram demonstrates the bullet fragment in the spinal canal within the dura that is compressing the spinal cord. Removal is required.

the normal anatomy. The goals are to remove all the obscuring blood, identify the spinal cord and nerves so that no further injuries occur during dissection, and remove all bullet fragments and bone that may be compromising the spinal contents. Once the blood is washed away, this is best done under high magnification. The fragments usually lift out of the cord. Gentle blunt dissection may be necessary. Hemostasis should be complete and may require the use of hemostatic agents over the injured spinal cord. The dura should then be repaired with or without grafting as necessary. Once this is accomplished, the wound can be closed without special considerations.

The surgical treatment of gunshot wounds of the spinal canal remains undefined. There are two schools of thought. The first follows the time-honored dictum of war experience, which recommends exploration of virtually all wounds. More recently, an increasing number of surgeons have suggested that routine exploration is not necessary and that surgery is required only in specific circumstances. It is not the purpose of this atlas to debate the merits of differing approaches to the management of these injuries. There is general agreement on the approaches to certain specific problems, and these are described.

Persisting Cerebrospinal Fluid Leak

Gunshot wounds of the spine may result in cerebrospinal fluid (CSF) fistulae to the outside, in the abdomen, or in the chest. These should be repaired if they persist for more than a short period of time. There are no specific guidelines, but the general range

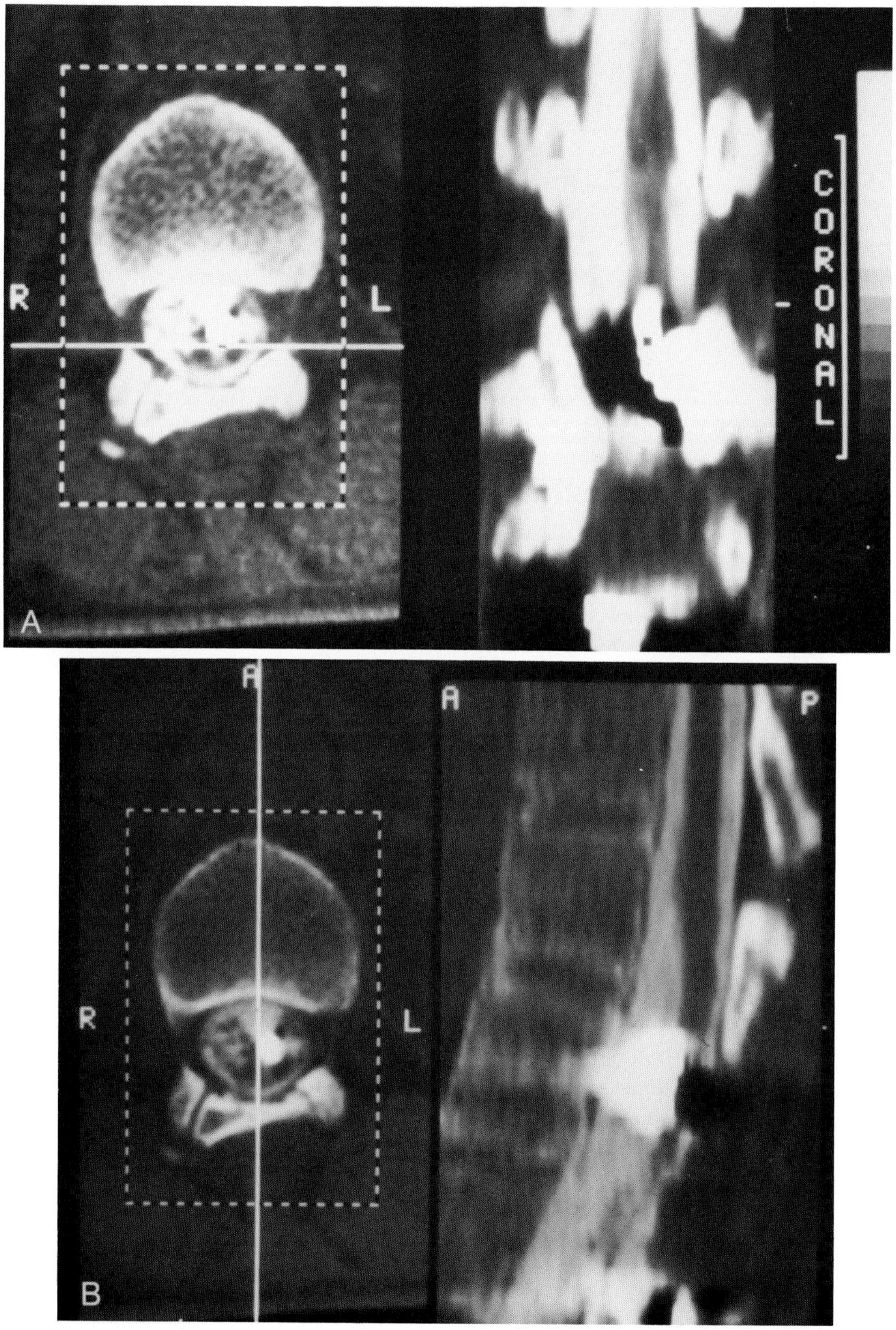

Figure 32.2. CT myelogram demonstrates a gunshot wound with the bullet fragment within the canal at the level of posterior bony disruption. Posterior laminectomy with removal of the fragment and restoration of stability is the procedure of choice.

of tolerance is 24–72 hours. Use of a spinal drain to stop a persisting leak is always worth considering. Of course, if the bullet has traversed chest or abdomen and exploration of those body cavities is required, a spinal surgeon should be called to explore the spinal wound and take measures to stop possible CSF fistulae. When a persisting leak is present, the first step should be to identify the source. CT myelography will do so and will accurately delineate the repair that may be necessary. The operation should then be planned according to the problem.

In the cervical region the approach may be anterior or posterior, depending on the location of the leak and the configuration of any associated bony injury. Whenever possible, the course of the bullet should be included in the incision, and the entire track explored, debrided, and cleansed of all dead and foreign material. The exposure otherwise does not differ from that described for the anterior and posterior approaches to the spine, nor does the surgical procedure. The goal of the operation is adequate exposure of the dural laceration, repair of the laceration, or if repair is not feasible, packing the area with fat. Whether the posterior or anterior approach is used depends on the ease with which the repair can be effected. Secondary goals include removal of all foreign bodies, potential decompression of root and spinal cord if compression occurs, and debridement of the bullet track. The reason for surgery is the fistula, and operation is not required for the other features of the injury, except in unusual circumstances.

In the thoracic region, the decision is usually whether to approach the problem through the costotransverse route or by posterior laminectomy. If the bullet wound has been explored through the chest, then appropriate measures to stop a fistula should have been taken. Exploration through the chest will not provide adequate exposure to repair the dura. Packing is the best that can be accomplished. Therefore, the surgeon usually approaches by the posterior or posterior lateral route. There is nothing unique in the approach required. It will be the same as that utilized for a traumatic fracture in the same area. Again, the goals as described for cervical injuries obtain.

In the lumbar region, the decisions relate to transabdominal, retroperitoneal, or posterior approaches. The transabdominal approach rarely will allow adequate exposure, and the surgeon must be satisfied with packing a leaking bullet hole in disc or body. This is less satisfactory and is most commonly done with the primary abdominal exploration. The decision for a posterior or posterior lateral approach is dependent on the anatomical configuration and the location of the leak. The operation should also include repair of damage and ensurance of stability. Theoretically, injured roots might be repaired. While the microsurgical techniques are now adequate to allow this to be done, the disruption by the missile usually precludes primary repair, but the surgeon should keep this in mind as a potential. Peripheral nerve repair is even more feasible, and if components of the lumbosacral plexus that are injured are to be exposed in the debridement and dural repair, then primary anastomosis of severed nerves can accompany the primary procedure.

These operative procedures are no different from those required for traumatic fractures, and the same principles and techniques should be used.

Gunshot Wound of Cord or Cauda Equina with Partial Dysfunction and Mass Effect

One indication for immediate exploration of a gunshot wound to the spinal cord is partial injury coupled with a demonstrated mass effect. The mass may be the bullet, blood, or bone. The principles are the same as those used for choosing an approach and a procedure in traumatic fracture. The only significant difference is that the bullet track should be debrided with the procedure. Usually, this is best done by including it in the operative incision. Sometimes, a bullet wound may have occurred from an anterior route, and posterior or posterior lateral exposure is appropriate. In such an instance, the track can be ignored unless there are other indications for its exploration.

Restoration of Stability

Another reason for exploration of gunshot wounds from large caliber weapons may be the associated fracture. Aside from the need to debride, there are no differences from other types of traumatic fractures, and the same surgical procedures and principles should be employed.

SECTION 10

Procedures for Pain

33 Spinal Operations for Pain

Open Cordotomy

Percutaneous cordotomy has almost eliminated the need for operative section of the spinothalamic tract. There are still some patients who are not candidates for percutaneous cordotomy or situations where bilateral cordotomy is required and a bilateral upper cervical cordotomy is not feasible. This once-important neurosurgical operation is now done very infrequently. It was always a procedure done by a relatively small number of skilled surgeons with special interest in this field.

The operation requires use of general anesthesia and may be carried out with the patient in either the sitting or the prone position. Typical bilateral upper cervical cordotomy requires an incision at C1-C2 on one side and at C5-C6 on the other. The higher cut is made opposite the side where the highest level is required for pain relief. A midline skin incision is made from the occiput to the spinous process of C6 or C7. The usual subperiosteal dissection is carried out at C1-C2, exposing the arch of C1 and the lamina of C2 on the side to be sectioned. A subperiosteal dissection is carried out on the opposite side to expose the laminae of C5 and C6. Especially at C1-C2, it is very easy to enter the vertebral plexus laterally with the attendant risk of air embolism. Should venous bleeding occur, the area must be packed immediately. Unilateral laminectomy at C2 is performed, and the dura is then opened through the length of the exposure laterally enough that the lateral margin of the cord can be seen but not so far laterally as to compromise the integrity of the dural closure. Before the dura is opened, a partial laminectomy of C5 and C6 that exposes 1–2 cm of dura is performed. Although the skin incision is relatively long, the amount of muscular disruption that occurs as a result of these exposures is small. The dura is then opened at the C1-C2 level and sutured laterally out of the way to provide good access to the cord. The arachnoid is opened separately, and cerebrospinal fluid (CSF) is allowed to drain until it stops spontaneously. The arachnoid must be dissected free from the posterior portion of the cord and be excised. The dentate ligament between C1 and C2 is identified and cut at its attachment to the dura laterally. The dentate ligament is then grasped with fine forceps or a straight clamp made for this purpose. The Adson clamp is an excellent tool. The cord is then gently rotated until the anterior quadrant comes into view. A place on the anterior surface of the cord that has few blood vessels is chosen, and the anterior quadrant is cut with a fine knife. Because the cord is distorted by rotation, it is necessary to keep in mind the extent of the cut and the direction of the knife blade. If a high level is required and if sacral analgesia is to be obtained, the blade must enter just at the anterior margin of the dentate ligament, and the cut be carried directly in parallel to the imaginary plane between the two ligaments for 5–6 mm. It is then swept forward to the exit of the anterior roots, which is the limit of the cut anteriorly. The completeness of the cut is judged by sweeping a blunt hook through the sectioned cord. The height of the level is determined by the anterior and medial portion of the cut. To avoid any risk of cutting the anterior spinal artery, it is usually better to crush the fibers beyond the origin of the ventral roots. This is performed with a fine straight clamp inserted under direct vision to crush the last few millimeters of the cord.

The somatotopic arrangements within the spinal thalamic tract make it possible to obtain differential sections. The whole quadrant does not have to be destroyed in every patient. When pelvic pain is the problem, the cut can traverse the portion of the anterior quadrant nearest to the dentate ligament and stop with the exit of the root. Anterior destruction is not required. If a high level is required or if the pain is in the trunk or upper extremity, the anterior and medial portion of the quadrant is sectioned, and lower extremity and sacral sparing can be accomplished. Once the cord section is complete, the area is packed with moist cotton, and the procedure is repeated on the opposite side at the lower level previously exposed. The operation is identical in that region. The dura is then closed in a watertight fashion at both levels. The ligamentum nuchae is closed in the midline, and the subcutaneous tissues and skin require no special closure.

High Thoracic Cordotomy

An identical procedure is carried out in the high thoracic region. These operations are usually performed with the patient in the prone position, but they may be done quite well with the patient on his or her side. In this case, the side of the cord to be sectioned is up. When a successful percutaneous or high cervical cordotomy has been accomplished at an earlier operation, it may be feasible to perform the thoracic cordotomy with the patient under local anesthesia, taking advantage of the anesthetic skin. In this case, the skin incision is made off the midline approximately 1 cm in the anesthetic skin, and then the appropriate side is exposed, with local anesthesia being used in ligament and muscle. The thoracic operation is identical with the cervical operation, but it must be remembered that the thoracic cord is significantly smaller than the cervical cord. Therefore, the cord incision must be appropriately sized. In general, the anterior quadrant at the T1-T2 level will be 3–4 mm, so the cord incision must be approximately this size. It is better to visualize the anterior roots by rotating the cord and use them as the guideline rather than cutting any predetermined distance. Otherwise, the thoracic procedure is identical with that described for cervical laminectomy, and no other special precautions need be taken.

Midline Myelotomy

Midline myelotomy is done for the relief of intractable pelvic pain. It is most appropriate in patients who have loss of bowel and bladder function, so that this need not be considered a risk of the operation. However, it can be done in patients with normal or reasonably normal function without great risk of prolonged impairment. The operation is designed to relieve the midline pelvic pain that so often complicates lumbosacral invasion from colon, uterine, or ovarian cancer. The operation is done with the patient in the prone position under general anesthesia. A skin incision is made from approximately the spine of T10 to the L1-L2 interspace. A subperiosteal dissection of the muscles is performed, and laminectomy retractors are employed to expose T11, T12, and L1. The goal of surgery is to divide crossing fibers carrying pain from lowest thoracic, lumbar, and sacral segments. The sacral segments are found over the body of L1 and the L1-L2 interspace. The lumbar segments are virtually all over the body of T12 and L1, and the lowest thoracic fibers will be no higher than the body of T11. A laminectomy of T11, T12, and L1 will be sufficient to expose all of these fibers. The spine should be removed with large bone-cutting rongeurs, and a complete laminectomy of the three levels to be exposed is carried out. The dura should be opened in the midline and should be retracted out of the way with 4-0 sutures (Fig. 33.1). There is no reason to expose the cord widely, since only the midline needs to be sought. The cord should be seen from the tip of the conus to the body of T11. The operating microscope is required for the myelotomy. The first step is to identify the midline. The median sulcus is usually obvious, and identification of the midline is not difficult. There are small veins that crisscross the midline and must be moved out of the way. It is best not to coagulate any veins, and it usually is possible to open the pia and push these veins to one side or the other without either breaking or coagulating them. The pia along the midline should be opened with a #11 knife. This sharp point makes it easy to cut the pia without entering the posterior columns. The angled disposable knives currently available are extremely sharp and are useful for this purpose. The actual division in the cord is done with semisharp instruments. The large Rosen knife is an ideal tool (Fig. 33.2). With a blunt dissector and a Rosen knife or a pair of Rosen knives, the cord should be divided in the midline from back to front. The length of the myelotomy is approximately 2 cm and should cover the cord from near the tip of the conus to the lower thoracic segments, at least the lower border of T11. It is important to retain the relationships of the cord in as near an anatomical configuration as possible. The cord should not be retracted or distorted so that the myelotomy can remain exactly in the midline. When this is done, the anterior and posterior median septae define avascular planes, and the myelotomy can be carried out without disturbing anything except the crossing commissural fibers. The Rosen knife is gently swept along the length of the myelotomy in ever-deepening cuts, through the central canal, through the anterior commissural fibers, and on along the anterior median septum until the cord is completely divided. Sometimes, a large anterior spinal artery will pop into view as the first sign that the cord has been completely transected. Using the semisharp instruments reduces the chance that the anterior spinal artery can be injured. The myelotomy is then continued, exposing the artery until the entire cord is divided. Sometimes, the artery is not visualized, and it is simply apparent that the cord has been transected, since the two pial covered anterior quadrants are more easily divided than the crossing commissural fibers. It is important to be certain that the anterior fibers are divided throughout the length of the myelotomy. Little bleeding occurs during this maneuver, and if bleeding is apparent, packing with a hemostatic agent such as Avitene or thrombin-soaked Gelfoam will stop it promptly. The dura should then be closed in a watertight fashion. The muscular and subcutaneous skin closures are approximated routinely.

Rhizotomy

There are very few indications for rhizotomy for pain. Trigeminal and upper cervical nerve section for relief of pain from infiltrative cancer can be a successful operation. Thoracic rhizotomy to relieve the pain of an unhealed rib fracture or to treat postthoracotomy syndromes may occasionally be necessary. Radiofrequency techniques have virtually eliminated the need for open operations. The low success rate for lumbar rhizotomy as a beneficial procedure to relieve leg pain in the patient with failed back syndrome has led to the virtual abandonment of the operation. Dorsal ganglionectomy appears to be more successful in the unusual circumstance in which such a procedure is contemplated. The operations are used infrequently enough that the various spinal rhizotomies really do not require separate description.

These operations are performed with the patient under general anesthesia in the prone position. Accurate localization of the bony landmarks is required to be certain that the appropriate roots are being sectioned. When the bony anatomy is not absolutely localizing, a film during surgery is required. The operation can be done through a hemilaminectomy, so disruption of the spinal anatomy is minimized. The

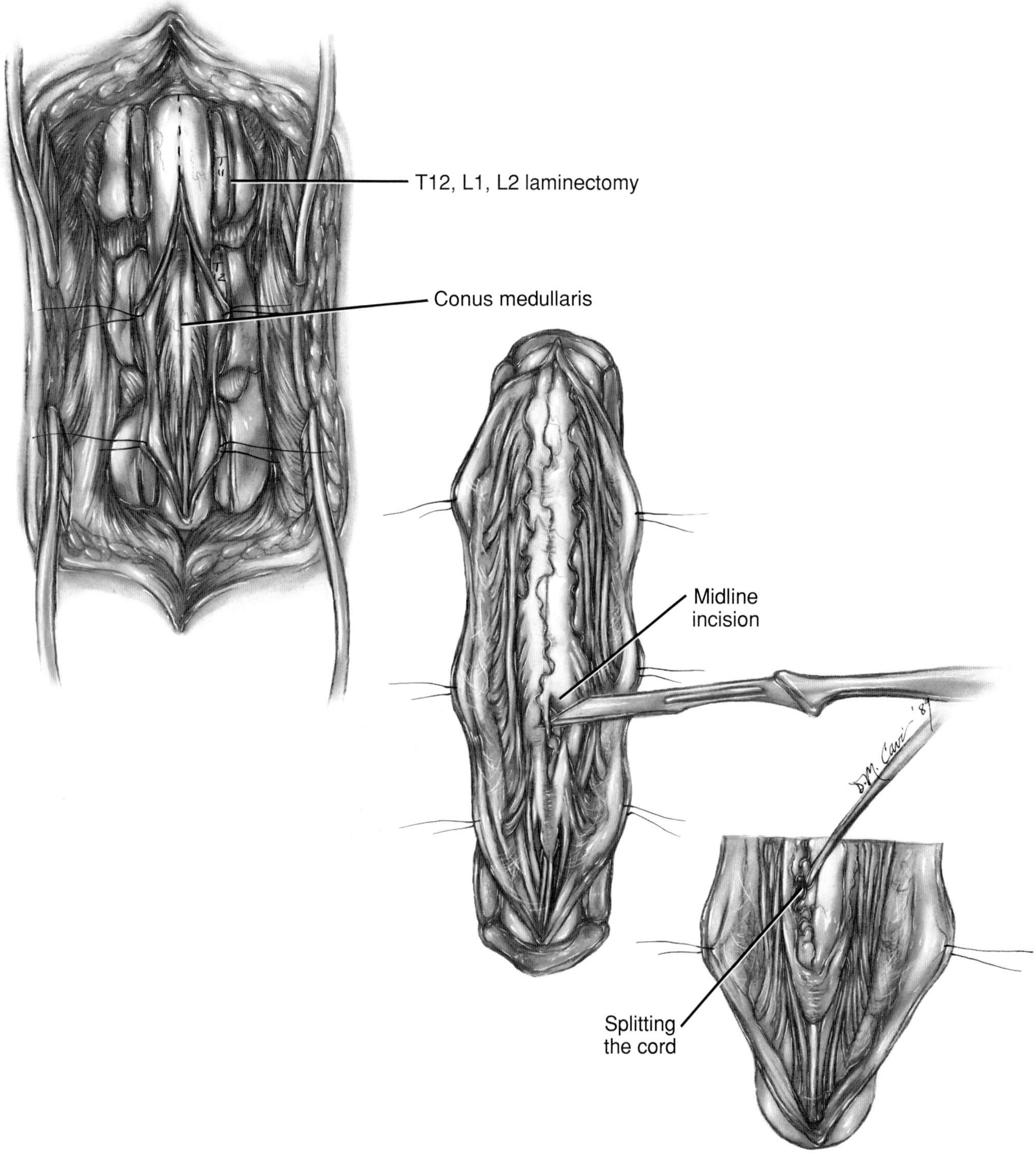
T12, L1, L2 laminectomy
Conus medullaris
Midline incision
Splitting the cord

Figure 33.1.

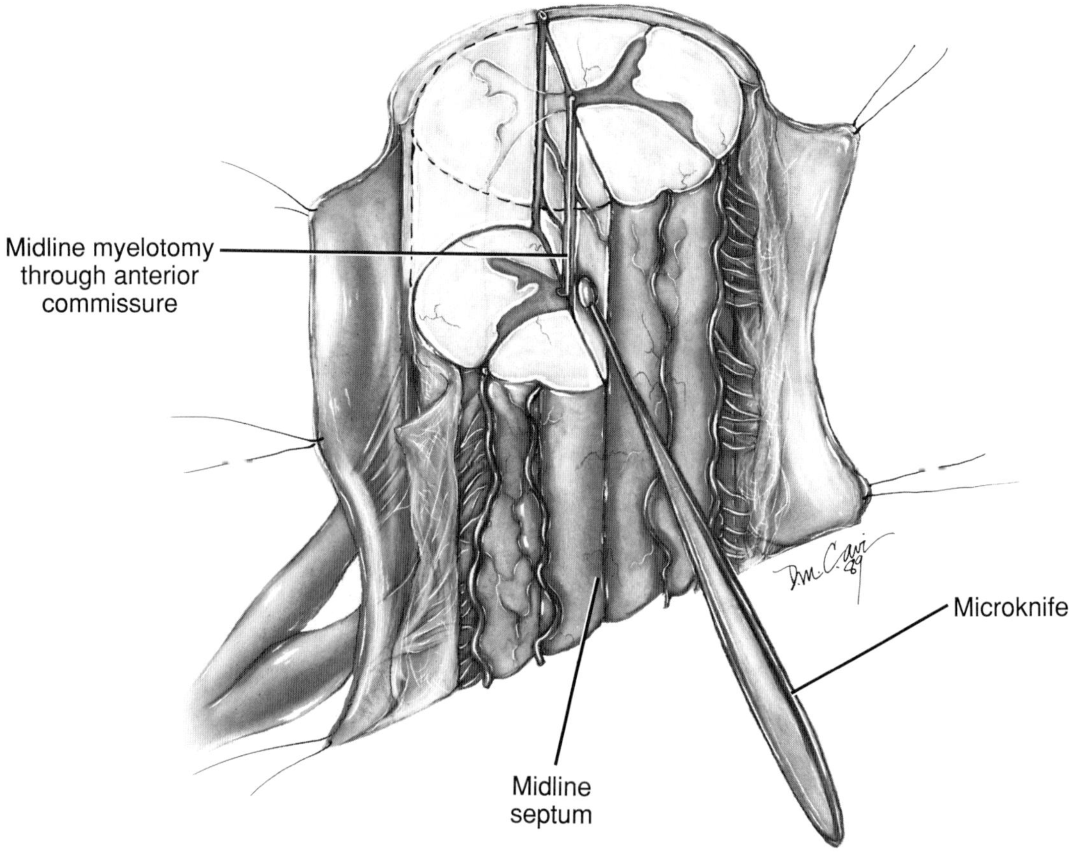

Figure 33.2.

dura should be opened laterally at the junction of the root sheath with the main dural tube. At least 1 mm of dura should be left medial to the root sheath so that the closing sutures can be placed without distorting the root. The dura should be retracted out of the way, with retention sutures and the arachnoid opened. The roots to section should be identified, and if there is any question about localization, a film should be taken either just before the dura is opened or after the roots are adequately identified. Posterior rhizotomy is the usual goal. The indications for anterior rhizotomy are few. In the cervical and thoracic region, differentiation of the posterior roots is made possible by their relationship to the dentate ligament. All the roots that are behind the dentate ligament can be isolated, inspected under magnification, and then crushed with a small clamp and cut. Some intrinsic vessels that are actually contained by the covering of the root are crushed and sectioned with the root. Larger radicular vessels that are separable should not be sacrificed. Blunt dissection will suffice to free them from their adherence to the roots so that the roots can be crushed separately and the vessels left intact. The actual rhizotomy technique requires a fine microclamp that can be used to crush the root, and then the root can be sectioned without bleeding through the crushed area. Hemostasis should be perfect when the procedure is complete. The dura is then closed in a watertight fashion. The remainder of the closure requires no special precautions.

Cervical and Trigeminal Rhizotomy for Head and Neck Cancer Pain

For cervical and trigeminal rhizotomy, the patient is placed in the parkbench position with the side to be sectioned uppermost. General anesthesia is required. The incision is a variation of that utilized for exposure of the posterior fossa for microvascular decompression. The incision is made at the midpoint of the posterior fossa and angled from behind the ear toward the midline. The midline should be reached at approximately C2 or C3, and then the incision turned to extend downward for a short ways. The incision should be taken to the occipital bone and to the midline to expose C3 and C4 spinous processes and laminae. The muscle is scraped away from the bone to expose an area of the occiput from the origin of the sigmoid sinus to the foramen magnum. Laterally, the exposure should be to the mastoid. Medially, it is not necessary to extend the exposure to the midline. Next, subperiosteal dissection of muscles from one half of C1 and the spinous processes and laminae of C2 and C3 on the side to be exposed is carried out. Only a hemilaminectomy will be required. The posterior fossa exposure is a variation of that used to obtain exposure of the fifth or seventh and eighth cranial nerves for microvascular decompression. Envision the bony incisions described for those operations superimposed to provide the proper exposure. Self-retaining retractors should be put in place to expose one half of the occipital bone in the area of the foramen magnum and one side of the cervical spine, including the laminae out to the zygapophyseal joints. The posterior fossa bone should be removed first. A single burr hole placed between the exposure for the fifth nerve and the cerebellopontine angle will allow a small craniectomy to be performed. The bony removal does not have to include the entire hemioccipital bone. An ellipse of bone should be taken out that exposes the junction of the transverse with the sigmoid sinus and extends down along the mastoid bone to the level of the jugular bulb. The medial extent of the bony removal does not have to be large. All that is required is that enough bone be removed to allow a dural incision that will expose the fifth and the ninth nerves. It is not necessary to remove the rim of the foramen magnum. Then the arch of C1 and the lamina of C2 should be removed. This will provide adequate exposure for division of first, second, and third cranial nerves. The dura should be opened parallel to the lateral aspect of the bony incision, at least 2–3 mm from the sinus. The cut edges of the lateral dura can be retracted out of the field with sutures. A medium brain retractor is employed to expose the fifth nerve by approaching its entrance into the dura along the superior lateral margin of the cerebellum. Undue retraction may tear the petrosal vein and cause an annoying, though not dangerous, hemorrhage. Gentle retraction in this plane spares hearing. As the cerebellum falls away, the fifth nerve will come into view. The large fifth nerve is unmistakable, and its entrance into Meckel's cave is visualized without difficulty. All blood vessels should be carefully dissected away from it, and if possible, the motor branch should be identified. It probably will not be seen from this posterior approach, but careful dissection anteriorly may bring it into view. Much has been made about the divisions of the fifth nerve and the possibility of differential sections for pain. In cancer, this is not an important consideration, and it is safer to cut the entire nerve. The nerve should be crushed with a fine cramp. Preferably, this is done in increments so the motor root can be identified and saved. After a small visualized section is clamped, it should be cut, and any small bleeders that persist can be coagulated with the bipolar cautery. The nerve should be totally divided in this way. It should be possible to save the motor branch. The retractor is then withdrawn and moved to the lower margin of the incision. The jugular bulb should be exposed by lifting the cerebellum somewhat up and medially. This will usually show both the jugular bulb and the seventh and eighth nerves. Again, the anatomy is unmistakable to the experienced surgeon. The seventh and eighth complex is recognized by the typical appearance of porus acusticus, its relationship to the fifth nerve, and the nervous anatomy. The jugular bulb is recognized by its relationship with the sinus and the neural anatomy of the ninth-tenth-eleventh nerve complex. The ninth nerve is seen entering the neural compartment of the jugular bulb most superiorly. It is a single well-defined fiber, and there is no problem in differentiating it from the tenth nerve. The ninth nerve should be crushed and divided. The upper two filaments of the tenth nerve should also be crushed and cut. This is not because of difficulty in recognizing the ninth nerve but relates to the overlap of the innervation. The upper dura should then be closed in a watertight fashion. The upper cervical dura has been exposed by the hemilaminectomy of the first and second levels. This dura should be opened in the midline of its exposure, and the flaps retracted out of the way. This will show the posterior roots of C1, C2, and C3. C1 frequently has no roots or, at best, rudimentary filaments. These should be identified, if present, crushed, and divided.

The large root is C2. Its exit between C1 and C2 is easily identified. The roots are sequentially crushed and divided, sparing any large radicular blood vessels that are not intrinsic to the roots. The C3 root can be seen as it exits between C2 and C3 without lower bony removal in most situations. Again, the roots posterior to the dentate ligament are isolated, crushed, and divided. The dura is closed in a watertight fashion, with closure requiring no special care otherwise.

Operation for Dorsal Root Entry Zone Lesions

The operation for dorsal root entry zone (DREZ) lesions may be done for avulsion of the brachial plexus for treatment of pain. It may also be done for phantom pain and postherpetic neuralgia, although its efficacy in treatment of these latter conditions is not clear. The acronym DREZ refers to the location of microlesions in the region where the dorsal root enters the spinal cord. The patient is placed in the prone position under general anesthesia. The sitting position is not necessary and only adds to the possibility of anesthetic complications. A standard laminectomy procedure is done to include the segments avulsed. In cases where there is complete avulsion of the brachial plexus the cervical plexus may also be avulsed, and in this case the laminectomy should proceed from C3 through and including T2. The laminectomy can be a narrow one with careful preservation of the zygapophyseal joints (Fig. 33.3). A wide laminectomy may jeopardize stability and does not enhance the exposure of the relevant areas of the spinal cord. The microscope is always used in this operation and is brought at the point that the dura is opened. Frequently, there is considerable arachnoiditis associated with the trauma of the avulsion. On the dorsal surface of the cord there are three sulci. The median sulcus represents the midline and separates the two dorsal columns. The fasciculus cuneatus and fasciculus gracilis are separated by the posterior intermediate sulcus, while the posterolateral sulcus represents the lateral border of the dorsal columns, viz., the DREZ. The posterolateral sulcus is the most prominent of the sulci. If the cord is balloted with a sharp tip needle, a clear indentation occurs only in the posterolateral sulcus. Correct localization of this sulcus is essential to avoid damage to the posterior column, the cortical spinal tract, and other long tracts. As further assurance of the location of the posterolateral sulcus, it is well to visualize the intact dorsal root fibers either above or below the avulsion (Fig. 33.4). When the cervical plexus has been avulsed along with the brachial plexus, intact dorsal root fibers may not be seen up through C3. In this case, it is well to observe the T2 fibers below and work up from this point. The lesions themselves may be made with CO_2 laser or with more traditional radiofrequency techniques. The actual area to be injured is not known except by implication that it must be some part of the posterior horn. In this author's hands excellent relief of pain has been obtained by using the radiofrequency technique, and no notable neurological complications have occurred. Although temperature control of the needle tip is theoretically advantageous, this author has chosen to use visual control of the lesion size, maintaining a constant current level. Two or three cordotomy needles are examined, and the sharpest one is picked for performing the lesions. It is well to do this prior to surgery in order to make sure that an adequately sharp needle is available. Practice lesions are made in the muscle tissue to ensure that the assistants know how to make the lesions and that the equipment is working satisfactorily. The needle is placed into muscle tissue, and the current is brought up to 50 mA for 5–10 seconds when under the microscope a small contraction of the muscle tissue is visible, indicating coagulation of the muscle fibers (Fig. 33.5). The lesions are made in the DREZ region, contiguously beginning at the low end and proceeding cephalad until intact dorsal root fibers are encountered. The needle is placed 2 mm into the DREZ at an angle of 30°. The radiofrequency current is increased to 40–45 mA, and the lesion is made from any point for 5–8 seconds. It is important that the pia be sufficiently dissected to ensure that the lesion is being made in the spinal cord and not the pia. The needle is hand held and is withdrawn at the point when under 10 × magnification a contraction of the tissues is noted. A small eschar will form on the pia, further substantiating the placement of the lesion. Each lesion is done in this way, and at the completion of the procedure a faintly visible eschar is observed in a straight line longitudinally extending from intact dorsal root fibers below to intact dorsal root fibers above. The dura and wound are closed in routine fashion, and a neurological examination is done immediately postoperatively to serve as a baseline. The patient may develop an ipsilateral increase in the lower extremity reflexes, but this does not normally interfere with gait.

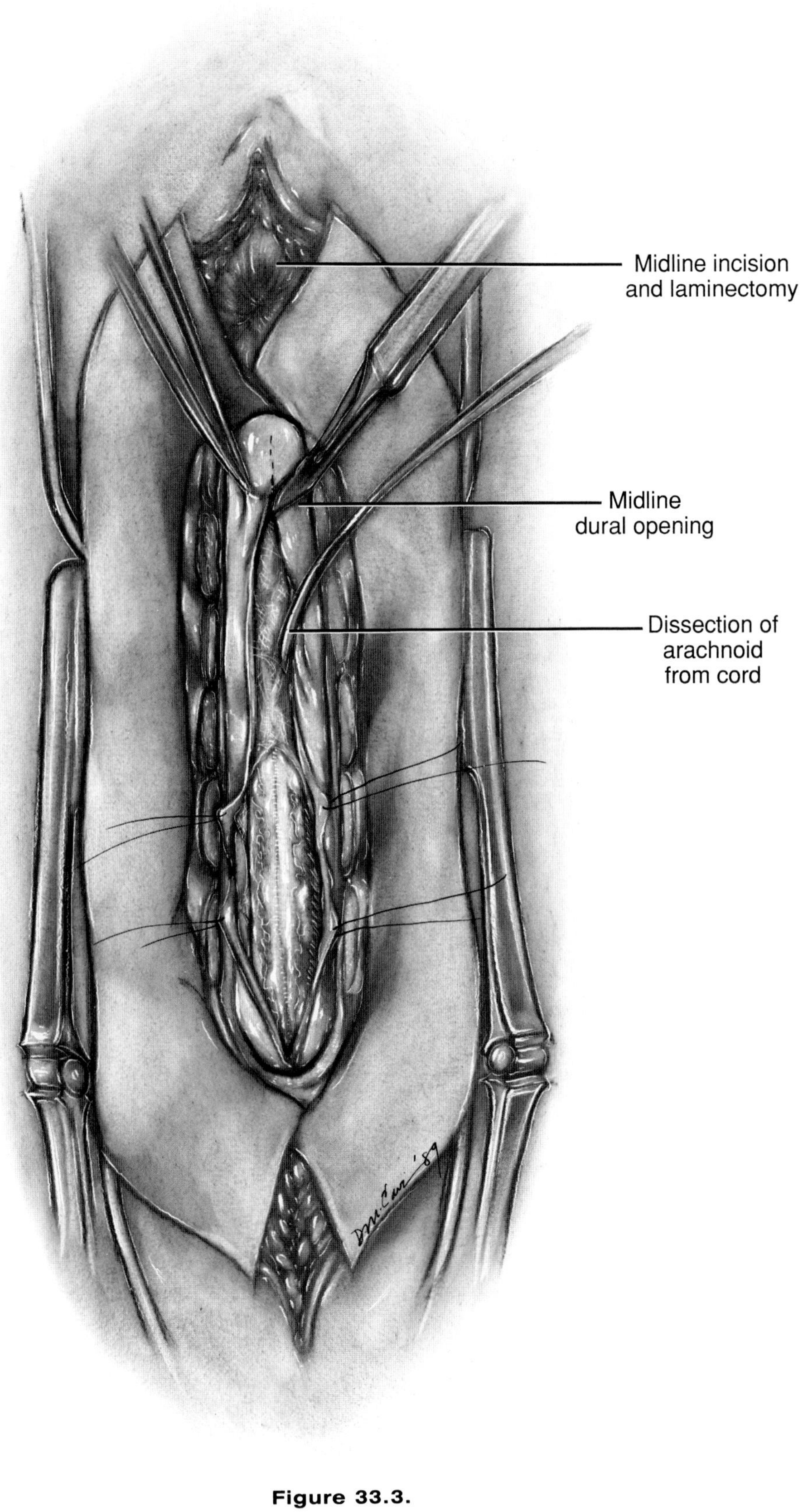
Midline incision
and laminectomy
Midline
dural opening
Dissection of
arachnoid
from cord

Figure 33.3.

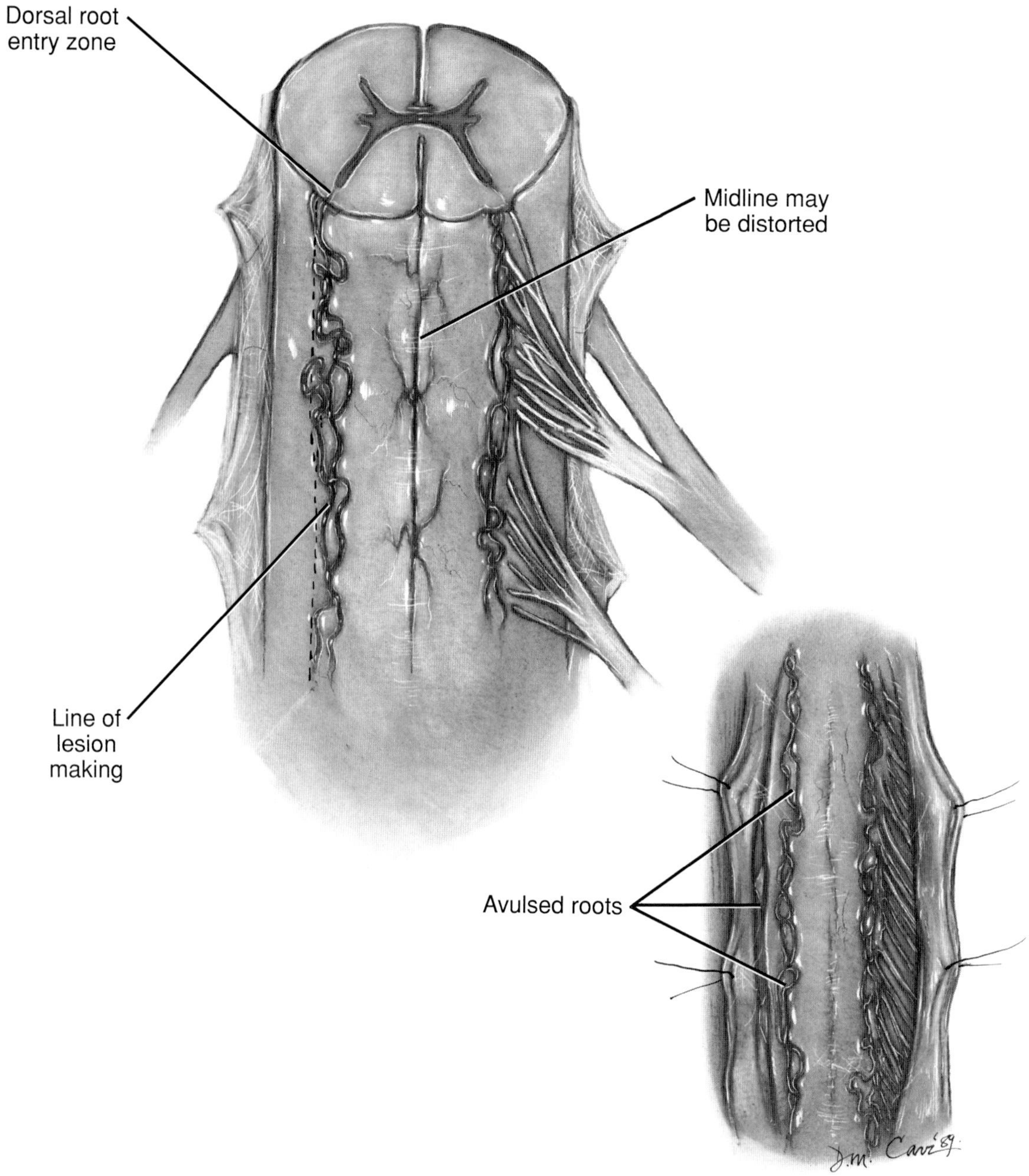
Dorsal root
entry zone
Midline may
be distorted
Line of
lesion
making
Avulsed roots

Figure 33.4.

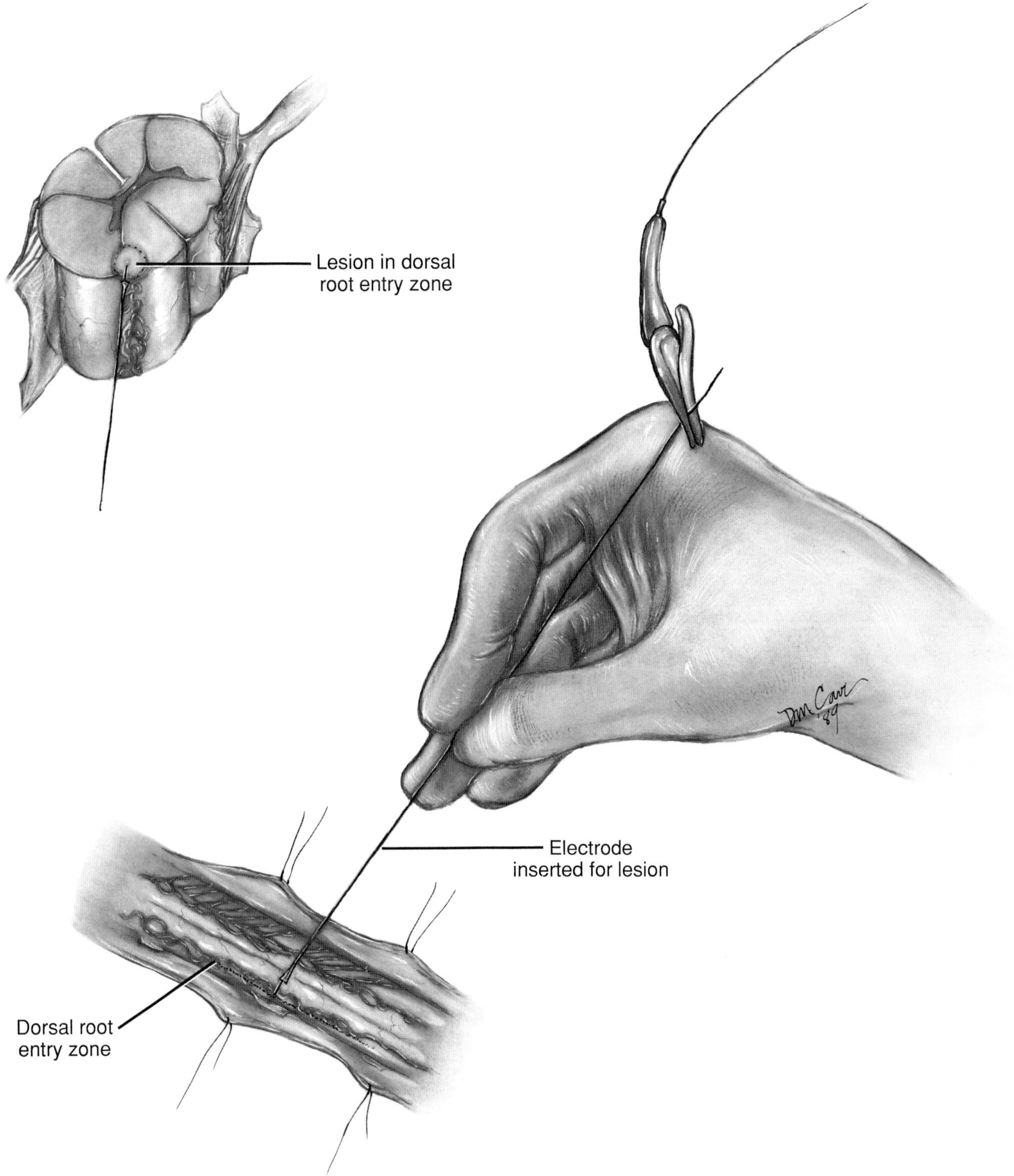

Lesion in dorsal root entry zone
Electrode inserted for lesion
Dorsal root entry zone

Figure 33.5.

Bibliography

Primary Operations on Lumbar Disc *(Chapter 1)*

Finneson BE: A lumbar disc surgery predictive score card. *Spine* 3(2):186–188, 1978.

Gado M, Patel J, Hodges FJ III: High resolution CT of the spine in lumbar disc disease. *Clin Neurosurg* 30:654–676, 1983.

Godersky JC, Erickson DL, Seljeskog EL: Extreme lateral disc herniation: diagnosis by computed tomographic scanning. *Neurosurgery* 14(5):549–552, 1984.

Loew F: Different operative possibilities for treatment of lumbar disc herniations—how to choose the best method for the individual patient. *Neurosurg Rev* 9(1–2):109–111, 1986.

Pheasant HC, Dyck P: Failed lumbar disc surgery: cause, assessment, treatment. *Clin Orthop* 164:93–109, 1982.

Salenius P, Laurent LE: Results of operative treatment of lumbar disc herniation. A survey of 886 patients. *Acta Orthop Scand* 48(6):630–634, 1977.

Weber H: Lumbar disc herniation. A controlled, prospective study with ten years of observation. *Spine* 8(2):131–140, 1983.

Weinstein J, Spratt KF, Lehmann T, McNeill T, Hejna W: Lumbar disc herniation. A comparison of the results of chemonucleolysis and open discectomy after ten years. *J Bone Joint Surg [Am]* 68(1):43–54, 1986.

Failed Back Syndrome and Disc Space Infections *(Chapter 2)*

Boston HC Jr, Bianco AJ Jr, Rhodes KH: Disk space infections in children. *Orthop Clin North Am* 6(4):953–964, 1975.

Heithoff KB, Burton CV: CT evaluation of the failed back surgery syndrome. *Orthop Clin North Am* 16(3):417–444, 1985.

Lang EF: Postoperative infection of the intervertebral disk space. *Surg Clin North Am* 48(3):649–660, 1968.

Aneurysmal Bone Cyst *(Chapter 3)*

Campanacci M, Cervellati C, Donati U, Bertoni F: Aneurysmal bone cyst (a study of 127 cases, 72 with long-term follow-up). *Ital J Orthop Traumatol* 2(3):341–353, 1976.

Haney P, Gellad F, Swartz J: Aneurysmal bone cyst of the spine: computed tomographic appearance. *J Comput Tomogr* 7(3):319–322, 1983.

Morton KS: Aneurysmal bone cyst: a review of 26 cases. *Can J Surg* 29(2):110–115, 1986.

Nicastro JF, Leatherman KD: Two-stage resection and spinal stabilization for aneurysmal bone cyst. A report of two cases. *Clin Orthop* 180:173–178, 1983.

Lumbar Pedicle Screw Fixation and Fusion *(Chapter 5)*

Akbarnia B, Gaines R, Keppler L, Lorenz M, Merenda J, Zindrick M, Niemann P: Surgical treatment of fracture dislocations of the thoracolumbar and lumbar spine using pedicular screw and plate fixation. Presented at the 23rd Annual Meeting of the Scoliosis Research Society, Baltimore, Maryland, 1988.

Berry J, Moran J, Berg W, Steffee A: A morphometric study of human lumbar and selected thoracic vertebrae. *Spine* 12(4):362–367, 1987.

Gaines R, Henstorf J, Steffee A: Transpedicular fixation of spinal disorders with Steffee plates. *Surg Rounds* 35–43, March 1987.

Goel V, Kim Y, Lim T, Weinstein J: An analytical investigation of the mechanics of spinal instrumentation. *Spine* 13(9):1003–1011, 1988.

Gurr KR, McAfee PC, Shih CM: Biomechanical analysis of posterior instrumentation systems after decompressive laminectomy. *J Bone Joint Surg* 70A:680–691, 1988.

Gurr KR, McAfee PC, Shih CM: Biomechanical analysis of anterior and posterior instrumentation systems after corpectomy. *J Bone Joint Surg* 70A:1182–1191, 1988.

Steffee A, Biscup R, Sitkowski D: Segmental spine plates with pedicle screw fixation. *Clin Orthop* 203:45–53, 1986.

Steffee A, Sitkowski D: Reduction and stabilization of grade IV spondylolisthesis. *Clin Orthop* 227:82–89, 1988.

Steffee A, Sitkowski D: Posterior lumbar interbody fusion and plates. *Clin Orthop* 227:99–102, 1988.

Weinstein J, Spratt K, Spengler D, Brick C, Reid S: Spinal pedicle fixation: reliability and validity of roentgenogram-based assessment and surgical factors on successful screw placement. *Spine* 13(9):1012–1018, 1988.

Zindrick M, Wiltse L, Coornik A, Widell E, Knight G, Patwardhan A, Thomas J, Rothman S, Fields B: Analysis of the morphometric characteristics of the thoracic and lumbar pedicles. *Spine* 12(2):160–166, 1987.

Zindrick M, Wiltse L, Widell E, Thomas J, Holland W, Field B, Spencer C: A biomechanical study of the intrapeduncular screw fixation in the lumbosacral spine. *Clin Orthop* 203:99–112, 1986.

Spinal Metastasis *(Chapter 7)*

Boland PJ, Lane JM, Sundaresan N: Metastatic disease of the spine. *Clin Orthop* 169:95–102, 1982.

Giannotta SL, Kindt GW: Metastatic spinal cord tumors. *Clin Neurosurg* 25:495–503, 1978.

Siegal T, Siegal T: Surgical decompression of anterior and posterior malignant epidural tumors compressing the spinal cord: a prospective study. *Neurosurgery* 17(3):424–432, 1985.

Slatkin NE, Posner JB: Management of spinal epidural metastases. *Clin Neurosurg* 30:698–716, 1983.

Solini A, Paschero B: Surgical management of spinal cord lesions due to metastases. *J Neurosurg Sci* 28(3–4):201–212, 1984.

Sundaresan N, Digiacinto GV, Hughes JE: Surgical treatment of spinal metastases. *Clin Neurosurg* 33:503–522, 1986.

Sundaresan N, Galicich JH, Bains MS, Martini N, Beattie EJ Jr: Vertebral body resection in the treatment of cancer involving the spine. *Cancer* 53(6):1393–1396, 1984.

Spinal Fusion *(Chapter 16)*

Cahill DW, Bellegarrigue R, Dubker TB: Bilateral facet to spinous process fusion: a new technique for posterior spinal fusion after trauma. *Neurosurgery* 13(1):1–4, 1983.

Capen DA, Garland DE, Waters RL: Surgical stabilization of the cervical spine. A comparative analysis of anterior and posterior spine fusions. *Clin Orthop* 196:229–237, 1985.

Collis JS: Total disc replacement: a modified posterior lumbar interbody fusion. Report of 750 cases. *Clin Orthop* 193:64–67, 1985.

Crock HV: Anterior lumbar interbody fusion: indications for its use and notes on surgical technique. *Clin Orthop* 165:157–163, 1982.

Flynn TB: Neurologic complications of anterior cervical interbody fusion. *Spine* 7(6):536–539, 1982.

Gore DR, Sepic SB: Anterior cervical fusion for degenerated or protruded discs. A review of one hundred forty-six patients. *Spine* 9(7):667–671, 1984.

Lin PM: Posterior lumbar interbody fusion technique: complications and pitfalls. *Clin Orthop* 193:90–102, 1985.

Lin PM, Cautilli RA, Joyce MF: Posterior lumbar interbody fusion. *Clin Orthop* 180:154–168, 1983.

Murphy MJ, Daniaux H, Southwick WO: Posterior cervical fusion with rigid internal fixation. *Orthop Clin North Am* 17(1):55–65, 1986.

O'Brien JP, Dawson MH, Heard CW, Momberger G, Speck G, Weatherly CR: Simultaneous combined anterior and posterior fusion. A surgical solution for failed spinal surgery with a brief review of the first 150 patients. *Clin Orthop* 203:191–195, 1986.

Prolo DJ, Oklund SA, Butcher M: Toward uniformity in evaluating results of lumbar spine operations. A paradigm applied to posterior lumbar interbody fusions. *Spine* 11(6):601–660, 1986.

Rosenrn J, Hansen EB, Rosenrn MA: Anterior cervical discectomy with and without fusion. A prospective study. *J Neurosurg* 59(2):252–255, 1983.

Sherk HH, Snyder B: Posterior fusions of the upper cervical spine: indications, techniques, and prognosis. *Orthop Clin North Am* 9(4):1091–1099, 1978.

Tunturi T, Kataja M, Keski-Nusula L, Lapinsuo M, Lepisto P, Paakkala T, Patiala H, Rokkanen P: Posterior fusion of the lumbosacral spine. Evaluation of the operative results and the factors influencing them. *Acta Orthop Scand* 50(4):415–425, 1979.

Cervical Cord Fusion *(Chapter 17)*

Jacobs B: Anterior cervical spine fusion. *Surg Ann* 8:413–446, 1976 (review).

Lesoin F, Combelles G, Bouasakao N, Cama A, Delandsheer JM, Jomin M: Use of acrylic prosthesis in cervical spine pathology (report of 45 cases). *Acta Neurochir (Wien)* 71(1–2):141–149, 1984.

Lesoin F, Jomin M, Pellerin P, Pruvo JP, Carini S, Servato R, Rousseaux M: Transclival transcervical approach to the upper cervical spine and clivus. *Acta Neurochir (Wien)* 80(3–4):100–104, 1986.

McWhorter JM, Alexander E, David CH, Kelly L: Posterior cervical fusion in children. *J Neurosurg* 45(2):211–215, 1976.

Murray JW, Seymour RJ: An anterior, extrapharyngeal, suprahyoid approach to the first, second and third cervical vertebrae. *Acta Orthop Scand* 45(1):45–49, 1974.

Pasztor E: Transoral approach for epidural craniocervical pathological processes. *Adv Tech Stand Neurosurg* 12:125–170, 1985.

Ranawat CS, O'Leary P, Pellicci P, Tsairis P, Marchisello P, Dorr L: Cervical spine fusion in rheumatoid arthritis. *J Bone Joint Surg [Am]* 61(7):1003–1010, 1979.

Robinson RA: Anterior and posterior cervical spine fusions. *Clin Orthop* 35:34–62, 1964.

Sim FH, Svien HJ, Bickel WH, Janes JM: Swan-neck deformity following extensive cervical laminectomy. A review of twenty-one cases. *J Bone Joint Surg [Am]* 56A(3):564–580, 1974.

Syringomyelia *(Chapter 20)*

Anderson NE, Willoughby EW, Wrightson P: The natural history and the influence of surgical treatment in syringomyelia. *Acta Neurol Scand* 71(6):472–479, 1985.

Barbaro NM, Wilson CB, Gutin PH, Edwards MS: Surgical treatment of syringomyelia. Favorable results with syringoperitoneal shunting. *J Neurosurg* 61(3):531–538, 1984.

Garcia-Uria J, Leunda G, Carrillo R, Bravo G: Syringomyelia: long-term results after posterior fossa decompression. *J Neurosurg* 54(3):380–383, 1981.

Suzuki M, Davis C, Symon L, Gentili F: Syringoperitoneal shunt for treatment of cord cavitation. *J Neurol Neurosurg Psychiatry* 48(7):620–627, 1985.

Tator CH, Meguro K, Rowed DW: Favorable results with syringosubarachnoid shunts for treatment of syringomyelia. *J Neurosurg* 56(4):517–523, 1982.

Williams B, Fahy G: A critical appraisal of "terminal ventriculostomy" for the treatment of syringomyelia. *J Neurosurg* 58(2):188–197, 1983.

Myelomeningocele and Lipoma *(Chapter 22)*

Guthkelch AN, Pang D, Vries JK: Influence of closure technique on results in myelomeningocele. *Childs Brain* 8(5):350–355, 1981.

Hoffman HJ, Taecholarn C, Hendrick EB, Humphreys RP: Management of lipomyelomeningoceles. Experience at the Hospital for Sick Children, Toronto. *J Neurosurg* 62(1):1–8, 1985.

Lehrmann A, Owen MP: Surgical repair of large meningomyeloceles. *Ann Plast Surg* 12(6):501–507, 1984.

Sutton LN, Charney EB, Bruce DA, Schut L: Myelomeningocele—the question of selection. *Clin Neurosurg* 33:371–381, 1986.

Lister J, Zachary RB, Brereton R: Open myelomeningocele—a ten-year review of 200 consecutive closures. *Prog Pediatr Surg* 10:161–176, 1977.

Luce EA, Walsh J: Wound closure of the myelomeningocoele defect. *Plast Reconstr Surg* 75(3):389–393, 1985.

Mazur J, Menelaus MB, Dickens DR, Doig WG: Efficacy of surgical management for scoliosis in myelomeningocele: correction of deformity and alteration of functional status. *J Pediatr Orthop* 6(5):568–575, 1986.

McLone DG: Technique for closure of myelomeningocele. *Childs Brain* 6(2):65–73, 1980.

McLone DG: Treatment of myelomeningocele: arguments against selection. *Clin Neurosurg* 33:359–370, 1986.

McLone DG, Naidich TP: Laser resection of fifty spinal lipomas. *Neurosurgery* 18(5):611–615, 1986.

Pierre-Kahn A, Lacombe J, Pichon J, Giudicelli Y, Renier D, Sainte-Rose C, Perrigot M, Hirsch JF: Intraspinal lipomas with spina bifida. Prognosis and treatment in 73 cases. *J Neurosurg* 65(6):756–761, 1986.

Schut L, Bruce DA, Sutton LN: The management of the child with a lipomyelomeningocele. *Clin Neurosurg* 30:464–476, 1983.

Intramedullary Spinal Cord Tumors *(Chapter 28)*

Alvisi C, Cerisoli M, Giulioni M: Intramedullary spinal gliomas: long-term results of surgical treatment. *Acta Neurochir (Wien)* 70(3–4):169–179, 1984.

Cooper PR, Epstein F: Radical resection of intramedullary spinal cord tumors in adults. Recent experience in 29 patients. *J Neurosurg* 63(4):492–499, 1985.

DiChiro G, Doppman JL, Dwyer AJ, Patronas NJ, Knop RH, Bairamian D, Vermess M, Oldfield EH: Tumors and arteriovenous malformations of the spinal cord: assessment using MR. *Radiology* 156(3):689–697, 1985.

Epstein F, Epstein N: Surgical treatment of spinal cord astrocytomas of childhood. A series of 19 patients. *J Neurosurg* 57(5):685–689, 1982.

Johnston CE II: Post laminectomy kyphoscoliosis following surgical treatment for spinal cord astrocytoma. *Orthopedics* 9(4):587–594, 1986.

Reimer R, Onofrio BM: Astrocytomas of the spinal cord in children and adolescents. *J Neurosurg* 63(5):669–675, 1985.

Schwade JG, Wara WM, Sheline GE, Sorgen S, Wilson CB: Management of primary spinal cord tumors. *Int J Radiat Oncol Biol Phys* 4(5–6):389–393, 1978.

Stein BM: Surgery of intramedullary spinal cord tumors. *Clin Neurosurg* 26:529–542, 1979.

Gunshot Wounds of Spine *(Chapter 32)*

Berman AT, Salter F: Low velocity gunshot wounds in police officers. *Clin Orthop* 192:113–119, 1985.

Ducker TB, Lucas JT, Wallace CA: Recovery from spinal cord injury. *Clin Neurosurg* 30:495–513, 1983.

Ducker TB, Bellegarrigue R, Salcman M, Walleck C: Timing of operative care in cervical spinal cord injury. *Spine* 9(5):525–531, 1984 (review).

Stauffer ES, Wood RW, Kelly EG: Gunshot wounds of the spine: the effects of laminectomy. *J Bone Joint Surg [Am]* 61(3):389–392, 1979.

Waters RL: Gunshot wounds to the spine: the effects of bullet fragments in the spinal canal. *J Am Paraplegia Soc* 7(2):30–33, 1974.

Wu WQ: Delayed effects from retained foreign bodies in the spine and spinal cord. *Surg Neurol* 25(3):214–218, 1986.

Index

Page numbers in *italics* denote figures.